The
ENERGETICS
of
WESTERN HERBS

Integrating Western and
Oriental Herbal Medicine Traditions

The
ENERGETICS
of
WESTERN HERBS

Integrating Western and Oriental Herbal Medicine Traditions

Peter Holmes

In Two Volumes
Vol. I

ARTEMIS ❧ Boulder

Important Notice

The information contained in this book is for educational purposes only. It is not intended to diagnose, treat or prescribe, and does not purport to replace the services of a duly trained practitioner. The information presented herein is correct and accurate to the author's knowledge up to the time of writing; however, since herbal medicine, like anything else, is in constant development, it is possible that new information may cause future modifications to become neccessary.

The only Chinese medical terms which have been retained in their original form is the word Qi, pronouced chee and meaning breath(s) or vital force(s), and the terms Yin and Yang.

Acknowledgement is made for permission to reprint the following:
From Henri Leclerc, *Précis de phytothérapie*, © 1983 Masson; reprinted by permission of Masson et Cie., Paris.
From Virgil Vogel, *American Indian Medicine*, © 1970 Virgil Vogel; reprinted by permission of the University of Oklahoma Press, Norman.
From Georg Harig, *Bestimmung der Intensität im Medizinischen System Galens,* © 1974 Georg Harig; reprinted by permission of the author, East Berlin.
From Merlin Stone, *Ancient Mirrors of Womanhood*, © 1979 Merlin Stone; reprinted by permission of Beacon Press, Boston.
From Daryl Kollman, unpublished transcript, © 1986 Daryl Kollman; reprinted by permission of the author, Klamath Falls.

Illustrations by Hazel Thornley and Daemian Masters
Cover design by Peter Holmes
Cover art by Ken Bernstein
Cover calligraphy by Li Ming Lee
Typesetting by Mountain Media & Graphic Center, Boulder, Colorado
Woodcut illustrations from Leonhardt Fuchs' *Kreuterbuch*

FIRST EDITION

Copyright © 1989 by Peter Holmes

All rights reserved. No part of this book may be reproduced or transmitted in any form or by any means, electronic or mechanical, including photocopying, recording or by any information storage or retrieval system, without written permission from the author, except for the inclusion of brief quotations in a review.

ISBN 0-9623477-6-0
Library of Congress Number 89-080816

Published by

ARTEMIS PRESS INCORPORATED
P.O.Box 4295
Boulder, Colorado 80306, U.S.A.

Manufactured in the United States of America

Written in memory of Nancy Salian

ه

Dedicated to Artemis,
Lady of the Wild Things

*As provider of the juniper and the hellebore that could be used for healing,
Artemis taught of the medicines of the woods.*

ACKNOWLEDGEMENTS

My teachers in all aspects of Chinese medicine, through the living word: Naburo Muramoto, Cecile Levin, John Hicks, David Lee, Jean Schatz, Elizabeth Rochat de la Vallée, Claude Larre, Ted Kaptchuk, Kathy Boisen; and through the written: Leung Kok Yuan, Henry Lu, Manfred Porkert.

My teachers in Western herbal medicine, through the living word: Christopher Hedley, Henri Verdier, Michael Moore; and through the written: Simon Mills, Maud Grieve, Jean Valnet, Charles Lichtenthäler, Werner Christian Simonis, Olivier Dezeimeris, Bernhard Aschner, Hans Funke, Finley Ellingwood, Edward Shook, John Quincy, John Floyer, Wilhelm Pelikan.

Not to forget numerous medical and herbal writers from the more distant past, in the Greek, Chinese, and Ayurvedic traditions—some of them illustrious, a few of them divine, and most of them unremembered.

The book itself came into being with contributions of various kinds from a number of people. I am grateful to many, too numerous to mention all, in the Chinese acupuncture and Western herbal medicine community in San Diego and Santa Fe: their hearts and spirits were open and inspirational. I owe especial thanks to certain individuals who were instrumental in helping me produce this text:

Randy Barolet, Gail Derin, Jonathan Clogstoun-Wilmot, Peter Stanton and Eric Kiener, who offered invaluable advice for this project at the onset;

Christopher Hedley, without whose invaluable insights on Western herbal medicine this text would certainly be a poorer one;

Willem Daems, Director of Pharmacy at Weleda A.G., Arlesheim, Switzerland, who generously made the excellent library available to me;

Govinda McRrostie, Linda Meloche, Maureen Sandler, Chana Frank, Valerie Hobbs, Jyoti Masters, Lore Freeman, Laurel Mage, Debra Nuzzi and Feather Jones who read through and imaginatively criticised certain sections of the text;

Jake Fratkin, who suggested some of the comparisons with Chinese herbs in the Materia Medica;

Jane Maier who, by patiently pruning redundant words and carefully cutting prolix sentences, helped produce a more readable text;

Shirley Weisz who, by bringing the punctuation up to the twentieth century idiom, edited the whole text;

Frank Gray who, by solving near impossible computer problems, made the production of this book possible;

Jyoti Masters, my publisher, who contributed valuable advice and much moral support;

And last but not least, my mother, who supported the project.

Contents

Foreword by Stephen Fulder, Ph.D. — xi
Preface: An Historical Overview, by Ted Kaptchuk, O.M.D. — xiii
Preface: The Value of Integration, by Randall Barolet, O.M.D. — xv

Part One

Prologue — 1

1 HERBAL MEDICINE EAST AND WEST: MEDICAL PHILOSOPHY — 11
Chinese and Western Thought: Complementary Paradigms
Chinese and Greek Medical Concepts

2 HERBAL MEDICINE EAST AND WEST: MEDICAL THEORIES — 21
The Two Paradigms
The Two Polarities
Essential Chinese and Greek Medical Terms

3 THE MEANING OF INTEGRATION — 31
The Need for Integrating both Paradigms
The Two Keys to Integration
Working with both Paradigms within a New Context
Integration and Localization

4 THE MATERIA MEDICA RECLASSIFIED — 41
Present and Past Classifications of the Materia Medica
Reclassifying the Materia Medica
The Twenty-Five Herb Classes

5 THE INTEGRAL PRESENTATION — 47
The Herb's Definition and Nomenclature
The Herb's Nature
The Herb's Functions and Uses
The Herb's Preparations
The Three Categories of Herbs

6 HISTORICAL ANTECEDENTS — 55
Historical and Modern Sources
Primary Historical Sources
Methodology

7 GUIDELINES TO PRESCRIBING — 67
Herb Selection
Duration
Preparation
Dosage
Herb Combining

The Energetics of Western Herbs

8	**PREPARATION FORMS AND USES**	**79**
	Preparations for Internal Use	
	Preparations for External Use	
	ENDNOTES	93

Part Two: the Materia Medica

GUIDELINES TO USING THE MATERIA MEDICA		**98c**

Eliminating 99

Class 1	**HERBS TO CAUSE SWEATING AND RELEASE EXTERNAL CONDITIONS**		**103**
	CAUSE SWEATING AND SCATTER WIND COLD		
	pungent warm circulatory stimulant diaphoretics		
	Peppermint		107
	Ginger		110
	Sassafras		112
	Oshá		114
	Butterbur		116
	Virginia snakeroot		118
	CAUSE SWEATING AND SCATTER WIND HEAT		
	pungent cool peripheral vasodilatory diaphoretics		
	Linden		119
	Elder flower		121
	Catnip		124
	Spearmint		126
	Eucalyptus		128
	Boneset		130
	Vervain		132
Class 2	**HERBS TO PROMOTE URINATION AND RELIEVE FLUID CONGESTION**		**135**
	seeping diuretics		
	Lovage		137
	Goldenrod		140
	Squills		142
	Wild carrot		144
	Dandelion leaf		146
	Elder bark		146
	Couch grass		148

Contents

Class 3 **HERBS TO PROMOTE BOWEL MOVEMENT AND RELIEVE CONSTIPATION** **151**
   STIMULATE THE LIVER AND GALL BLADDER, BREAK UP OBSTRUCTION AND PROMOTE BOWEL MOVEMENT
   choleretic and *cholagogue laxatives*
Celandine	156
Milk thistle	159
Culver's root	161
Blue flag	163
May apple	166
Fringe tree	168
Balmony	170
Fumitory	170

   CLEAR HEAT AND PROMOTE BOWEL MOVEMENT
   cold laxatives and *purgatives*
Rhurbarb	173
Cascara sagrada	176
Alder buckthorn	178
Senna	178
Aloes	180
Tamarind	182

Class 4 **HERBS TO EXPEL PHLEGM AND RELIEVE COUGHING** **185**
   GENERATE WARMTH AND EXPEL PHLEGM
   warm stimulant expectorants
Hyssop	187
Pine	190
Blood root	192
Yerba santa	194
Inmortal	196

   CLEAR HEAT, RESTRAIN INFECTION AND EXPEL PHLEGM
   cold antiseptic expectorants
Pleurisy root	198
Scabious	200
Grindelia	202
White horehound	203
Coltsfoot	206

Class 5 **HERBS TO PROMOTE THE MENSES AND CLEAR STAGNATION** **209**
   stimulant emmenagogues
Juniper	213
Wild ginger	216
Hazelwort	218
Pennyroyal	219
Oregano	221
Rue	223

Class 6	**HERBS TO CAUSE VOMITING**	**225**
	emetics	

Restoring 227

Class 7	**HERBS TO INCREASE THE QI, RESTORE AND REPLENISH DEFICIENCY**	**231**

INCREASE THE QI, RESTORE THE LUNGS AND NERVE, ENHANCE IMMUNE POTENTIAL AND CREATE STRENGTH

Qi, lung & nerve tonics

Licorice	238
American ginseng	241
Elecampane	243
Sage	246
Thyme	249
Cardamom	252

RESTORE, STRENGTHEN AND SUPPORT THE HEART, HARMONIZE THE CIRCULATION, LIFT THE SPIRIT AND RID DEPRESSION

cardiac tonics

Arnica	254
Hawthorn	257
Cereus	260
Lily of the valley	263
Valerian	265
Cowslip flower	269

RESTORE THE LIVER, STOMACH, SPLEEN AND INTESTINES, AWAKEN THE APPETITE, PROMOTE DIGESTION AND CREATE STRENGTH

bitter digestive & hepatic tonics

Calamus	272
Angelica	275
Holy thistle	278
Yarrow	280
Tansy	283
Feverfew	286
Barberry	287
Oregon grape	290

RESTORE AND STRENGTHEN THE UROGENITAL ORGANS

urogenital tonics

Fennel	291
Saw palmetto	294
Buchu	296
Jasmine	298
Damiana	300
Poplar	302
Gravel root	303
Sea holly	305

RESTORE THE UTERUS AND RETURN THE MENSES
uterine tonics

Helonias	308
Life root	311
White deadnettle	313
Mugwort	315

Class 8 — HERBS TO SUPPORT THE YANG, GENERATE WARMTH AND DISPEL COLD — 319
pungent hot circulatory stimulants

Cayenne	322
Horseradish	325
Black pepper	328
Rosemary	330
Prickly ash	333
Cinnamon	335
Camphor	338
Bayberry	340

Class 9 — HERBS TO RESTORE THE BLOOD, NOURISH AND REPLENISH DEFICIENCY — 343
nutritive blood tonics

Flower pollen	345
Microalgae	349
Wheatgrass	354
Asparagus	357
Oats	359
Parsley root	362
Iceland moss	364
Kelp	366
Bladderwrack	369
Alfalfa	370
Nettle	372
Watercress	375

Class 10 — HERBS TO FOSTER THE YIN, PROVIDE MOISTURE AND LENIFY DRYNESS — 379
sweet bland demulcents

Marsh mallow	381
Blue mallow	383
Slippery elm	384
Comfrey	385
Mullein	388
Borage	390
Chickweed	393
Irish moss	395
Lungwort lichen	396

The Energetics of Western Herbs

	Aloe gel	397
	Balm of Gilead	399

Class 11 — HERBS TO CAUSE ASTRICTION, DRY MUCOUS DAMP, ARREST DISCHARGE AND STOP BLEEDING — 401

astringents

Tormentil	403
Cranesbill	405
Oak bark	407
Geranium	408
Eyebright	410
Turpentine	412
Walnut	415
Canadian fleabane	418
Sumac	420

VOLUME II — Draining — 423

Class 12 — HERBS TO CIRCULATE THE QI, RELAX AND LOOSEN CONSTRAINT — 425

relaxants

Lobelia	429
Pasque flower	433
Black cohosh	436
Parsley seed	439
Motherwort	441
Marjoram	444
Skullcap	447
Bugleweed	449
Wood betony	451
St. John's wort	454
Lady's slipper	457
Wild cherry	459
Wild yam	460
Camomile	462
Bergamot (Bitter orange rind)	466
Aniseed	468
Caraway	470
Chasteberry	471

Class 13 — HERBS TO CLEAR HEAT, RESOLVE FEVER AND REDUCE INFLAMMATION — 475

RESOLVE FEVER AND CLEAR HEAT ON THE QI LEVEL

bitter cold febrifuges

Gentian	483
Bogbean	485
Centaury	487
Wormwood	489

Chicory	492
Melissa	494
Lavender	498
Melilot	501
Selfheal	503

REMOVE CONGESTION, RESOLVE INFLAMMATION AND CLEAR HEAT ON THE BLOOD LEVEL
sour astringent cold anti-inflammatory decongestants

Wood sorrel	505
Grapevine	508
Rose	510
Lady's mantle	513
Sanicle	515

RESTRAIN INFECTION, RESOLVE INFLAMMATION AND CLEAR DAMP HEAT
bitter astringent cold antiseptics

Horsetail	517
Sandalwood	520
Agrimony	522
Willow	524
Loosestrife	526
Bearberry	528
Blackberry	531
Bilberry	533
Cornsilk	536

CLEAR TOXEMIA, RESOLVE INFLAMMATION AND CLEAR FIRE TOXIN
cool detoxifying antiseptics

Lemon	538
Purslane	541
Ribwort plantain	543
Meadowsweet	547

Class 14 HERBS TO ENLIVEN THE BLOOD, RELIEVE CONGESTION AND MODERATE THE MENSES — **551**
astringent venous & uterine blood decongestants

Goldenseal	553
Red root	557
Shepherd's purse	559
Horse chestnut	561
Witch hazel	563
Marigold	565
Cypress	567
Stoneroot	570

The Energetics of Western Herbs

Altering & Regulating — 573

Class 15 HERBS TO PROMOTE CLEANSING, CLEAR TOXINS AND RESOLVE TOXEMIA — 574
cleansers

Dandelion	580
Artichoke	583
Cleavers	584
Yellow dock	586
Pipsissewa (Wintergreen)	588
Speedwell	591
Birch	592
Figwort	594
Burdock	596
Celery	599
Sarsaparilla	601
Poke root	603
Hydrangea	606
Heartsease	608
Red clover	610
Cowslip root	613
Bittersweet	615

Class 16 HERBS TO REGULATE THE YIN AND THE YANG — 619
systemic Yin/Yang or CNS regulators

Class 17 HERBS TO REGULATE HORMONES — 623
hormonal regulators

Symptom Treatment — 625

Class 18 HERBS TO ENHANCE PREGNANCY AND CHILDBIRTH — 627
pregnancy enhancers

Raspberry	630
Black haw	632
Cramp bark	634
Squaw vine	635
Blue cohosh	637
Birthroot	640
Birthwort	642

Class 19 HERBS TO RELIEVE INDIGESTION — 645
digestives

Class 20 HERBS TO CALM THE SPIRIT — 647
nerve sedatives

Mistletoe	649

		Contents
	Hops	652
	Passionflower	655
	Neroli (Bitter orange flower)	657

Class 21 **HERBS TO LIFT THE SPIRIT** **659**
antidepressants
    Basil   660
    Savory   662

Class 22 **HERBS TO RELIEVE PAIN** **665**
anodynes

Class 23 **HERBS TO PROMOTE TISSUE REPAIR** **669**
vulneraries

Class 24 **HERBS TO ACTIVATE IMMUNITY, RESTRAIN INFECTION AND CLEAR TOXINS** **671**
anti-infectives
    Garlic   673
    Myrrh   676
    Cajeput   678
    Tea tree   680
    Echinacea   681
    Wild indigo   684
    Chaparral   686

Class 25 **HERBS TO KILL AND EXPEL PARASITES** **689**
anthelmintics & parasiticides

Classification of Remedies according to Treatment Methods and Herb Actions   691
Classification of Remedies according to Organ Syndromes   715

APPENDIXES   729
A The Greek Four Element System
B Synthesis of the Greek and Chinese Element Systems
C The Organs and the Four Organisms
D The Eight Krases (Temperaments) and the Eight Biotypes
E The Three Constitutions

BIBLIOGRAPHY   735
  Source books
  Works on Chinese Herbal and General Medicine
  Works on the History of Herbal Medicine
  Works on Lexicography

Glossary of Terms   745
Pharmaceutical Name Index   751
Botanical Name Index   755
Common Name Index   765
Repertory   775
General Index   787

FOREWORD

There is a plethora of books available today on herbs. They cover uses, constituents, botany, history and so on. At first sight this appears to be as full a literature as at any time since the seventeenth century. However, a closer look shows that almost all of this literature is derivative, based on a few well known books that have been published over the last few years. Unfortunately these main sources are also not themselves original works of major importance. They too are haphazard collections of early literature and some practical experience. They do not bear the ancient herbal tradition intact across a century of herbal amnesia. Nor can they attempt the synthesis of traditions that is necessary and possible today. One cannot integrate fragments. Yet this integration is urgently required.

Partly for historical reasons, modern herbalism is not a full and coherent medical system. It is more a patchwork of ill-defined and semi-systematic therapeutic guidelines. The herbal lineage has zig-zagged its way from Greece to Arabia, to Europe, to America and back to Europe again, picking up and loosing things on the way, and arriving in the 20th century as an eclectic mixture of Galenic flotsam, folk medicine, early Victorian therapeutic classifications and language, and a little chemistry and pharmacology. This does not denigrate its value, which is unquestionable. But instead of taking its place as the exemplary and primary complementary medical system, alongside conventional medicine, as in India, it is still struggling to find its roots. True and complete herbal medical systems do exist and have existed. Both Chinese and Ayurvedic medicine represent vast bodies of knowledge, with a philosophical basis sublime and deep as the oceans, with well constructed classifications, systems of diagnosis and treatment, rational and universal principles for the cure of mind, body and spirit, and with astonishing and potent therapeutic discoveries. It is not only on the other side of the globe that we need to look for herbal erudition. In the Western tradition there is also a systematic body of knowledge, originally from the Greeks. It has undergone testing, development and refinement since Galen, and also much interruption, distortion and obscuration. These are our building blocks. We haven't understood them properly.

Recognising this, Peter Holmes has begun the work towards the reconstruction of the living herbal medical tradition. This can only be done by a painstaking restoration of the original picture, followed by a creative matching of herbal medical systems of East and West. This was the task he set himself, and this book is his offering. It is the original work that is sorely needed in the Western herbal tradition, and perhaps we didn't know how much we missed it until it arrived.

Like the herbal masters to whom Holmes pays respect, his work is not merely one of refined scholarship. It is also full of insight and practical application. He identifies the therapeutic properties of herbs as much by their taste and their clinical use as by the evidence from sources. The result is a fundamental classification that is a foundation upon which can be built a much more solid and self-consistent structure of theory and practice. It is a very important text, and I hope it becomes a landmark, an historical breakthrough, on the way to an authentic modern herbal medical system.

Stephen Fulder, M.A., Ph.D.
Oxford, 1988

Preface: An Historical Overview

The breakthroughs into new frontiers of knowledge that marked the west's scientific revolution reshaped our consciousness of what illness and health mean. Vesalius' anatomical studies (1543 A.D.) and Harvey's discovery of circulation (1628 A.D.) forever overthrew older notions of what is verifiable information and how to proceed to uncover new truth.

While such new theoretical knowledge continued to develop, little useful clinical therapeutics was discovered for centuries. Vesalius and Harvey never abandoned their herbal repetoire because of the new science, but the later generations of university trained doctors began to feel uncomfortable using the herbal knowledge of the prescientific Greco-Muslim traditions. The university trained elites felt that traditional herbalism was "tainted" by association with "archaic" ideas. The revolution in science began to zealously attack any "contamination" of the old order. An era of therapeutic chaos resulted which completely abandoned the old herbalism. Educated elite doctors infused with science would not be soiled with the past; herbalism was purged from the august halls of scientific universities. This nihilism reached its peak with the eighteenth and nineteenth centuries' madness of bleeding (raised to a new fervor by Harvey's discoveries) and calomel poisoning (inspired by the technology of the times). Traditional western herbalism was exiled from the universities into the folk practices of uneducated practitioners. The richness of the tradition was buried in rare book collections out of harm's way in inaccessible European libraries.

China never experienced a scientific revolution. Although its political revolutions have brought modernity and the scientific revolution itself to China, the older "archaic" therapeutics, for various reasons, still has a claim on its health care and its soul. The traditional medicine of China has been an inspiration to many of us in the west looking for an effective and rational way to be sophisticated herbalists. The Oriental herbal tradition has challenged many of us to ask Joseph Needham's question in reverse: "How is it that herbalism has become such an elegant and powerful tradition in the east and not in the west?" Peter Holmes in this important volume has accepted this challenge, gone to the libraries and shown that there is a rich herbal tradition in the west that was discarded by the enthusiasm and ideology of the scientific revolution. Peter Holmes has creatively engaged the best of the buried western herbal tradition in a dialogue with the rich tradition of the east. *The Energetics of Western Herbs* is an important discussion that can only enhance the creativity, depth, intelligence and clinical skills of all herbalists both in the east and in the west.

Ted Kaptchuk, O.M.D.
Cambridge, Massachusetts
May, 1989

PREFACE: THE VALUE OF INTEGRATION

Peter Holmes' work, *The Energetics of Western Herbs,* serves as a strong and thorough foundation for an integrated system of energetic herbal healing. It offers us a synthesis of Galenic and Chinese herbal concepts, and establishes a classification scheme which, although possessing slight distinctions from that used in Chinese herbal healing, is essentially the same.

Peter Holmes has achieved something of significance. He has not acted merely as a scholarly intellectual or historian, though his work may certainly be appreciated at that level. Rather, he has moved on a path through the literature of the western herbal tradition using the scholarly mind as a vehicle, but ever watchful with the eye of a sensitive artist, in order to bring to us the product of his creative imagination. His journey has been a path of integration within and without. In reading his work, I feel both the focus of the dedicated scholar and the spark of the committed visionary. The careful literary archaeology and analytical thinking is admirable from the scholarly perspective; however, it is not used here as an end in itself, but rather as a means for the creative realization of an expanded and revitalized herbal healing system.

The foundation upon which this all takes place is the spirit of the quest: searching—discovering—testing—and creating. It seems that he has used this work to share with us a vision of global herbal healing which recovers the treasures of the European and Near Eastern herbalists and medical philosophers, recombines these with the guiding light of systematic energetics provided by the Chinese herbal tradition, and thus arrives at an entirely new destination. That destination is the place of further integration. It is neither a singular product of the western mind, nor is it solely characteristic of the eastern mind, but is instead a manifestation of the search for Global Mind. The mystics, monks, and yoga masters tell us that "Truth is one, paths are many." Each step we take along the path of creative integration may bring us just a little closer to practicing in accord with that one Truth. It is for that step along the path which Peter Holmes is daring to take, and for the increment of global insight which it may offer, that I believe we should be grateful to the Spirit which is moving him.

Although Peter Holmes' work is based on careful research and clinical experience, we do not have to assume that his classifications are definitive and final. Naturally, we may feel the need to make modifications in light of our own experience. As practitioners and scholars, we need to critically evaluate this work and apply it in clinical practice in order to bring this synthesis of two major energetic traditions into full play in the world. Until Peter's book, we lacked a systematic theoretical knowledge of how to align western herbs with their counterparts in the Chinese materia medica. Now we have a firm footing from which to start building our practical knowledge.

Honoring the ancestors, the Chinese cultural gaze rarely stops looking backward. In doing so, it preserves traditions and its feeling of continuity in time. Pioneering with the analytical mind, the European cultural gaze rarely stops looking forward. In doing so, it sees itself as blazing a trail into space. Peter's task has been to pick up the forgotten threads of our western herbal healing art so that it may regain its sense of continuity, become historically self-reflective, and in that sense become an equal partner with the Chinese herbal healing art. Peter is a creative and synthetic thinker who, like an archaeologist, is digging up the priceless relics of our discarded healing lineage, carefully dusting them off, and examining every detail in light of the cross-cultural insight provided by comparison with another rich tradition—the energetic and vitalistic tradition of Chinese herbal

The Energetics of Western Herbs

healing. By paying respects to the healing ancestors, the modern healing mind is reconnecting itself to another source of wisdom. In this manner—looking backward in time, moving foward in space, but always in the present moment—the collective global healing consciousness evolves.

As you move along with Peter through this text, you will not only be offered a new integrated methodology for using herbs, but you will also have the enjoyment of joining in his quest to recover the past, be delighted by the stories he has to tell, and be enlightened by the insightful commentaries he has carefully crafted for us.

Randall Barolet, Lic. Ac., O.M.D.
Martha's Vineyard, Massachusetts
June, 1989

PART ONE

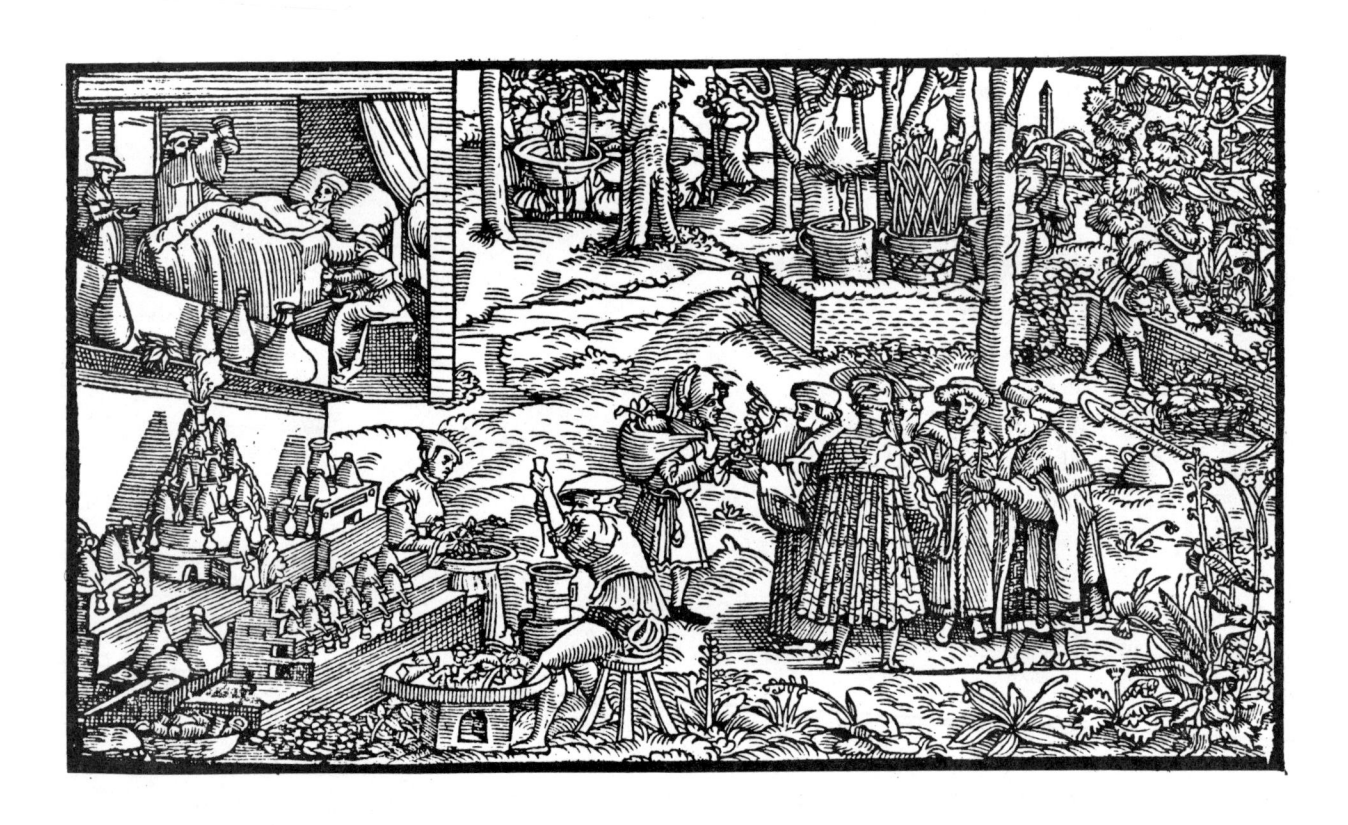

From an old German herbal, ca. 1550.

PROLOGUE

This book was begun many years ago in a small blue notebook bought in one of those wholesale stationers that line Clerkenwell Road in London. "*Circulates the meridians and clears obstructions, benefits the Spleen and clears damp,*" begins the entry for Lovage root. Over the years this booklet grew and grew, becoming a favorite handbook of herbal notes and jottings, until they outgrew its size. Another notebook was started, this time a thick black one obtained from one of the better office supplies in Hollywood. It rapidly became filled with the herb classes of Chinese medicine with listings of the corresponding Western herbs: "*Relieve the surface and disperse, clear heat and quell fire ...*" and so on.

At that point it became clear to me that I was faced with a decision: to write, or not to write. It was a difficult one. After all, my only aim in keeping these notes had been to make botanical remedies understandable to me and useable in my own practice, alongside the use of acupuncture and Chinese herbal formulas. I was disappointed with long lists of near meaningless adjectives found in all the available books on herbal medicine or phytotherapy. I wanted to get to know the plants that grew in the areas where I lived in the simple, functional, energetic and vitalist-based way of Chinese medicine, which had been my initial training. As a result, I decided to familiarize myself with Western herbs in the empirical way of all traditions—namely, by tasting them for their actual taste, by noticing any warming, cooling or other effect they might have, and by trying them out with actual ailments, according to their energetic properties. This learning was not an overnight affair. On the contrary, it was a process that dominated my life over many years and that demanded endless patience. My conclusions kept shifting, as my experience with herbs evolved, and finally settled to their present state. In this way my perspective of the common wild plants of Hampstead Heath in London, of the Penwyth penninsula in Cornwall and, later, of the Sangre de Cristo mountains in New Mexico gradually became transformed.

At the same time, through clues provided by reprints of popular writings such as NICHOLAS CULPEPER's *Herball,* it began to dawn on me that possibly Greek-Galenic medicine had for over two thousand years regarded plants in the same way as Chinese medicine. Having spent years of extensive trial and error investigations applying energetic principles, there was now no alternative but to begin to find out what lay hidden in the dust laden annals of Western medicine itself. I was determined to pry open the connections between Chinese and traditional European herbal energetics. When I met a colleague in a Chinese pharmacy in Soho (obtaining such essential supplies as *Shou di, Dang gui* and the like) and told him of my research in the British Library, he exclaimed, "You mean there's a sunken Atlantis of information in there?"

The records and testimonies of writers from Hippokrates up to the present day were indeed impressive and rewarding. Each of the libraries I visited in European cities yielded a treasure trove of little known—and, to me, novel—information. Of the libraries I visited, the richest of all was the Richard Banks collection in the British Library itself. Through physicians and compilers writing in a variety of languages, the whole breadth and depth of Galenic medicine came alive in its many variations, as it passed from its Greek origins over to Alexandria, then to Bagdhad, back to Italy and central Europe and, finally, over to the New World.

In taking in this depth of material I felt confirmed about certain conclusions I had reached, while having to let go of others. Through this research, my initial foundation in the practice of

The Energetics of Western Herbs

Chinese medicine and my original enthusiasm for herbal energetics now became consolidated with an inspiration to present Western botanicals as they had always been historically employed, namely in the functional and energetic way. In the vitalist Galenic tradition, herbal remedies are consistently described in a way that includes their qualitative aspects such as taste, warmth, and moisture—in other words, their energetics. The word energetics itself derives from the Greek word *energeia,* meaning force or energy. In Oriental medicine herbs are classified according to the treatment method that they serve, such as those that bring about tonification, draining, cooling, etc. They are also described according to the whole pattern or configuration of signs and symptoms that they treat. Essentially the same approach was taken in Greek-Galenic medicine, though the language in which this was expressed was that of Greco-Roman philosophy of GALEN's day (late second century). Whereas the recurrent theme in Chinese medicine is a rebalancing of a whole pattern of disharmony in order to re-establish harmonious Qi and blood flow throughout the meridians, the medical writings of Greek medicine speak rather of rebalancing the individual ground according to his or her innate natural constitution so that the four qualities and the four fluids become once more harmonious. While reading this source material, it was clear again and again that what was needed was an unbiased evaluation of Galenic herbal energetics, not only in the light of Chinese energetics, but also based on our present-day trial and error empirical conclusions.

After years of feeling alienated from Western medicine, through this process of research and discovery I began to feel deeply linked with the Western medical tradition. The feeling of belonging to an authentic historical tradition was empowering and grounding for me as a practitioner of herbal medicine. It was clear that the herbalist had played the most important role within the Galenic tradition as a whole and that his training and practice had not been all that different from my own.

After discovering the real threads of our European medical tradition, I felt the need to understand why vitalistic Greek-Galenic medicine collapsed as it did. From written medical histories I was unable to find an adequate account of this. From my studies of Greek-Galenic medicine itself, however, I could hypothesize how the initial vital theories had increasingly fossilized, becoming turgid dogma and meaningless mannerisms divorced of any empirically based understanding of energetics. Exploring this question has led me into some unexpected byways and surprising conclusions that have fostered the unfolding of parts of this book.

Unfortunately, in the modern practice of herbal medicine we have not had access to the depth from which its skill arose, which is none other than the energetic qualities of botanicals properly applied to the energetic imbalance of the individual. Because of this, scientific pharmacology, for example, only became understandable to me once I realized that it was the modern analytical version of energetic pharmacology which had been in use for over two milleniums.

The closer I looked, the more two things dawned on me. First, I would never be able to look at any modern information about an herbal remedy in the same way again. Knowing that the origin of the current terminology and content of botanical medicine was an energetic approach, I was able to see through what are today mere relics of its past. This has provided me with a basis to evaluate the creative and living elements of herbalism today, as well as to recognize the empty shells from the past.

Secondly, and more importantly, I realized that an attempt to simply recreate an herbal text in the traditional Chinese or Greek style was in itself not sufficient at the present day. It is not enough to merely reconstruct herbal medicine according to a phenomenological (i.e. observation based) orientation and one based on more holistic concepts of the human organism, such as existed even three hundred years ago and still exists in the form of current Chinese medicine. Materialistic

Prologue

quantitative experimental science based on analysis has irrevocably changed our consciousness and is the only widely accepted currency of value today. There seemed little point then in recreating an isolated polynia of a holistic, qualitative system in this type of landscape, however fashionable at the present time.

It became clear to me that the key lay in the **integration** of the two styles of herbal medicine, the holistic and the analytical, each based on its own values. The Eastern holistic approach from the past had to harmonize with the Western analytical method of the present. How can this seemingly impossible integration be achieved? To answer that, we need to understand the process of consciousness underlying these very different approaches.

The challenge of our time is nothing less than to include the divergent elements that make up our present-day consciousness. The essential reason that we can no longer bring forward Galenic herbalism, however appealing the idea, is that it comes from a much simpler time and state of consciousness. As part of a necessary stage in his process of individuation, Western man has developed a highly individualized consciousness, in which analytical aspects of thinking and perceiving are brought to the fore. It is this shift of consciousness which lies at the base of the development of analytical Western medicine.

Today, we can readily admit that the reductionistic, analytic paradigm that has developed as part of our scientific age has many drawbacks for the discovery of health and well-being. By the same token, however, we can also see how taking the analytical approach as we have has led us to the very threshold of the great ancient holistic traditions of the East. It is because of that insatiable hunger of the analytical mind itself that we have sought a deeper wisdom. Through the current emergent meeting of these traditions with what appears to be a very limited modern paradigm, we have a potent cross-fertilization of ancient wisdom and modern consciousness.

We have opened to a foreign ancient system such as Chinese medicine because of its proven efficacy in effecting cure. In linking to those perennial wisdom-based principles of healing within the Chinese tradition, we are given the means to turn back to our own traditional roots and to recognize what similar wisdom and depth may lie behind its healing methods. As a result, we are now in a position to include this wisdom in creating a present-day integrated approach, a paradigm based on principles of holism. In this way the ancient wisdom itself is redeemed: it develops and moves forward in a new setting, becoming the all-integrating foundation that it is, rather than the empty theoretical superstructure it always tends to become.

In allowing in the words of that traditional Oriental paradigm, the language of our culture is being enriched and molded by nonanalytic, nonlinear concepts such as *qi, karma, dao, dharma*. Even everyday words such as "energy" and "balance" have in the process taken on deeper meanings. Therefore, rather than throwing out lock, stock and barrel the entire modern analytical approach to curing, we need to permeate this current knowledge with the principles of healing that have served mankind for millenniums, be they Chinese, Greek or any other. In short, we need to allow these holistic principles to be in charge, while allowing analytical knowledge simply to serve their holistic goals. This, in a nutshell, is how the two styles of herbal medicine may be integrated.

Including the analytical approach serves to confirm and make precise these holistic traditional principles of medicine. If, for example, one can determine that a person's right flank pain is due to gall bladder stones, then this is a great asset in the diagnosis and treatment of the Chinese syndrome liver Qi stagnation. It is my belief that the value of including analytical information not only provides a means to communicate to a Western audience, but also opens a doorway to using that information in a deeper, wisdom-based context. The analytical method thereby becomes grounded, and is able to fully come into its own as the practical and useful tool that it actually is.

At the same time, I realized that any holistic presentation of herbal remedies could not rely exclusively on either traditional Greek **or** Chinese systems. I discovered that certain aspects of botanical therapeutics in the Greek tradition opened a perspective not found in Chinese medicine. The well-developed energetic understanding of herbs based on the four primary qualities of hot/cold, dry/damp is a case in point. The great attention paid to the *physis,* the natural balance innate to every individual, and the **ground** of disharmony, the underlying tendencies to imbalance in every disease condition, is another example. Clearly, here also a meeting between the Chinese and the Greek holistic systems had to be arranged, and a synthesis—however experimental—essayed. It would have been a mistake to attempt a recreation of a latter-day Galenic herbal or a mere emulation of Chinese texts, however tempting these propositions. The former would plunge us into a strangely familiar yet highly unfashionable past, whereas the latter would immerse us into a very unfamiliar, though stylish present. Instead, the essential holism of each had to be extracted and applied to our present-day use of Western herbs, in order to create a pharmacopoeia grounded in the past, but written in the present as an offering to the future.

Having reached this point, the decision I had been faced with much earlier, to write a book, was finally made. And several years down the road, this is the result.

My search for a way of integrating Oriental and Western herbology and my understanding of the paradigms that underpin them, have resulted in a book that is clearly a gathering of various elements. Four separate strands have gone into the weaving of the present text, the first two being major, the second two minor. They are, first, the teachings of Chinese medicine; second, the comparable body of wisdom from Greek-Galenic medicine; third, the empirical wisdom of the European wise woman tradition and the Native American tradition; and fourth, the analytic-scientific medicine of the last century or so.

My predilection for Chinese medicine rests on the fact that at this time it represents the clearest example of an observation-based and therapeutics-oriented system of healing. As a model of a vitalistic system of herbology, with its axis on the concept of **Qi**, it is unsurpassed and, indeed, unique. Throughout Chinese medicine, functions take priority over structure, and processes over fixed entities. As a result, with the use of Chinese medicine a complete articulation from plant pharmacology to human pathology becomes possible. Consequently this text emphasizes the clinical uses of herbal energetics, indicating not only the syndromes, or patterns of disharmony, that each botanical is typically used for, but also the specific symptoms that it treats within each syndrome.

My predilection for the strand of Greek medicine is no less influential on this Materia Medica. In addition to developing a system of qualitative pharmacology similar to that of Chinese medicine, the Greek medical heritage is fairly unique in developing the concepts of **physis** and **ground** as major therapeutic factors. Here it is the individual in all his idiosyncrasies, both in health and sickness, that is considered the focus of attention. As a result, prevention becomes even more weighty than treatment. Moreover, that delicate dialectic between a person's ability to effectively respond to disease, between his **vital spirit** and pathogenic factors, is given more careful consideration than in any other medical literature. As a result, in this Materia Medica the *krases* (temperaments), biotypes and constitutions most suited to being treated by a certain herb are indicated; and elements such as disease stages in the progression of fevers are fully discussed in the introduction to each treatment method.

Although precious little information has been handed down to us concerning the use of herbs by wise women practitioners, this secondary strand was woven into the tapestry of the Materia Medica nevertheless. What commends it above all is the empirical foundation of its tradition. Over many centuries, certain herbs, in certain combinations, were used time and again for certain conditions with unfailing success. The same is true for another major empirical tradition, that of the Native Americans. The most influential Greek medical herbal, that of DIOSKURIDES, is essentially a compilation of the empirical wisdom of his day. This attests not only to the significance of the empirical approach in healing, but also to the fact that the largest part of herbal treatment was, and still is, a practical service to the community. In the past this was carried out first and foremost by women practitioners of various kinds. Today, although both the wise woman and the Native American traditions are almost defunct, they can live on if we make use of the expertise acquired over millenniums, and develop it according to actual present-day needs. This element, too, is incorporated into the Materia Medica.

Finally, the use of analysis-based information from Western medicine in any herbal text today is not only unavoidable, but also positive. As important as the fact that the applications of herbal remedies include Western disease concepts such as infectious diseases and tissue pathology is the fact that biochemistry has brought some interesting clarifications to traditional energetic pharmacology. When used to further more holistic, integrated therapeutic concepts such as we find in Greek and Chinese medicine, a knowledge of plant chemical constituents and their theoretical action on human tissue is often an invaluable support. This kind of information then serves to make substantial and specific the insights gleaned through the observational or empirical methods. Holistic qualitative knowledge becomes enhanced by analytical precision and clarity in the process. For this reason, in the Materia Medica section plant constituents are given with every botanical and in the Notes are related to the overall energetic picture of both herb and illness, where this is possible.

The four strands of this book can be reduced to three basic elements. They are vital for the continuance of an effective, authentic and humane system of herbal medicine based on the integrity of the human being, not on technology. These elements are the **holistic context**, provided by traditional systems such as the Chinese and Greek; the **empirical content**, as embodied in the wise woman and the Native American traditions; and the **analytical back-up** provided by biochemistry. It is the use of these three in concert that goes to make a truly integrated, dynamic herbal medicine.

Clearly, my aim in writing this eclectic Materia Medica is not simply to revamp Galenism or to duplicate Chinese herbalism, holistic and wisdom-based though these are. Nor is it another attempt to squeeze yet more information out of past herbals. Neither is it an attempt to find new uses for common herbs under the sanction of biochemistry. All these approaches are fully represented in currently available books on herbs. Instead, in this book I attempt to present a **new context** for herbal medicine. The intoductory chapters, as well as the presentation of each botanical, purport to show how the real need today is not for more herbal uses or applications but, more fundamentally, for that new context. This allows much of the confusion between the various styles of herbalism to be clarified and the endless search for novelty—so endemic to our culture—to be pacified.

A new context is created when we understand systems of herbal medicine as emblematic expressions of paradigms rather than as absolute, immutable truths. In this way, the new context here proposed allows us to make use of the information passed on in Chinese and Galenic medicine as a model of these traditions. Rather than remaining dead theoretical knowledge, this information then becomes alive, malleable and extremely workable. As a result, it can begin to serve the needs of both present-day consciousness and current health concerns, addressing problems inherent in modern medicine, as well as contemporary illnesses and ways of being dis-eased themselves.

When the context in which we use botanical remedies changes, then everything within it changes, from herb selection to treatment methods. This may be described as an integral approach. As far as we can see, this is the only way that these very divergent styles that dominate herbal medicine today can be reconciled and put to advantageous use simultaneously. In this way, the very

The Energetics of Western Herbs

specific advantages that each has to offer in clinical practice are culled, while their disadvantages are spontaneously, and painlessly, shed.

That there is a real need in herbal medicine today for a system that exhibits the characteristics of balance, authenticity, rationality and efficacy in full measure is, I hope, an obvious one. Western phytotherapy is fragmented into a variety of sects, arising largely from the turmoil of the years 1450 to 1850. This period saw the decadent phase of the Galenic tradition, culminating in its complete overthrow with the establishment of FRANCOIS MAGENDIE's experimental scientific method. By 1900, herbal medicine, as the most essential part of Galenism, was effectively declared dead. It lost the ground beneath its feet and the grounding in its own tradition as a result. In this connection, it is ironic to consider that it was not experimental science alone that led to the demise of traditional Galenic herbalism. The search for new ways of employing herbs has always been very much part of the Western style.[2] As Chapter 1 explains, it is the perpetual cycle of new theory/old theory inherent in the process of Western knowledge that essentially sabotaged the Greek medical tradition.

This lack of connection with past practice, this lack of continuity from the ancients to the moderns, has been a singularly debilitating factor in herbal medicine since that time. It lends to all our endeavours in this branch of healing an unfortunate ephemeral, superficial quality which no amount of sophisticated scientific language can ever mask, however well-intentioned. As a result, there is no real agreement today, for example, as to the nature and functions of remedies from either a terminological or a practical viewpoint. Even simple terms such as *diuretic* and *astringent* are used with different connotations and implications by different schools and individuals. Again, the same herb may be used in quite different ways from one country to another, as the remnants of regional traditions intermingle with newer ideas spawned in laboratories.

In this setting, it is not surprising that complementary medicine as a force in its own right has come to the fore. Its focus has increasingly been traditional medical systems that have retained some kind of authenticity of tradition and holism of approach, in recent decades Chinese medicine especially. Here, not only are terminology and teaching absolutely standardized and clear, but they carry with them the considerable weight of at least four thousand years of uninterrupted accumulated experience.

Clearly, the need at this time is to link up once again with our own broken tradition, in order to better be able to work with Chinese medicine. Only by understanding the basis of our own Western tradition from both a historical and philosophical perspective can we become grounded enough to have a fruitful exchange with Chinese herbalism.[3] If any headway in this direction is to be made, then the roots of Greek/Galenic/Tibb Unani medicine (all elements of a single continuous tradition) have to be explored and interpreted afresh, and its system of herbology and therapeutics directly compared to the Chinese system. Chapter 1 is an attempt in this direction.[4] Only in this way can the new context be created which is able to encompass both the phenomenon orientation of Chinese medicine and the analysis orientation of Western. Moreover, if we are to pretend that we are on anything but slippery ground, then an exploration of herbal writings in the West, in both the natural scientific and medical streams, is unavoidable. Clearly, the different types of herbal classifications used, the variations in the presentation of remedies, as well as their underlying paradigms, all need due examination. This is the object of Chapters 3 and 5.

At the moment, as practitioners of Western herbalism without this grounding in the past, we have precious little to offer in exchange; hence our sponge-like eagerness to absorb holistic systems from elsewhere. Yet with a little exploration this situation can be remedied, although an equal exchange may never be possible due to the recent loss of a continuous tradition. Still, any exchange at this point is better than none, and the picture that may result from this interchange is

Prologue

guaranteed to be a highly stimulating one for both sides.

In this light, the present work is an attempt to bring about a more current, integrated herbal medicine guided by the time-tested principles of energetics. I emphasize these principles because they come from traditions whose vision of the human being is one of depth, complexity and interrelatedness, involving a waking of the body, the mind and the spirit as vital elements of well-being.

I should single out certain practitioners of Greek medicine that have been a continued source of inspiration, and that have confirmed my own search. The late-Greek physician CLAUDIOS GALENOS, known as GALEN for short, and his eleventh century Persian successor IBN SINA, heve definitely been outstanding in this respect. The work of both these practitioners has made it clear to me that if a Western energetics-based herbal medicine was able to thrive in the past, then it should be possible to initiate (with the assistance of Chinese medicine) and develop such a system once again today. Specifically, GALEN's way of assimilating and reorganizing disparate medical theories, and then transforming them on the basis of an energetic context—his lifetime's work—has no parallel. His example heartened me in bringing forth a Materia Medica not only based on energetic principles as in Chinese herbalism, but one which also uses as its working material a variety of strands of herbal practice traditional and modern. The work of IBN SINA, on the other hand, is the clearest model of a fine elaboration and an in-depth integration of herbal medicine. It was genius such as his which motivated my attempt to weave these various strands into an articulated coherent whole.

There are also other practitioners who have inspired me to emulate their example in my own time. They are herbalists such as HILDEGARD VON BINGEN, OTTO BRUNFELS, HIERONYMUS BOCK and PIERANDREA MATTIOLI. The impulse they embody is simply a devotion to using plant remedies that are native rather than those from abroad, and mild herbs rather than more toxic ones. In the introduction to their herbals, for example, both BRUNFELS and BOCK decry the prevailing fashion of their day for prescribing page-long formulas of Middle Eastern remedies from dispensatories such the *Antidotarium* of AR-RAZI and PSEUDO-YUHANNA. Local plants are what they want to see used, the same common plants used by the wise women, in fact, and write about them in their herbals they do. Their wisdom not only confirmed me in my own approach, but also awakened in me a deeper conviction that the use of gentle and easily available plant remedies can be equally successful in clinical practice. The historical parallel between then and now, in this regard, became very clear to me.

Because this book is also a pragmatic attempt to put some of the above ideas into practice, the Materia Medica forms its core. Some difficult decisions had to be made: which herbs to include, which to leave out, which classes to place them in, etc. The choice of botanicals, for example, was not guided by any arbritrary decision about their importance. Every remedy is important when used effectively. This is a pragmatic truth, whether it is a kitchen remedy like raw Ginger, or a professional remedy like Aconite. Herbs were chosen which are known to be effective, regardless of whether they have a wide or a narrow spectrum of uses, or whether they are widely used today or were more popular in the past and are now neglected. The selection was further guided by considering which plants grow both in Europe and America. Finally it was moderated by the simple availability, or non availability, of certain herbs. Rupturewort, for example, is a superlative remedy in almost all urinary conditions, but is not included due to the difficulty of obtaining it, especially in America. Hedge hyssop, Water germander and Parsley piert found in Europe, and Yellow jasmine, Seneca snakeroot and Ipecac found in the States, are all brilliantly tried and tested

The Energetics of Western Herbs

botanicals, but are omitted for the same reason. Nevertheless, these and many others are included in the two synopses found at the end of the Materia Medica.

There are at least two ways in which the Materia Medica may be viewed. From one perspective, it is a suggestion of a way in which Western herbs can be incorporated into the practice of Chinese medicine, i.e. by cataloging the treatment strategies that they serve and the syndromes that they treat. From the other viewpoint, the Materia Medica is a compilation of the nature, function and use of herbal remedies from the Western pharmacological perspective both traditional and modern.

Insofar as the Materia Medica consists of treatment methods based on Chinese pharmacology, and insofar as Chinese syndromes of disharmony are presented, the Materia Medica is the result of what could be called creative craftsmanship. This is not altered by the fact that some treatment methods and syndromes (as well as the overall five-fold organization) are distinctly Galenic in conception. It is impossible to ascertain the patterns of disharmony Chinese doctors would have assigned these plants to. Fortunately, this is not the issue. The question we are faced with is, *how are we, as Western practitioners going to benefit from the principles of Chinese herbal medicine today?* And more specifically, *how are we going to use Western herbs in the light of the Chinese influence?* These questions are open ones. The answers will evolve from the experience of many practitioners over many years, as the interaction between Chinese and Western medical systems continues. In this field, we are all beginners and experimenters. This book is written as a suggestion, a working proposition in this direction. While it provides a precedent and represents a new development, it does not pretend to be the final word or even propose the *dernier cri*. It aims instead simply to inspire further trials, reasearch and conclusions.

Seen from another perspective, the Materia Medica represents both a compilation and re-creation of some (not all) received traditional uses of botanical remedies. In more ways than one it tries to define the ways that herbal medicines were thought about and used in the past by the many individuals who were connected to them. It attempts not only to give credit to the masses of educated, literate physicians going back to HIPPOKRATES in the 4th century B.C., but also to acknowledge the unrecorded illiterate healers, most of them women, who practiced the herbal art since prehistoric times. Through their intimate contact with the living Earth, Gaia, and the mysteries of goddesses such as Artemis and Cerridwen who were its physical and spiritual expression, the empirical practitioners of the past developed highly evolved and intuitive knowledge of natural healing. Certainly, the distinction between these two types of healers became blurred at times. Throughout Greek culture and up to the early Middle Ages, for example, women physicians, including midwives, were sometimes even more common than male physicians. Far from being the sole domain of an elite legislated group of practitioners as at present, medicine in the past was always practiced by a motley assortment of healers, ranging from wise women, midwives and wildcrafters to monks, theologians, pharmacists and naturalists. The present Materia Medica thus is an attempt to reclaim this Western herbal heritage, to present a case for the traditional Western practitioner.

It would be a mistake to assume that this rich fabric of traditional medical practice is not worthy of our consideration. On the contrary: it represents a content of inestimable value, since each practitioner was a true specialist in her or his particular skill. In the unrecorded traditions of herbal medicine, for example, each healer was a link in a chain that went from mother to daughter or, less frequently, from father to son, and as such embodied a font of accumulated empirical practice. The skill that individual practitioners achieved in *tonic herbal medication*, midwifery, bone setting and so on must have been very high. Certainly this knowledge was significant enough to represent a threat to the university trained healers, who by the fourteenth century conspired with Church and state to eradicate it once and for all.[5]

Prologue

Obtaining information on the herbal practices of the literate practitioners within Galenic medicine proper is comparatively straightforward—although not without its own difficulties, as Chapter 5 explains. On the other hand, accessing the ways in which the unlegislated women practitioners utilized herbal medicines is another question entirely. It is a tricky task, since almost nothing of their experiences was ever written down, except for what was recorded secondhand during the Renaissance by herbalists such as BOCK and BRUNFELS. While some of their practices still survive in very diluted form in European country areas today, many of these are definitely lost.

Reclaiming our heritage is nothing less than an act of self-empowerment. A big question, however, remains, namely, *how as healers can we reclaim this heritage?* Specifically, *how do we integrate the knowledge from the past with our current state of knowledge today and use it in a practical way?* Here again there are no pat answers, since the questions are part of the current process, one of many processes that complementary medicine is undergoing.

To sum up: the Materia Medica in this book raises as many questions as it proposes answers. It opens a discussion which hinges around how traditional, vitalistic and energetics based uses of herbal remedies may be integrated with the current Western understanding of them. The traditional uses include both those of "literate" Chinese and Greek medicine and Western folk use, and since there is a definite link between the two aspects of traditional herb usage, the process of elucidating one will also help shed light on the other. This Materia Medica is a first step in suggesting working answers.

The basic message of this book is that we need to develop a new attitude towards the use of herbal remedies. We are all to some extent in the process of finding answers to these issues. We ourselves are the creators of that all-embracing new context which sees the Western and Oriental systems as expressions of paradigms. We ourselves are the facilitators for the unfolding of herbal medicine by allowing an integration of these systems to occur. This places integration in its largest, most creative context—the human being him/herself. And we can continue the renewal of integrated vitalistic Western and Chinese traditions in the manner that seems most appropriate to us.

Notes

1   It is precisely the lack of these creative processes that keeps each system disconnected, while accentuating the other system's weaknesses to the point of manifest absurdity: the holistic approach floundering in its own "eternal now", lack of content, overrelativity and ungroundedness; the analytical approach ever out on a limb with its never-ending search for insight and understanding.

2   This search has taken an interesting twist today in the attempt to find medicinal properties in Western plants identical to their botanical counterparts in China. Although innocent enough in its basic conception, this approach has two inherent dangers. First, the search for new therapeutic properties can easily turn into a justification for novelty seeking—all the more so as it is therapeutically unused agents such as Privet (*Ligustrum vulgare*) and Locoweed (*Astragalus* spp.) that are being investigated.

Secondly, it is a fact of plant chemistry that although botanical relationship is a useful indication of therapeutic similarity of a very general kind, it does not guarantee identical biochemical constituents, let alone even similar medicinal properties, in plants grown in different countries. The reasons for this are to be found in microvariations at the genetic level as well as in external factors such as climate, soil and disease. As a result, the fact that types of *Astragalus* are found growing in America does not automatically make tham Qi tonics like the types of *Astragalus* grown and used

The Energetics of Western Herbs

America does not automatically make tham Qi tonics like the types of *Astragalus* grown and used in China. Nor does it even guarantee any other kind of therapeutic action. In fact, as far as the author can determine, American varieties of *Astragalus* have not been used in herbal medicine at all! Botanical similarity simply cannot guarantee therapeutic similarity. This fact alone undermines the whole basis on which the approach rests, since it introduces a very fundamental aleatory element.

In view of these limiting factors, it is clear that we are on much firmer ground if we search for **therapeutic equivalents** to Chinese remedies rather than botanical equivalents.

3   If Western phytotherapy fails to become grounded in its own roots, then it may well become co-opted by the other system and turn into a purely one-sided phenomenological skill, thus replacing the analytical extreme with the phenomenological one.

4   Aspects of Hippokratic Greek medicine are brilliantly exposed in the works of CHARLES LICHTENTHAELER, and to some extent those of FRIDOLF KUDLIEN and HEINRICH SCHIPPERGES.

5   For reliable, sober (and sobering) historical accounts of the supression of women healers see in particular *Dreaming the Dark* by STARHAWK, p. 183, (Harper & Row, San Francisco, 1989) and *Witches, Midwives and Nurses* by BARBARA EHRENREICH and DEIDRE ENGLISH.

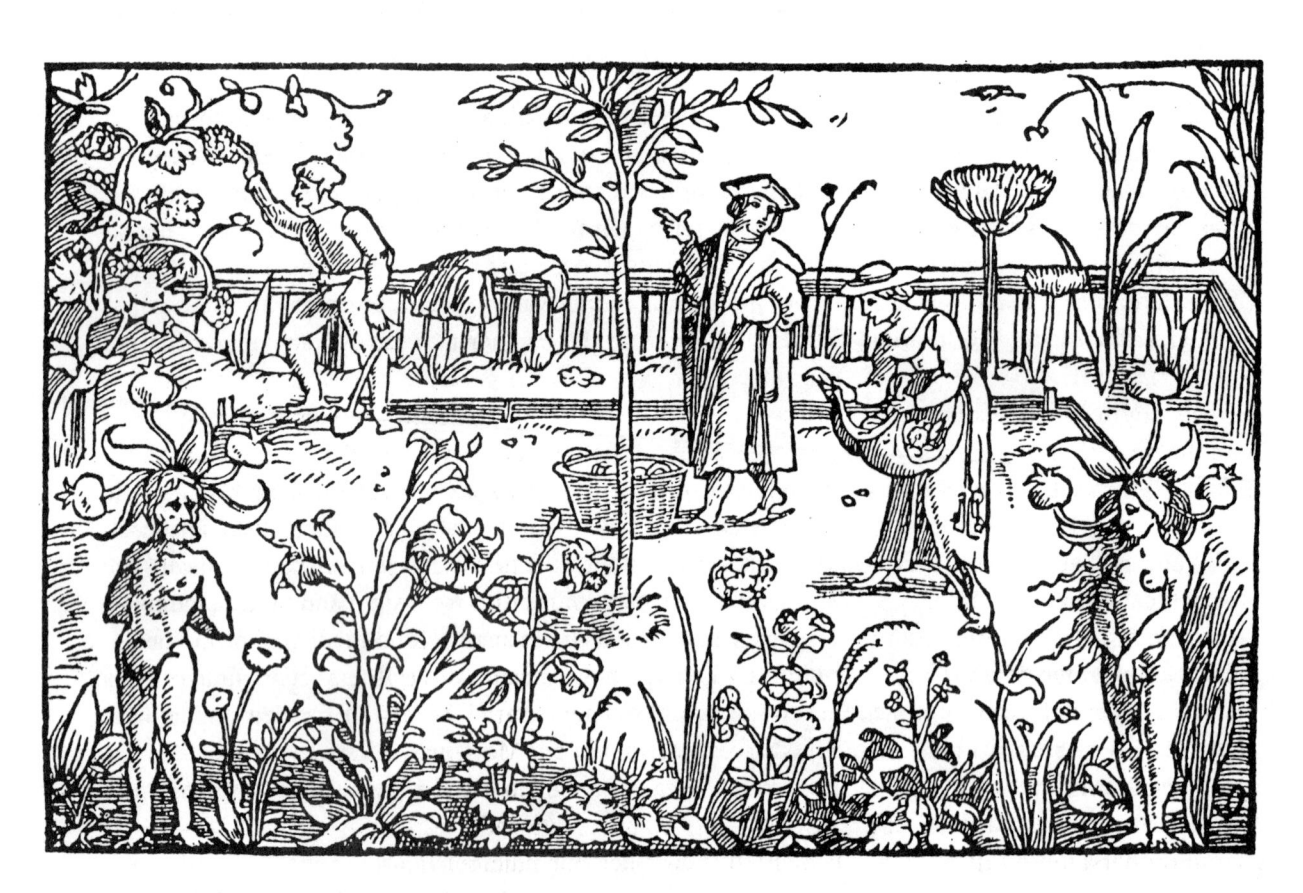

From Gart der Gesundeit, *Antwerp, 1533.*

1
HERBAL MEDICINE EAST & WEST: MEDICAL PHILOSOPHIES

> *The Yellow Emperor asked:*
> "Why is it that people these days cannot always recover from their illnesses by drinking cereal broths and wine delicacies?"
> *Qi Bo replied:*
> "Today, people can only recover from their illnesses through the internal treatment with herbs, and the external treatment of sharp stone needles and moxibustion."
>
> Huang di nei jing *(The Yellow Emperor's Classic of Internal Medicine)*, chapter 14, 5th century B.C.

In the world of Western and Oriental herbal medicine today there are several themes that recur time and again, that run deeply through these healing arts as they are currently practiced. These themes concern the assumptions on which the practice of herbal medicine rests, affecting its very rationale and basic ways of proceeding. Seeing they are very much at the forefront of present-day developments, at a time when we are witnessing nothing less than a renaissance of natural healing methods, we feel it necessary to explore these interlinked themes at the outset. Consequently, this chapter probes issues that have deep historical and philosophical roots, issues whose branches occupy a great deal of the energy of practitioners of both Western and Oriental medicine today.

In sounding these issue to their root we will begin to suggest answers to such questions as *What makes Western and Chinese herbology so fundamentally different from each other? Why is herbal medicine in the West almost a forgotten art, whereas in the East it is still a flourishing tradition?* We may begin our approach to answering these questions by noticing their common pull. Evidently, underlying questions such as these is a fundamental curiosity about the relationship of different parts to a larger whole. *How do different systems of herbal medicine relate?* is perhaps the most basic query being put today.

However, if we are to obtain concrete answers to these questions, the general historical and philosophical terrain in which they lie needs to be explored. Specifically, we need to take a closer look at the significant points of similarity and difference between two of the major systems of herbal medicine, the Western and the Chinese. In so doing we can lay the foundation for a new holistic context that can encompass both systems, one that not only illuminates their interconnections, but also provides a greater insight into each. Moreover, establishment of this fundamental holistic context will be instrumental in allowing us to explore the ways in which the most refined and useful aspects of each system may be integrated and used to mutual advantage, in order to further a more authentic, whole and efficacious herbal medicine.

There are essential points of contact among Chinese, Greek-Galenic and modern herbal medicine. First, Chinese and traditional Greek herbalism share as a common basis the **phenomenological**, or **observational**, method. This similarity is a very strong one, as will shortly be seen. Secondly, Greek medicine and modern herbal medicine have the same **exploratory**, **analytical** bias. However, the common ground of Chinese and Greek herbal systems vis-à-vis

The Energetics of Western Herbs

modern herbalism is a much stronger link than the common ground of the Greek and modern systems vis-à-vis the Chinese.

It is the **common ground** of the phenomenological approach, as expressed by both Greek and Chinese medicine, which is presented in the Materia Medica in this text. Phenomenological thinking is simply based on **observing phenomena closely**, rather than on speculating through general theories, and, for this reason, is also called observational thinking. It places more emphasis on the **sensible qualities** that herbs possess, such as taste, warmth, texture, color, etc.; the **human biotypes**, i.e., psycho-somatic character types that they serve; and the **syndromes of disharmony** that are their indications. The phenomenological method is less concerned with quantifiable aspects such as the biochemical constituents and mechanisms of plants, the treatment of disease mechanisms with these, and symptom removal. If a text on herbalism is to be holistic in more than just name, and use expressions such as "patterns of disharmony" in a way more meaningful than a trendy cliché, then it should live up to its purported aim by a holism of content and method, not merely by a holism of idealistic intent. Phenomenology, as a result, as best exemplified by the botanical systems developed in the Greek and Chinese traditions, has been built into this Materia Medica as the fundamental method at its very roots. Moreover, the analytical approach rooted in Greek medicine and most clearly represented by modern herbalism is also integrated into the present Materia Medica. In discussing an herb's nature, for example, not only its traditional qualities of **taste**, **warmth** and **moisture** are given, but its quantifiable **chemical constituents** as well. The section on each herb's functions and indications, for example, list not only the traditional Chinese and Greek syndromes, but also the Western disease entities for which it has been found useful.

Clearly, these points of contact between the two systems need further investigation if their relative similarities and differences are truly to be appreciated.

Chinese and Western Thought: Complementary Paradigms

What is it that fundamentally determines any system's medical theory, in its conceptual or linguistic aspect? Here we observe that it is a culture's philosophy, as an expression of its ontology, which is all-determining. Its philosophy informs the paradigms, or basic organization of concepts, on which all its theories rest. Moreover, medical language is no exception in reflecting the philosophical heritage of any given culture. Examining this language allows us to pinpoint, more or less specifically, the difference of approach to health, disease and healing between Oriental and Western thinking.

Before embarking on an exploration of the similarities of philosophy and medical thought between East and West, we may first of all usefully define their differences.

Speaking in general terms, whereas Western thinking is more based on logic, linear causality and isolation, Oriental thinking is based on patterns, relations and synthesis (or holism). Western thought is analytical, positivist and reductionist; Oriental thinking manifests dialectic and phenomenological qualities.

Western thought is based on empirical observation, which leads to the creation of a theory. Truth undergoes a life cycle of knowledge characterized by a long, slow phase of development, followed by a sudden, short, revolutionary change, which then makes way for the germ of a new theory.[1] Truth is a transcendant established paradigm or set of beliefs behind a theory, which, by dominating all knowledge tends to create a rigid, structured monopoly, in which other truths are incompatible, and therefore necessarily inadmissible. Historically this has been the case of secular truths such as natural scientific theories, and also of religious truths. Truth in the West has the character of the masculine principle, authoritarian and exclusive as reflected in any society dominated by the patriarchal archetype.

Oriental thought, on the other hand, remains more closely connected to eidetic, precognitive experience and therefore observes differently, seeing universal models or emblems of laws in these observations.[2] Truth is an immanent pool of knowledge which allows for continuous dialogue, ongoing cyclic changes and innumerable variations without altering the contextual structure of the universal models of knowledge itself.[3] This may be seen in the religions, arts and natural sciences throughout China's history. Truth in the Orient is very much like the feminine principle, all-embracing without being dominating, hidden yet everywhere immanent, and is seen in societies past and present with a matrifocal bias.

Examples of this immediately spring to mind. In the West, both ARISTOTLE's concept of the four elements, namely, water, earth, air, and fire, and GALEN's theory of the four fluids were slow in developing and only gradually evolved and changed to accomodate new facts over a period of one and a half milleniums. During this time, these two theories held absolute sway over thinking in medicine and the natural sciences. However, the first came to a rapid end in the heady fumes of the Iatrochemists' laboratories of the sixteenth century when they primitively discovered chemical elements; while the second came crashing down in the experiments of the French biochemist FRANCOIS MAGENDIE in the firtst decade of the 1800's. Both theories have since been replaced by the atomic elements and cellular pathology, and more recently by other theories such as electrical biomedicine. The point is that, although autocratic while they exist, the theories all have predictable, limited life cycles, like those of biological phenomena. Like biological phenomena, they evolve and fall.

The situation is quite different with the Oriental type of thinking. Here patterns of thought such as Yin/Yang, the five elements and the six divisions of Yin/Yang have endured from prehistoric times without any development or radical fall; they are still as important in the East as they have always been. Not being theories in the Western sense, but universal models of knowledge and repositories of information, they have been interpreted, utilized and modified in countless ways. They have been applied to every conceivable human enterprise, including geomancy, medicine, art and historical interpretation, to cooking, warfare and fortunetelling. The validity, let alone the existence, of these giant models or emblems themselves has never been questioned. This would be as meaningless as questioning the existence of sunlight, or of life itself. Yin/Yang simply is, and can be experienced in life itself—that is all there is to it—hence the stability and endurance of these emblems, in spite of the innumerable variations and presentations in which they are to be found. Their constancy and endurance very much resemble the permanence of the cosmos itself, with its ever present (although ever changing) sun, moon and stars.

In the West, truth is **becoming.** In the East truth is **given**.

Turning now to the healing arts specifically, we see the Western paradigm exemplified by the dominance of **one medical theory** above all, whether based on fluids, vital force, tissue tone, cells, atoms or whatever. In early Greek medicine, for example, each medical school (Dogmatic, Pneumatic, Hippocratic, etc.) had its dominant theory to the exclusion of all other theories. GALEN's brilliant eclectic synthesis of these divergent Greek theories itself became the paramount theoretical paradigm in the hands of later practitioners up to the seventeenth century. The Oriental way, in contrast, is characterized by **several medical models** simultaneously. This allows, for example, both the eight principles (*ba gang*) and the five elements (*wu xing*) to be used as working models of pathology, depending on which best fits the need of any given case. Another example is

The Energetics of Western Herbs

the concurrent use as diagnostic models of both the theory of the six stages of disease according to the six channels (*liu jing*), as set out in the *Shang han lun* (*Treatise on Cold Diseases*), and the theory of the four stages of disease according to the four levels (*si fen*), as presented in the *Wen bing lun* (*Treatise on Warm Diseases*).

It is clear that a culture's basic thinking processes, the paradigms that it develops and the medical theories that follow, are inextricably linked. The theories that Oriental medicine and Greek medicine developed over thousands of years are clearly expressions of these paradigms.

The implications for medicine itself of these two paradigms are very far-reaching. They fully characterize the most fundamental processes involved in describing and diagnosing a disharmony (i.e. a dis-ease), as will shortly become clear. Western medicine essentially goes about looking at a **part in isolation** (of a disease, person or body; it tends also to look at a fixed, somatic structure. The purpose of the Western biomedical approach is to discover by analytical means the **cause** or **mechanism** of a disharmony, on the basis of a disease theory, in order to then be able to name a certain illness. The parallel process in Chinese medicine, on the other hand, involves looking at a **whole, consisting of relationships** (of a person, symptom-sign complex, etc.) in a functional, dialectic way. Here the aim is to synthesize different aspects, to arrive at the **pattern** of a disharmony purely through the act of observation, and to describe the disharmony using a model appropriate to that observation.

Both the Western and the Oriental way of going about things have a place. Neither is correct or wrong. Both simply have advantages and disadvantages. The disadvantages are more obvious. In the West, the problem is that theory so often turns into dogma and inflexibility. This has been shown throughout Western history, in which the forces of the rulers and the Church empower a secular or religious theory with universal and transcendant validity. Not only Christian dogma, but also Galenic medical dogma, e.g. the four fluids theory, the eliminating treatment methods of purging, vomiting, etc., are outstanding cases in point.In the East, on the other hand, models of knowledge can become too numerous and meaningless. In multiplying and undergoing innumerable variations, they become more speculative and lose their original power and effectiveness. This occurred classically in the art of geomancy, in which thirty-two sets of variables eventually came to be used to describe the energetic configuration of a locality, simultaneously applying models such as Yin/Yang, five elements, four directions, six phases, many times over in different ways.

The advantages, however, are more difficult to accurately define, yet are self-evident to the individuals using one or the other modality of knowledge. They will be examined in Chapter 3. Moreover, it is becoming evident that the paradigms generated by Chinese and Western styles of thinking are, in fact, complementary. They are so perfectly polarized that they actually complement each other. The evolutionary, directional, analytical, masculine character of Western thought is complemented by the circular, timeless, synthetic, feminine nature of Chinese thought. Moreover, since they are complementary paradigms, it is evident that they can also be grasped **as a whole**, understood as two parts of a single entity. In fact, seeing them in this way suggests the question of whether they could not be used simultaneously in some way.

If indeed our objective is to cull the advantages that both the Chinese and Western paradigms have to offer, we need to resolve the dichotomy of radically different philosophical paradigms when engaging them in the actual practice of herbal medicine. A way of working must be found which utilizes the advantages of both systems while minimizing their disadvantages. Such a solution will also be offered in Chapter 3.

Chinese and Greek Medical Concepts

The similarity between the traditional world views of ancient Greek and Chinese culture long ago established a relationship between their medical systems. This is evident, for example, from the fact that a college of Greek medicine was established in Peking by a group of Muslim practitioners of Greek medicine in the twelfth century. However, neither medical tradition recorded anything worth speaking of about the other. There are two reasons for this. The first is the proximty of the Indian subcontinent with its vastly influential Ayurvedic medical system. The other reason is that communication from the Northeast of the Arabian territories, where Greek/Tibb Unani medicine was practised, was blocked by the three gigantic Central Asian mountain chains, on the other side of which Tibetan medicine alone was practiced. As a result, both Greek and Chinese medicine had more direct medical exchanges with neighboring Ayurvedic medicine in the west and east of India than they did with each other. The links found between them, therefore, are due, more than anything else, to the similarities in their world view.

Generally speaking, most of the characteristics of Chinese thinking were shared to some extent by Greek culture and its healing arts. Like Chinese medicine, Greek medicine for over seven centuries up to the time of GALEN was typified by thinking in terms of **patterns**, **relationships**, and **synthesis**. By the fourth century B.C., when the Hippokratic writings were set down, Greece was very much a jacuzzi pool of ideas where philosophies jostled for attention and came and went in a very liberal ambiance. Observation, dialogue and phenomenology were their main features, like those of the best Chinese philosophies. The more close-circuited life cycle of Western knowledge had not yet taken shape. The greatest empiricist, HIPPOKRATES, in *De veteri medicina* (4th cent. B.C.), was able to say in all sincerity that "all thought which is founded on observation leads to truth...every skill owes its original results to the observation of every phenomenon, reflected upon and then reduced to general principles."

Looking at the way in which the relations between the human and the environment are described and developed in both medical systems reveals an underlying similarity. Natural elements such as earth, water, fire, air (metal in China), are portrayed, in both, with qualities (*dynameis* or *qi*) such as heat, cold, dryness, damp and wind arising from their interaction. The mutually generative and restraining interactions of the Chinese five elements (*wu xin*) is different from the more structural Greek approach; nevertheless, both are emblems of knowledge which allow a system of inductive correspondences to be established, linking the cosmic and the particular, the universal and the individual (see Appendix A). In both medical systems these terms are used not only to explain the origins of disease, but also to describe it diagnostically. Greek medicine uses both the four qualities (*tessares dynameis*) just mentioned, and the four fluids (*tessara chumoi*). The former, of course, include two of the eight principles (*ba fa*) used in Chinese medicine, namely hot/cold. Using the four qualities, both Greek and Chinese medicine classify illnesses into hot diseases, cold diseases, dry diseases and damp diseases, and, using the four fluids model, into diseases due to yellow bile, black bile, phlegm and blood. Hence it comes as no surprise to learn that herbal remedies themselves are also categorized according to their effect on the four qualities and the four fluids, and may increase, decrease, or qualitatively alter these. In addition, when it comes to therapy, much emphasis is given to adjusting treatment according to the changing circumstances of time (of day, month, season and even year), of place (or region), and of the human (i.e. the ground) affected. Clearly, the human being, the natural environment which nurtures him/her, illness and the remedies to cure them are all related and hence unified through these natural elements.

Wholeness is another hallmark of the common ground of both systems. Primary in traditional Greek medicine, for example, (especially for practitioners of the Kos school) is treatment according to the axiom *holon tou somatos*—the whole person. This is not the cliché it now sounds but simply points to the importance of observing the whole person and condition before inspecting any part. Chinese practitioners have also taken this principle for granted. Both invariably read the pulse; examine the tongue; look at or enquire about the patient's excretions, such as urine, stool, phlegm; and take careful note of every sign or symptom, however minor. Moreover, they want to know about the natural, social and personal environment of the patient. Through this comprehensive diagnostic approach they were able to assess the gestalt of the disease, spanning mental, emotional and physical ailments.

Likewise, both Greek and Chinese medicine regard the re-establishment of **balance**, or *mesotes* in Greek, as the fundamental principle of all therapy. Whether talking in terms of qualities (*dynameis*), fluids (*jin ye* or *chumoi*), breaths (*Qi* or *pneuma*), blood (*xue* or *haima*) or spirit (*shen* or *spiritus vitalis*), both practitioners sought to bring about that delicate, dynamic state of balance according to each individual's *physis* or innate, natural condition. This balance was assessed by Greek physicians as a person's particular natural *krasis*, or mixture of fluids, which for that individual represented a *eukrasia*, a positive fluid mixture. Preventive treatment whose objective was to rebalance a person's entire innate condition, succinctly expressed in the two Greek words *kata physis*, was the highest form of therapy in both Greek and Chinese medicine.

In their treatment objectives also, Greek and Chinese medicine are on common ground. Both treat **whole patterns of disharmony** rather than isolated ailing body parts. Before treating any certain symptom or ailment (and barring emergencies), in order to rebalance the whole individual in all his/her capacities, they specifically advise lifestyle and dietary adjustments, exercises, and changes of attitude, in addition to prescribing botanical medicines. Over centuries and milenniums both systems developed herbal prescriptions which address the entire energetic state of imbalance rather than relieve the symptoms alone. While not neglecting to treat the symptoms, the part of the disease, especially when acute, they always do so in the context of rebalancing the whole disharmony. In this connection Chinese medicine talks about treating the **root** of illness rather than its **branches** (*biao ben guan nian*), focusing more on the unique disharmony brought about by a particular imbalance of Qi and blood, Yin and Yang. Likewise, to Greek practitioners, finding the underlying ***diathesis***, or tendency to imbalance, from which a multitude of symptoms may arise, was a more worthwhile goal than merely relieving the more manifest symptoms separately. Moreover, in focusing more on the individual **ground of disharmony**, by observing how an imbalance of the fluids and qualities, a *dyskrasia* or *kakochumia*, arose from constitutional potentials (*katastasis*), Greek physicians were able go on to define the particular **biotypes**, such as lymphatic, sanguine and melancholic, that these *dyskrasias* typically generated. Even though the language and method used differs somewhat in Greek and Chinese systems, in both cases it is the entire, unique, and individual configuration of imbalance that is assessed and treated.

The specific **principles and methods of treatment** are also very close in both medical systems. Essentially, the treatment principles boil down to either "supporting nature and conserving forces by treating *kata physis*" (GALEN), i.e. supporting the righteous Qi (*zheng zhi*), in Chinese medicine in deficiency conditions; or "chasing illness by treating *kata diathesis*" (GALEN), known as confronting the injurious Qi (*fan zhi*), in Chinese medicine, in the case of excess conditions. In the first case, the treatment strategy chosen is one of *plerosis*, replenishing, or *bu*, restoring, the deficiency; while in the second case the objective is *kenosis* or *xie*, draining the excess. Since botanical remedies were the agents of choice used to effect these changes, in both Greek and

Herbal Medicine East and West: Medical Philosophies

Chinese herbology they were organized in herbals and dispensatories according to these broad methods. Here they were further subdivided into more specific restoring methods such as increasing the Qi, the blood, the Yang and the Yin, as well as draining or dispersing methods such as "penetrating the evils" (*tou xie*), "draining the blockages" (*tong wu yu*), and "chasing winds" (*qu feng*), using means such as causing sweating, urination, bowel movement, clearing heat, activating the blood, etc. It is the common ground of Greek and Chinese therapeutic categories, in fact, that allows an integrated presentation of herb classes in this Materia Medica (see chapter 4).

In their theoretical constructs, furthermore, both Greek and Chinese systems are distinguished by typically **qualitative** and **dialectic** value and methods of working, as opposed to the **quantitative** and **theoretical** ones of Western medicine. Both medical systems rely for their philosophical framework on paradigms such as the four elements (*tessara stoicheia*) in Greece and the five elements (*wu xing*—better translated as *five effective principles*) in China. These cannot be given any purely quantitative value in terms of modern science, nor, indeed, were they designed for such reductionism. Their purpose, being defined by **qualitative** criteria, is much larger, deeper, and more authentically human than anything the limited quantitative approach can define. Likewise, both Greek and Chinese medicine share purely qualitative principles and systems of etiology, diagnostics and therapeutics, such as the four effective qualities used in Greece and the six Yin Yang qualities used in China.

Moreover, these philosophical-medical models are also **dialectic** by nature. When a Yin function or process is observed in physiology, for example, then its opposite-complementary Yang function also needs to be taken into account. When the relative proportion and intensity of the qualities such as heat and cold, dryness and damp, and excess and deficiency are assessed in different parts of the body, once again this is carried out on the basis of dialectic principles. All aspects of Greek and Chinese medicine, from pharmacognosy to therapeutics, are stamped with qualitative and dialectic characteristics.

Clearly, these models cannot be reduced to mere theory, in the sense of a scientific theory. They are both theory and practice in one, indivisibly. Their only theoretical value is in being exercised in clinical, real-life practice.

In particular, it is GALEN's brilliant synthesis of various conflicting medical theories which bears a striking resemblance to the corpus of Chinese medicine. GALEN was able to make a unique amalgam of the teachings of the Greek medical schools from Alexandria, namely the Empiricists, Experimentalists, Methodists, Pneumatists and Dogmatists. While the systems of both GALEN and Chinese medicine contain roughly the same knowledge, their organization and presentation concerning both terminology and methodology are somewhat different. This is true in spite of the fact that they in places seem identical. A whole study presenting one system with reference to the other would be required if one wanted to adequately define their intersecting points. It certainly would be a long study.

Nevertheless, we may still fruitfully take a few concrete examples from Chinese and Greek medical philosophy and physiology to illuminate their common ground.

a) One of the bases of Chinese medicine is what is called the **three treasures** (*san bao*). These are **spirit** (*shen*), **breaths** (*qi*) and **essence** (*jing*).

The idea of spirit (*shen*) is paralleled in Greek medicine by the concept *pneuma*, or by ruh in Arabic or *prana* in Ayurvedic. These words describe a configurative force of cosmic origin whose function is to create and maintain all active physiological forces.[4] Qi is a type of spirit which best translates as *breaths*, and which equates with the Greek *pneuma*. Essence is found in Greek

The Energetics of Western Herbs

medicine as the concept **ground fluid**.

Both Chinese and Greek medicine stress that the fundamental balance in the individual is between the spirit (*shen, pneuma*) and the essence or ground fluid (*jing*). On the basis of this assumption, GALEN emphasizes that when the spirit and the fluids are in harmony a state of *eukrasia*, a harmonious balance of the fluids, can result. When in disharmony they create an unhealthy mixture between them, a *dyskrasia*.

That the concept of the three treasures also reached the European West is evinced, for example, by a 1570 text of LEVINE LEMNIE entitled *The Touchstone of Complexions*. Undoubtedly drawing on an unknown Persian or Arab author, LEMNIE calls them the "three especiall things." In a discussion of "krasis and diskrasis" he launches into the subject with the words "for seeing as there be three especiall thinges in whose Temperature and moderation the health of man's body doth principally consist, *viz*. vitall moysture, natural heate, and Spirite, which combineth all things, and imparteth his force, virtue and nature unto them..." The descriptions of these three elements that follow are unfortunately too long to quote; however, they leave no doubt as to the object of LEMNIE's discussion. He closes by observing that "these three do inseparably cleave together and mutually helpe one another, and cannot be sundered, wythout present death of the party, and for this cause do wee thus in one definition expresse, conclude and comprehend, theyr force and nature within one definition."[5]

b) According to Greek medicine, spirit, *shen* or *pneuma*, then creates three physiological forces:

(i) **physiological spirit** or *shen*, also known as **vital spirit**, which resides in the heart and warmth organism. It begets consciousness of the self, is responsible for ancestral Qi, or *zong qi* in the chest, which regulates heart and lung functions, and also "preserves the integrity of all spirits" (IBN SINA). The vital spirit oversees all uptake, transformation, storage and elimination of physical and non-material nourishment.

(ii) **soul spirit** or **Qi**, (formerly known as **animal spirit** from the Latin word *anima* meaning soul) residing in the brain and the air organism. It allows consciousness, sensation, feeling and movement and also underlies nervous and sensory functioning.[6]

(iii) **natural spirit** or **nutritive Qi** (*yong qi*) housed in the liver and the fluid organism. They allow transformation, nutrition and regeneration to take place and are the basis for vitality, growth and reproduction.

c) As a result of the activities of the three spirits, many aspects of organ functions and their pathology are very similar or identical in the Greek and Chinese systems. Lists of the Galenic syndromes of the liver and stomach, drawn from sample late Renaissance texts, will illustrate this.

liver weakness
liver stoppage
liver heat
liver cold
liver dryness
liver damp
liver jaundice
liver fluid congestion
       O.BRUNFELS, *Contrafayt Kreutterbuch*, 1532
and
stomach heat & ulcer

stomach cold
stomach steam
stomach phlegm
stomach rotten fever
W.RYFF, *Reformierte Deutsche Apotheck,* 1573

The similarity and overlays with the currently-used Chinese syndromes of these organs is striking, and it would not have taken much imagination for a Chinese physician to recognize these Galenic syndromes—nor vice versa. The entire corpus of Galenic and Chinese terminologies, drawn as they are from the natural elements, is essentially the same.

Both Greek and Chinese medicine also developed sophisticated systems of pulse diagnosis—again another comparative study that could fill many pages.[7] GALEN in the second century standardized 27 pulse qualities in his *De pulsibus*, exactly the same number arrived at by LI SHI ZHEN only 400 years ago! Similarly to the Chinese system, the basic six pulses from which all others are derived are the large and small, strong and weak, quick and slow. Again, many pulse qualities are identical in both systems, in fact if not in name. Some examples are:

- the Galenic bowstring pulse (*pulsus nervosus*) = the Chinese bowstring or wiry pulse (*xuan mai*);
- the Galenic surging pulse (*pulsus undosus*) = the Chinese flooding pulse (*hong mai*);
- the Galenic vibrating pulse (*pulsus vibrans*) = the Chinese tight pulse (*jin mai*).

In general, excellent pulse studies were written by medical authors both before GALEN (CORNELIUS CELSUS, RUFUS of EPHESOS,[8] ARCHIGENES) and after him (ARETAIOS, JEAN FERNEL). Works such as GILLES DE CORBEIL's *Liber de pulsibus*, 1484, and JOSEPH STRUTHIUS' *Sphygmicae artis…* of 1555 only added to this already solid corpus.

Whereas Chinese diagnostics relies on the observation of the tongue for its main visual technique, Greek diagnostics turned to urine inspection with as much systematic fervor. This was natural for a system based on fluids and their *dyskrasia*, since urine is the most important fluid excretion. Pulse and urine diagnosis was the cornerstone of Galenic medicine for sixteen centuries and was depicted in many illustrations and paintings throughout this time. Important texts on urine diagnosis are those of THEOPHILOS of the sixth century, PAUL of AEGINA of the seventh and GILES DE CORBEIL of the twelfth. The classic, however, is IOANNES AKTUARIOS' *De urinis* of about 1300. As late as 1891 FINLEY ELLINGWOOD (an American, not a Greek Eclectic physician) wrote a *Manual of Urinalysis*. The quantity, color, consistency and contents of the urine were all aspects taken into consideration; they were then related directly to pathological conditions or syndromes based on the four fluids and the four qualities.

Turning to the practice of herbal medicine itself, once more the similarities between the two systems are outstanding. Both systems have an emphasis on using the **roots** of plants rather than the herbal part above ground, whereas the opposite is true of Western herbalism today. The *rhizotomoi* and the *rhizotomachia* who specialized in collecting, juicing and vending medicinal roots were an essential part of the healing scene in ancient Greece. Both the Greek and the Chinese systems also emphasize the use of mild and medium-strength remedies in preference to more toxic ones. Both have in common simple preparation forms such as infusion, decoction, honey-ball, pill, electuary, rather than the more complex preparations of the Persian and later Western pharmacists; and both use animal and mineral products to supplement their larger body of botanical substances.

The differences between Greek and Chinese herbal medicine take a secondary place to their common ground, and only evolved gradually as Greek medicine was introduced and developed in Muslim countries with the expansion of the Arabian empire from the seventh century onwards.

The Energetics of Western Herbs

Here Greek medicine became known (and correctly so) as *Tibb unani*, i.e. Unani medicine (that is, Ionian medicine), a name under which in some quarters it still goes today. At this point its theoretical component was developed in a more analytical, linear vein by the genius of several stellar Persian physicians such as AR-RAZI (know as the "Arabian Galen" in his day), and IBN SINA (dubbed the "Arabian Hippokrates"). Practically speaking, since both these doctors were philosophers and alchemists primarily, they and their acolytes heavily influenced Greek medicine with Persian alchemy[9] (itself originally from Greece and Egypt). Thus pharmacy as we know it today arose as herbalism acquired more complex preparation techniques such as essential oil distillation, tincturing, preparing distilled waters, and a variety of other lengthy extraction processes. Greek medicine at this time was also influenced by Ayurvedic medicine from India, both in its theory and its choice of remedies. Moreover, its prescribing habits became more lengthy and began to fill a whole page rather than just a corner. Although the Chinese Tang period also saw such a trend to complexity, which was later cancelled out by other trends toward simplification, it never altered the basic structure of its herbal system. After settling back in Europe during the Middle Ages, Greek medicine from about 1500 to 1800—the period of decline and transition before the arrival of materialistic experimental medicine—developed its own offshoots such as iatrochemistry, iatromathematics and vitalism, which showed more differences than similarities with the Chinese system.

We have followed our curiosity and explored the ways in which, at the deepest levels, Western and Chinese medicine relate. Having examined their theoretical and practical points of contact, we are now provided with the necessary background with which to look more closely at their systems of herbal medicine. Even more importantly, however, having established a common context of phenomenology East and West, we have taken the first step in our process of realizing an integrated, energetics-based Western materia medica, the practical aim of this book. Linking up with our own holistic tradition—so decisively cut off by experimental science—is the first step of empowerment that we can take towards our objective. Western herbal medicine must find its own roots first—as holistic as those of Chinese medicine—before being able to benefit creatively from its present contact with Chinese herbalism. Only then will it be able to develop along new, more integrated lines.

2 HERBAL MEDICINE EAST & WEST: MEDICAL THEORIES

When the several Compositions of Tastes, and sometimes Odors, in the same Plant, are well considered..., I question not, but that the Artificial Jumbles of many Medicines together, will be rejected; and every Ingeneous Practicer will chiefly make use of Simple Medicines; by which his Patient will be more suddenly, safely and pleasantly Cured.

John Floyer, *Pharmaco-Basanos: or, the Touchstone of Medecines*, 1687

Having seen the ways in which traditional Greek and Chinese medicine generally intersect, we may now focus more specifically on aspects of herbalism such as pharmacology and therapeutics. Our aim here is to clarify the fundamental differences between these traditional systems as they were, and still are, practiced and modern herbal medicine as it is practied today. To do this, certain generic approaches to herbal therapy, used throughout history, have also been selected for closer examination. Understanding these common orientations, which usually fall into polar pairs, allows us to pursue our objective of selecting aspects of Chinese and Greek, traditional and modern herbal systems and of integrating certain of their elements in a new holistic context. Getting to grips with the content of various herbal practices will provide us with a matrix for creating a synthetic, historically-based herb remedy description and materia medica, allowing us to put these theoretical considerations to actual use in the following chapters.

The Two Paradigms

Picking up the thread of the two complementary paradigms that dominate Western and Oriental thinking, i.e. the phenomenological and the analytical, we may now examine how they are put into practice in specific areas of herbal medicine, namely pharmacognosy[1] and therapeutics.[2]

PHARMACOGNOSY

Pharmacognosy, which studies the nature of medicinal plants, provides us with very clear examples of the phenomenological and the analytical approaches put into practice. Here more than anywhere else perhaps, their polarity becomes absolutely clear and far-reaching.

Being based on holism and phenomenology and still deeply connected to both physical and spiritual phenomena of the Earth (*Gaia*), Greek and Chinese descriptions of an herb's nature show identical hallmarks. Using the simple but powerful elemental language that has been used ever since Neolithic times by shaman healers, they describe the nature of vegetable remedies in purely experiential terms. Directly sense-perceptible qualities such as aroma, heat and coldness, moisture and dryness, sweetness, spiciness, sourness, bitterness, etc. are invariably used, covering the many aspects of a plant such as its scent, color, taste, texture, warming or cooling effect, etc. These terms

The Energetics of Western Herbs

are clearly qualitative, not quantitative, terms and energetic, not substantive—hence the general term *energetics* for this approach. In addition, the further back we go, the more we see the spirititual energetic qualities of plants recognized and the connection with spirits and elementals described, as in the shamanism based healing practices of the Native American and the Wicca traditions in the West.

In addition, Greek and Chinese herbalism make no real distinction between the quality of a medicinal plant *per se* and its functional effects. This is a more analytical distinction belonging to the modern era. In Greek pharmacognosy the above-mentioned qualities are called *dynameis* and their functional effects *energeia*. *Dynamis* is best translated as "effective quality", although calling it a "dynamic" or "dynamic quality" would not be wrong either. *Energeia* directly translates as "energy" in the current general, non-scientific usage of that term, and hence the term "energetics" for a qualitative-based pharmacognosy is historically and semantically quite correct. The classics scholar THOMAS LINNACRE's translation (1519) of *dynameis* was faculties, a word that has unfortunately lost precisely the meaning of "power", "energy" and "effectiveness" that it once conveyed in its Latin original, *facultates*, which GALEN used. Today, the qualifier "effective" is needed to show that these plant characteristics are not passive attributes, but active in causing physiological effects. *Dynameis* or effective qualities are therefore actually usable in medicine: they embody *energeia* or energy. They are dynamic and energetic qualities.

The recognition and use of effective qualities are the result of a deep eidetic contact with the natural world and its forces; a recognition of nature as being alive and powerful and of the human being as an inextricable part of this ongoing, ever-changing and beautiful play of forces involving all forms of life without exception. Hence, it is understandable that in every culture's traditional herbal system, the healing potential of plants' effective qualities—both sensory and spiritual—has been explored, developed and refined over millenniums. They have been shown consistently through empirical usage to produce predictable and reliable results in both the prevention and treatment of illness. It is through the use of these energetic qualities that both Greek and Chinese medicine, being simply the sophisticated results of extensive accumulated clinical experience, are able to directly link up an herb's inherent properties with the disharmonies it treats. The **pungent** taste, for example, is known to cause sweating, and is therefore used in external conditions with fever, chills, etc. Plants containing much **moisture** are known to moisten, lenify and calm, and are thus used in dry, irritable or constraint conditions. Those that have a **cooling** effect locally or systemically are used to clear heat, resolve inflammation, move Qi downwards, etc. Moreover, the specific combination of qualities found in a botanical are used to treat a correspondingly specific configuration of disease qualities, a *dyskrasia*—also described by the very same terms. On the simplest level, therefore, plant qualities which directly oppose those of the disease are used in treatment. The level of complexity reached using such an essentially simple energetic system can be very great. The amazing efficacy of Chinese herbal formulations, which have been empirically developed over millenniums by thousands of practicing herbalists, is an outstanding example.

A lovely and unusual example of herbal energetics in a popular vein may be found in some of the writings of THOMAS TRYON, one of the popularizers of Galenic medicine during its final, decadent phase in Europe. *The Good Housewife Made a Doctor* of 1692, for example, contains lengthy descriptions of the actions of the six tastes, in addition to discussing dietary theory and presenting the nature, effects and medicinal uses of countless foods. He calls the sweet taste "an amiable, blessed and pleasant Property, comforting and refreshing every thing; 'tis an Assuager of wrath and fierceness, a calmer of storms and tempest..." Further on he declares that "when it is temperate and moderate in any thing, bearing a gentle sway over the Martial [Bitter] and Saturnine [Salty] Properties, then such creatures are Sanguine, of friendly dispositions and temperaments, of tractable human Inclinations, and all meats and drinks in which it does a little predominate, are enbued with Concord and Equality, as Bread, Milk, mild Ale..." He goes on to describe the "fierce wrathful Poyson" which is engendered "when this quality shall too violently bear sway in Foods and Drinks...They thereby become heavy and dull, apt to cloy both the Appetite and the Stomach, hot in operation, making the Blood thick and sharp, and consequently the Spirits impure, the Senses stupefied, the Understanding clouded, the Joynts loaded with pernicious Juices, &c."

Somewhat less imagistic and more clinical in his descriptions is the physician JOHN FLOYER, writing a few years earlier in 1687. His *Pharmaco-Basanos: Or, the Touchstone of Medicines* in fact is a rare, late flowering of Galenic herbal energetics. It is a brilliant, pithy synopsis of pharmacology based on the phenomenological paradigm. His introduction makes this plain.

> The Design of this *Essay*, is, to vindicate the Art of curing *Diseases*, from the common Scandal of being too Conjectural, by describing the *TASTES & ODORS* of *Medicines*, and also of *Animal Humors*: for by these, *Medecines* were first discover'd, and the Humors of the *Body* examin'd; and from the Observation of the Agreement & Conformities behind the *TASTE* of *Humors* in the *Body*, and the *Medicine*, it was easy for *Physicians* to infer, that by a Medicine of the same *Taste*, the *Humours* of the *Body* are preserv'd; and by the contrary *Taste* in the *Medicine*, they are altered and corrected. These are the true Fundamental rules of *Physick*, built on the Testimony of our Senses, and not on the Whims of *Chymists*, or the Fanaticisms of *Occult Qualities*, by which the *medicines* work, like Charms, insensibly...[original italics].

In pharmacology as in sphygmology (the study of the pulse) and hydrotherapy, JOHN FLOYER shows his original, creative observational bent. Although in *The Touchstone* he could be pigeonholed as yet another neo-Hippokratic practitioner in the footsteps of THOMAS SYDENHAM, closer inspection does not actually bear this out. The thorough and innovative way in which he develops his entirely empirical energetic system of pharmacology, based on the taste and smell of botanicals, is not found anywhere else in mainstream Galenic medicine;[3] nor has it been bettered since. Indeed, it stands unique, both in the historical time-frame and in sheer content—quite as unique as another energetic system developed a hundred years later, Homeopathy. FLOYER's energetic herbal medicine is only paralleled by the much earlier pharmacological writings of Persian, Indian, and Chinese authors.

Pharmacognosy viewed from the analytical approach is most fully embodied in modern experimental pharmacology. It has become so pervasive that it is usually known as pharmacology for short—as if no other type existed. That there is another kind should now be clear.

Although the analytical understanding of plant remedies has its roots in Greece and was fostered by the Arabian natural sciences, this trend only properly grew when knowledge was increasingly appropriated by the rising professional classes (including doctors) during the late Middle Ages. By the eighteenth century it was able to displace the traditional Galenic approach in the form of a new biochemistry, and with the beginnings of organic chemistry in 1828 when FRIEDRICH WOEHLER synthesized urea, scientific pharmacology was born. Analytical pharmacognosy describes herbs in objective, measurable, quantitative terms only. As a result of its analytical bias it has developed a specialized, cultish language (as opposed to using everyday terms) intelligible only to the trained and initiated few.

Rather than describing a plant's sense-perceptible qualities, the analytical approach is only interested in seeking out its mechanisms of action. Not satisfied with **describing** phenomena, it wants

The Energetics of Western Herbs

to know **how** phenomena **work**. Moreover, being materialistic and not energetic or vitalist, it looks for actual physical substances which might account for the healing properties of plants. Further, being reductionist and out of touch with the larger spiritual context of living things, it confines the explanation of their whole healing potential to just these few substances. Finally, being fundamentally against matter and spiritual immanence (in the Judaeo-Christian tradition), it then goes on to call these substances "active principles". This is another misnomer, since it is concrete physical substances that it investigates and defines, not abstract principles. In short: the nature and effects of plant remedies are reduced to the action *in vitro* of its supposed main "active" constituent substances.

The reductionist and abstract nature of the analytical approach to herbs is clear. Here the key "active" substances are chemically defined, isolated and then synthetically reproduced; experimented with in laboratories to understand their action on living tissue; and finally neatly classified according to these findings.

The net result today is a form of herbal therapy originating entirely in the theoretical experimental effect on tissue of chemical compounds in isolation. Substances such as tannins, mucilages, alkaloids, glycosides, etc., are said to have predictable effects in those plants in which they are found in significant amounts. Plants containing over a certain percentage of tannins, for example, are said to have *astrictive* or *astringent* effects; those with mucilage, a *protective* coating and *relaxant* effect, and so on.

From the historical perspective, analytical pharmacology is a recent variation on the remedy-oriented approach (discussed below) to herbal medicine which has dominated Western natural sciences as a whole. It is a development of the logic and analysis of the Greek ALKMAION (seventh century B.C.) and of the cool formal systematics of ARISTOTLE, which flourished with both Persian-Arabic and French scholastic philosopher-physicians from the tenth to the fouteenth centuries. It is a search that was vigorously joined during the fifteenth and sixteenth century Renaissance—albeit in a more speculative, analogical vein—by the new breed of chemical alchemists such as BASILIUS VALENTINUS, PARACELSUS and their many acolytes throughout Europe.

Seen in this light, the speculations of FRANCIS BACON, RENÉ DESCARTES and ROBERT BOYLE in the early 1600's, which pioneered this quantitative-mechanistic approach, were simply further variations on the philosophical musings of ARISTOTLE, GALEN and IBN SINA. The experiments of MICHAEL KLAPROTH and ANTOINE LAVOISIER, who perfected the quantitative method of chemical analysis in the 1780s, and later of NEUMAN and S. F. HERMBSTAEDT, who initiated pharmaceutical chemistry proper, can be seen as a metamorphosis of the endless trials of earlier alchemists such as the Islamic Greek GABIR (JAFAR AL SUFI), the Persian AL-KINDI and the Swiss PARACELSUS.[4]

THERAPEUTICS

In therapeutics also, the polarity phenomenological-analytical is evident. In the phenomenological herbal practices of Greek and Chinese medicine, for example, botanicals always subserve specific treatment methods. Since herbs are already described in the energetic, qualitative terms of their effective qualities such as *cooling, warming, restoring, draining,* they implicitly evoke the kind of conditions and disharmonies that they are used for. For example, herbs with *warm spicy* qualities such as Rosemary and Juniper have a *warming, restoring,* or *stimulating* effect, and by definition are used in **cold deficiency** conditions; while *cool, bitter* herbs, such as Melissa and Marjoram, exert a *relaxing, draining effect,* addressing conditions with **heat** and **excess**. Hence it is the herbs' actual qualities that are used as treatment methods. A *pungent, stimulating* herb is naturally used to *promote warmth* and *clear cold*, an *astringent* herb to *eliminate excess damp*, a *relaxing* herb to *loosen constraint*, etc.

Herbal Medicine East and West: Medical Philosophies

Moreover, since the qualities of herbs are able to carry out the effects intended by certain treatment methods, and since these methods usually address systemic imbalances, herbal remedis actually directly treat these imbalances. Rather than address specific dysfunctions, they address syndromes of disharmony as a whole. Fumitory, for example, was said by GALEN to treat the systemic syndrome called blood heat; likewise, *Xuan shen, Scrophularia ningpoensis*, is used in China for the same condition.

Another hallmark of the phenomenological approach is the use of entire plant materials rather than the refined, partial, or synthesized products. Besides, an herb is usually combined with others to create a formula of several (often up to eight and occasionally up to eighteen) ingredients. Both factors allow them to more effectively achieve a global rebalancing of systemic conditions rather than simply bring about symptom relief (good though this is in itself).

Since the rise of post-Galenic medical movements in the early 1500s, the nature of therapeutics has changed fundamentally. It has resulted in what may be called the **analytic** approach, still paramount today.

Since the Renaissance, trends such as iatrochemistry (DE LA BOE, GLAUBER, BOYLE), Galenic chemistry (CROLL, LIBAVIUS, LÉMERY), Vitalism (PARACELSUS, VAN HELMONT, STAHL) and Homeopathy (HAHNEMANN), as well as more analytical developments such as BICHAT's tissue pathology, BROWN's "irritability" theory, and VIRCHOW's cellular pathology, have narrowed the understanding of the mechanism or "cause" of disharmony to increasingly smaller and narrower factors. As a result, therapeutics has also become analytical, theoretical and isolational, based on the rational search for universally valid laws using quantitative scientific value standards. This is clear from the basic paradigm within Western thinking, which was discussed in the previous chapter.

Consequently, the aim of modern herbal treatment is to correct a specific mechanical failure in human physiology, using a single specific remedy to do so.[5] The correction of faulty mechanisms then relies on a direct link between the mechanism of action of a remedy and the mechanical dysfunction in the body. The logical endresult of this way of thinking is to use the supposed biochemically "active ingredient" of a botanical alone, stripped of its buffering components, which are held to be worthless. Based on this premise, synthetic chemistry has succeeded admirably in doing just this.

In this mechanistic, reductionist, analytical approach, therapeutics is defined simply according to a knowlege of the physically quantifiable properties and effects of an herb, called its "action" (and often its pharmacokinetics). For this reason, rather than serving larger contextual methods of treatment addressing larger syndromes, the treatment approach of modern herbalism is bound to consist of no more than a sole reliance on a detailed, in-depth analysis of the plant remedy itself. The modern herbalist therefore tends to rely more on his analytical knowledge of, say, Barberry bark, rather than on broader experiental information he might have gained. He knows that Barberry contains chemical constituents called tannins, and will therefore help clear infections with discharge, since tannins are *antiseptic, anti-inflammatory*, and *astringing* on the mucosal cells which cause discharge. Unlike the traditional women healers and Greek physicians, he will not use Barberry as a *bitter, astringent* tasting herb with *cooling* effects to cause astriction, clear infection and stop discharge in conditions of damp heat. In this analytical approach the remedies themselves are the beginning and end of all treatment. There is no treatment method as such. Herbs are defined purely in biochemical terms that infer the specific mechanical disorders they are used for, and are classified accordingly. Hence the existence of botanicals containing tannins, those containing alkaloids, those with essential oils, those with organic acids, those with mucilages, those with bitters, etc.

The analytical approach includes nineteenth century Eclectic therapy that was practiced in the

The Energetics of Western Herbs

U.S. However, it is most fully and logically embodied in synthetic chemical medicine. The latter and the modern biochemical style of herbal therapy together form a polar opposite to Chinese and Greek herbal medicine.

Although traditional systems of healing are orientated to therapeutic methods and modern systems to remedy actions, they may well seem to produce herb classifications that are effectively identical. **Herbs that purge downwards** (*xia*) from the Chinese pharmacopoeia, for example, seem to equate with Western *laxatives*. After all, both types of herbs actually cause bowel movement. However, although they may well overlap in the sense of producing similar results, they certainly do not equate. Whereas *xia* defines a downward moving **treatment method**, *laxative* refers to the **action of an herb** in the bowels. Clearly, they are two different things. Hence the resemblance is superficial, and coincidental. The Western and Chinese herb classes are not at all on the same level and cannot simply be equated across the board. Cross-wiring and short-circuits have all too often been the unfortunate results of such attempts—on both sides of the Pacific.[6]

All Chinese and, for that matter, Greek herb classes, then, have no **equivalents** today: they must be accepted and understood in their own terms or not at all. Moreover, even in the case where the result of a botanical's effect is absolutely identical, the terminology is still different. For example, where Western herbology speaks of **causing sweating** with *diaphoretics*, a Chinese doctor will refer to **releasing the exterior** (*jie biao*) with *pungent warm/cool* herbs. Although the sweating produced is the same in both cases, the Chinese term expresses the **treatment intention** involved and points forwards to the **condition being treated** (in this case external conditions). The Western expression, on the other hand, points back to the **herb itself** with respect to its **mechanism of action.** Here the intent is nothing more than to cause sweating using a remedy that has the right constituents to do so.

As a result, it becomes more understandable why, in the history of Western/Greek medicine, treatment methods such as causing sweating, causing bowel movement, bloodletting and so on, once freed from their larger therapeutic context of treatment intentions, tended to become misused. From the Renaissance onwards they tended to become ends in themselves, divorced of any understanding of the therapeutic principles behind them and the vitalistic context which originally gave rise to them. By the time of the eighteenth century heroic phase of medicine in America, these Galenic methods had become entirely devoid of meaning, emptied of any content, and their use often dangerous or fatal. Carried out simply for their own sake in the blind hope that they might work, they failed to account for and respect the individual's vital force or *zheng qi* and hence were unable to treat *kata physis*. In the hands of mechanically acting medics, regular or popular, these methods became totally abused, whether Calomel or Cayenne, Jalap or Lobelia were used: all became literally irritating mannerisms, obsessively foisted on a bewildered and increasingly fed-up populace. Hence the disrepute into which a safe and effective method such as bloodletting has fallen, a status it has still been unable to shake off (see p.481).

The Two Polarities

Two polar approaches have underpinned the practice of herbal medicine since earliest days. They are the remedy versus the clinical approach and the systemic disharmony versus the specific dysfunction approach. Examining these in turn will bring greater clarity to the issues involved in establishing a new presentation for the Materia Medica. They will illuminate universal trends in pharmacology and therapy that run across centuries and continents, spanning both the most simple and the most complex forms of herbal medicine, involving herbal therapists from every culture, society and social standing. The first polarity of approach concerns pharmacognosy, and the second concerns therapeutics.

THE FIRST POLARITY

The first polarity of approach results from the difference of emphasis in Greek and Chinese pharmacology. Greek herbal medicine, and also its descendant, modern Western herbalism, is typified by a reliance on understanding the nature and functions of a **remedy**, i.e. on pharmacognosy and pharmacology. It is a remedy-oriented system, taking as its criterion for treatment a thorough knowledge of medicinal plants themselves. What counts in this approach is plant qualities, properties, or active principles. This is as true of the more holistic and phenomenological systems such as the Hippokratic and Vitalist (e.g. HIPPOKRATES, PARACELSUS, VAN HELMONT, HELVETIUS), as it is of the more analytical systems practised by Persian physicians such as AL KINDI and IBN SINA, French scholastics such as GERARD OF CREMONA, humanist doctors such as FUCHS and DODOENS, Dutch and German iatrochemists such as DE LA BOE and GLAUBER, Galenic pharmacists such as LÉMERY, HORSTIUS and HOFFMAN, later experimental biochemists such as LAVOISIER and FLÜCKINGER, and American Eclectics such as SCUDDER, LLOYD and ELLINGWOOD. The point is that both systems rely on pharmacology rather than on therapeutics for their practice, the holistic school using qualitative-dialectic standards of value and the analytical school using quantitative-theoretical ones.

In contrast, Chinese medicine has a **clinical** orientation. By its very nature it relies on knowing the practical or clinical uses of a remedy, i.e. the exact signs and symptoms that call for its use. In Chinese medicine, the yardstick for successful treatment is simply a knowledge of the symptoms, conditions, and diseases that indicate the use of a botanical. Again, this holds true both for more holistic systems such as Hippokratic medicine, homeopathy, Japanese conformation-style herbalism, monastic medicine in the Middle Ages (including the work of HILDEGARD OF BINGEN), nineteenth century French clinical medicine, wise-women's medicine up to the Renaissance, and Native American medicine, and for more analytical systems, like those practiced by Persian physicians such as AR–RAZI and IBN SINA, humanistic Renaissance doctors including POTERIUS, RIVIERE and SYDENHAM, and later Eclectic practitioners such as KING, WEBSTER and ELLINGWOOD. All these medical systems rely for their treatment on a therapeutic approach rather than on a pharmacological one.

Of course, in practice many physicians and even medical movements such as the Eclectic school were able to find a nice balance between these two approaches; yet this distinction serves to clarify a basic polarity between ancient Greek and Chinese medicine. While the orientation of Greek herbalism, on the whole, is towards the **plant remedy**, the approach that Chinese herbalism generally pursues is a **clinical one**. The remedy-based approach is somewhat dependant on the prevailing cultural world view in a given historical period, while the clinic-based approach is more universal and independant of reigning philosophies. Examples of these polar orientations throughout history are given in the following chapters where the content of herbal medicine is more developed.

THE SECOND POLARITY

The second polarity of approaches in herbal medicine concerns the field of therapeutics. The first may be called a systemic disharmony orientation, the second a specific dysfunction approach.

In certain schools of herbal medicine (whether Greek, Chinese or more modern) therapeutics is oriented specifically to assessing and treating a **systemic imbalance**. In these systems the

The Energetics of Western Herbs

fundamental aim of all therapy is to rebalance an overall disharmony, whether this involves the Qi, the blood, the four fluids or the four effective qualities. This approach relies heavily on a very comprehensive and accurate assessment of the systemic disease state. The criterion it uses is a good knowledge of disease manifestation through signs and symptoms, their periodicity, intensity, quality, etc. Again, this is as true of more holistic schools such as Chinese, Hippokratic Greek and current homeopathic medicine as it is of the more analytical style as practiced by SYDENHAM, HUFELAND and American Eclectic physicians such as KING and WEBSTER. The point is that both these approaches rely on symptomatology and nosology for their success, the first using more phenomenology, the second more analysis.

In contrast, certain other schools, such as those of herbal medicine during the last 400 years, definitely have an orientation towards **specific dysfunctions**. Here the gravity of interest is an in-depth analysis of specific physiological failures. The criterion for successful diagnosis here is a thorough knowledge of specific body dysfunctions causing disease. As before, this is as true of the more holistic systems such as Galenic medicine and certain Japanese schools of Oriental medicine, as it is of more analytical schools found in medieval Muslim countries as well as in contemporary medicine as practiced worldwide today.

From this review it becomes clear that in every aspect of herbal medicine, namely pharmacognosy, pharmacology, and therapeutics, fundamental polarities are at play. These polarities hold true for Greek medicine as well as Chinese, and modern as well as traditional herbal therapy. Understanding these distinctions of approaches is fundamental if an appreciation is to be gained of the integration of elements from Chinese, Greek and contemporary systems of herbalism, so that today's health-care needs may be adequately addressed. These distinctions provide a basis for creating not only a new, integral presentation for each botanical in the Materia Medica, but also a more comprehensive reorganization of the Materia Medica itself.

Essential Chinese and Greek Medical Terms

YIN/YANG

This dyad is used throughout medical literature in various ways. It designates polar yet complementary positions between any two structures, functions or processes. In other words, Yin/Yang as a dyad defines relationships.

Yin is the **structive** aspect of an effective position;

Yang is its **active** aspect.

Both together are needed to describe an effective possition adequatesly.

Yin is associated with completion, confirmation, substantialization, consolidation, concentration, an awaiting organization.

Yang is associanted with inicpience, setting loose, dynamization, inducing change, development, and determination.[7]

The solid orgons, for example, are considered yin, while the hollow, active ones are said to be yang.

The most common usage, and the main one found in the Materia Medica, is the use of Yin/Yang in physiopathology. Here Yin/Yang describe physiological forces which may be in excess or insufficiency. Yin deficiency, for example, describes a syndrome where the Yin Qi is insufficient or weak. (See p. 619 for the syndromes of Yin/Yang.)

QI, BLOOD AND FLUIDS

Qi, blood and fluids are the fundamental physiological entities of Chinese medicine. They are the substances of human pathology from both a material and an energeticic point of view.

Qi is best translated as *breaths*. They direct and activate all physiological processes.

Blood is used here not only to describe the red circulating fluid; blood also carries out and manifests all physiological processes. Qi and blood, being an active/structive dyad like Yin/Yang, together bring about all physiological events.

Fluids refers to the entire inner fluid environment, and is synonymous with the Fluid organism. In the sense of traditional Greek medicine fluids includes blood, phlegm and bile in addition to interstitial fluid.

Various organs, systems or body parts possess varying amounts of Qi, blood and fluids. If they are not harmonious, imbalances of the affected part occur, such as Spleen Qi deficiency, lung Qi constraint and liver blood deficiency. Intestines dryness, conversely also indicates a lack of fluids.

On the other hand, the imbalance of Qi, blood or fluids may be global, systemic; in which case patterns such as Qi deficiency, Qi constraint, fluids depletion, general fluids dyskrasia come about.

The treatment of Qi, blood or fluids disharmonies varies greatly with the organ or part concerned and with the type of condition.

HOT/COLD, DRYNESS/DAMP

These terms belong to the fundamental effective qualities. (see p. 48). They are used both to describe the nature of botanicals themselves and to define certain pathological conditions.

Hot/cold define qualitative aspects both of an objective and subjective nature, of both signs and symptoms. Both the person who feels hot and the person who has an inflammation are said to have a hot condition.

Dryness/damp are used in a similar way to define both herbal qualities and pathological conditions.

These qualitative terms are favored because they describe phenomena in terms very close to our daily experience. Intestines dryness for example is a syndrome whose nature is not difficult to imagine. Certain combinations crop up frequently, such as damp heat and damp cold. Here two qualities simply combine, as in head damp cold.

At times the word fire is used to indicate a very manifest type of heat, as in the syndromes stomach fire and liver fire.

Hot conditions are treated by the method of clearing heat (Class 13); cold conditions by generating warmth (Class 8).

Dry conditions are treated by providing moisture (Class 10); damp conditions by causing astriction (Class 11).

DEFICIENCY/EXCESS

These terms are used in pathology only, and indicate either a lack or insufficiency, or a superfluity of some substance or process. Deficiency refers to a lack of some positive quality or quantity, as in lung Qi deficiency, for example; excess always refers to a redundancy of any kind, whether of a waste fluid causing an obstruction, as in liver fluid congestion, or an energetic one, as in Yang excess. Usually the excess nature of a condition is implied in a syndrome, but not spelled out. Liver Qi stagnation, liver damp heat are both excess type liver syndromes, for example.

Deficiency conditions by definition are treated by *restoring* methods of treatment (Classes 7 through 11, p. 227).

The Energetics of Western Herbs

Excess conditions are treated either by *eliminating* (Classes 1 through 6, p. 99) or *draining* (Classes 12 through 14, p. 423) methods.

EXTERNAL/INTERNAL

These terms describe the location of a condition in both time and space.

External conditions are said to be in the initial stages of conflict between pathogenic factors and the body's "defensive Qi", i.e. active defense responses. They are acute conditions. At the same time they are said to occupy the superficial, exterior aspects of the body: the skin and muscles. External conditions such as external wind cold are usually treated by causing sweating (Class 1).

Internal conditions are defined as being established and usually chronic, entailing as they do some degree of collapse of defense response, and a nesting of pathogenic elements. They are located in the internal areas of the body, even if they manifest on the exterior (through skin rashes, bleeding, pulse, tongue, and urine changes for example). Any syndrome that does not start with the word external automatically describes an internal condition. Internal conditions are treated variously, according to the further nature of the condition, which might be hot or cold, deficient or excess.

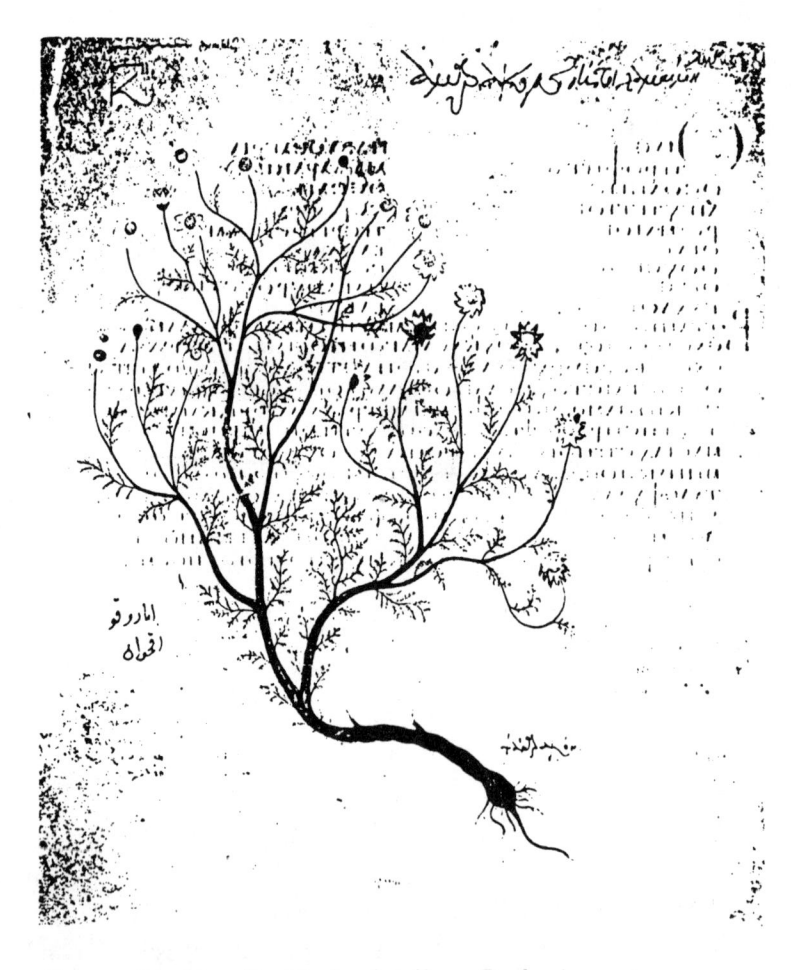

Camomile, from Peri hyles iatrikes, *Pedanios Dioskurides, ca. 77 A.D.*

3 THE MEANING OF INTEGRATION

It were to be wished, that Simples of the Growth of our own Country were more used, and the knowledge of their Virtues better improved...
Marchamont Nedham, *Medelae Medicinae*, 1665

In our exploration of traditional Greek and Chinese and modern Western herbal medicine, we established that the root of Western medicine, namely the Greek medical system set up by HIPPOKRATES and GALEN, has significant aspects of similarity with Chinese medicine. In terms of their underlying philosophies, both were seen to be based on the common ground of the phenomenological paradigm and, as a result, to be both opposed and complemented by the analytical paradigm underpinning contemporary herbal medicine. This became clear in the last section especially, where the polarities inherent in the two traditional systems were elucidated.

Having established the similarities between Greek and Chinese medicine we can now go on to the next step: an integration of the traditional phenomenological and the modern analytical approaches in herbal medicine. This implies integrating both energetic systems, the traditional Greek and Chinese, with the modern mechanistic system.

In keeping with the holistic paradigm emerging at the present time and because of the overwhelming need of today's health problems, herbal medicine, or indeed any healing modality, should have both these perspectives in order to be complete in theory and successful in practice. In this way herbal medicine becomes not only more universal, holistic and truly human centered, but also more rational, presenting a solution to the dilemma of the apparent antagonisms between radically different philosophical paradigms. Furthermore, on the practical level, this integration produces a more effective art of natural healing using herbal substances that draws on the positive advantages of each system, while letting go of both their weaknesses. In the actual process of working with both systems, the potential for new insights and connections is immediately opened up. This generates not only greater freedom and creative development, but also fulfills the need for a holistic, human being centered medicine. The benefits to actual practice, as will be seen below, cannot be underestimated and represent an increase in therapeutic efficacy, economy and elegance that was sought after, and often achieved, by all major past herbal schools, such as the the early Galenic, the humanistic Renaissance or the American Eclectic.

The Need for Integrating both Paradigms

A basic insight inherent in our approach is that the analytical Western and the energetic Greek and Oriental medical paradigms can supply what is lacking in each other's viewpoint and methods. Each has definite and precise advantages which are based on its own standards of value—superior elements, theoretical or applied, which are not found in the other. Moreover, the corollary to gaining the advantages of each paradigm is that their weak areas tend to become minimized and self-correcting, always being put to the test as they are by the other. In short, when put into

The Energetics of Western Herbs

practice, both systems restrain and correct as well as confirm and complete each other.

The more pragmatic and synthesis oriented Chinese paradigm can put a check on the tendency in Western herbalism to **endless conceptual fragmention**. The increasing subdivision of herb action is a case in point: some authors now define up to four types of *diuretics*. Other signs of this increasing fragmentation are the limited practical difference between *cholagogues* and *choleretics* and the vain distinction, advanced by some authors, between *antilithics* and *lithotriptics*. The therapeutic usefulness of such refined hairsplitting is virtually zero. The search for understanding pharmacodynamics in ever greater detail has led us to loose touch with phytotherapy as a **therapy**.

Conversely, the Western analytic modality can make a useful contribution by defining the limits of the Chinese medical tendency to **free flowing conceptual merging**. In Chinese medicine, the outlines of concepts may easily be blurred by use of a single term to denote several different concepts, resulting in a severe loss of definite meaning or an acquisition of a multiplicity of meanings. A prime example is the term **damp**, which may describe conditions as different as water retention, infectious catarrh, phlegm congestion, or indeed almost any condition, depending on the therapeutic context. Here the Western approach can make nice and useful distinctions, with the result that the Chinese class of herbs that *drain damp* can now be seen as treating conditions as varied as damp due to fluid congestion, damp due to phlegm congestion, damp due to inflammation, etc. Another example is the class of herbs that *support the Yang*, which in the Chinese materia medica consists not so much of systemic *Yang tonics*, as one would expect, but rather of *Kidney Yang tonics*, specifically treating urogenital disorders. In this case, the brilliant phenomenological concept of the Yang as a global physiological force is unfortunately reduced to botanicals used mainly for impotence and spermatorrhea, with miscellaneous other *Kidney Qi tonics* for asthma, weak sinews and ailing vision thrown in for good measure (compare p. 319). In both cases, the boundaries of the terms damp and Yang are quite open-ended and flowing, in the first instance leading to multiple meanings and in the second case resulting in a limited meaning.

It is important to remember that setting both paradigms side by side does not mean that Western conceptual fragmentation and Oriental conceptual merging are discarded. It simply means that as a result of clarifying and utilizing each system's strong points, their excessive tendencies, just described, are restrained and corrected.

Turning to the advantages that the two modalities of herbal medicine, the phenomenological and the analytical, have to offer when put to use, it is clear that the Oriental style of herb classification represents the more useful practical system from the perspective of the **clinical use** of herbal remedies. This classification results from the clinic based orientation discussed in Chapter 2. The linchpin in this pragmatic approach is simply a knowledge of the actual effects of botanicals in conditions of heat, cold, damp, stagnation, phlegm and so on. The advantage of this approach is that it allows one to link up pharmacology directly with Chinese internal pathology. As a result, any herb can immediately be located with reference to its therapeutic functions and uses. Its location in a particular herb class tells us by definition which types of patterns of disharmony it may be used for. Cranesbill, for example, in this Materia Medica belongs to the class of herbs that *cause astriction, dry damp and arrest discharge*, which automatically tells us that Cranesbill is used in conditions of damp entailing discharges.

Looking at the presentation of a botanical itself, it is clear that the Chinese, as also the Greek-Galenic, clinical orientation concerns the herb's nature, functions and uses all in one. Here the underlying assumption is that if the functions and uses of a remedy in terms of the eight principles (*ba gang*), the six injuries (*liu yu*), the six meridians (*liu jing*) or the four levels (*si fen*) are known, then its nature may be inferred. This is virtually the definition of a remedy's characteristics. All Chinese *ben cao* (herbals) up to the present day are based on this premise, which fosters the view that a botanical is no more than its therapeutic effects. The main and secondary qualities of a remedy (its warmth, taste, moisture, etc.) are viewed strictly from this pragmatic, clinical perspective. They are assesssed and described directly in terms of pathology, i.e. the syndromes and symptoms they can treat. There is no interest in exploring the intrinsic properties of a plant (either qualitative or quantitative) for their own sake, or abstracted from their manifest ability in dealing with pathogens. For example, the bitter taste of a plant is only relevant in the sense that it moves Qi downwards and has a heat clearing effect. Likewise, a botanical's functions are evaluated and described directly in terms of the syndromes that it treats[1]. This is a manner of thinking which views as the paramount factor function, not structure, and relationships between symptoms, not isolated symptoms themselves. As a result, this approach, which we called the systemic disharmony approach, is able to synthesize and unify. A problem is handled not by examining individual symptoms, but by viewing its constituent signs and symptoms as a gestalt, a whole syndrome or pattern of imbalance rather than a random set of symptoms each needing separate treatment. The final advantage for the therapist is that he/she can understand a remedy with direct reference to its practical usage.

At the same time, vitalistic systems of herbalism such as the Chinese and Greek lay an emphasis on the specific symptoms that an herb can treat within a syndrome. This is an important point, since every person's disharmony is individual, idiosyncratic, and rarely conforms to the normative textbook pattern of symptoms. In this sense, every clinical condition is always unique. The specific symptom-picture of an illness is therefore perfectly amenable to being treated by the specific symptom-picture of an herb, which matches it.[2] Like American Eclectic herbalism and Homeopathy, then, Chinese therapeutics deals with specific symptomatology.[3] Applied to Western herbs, this means that Barberry, for example, can treat liver fire specifically with constipation, whereas Linden and Melissa are for liver fire when palpitations and anxiety present. In short, the phenomenological modality allows us to make elegant direct links between an herb symptom-picture and an illness symptom-picture.

The Western therapeutic paradigm has advantages no less important than those offered by Chinese medicine. All systems of Western herb classification, whether based on modern pharmacology (biochemical constituents) or on traditional Galenic qualitative pharmacology (effective qualities), clearly afford the greatest insight into the nature of **botanicals themselves**. The classifications arise from the remedy based orientation which has underpinned Greek medicine since GALEN. In this more theoretical approach, the crucial thing is a knowledge of the **nature** of a medicinal plant itself. This may be described either in sensory and qualitative language or in analytical, quantitative terms. The advantage, then, of the remedy approach is that it allows one to focus directly on conditions and mechanisms of disease. In this style of classification, a botanical may easily be located with reference to its intrinsic properties. These automatically tell us what type of tissue conditions it may be used for. Since Cranesbill belongs to the herbs that *cause astriction, dry damp and arrest discharge,* we learn that it has an *astringent* nature.

In the presentation of each remedy, the traditional starting point is the sensory perception of the herb itself in terms of its taste, warmth, texture and so on. The fundamental premise is that if the effective qualities and tropism of an herb are known, then its functions and uses may largely be deduced. By definition, a remedy is essentially the same as what can be discovered of its intrinsic nature, which traditionally consisted of its qualities, tropism and ground. GALEN went so far as to define the functions of a remedy as its tertiary qualities! This approach produces the greatest understanding of a botanical's nature or character. It allows us to make extended use of traditional Galenic as well as Chinese and Ayurvedic pharmacognosy. The emphasis is on exploring the inner nature and properties of a remedy in any way possible and as far as possible. Arabian Galenism, Renaissance alchemy, Homoeopathy and experimental biochemistry are all examples of this search for the identity and power of a remedy. At the same time, there is a reluctance to admit the evidence, derived from actual observation, of the clinical orientation.

This remedy based approach still typifies modern pharmacology, where chemical analysis has simply extended and supplanted the use of our senses, and where the experiment has superseded our more informal empirical knowledge. Whether it is the traditional qualities such as taste, warmth and moisture of a remedy that are known, or whether it is its biochemical constituents, in both cases we are more informed about its functional effects. As a result, it can then be used with greater intelligence with respect to certain conditions or mechanisms of disharmony.

The Western therapeutic approach, then, focuses on the condition (as opposed to the pattern) of disharmony as it manifests in the physical body tissues. We called this fundamentally morphological orientation a **specific dysfunction** approach. Here, the thinking is purely in terms of structure. This approach also tends to isolate and analyse, similarly to the laboratory experiment (witness cellular and molecular pathology). Generally speaking, the condition refers to the tissue condition involved in the disharmony or illness (including all body substances), and is described in histopathological and nosological terms such as relaxation, tension, atonicity, inflammation and degeneration.

Nevertheless, a more whole, balanced perspective can be maintained in this approach as in the Chinese one, if, like the Eclectic physicians of the last century, we also single out the **specific symptoms** pertaining to a condition. In this case, the direct link is between a remedy's mechanism of action and the tissue condition it treats. For example, a remedy with an *astringent* quality will create tissue contraction in relaxed or catarrhal conditions. Symptomatology, then, like the functional effect of an herb, represents the common ground of both pattern and condition of disharmony.

The benefits of being able to use the methods of both herbal systems as complementary paradigms should now be clear: both patterns of disharmony (syndromes) and tissue conditions may be therapeutically addressed; both the ground of disharmony and the symptoms themselves may be treated. Diagnosis, treatment method, and herb selection are all equally affected. Diagnosis becomes more rational and precise, while treatment becomes more effective and recovery time is shortened. Moreover, new insights and possibilities in diagnostics, therapeutics and herbalism arise spontaneously, as greater freedom is experienced and as herbal medicine is developed in creative, untrammeled ways.

The Two Keys to Integration

Having seen the real need for taking advantage of the benefits that both Oriental and Western styles of therapeutics have to offer, we now turn to the question of how these benefits may be culled and engaged in actual practice. The approaches that will allow us to effectively integrate the disparate systems of natural healing can be summed up in two key phrases: multi-paradigm thinking and integrative thinking. Both approaches are general ways to view things; assimilating them will enable us to unlock the practical benefits of working with both types of herbal systems.

MULTI-PARADIGM THINKING

In a nutshell, multi-paradigm thinking means seeing paradigms as mental **models** or **emblems**

of reality rather than as **absolute, immutable** and **global truths**. In this way of thinking, both the traditional Chinese and Greek and the modern Western paradigms are understood as emblems of truth rather than as fixed, final truths. The current need for ths approach in the medical arts has been voiced for quite some time by authors such as SCHATZ, SCHNORRENBERGER, UNSCHULD and PORKERT. In a variety of ways they state that if Western medicine, including botanical medicine, is to become more rational, authentic and reliable, it needs to break out of its hoodwinked reliance on a single model, the analytical-mechanistic paradigm, and develop the complementary phenomenological approach using inductive synthesis.

Modern quantum physics has educated us to let go of the idea of the naive belief in the correctness of a single point of view. Writers from WERNER HEISENBERG and DAVID BOHM through to FRITJOF CAPRA have stressed that different models of reality can and should be applied to different situations, whether in daily life or with respect to a technical field. Equally, in the area of consciousness studies, the works of authors such as ALAN WATTS, TIMOTHY LEARY, KEN WILBER and CARLOS CASTANEDA have made it quite clear that a single, all-encompassing approach to reality simply does not exist; rather, a variety of views of reality need to be adopted if we are to do justice to its ever-changing, limitless and ungraspable nature. Clearly then, the fact that multiple models or theories of reality exist, many to be used equally and advantageously, points to the conclusion that here we are dealing with flexible particular emblems rather than fixed universal truths.

Chapter 1 reviewed the tendency of Western thinking to linearity, fixation, structuralism and monopolization. Theoretical models of thinking are seen in the West as having an absolute, fixed character rather than an emblematic, paradigmatic value. Today, now that the universal validity of a single approach to reality has been seen as a naive belief, it is of great importance to deal with reality models in a flexible way. We should now be prepared to exchange one theoretical model for another if and when reality requires it. Instead of letting us rely exclusively on a single dominant theory, the evolution of consciousness is encouraging us to balance a multiplicity of possible theories. Rather than blindly abide by a single truth, it is goading us to accept many perspectives on ineffable truth. It is presenting us with the opportunity to become **inclusive** in our ways rather than exclusive.

The point of multi-paradigm thinking is this: when using different paradigms of reality to assess any particular condition, we should remain aware at all times of their purely emblematic nature if we are to remain flexible, open and and nonexclusive in our approach. Only this will allow us to reap the benefits of working with several different paradigms rather than a single one alone.

INTEGRATIVE THINKING

Integrative thinking means both incorporating our intuitive faculties arising from the right brain with our rational thoughts from the left, and joining holistic thinking with inductive reasoning in our thinking as a whole.

From historical evidence, it apears that intuition and spiritual insight have alway played a significant role in all aspects of medicine. The basis for this is the close connection between healing and spiritual practice, seen in all cultures and in spiritual practices from Shamanism to Christianity.

Models of reality or paradigms have their intuitive side. Theories are not only elaborated rationally, but as often as not arise from the right brain, from intuitive perception. Indeed, many of the most significant discoveries in both physical and spiritual realms are known to have been triggered either by spiritual revelation or by sheer intuition. Although the intuitive experience is wonderful in itself, it does not have to remain an isolated polynia; it can be a doorway to other realities, realities which we need to view with an open mind and, if necessary, under a different paradigm. Intuitive information is integrated into logical linear left brain thinking, and in this way inductive links are made between the various levels of awareness. Finally, through repeated experience of links between different types of awareness, and by repeated observation of correspondences between natural events on physical and various energetic or spiritual levels, an integrated , unifying system of correspondences linking the human and the cosmos is established. The well-known Chinese, Hindu and Greek emblems of this type are outstanding cases in point. It is in this integrated way that intuitive thinking comes full circle to rational thought in setting up a certain paradigm.

Likewise, insight and intuition, based on the use of the right brain, have always had and always will have a strong bearing on the evaluation of an herbal remedy. Herbal medicine is the oldest empirical science, after all and empirical, phenomenological information is not obtained from the left brain through cold, logical analysis The traditional system of energetic pharmacology and its complex interactions with the individual's vital force is solidly based on a holistic understanding of nature, the plant and the human, an understanding which engages all our faculties conscious and unconscious as expressions of our continuity with all living things. Through inductive synthetic reasoning we set up a whole system of correspondences in which spiritual, energetic and material information are thoroughly articulated. Modern analytical pharmacology is also evaluated from the holistic perspective. The results of its experimental and theoretical investigations are not simply allowed to create new speculations and theories unrelated to the matrix of living connections; instead, they too are consciously evaluated and integrated into the whole realm of human experience.

The art of healing called medicine has been described as consisting of 90% quality and 10% quantity. In every aspect of medicine, including diagnosis, therapeutics and pharmacology, **quality**, not **quantity** is of decisive importance. Relying heavily on qualitative judgements, healing is an art that draws on the whole spectrum of human experience and judgement. It certainly is not limited exclusively to the left brain, to logical reasoning and to quantitative judgements, as the modern medical paradigm would have us believe.

PARADIM PRIORITIES

In practice, multi-paradigm and integrative thinking applied to herbal medicine means this: We need to think both in analytical ways and in terms of whole patterns; to see relationships between things (whether herb actions or symptoms) as well as to see things separately; to think in energetic or vibrational as well as in physical mechanistic terms. A materia medica which presented Chinese syndromes to the exclusion of everything else would be just as one-sided as the plethora of herbal texts which give Western illnesses and symptoms alone.

When both the phenomenological and analytical models of herbal therapy are used together, however, it is important to use them in the right way. This means establishing a correct relationship between them, one involving a definite priority. Since the former system is holistic or synthetic by nature (whereas the latter is isolational), the phenomenological approach should always form a larger context for the theoretical one. This is because functional thinking unifies, whereas structural thinking (as was seen above) separates. This is a complete reversal of the current Aristotelian-based scientific approach in which theoretical models dominate empirical findings. The largely speculative nature of current science is a prime example, and result, of the unbridled use of theoretical models freed from any grounding in empirical wisdom. A key error in this approach is a blind reductionistic reliance on analyzing mechanisms to explain phenomena (as was seen in Chapter 1), rather than allowing the phenomena themselves to count for us in a nonreductionist way. Science persists in this erroneous tack partly because it cannot admit the qualitative information gained by the phenomenological approach.

The reversal of priorities proposed here, i.e. making theoretical models of knowledge cede to phenomenological, empirical findings, is not a new one: it is an approach pursued by many original innovators past and present, producing great practical benefits as well as amazing insights. Thinkers that explored this method include the brilliant physicians THOMAS SYDENHAM and JOHN FLOYER, SAMUEL HAHNEMANN the initiator of homeopathic medicine, JOHANN W. GOETHE the natural scientist, RUDOLF STEINER the spiritual teacher, ALBERT EINSTEIN the formulator of relativity theory, LOUIS KEVRAN, who scientifically established biological transmutation, and EDWARD WHITMONT, who has investigated the energetics behind psychology and homeopathy, to mention just a few. This approach is all the more important in medicine where, out of all sciences, quality is by far more important than quantity.

In working with different systems as expressions of paradigms, in principle we should not limit ourselves to the two approaches used in the present text. Any two systems or set of principles may be seen as models and used in an integrated way, provided that the parameters, priorities and procedures used allow it. All integration, regardless of style or scope, can only bring advantages. Like inductive synthetic thinking itself, it may be seen as an aspect of negentropy or synergy, the priciple whereby individual parts tend to combine and create wholes. Entropy, or disintegration into randomness, would not exist without a process tending to its opposite, synergy—another example of Yin and Yang. It is the unity principle discussed by GREGORY BATESON, for example, who describes how the universe, in addition to falling apart, also comes together and creates larger wholes from smaller, separate parts. This is precisely the process involved when two or more systems are effectively used together, systems such as the phenomenological and the analytical underlying this Materia Medica.

Working with Both Systems within a New Context

Once Chinese and Western herbal systems are seen to be expressions of different paradigms, a neutral context is created. This context allows us to work with both systems in an integrated way, while the paradigmatic values and concepts informing them remain inviolate. This is an important point, since each system is authentic, internally consistent and scientific in its own right. Each can openly be used in its own terms, not in those of any other system. In this way we avoid the pitfall of creating **equivalence** between the two. An example of this would be to literally equate liver Qi stagnation with hepatic insufficiency. This is simply cross-wiring, since the first condition represents a syndrome of the phenomenological type, whereas the second represents an organ condition based on analysis. Even worse from the clinical point of view, for example, would be to equate herbs to clear wind from Chinese medicine with *carminatives* from Western, as has been common practice up to now. Because the term "wind" is involved in both types of remedies, it is assumed that the two can simply be equated, with no respect for the antipodean styles of thinking behind the application of this word.

In working with both herbal systems in an integral, dialectic context, **modulation** from one to the other is the key procedure. While the neutral context for the two systems does not permit word for word or conceptual equivalence, it will always allow dialectic modulation. The two operations are quite distinct. Modulation allows us to pass from either mode of thinking to the other; from syndrome to condition thinking, for example, or from traditional to biochemical pharmacognosy.

The Energetics of Western Herbs

Taking our example, we might modulate between the two pathological concepts "liver Qi stagnation" from Chinese medicine and "hepatic insufficiency". However, we are not limited to this: the syndrome liver Qi stagnation might as easily modulate with "hepatic cirrhosis", "portal congestion", or any number of other Western conditions in the same area.

Moreover, modulation is much facilitated through the presence of specific **semantic links**. These are key concepts which, although defined by the semantic criteria of only one system, effectively point to an identical phenomenon or series of phenomena in the other. Examples of such links are the concepts **damp, cold, heat** and so on. Damp (*shi*) from the Chinese medical perspective describes pathological qualities of heaviness, lingering, and moisture; it may modulate with certain Western concepts such as **catarrh, edema** and **phlegm**, depending on the context. The modulability of a concept is enhanced when it is qualified, as damp may be qualified, to give **mucus damp, water damp** and **phlegm damp**, for example. Damp as a semantic link then serves as an interface between Chinese damp and related Western concepts.

Since the pnenomenological paradigm forms a context for the analytical, it becomes clear that specific imbalanced physiological mechanisms or tissue conditions such as anemia, catarrh, infection, ulceration, etc., should be viewed in the context of, and as part of, the larger syndrome of disharmony. It is the overall picture, the larger systemic, energetic condition of imbalance which is primary and the specific, local, concrete mechanism of disease secondary. In the course of actual treatment, of course, the emphasis will vary with each case. In more acute, local and exogenous problems, priority may be given to the specific local condition, while with chronic, systemic and endogenous disharmonies priority may be given to the global syndrome. This does not undermine the *a priori* relationship between local condition and systemic disharmony, however. The latter should always have priority of consideration if this integral approach is to be successfully put into practice.

Moreover, this approach means that mental, emotional and behavioral signs and symptoms, such as depression, unrest, lack of motivation, etc., assume as much importance as purely physical ones. It is primarily whole person, as they are and present themselves, who are treated, not just the physical symptoms. The latter are now viewed as part of the condition presenting as a whole, not as isolated, unrelated phenomena requiring independent, objective fixing. This approach has a direct bearing on the presentation of plant remedies, in that the specific mental, emotional and behavioral symptoms treated by a remedy assume equal importance with the purely bodily signs. It also makes an assignment of the herbs to certain temperaments and biotypes, i.e. to a certain ground, all the more pertinent, since these are simply larger configurations of patterns of imbalance involving the body, the soul and spirit.

Two examples will illustrate the very real benefits from using the phenomenological and the analyical models of herbal medicine simultaneously in a new dialectic context. They are advantages accessible to anyone willing to use these systems in the sense of "both-and" rather than "either-or", adopting the modulation procedure and the priority just outlined.

A practitioner of Western medicine is visited by a person complaining of abdominal pains and diagnoses a gastric ulcer. He therefore prescribes one or several of a number of herbal remedies known to improve this local tissue condition. Had this practitioner been trained in Chinese medicine, he would in addition have been able to spot the **overall syndrome** afflicting the patient, not the stomach ulcer alone. In this case he might have diagnosed, e.g., Qi constraint, stomach fire, stomach cold or Spleen Yang deficiency as the contextual syndrome. As a result, not only would he have narrowed down his choice of botanical with far greater precision, but by treating the systemic imbalance in addition to the local one, his results would have been correspondingly superior.

Herbal Medicine East and West: Medical Philosophies

(However, a skilled therapist would make the simple differentiation between an ulcer due to excessive secretions and one due to insufficient ones, in which case the choice of herb is also reduced. Nevertheless, his selection of botanicals is still based on directly treating the ulcerated tissue).

The inverse is also true. A practitioner of Chinese medicine is visited by the same person with the same complaint. On the basis of his diagnosis he will prescribe an herbal formula according to the syndrome manifesting, thereby treating the condition as a whole. However, were he able at the same time to specifically diagnose an ulcer, his choice of remedies would then include those that are known to specifically heal ulcerated gastric lining. Here again, by treating the local condition in addition to the context, the global disharmony, his chances of therapeutic success would be greatly improved.

In a second example, a person visits a Western practitioner complaining of painful, frequent urination. He diagnoses a urinary infection and prescribes *urinary antiseptic* remedies. His choice is vast and includes a large range of different types of herbs. Not being trained in Chinese differential diagnosis, he cannot distinguish whether the underlying syndrome is, e.g., a Spleen Qi deficiency, a Kidney Qi infirmity or bladder damp heat. His remedy selection, therefore, is a comparatively general one, and the patient's recovery time longer than it need be. Had he diagnosed the systemic syndrome as well as the local condition, the patient's entire system would have been improved and recovery time greatly reduced.

Again the inverse is true. Being visited by the same patient, the practitioner of a traditional system makes a differential diagnosis and prescribes a formula addressing one of the syndromes named. Fine, but his results here also would be much improved were he able to consciously include in his selection one or more specific *urinary antiseptics* that would fit in with the overall energetics of the formula.

Unfortulnately, contradictions sometimes arise when working with both systems of phytotherapy simultaneously; there is no escaping this fact.[4] At times it may look as though the Oriental phenomenological and the Western analytical approach flatly contradict each other. However, what seems to be a contradiction usually turns out to be a paradox—a very different thing. Paradox is a hallmark of dialectic thinking. A striking example, taken from pharmacology, is that in Oriental medicine the bitter taste is said to cool and is thus applied to hot conditions; whereas in Galenic medicine bitter is said to be warm, implying a warming effect.

This contradiction may be resolved if we simply understand the intention behind the conclusions reached by the Chinese and the Greeks. The Chinese evaluation of bitter as *cool* refers to the *cooling, heat/fever/inflammation clearing* effect of herbs with a *bitter* taste, whereas the Galenic assessment of *bitter* as **warm** is based on the very active, energetic effects of bitterness on human physiology. Whereas the Chinese evaluation (in the best clinical tradition) is based on the **demonstrable effects** that bitter tasting botanicals manifest, the Galenic judgement is founded on the **active dynamics** that these exert. While Chinese medicine simply observes the *cooling, resolving* and *detoxifying* effects of a bitter herb, Galenic medicine analyses its *stimulation of digestion and bowel movement* by increasing salivary and gastric secretions, its reflex hormonal stimulation, and so on. No wonder the final assessment is *cool* in one case, and *warm* in the other. The Chinese intention is pragmatic **clinical usage**, whereas the Western one is **theoretical knowledge**. This is the kernel of the paradox.

To complete this discussion, it is interesting to note that the Western theoretical approach actually leaves the question of the clinical uses of bitter remedies entirely open. Proof of this is that most bitters in the Galenic tradition, such as Wormwood, Chicory, Centaury and Bogbean, which were considered *hot* in the 3rd degree, are typically described as "cooling fevers," or "abating hot

The Energetics of Western Herbs

distempers!" To the Galenic practitioner, this difference between the description of an herb's pharmacology and its actual clinical use, far from being considered a logical problem, was understood and accepted as a natural fact. Today, being equipped with the clearer, more objective perspective of seeing both approaches as informed by paradigms, we can understand this contradiction as a very fruitful paradox. In so doing we stand to benefit from both viewpoints: they can bring us greater understanding as well as greater freedom in actual usage.

Integration and Localization

The tendency toward localization is a paradoxical co-element of the more universal aspect of integration. While the general thrust of integration is to make things universal, its specific expression is to **localize**. In order to be applied at a certain time and place, integration requires a local expression. An integral approach to herbal medicine should therefore use the plants growing or available in the region where they are being used, and the preparation forms and methods suited to the inhabitants of that region and climate. In this way botanical medicine is better equipped to deal with the conditions arising in any given local population. It is in this sense, and in this sense only, of making maximum use of **local resources** that this text encourages the use of Western botanicals in the integral way proposed.

Local, indigenous natural medicines, no matter where our locality happens to be, have a direct connection with us. Plants are part of our local environment, part of our heritage and karma. We should acknowledge this connection by making full use of them for the benefit of ourselves and others. It is one way of acknowledging our interdependence with all of life. Besides, Western herbs are not superior or inferior to Oriental herbs, or herbs from any other part of our planet, for that matter. All depends on how we approach and use them and where we are when we use them. For many people, what matters most is the direct contact with the living plants that supply us with such a diversity of therapeutic effects. For these it is infinitely more satifying to collect herbs and roots in the wild themselves and to prepare and store them in readiness for use.

On a more pragmatic note, locally obtained herbs have certain very practical advantages over any dried, imported herbs. Quite apart from the obvious advantage that they grow wild and free for the picking (within judicious limits), they are also fresher and therefore usually more efficacious, although their effectiveness does to some extent depend on the type of use and preparation they are being put to. One thing is certain: fresh herbs win hands down when we need them for making fresh juices or tinctures. Certain herbs need this type of preparation for their full properties to unfold. Also, there is no substitute for immediate first aid application when it is required, as with Comfrey or Coltsfoot leaf, St.John's wort herb, Plantain leaf and Arnica flower.

Generally speaking, it is also true that herbs from one's region or continent are easier to obtain in dried, tincture, fluid extract or essential oil form. And last but not least, they are usually easier on the pocket than many imported herbs.

4 THE MATERIA MEDICA RECLASSIFIED

Every simple plant remedy is blessed and gifted by God and his handmaiden Nature to such an extent that, according to its own nature and way, it has the power to heal, strengthen, allay pain, cool, warm up, purge and sweat...

Hieronymus Bock, *Kreuterbuch*, 1532

The way that medicinal plant substances have been organized and classified, whether in written texts or in oral teaching, has always varied throughout the ages. The purpose of classification is simply to make plant remedies more accessible mentally and in written texts and therefore easier to use in therapy. This is done by introducing either a theoretical or structural criterion, as in botanical, pharmacological and alphabetical systems; or a practical, functional one, resulting in topographical and therapeutical classifications. Every method has its advantages and disadvantages, which depend on the nature of the text. Advantages are maximized when the classification reflects the intention of the author's work as seen in his or her treatment of herbs.

Every historical period has one or two dominant systems, and hybrid classifications have become more common in recent centuries. However all texts on botanical remedies follow one of six models. Examining these will provide us with the background necessary for a more complete understanding of the sytem chosen for the present Materia Medica.

Present and Past Classifications of the Materia Medica

NATURALISTIC OR BOTANICAL

Many important herbal compilations are organized according to plant families, a system known as *ton kata gene* in Greek. This method is inherent in all Western natural sciences, with its theoretical systematic approach initiated by ARISTOTLE. From the therapeutic point of view it can be better understood and justified when we consider that at certain periods for many authors there simply was no distinction between botany and herbal medicine as we know it. This was especially true for the classical authors such as ARISTOTLE and his pupil THEOPHRASTUS (*De historia plantarum*), PLINIUS SECUNDUS (*Historia naturalis*), as well as Persian philologists such as ABU HANIFA, whose works are cornerstones of both botany and herbalism. Their scientific and encyclopedic approach was eagerly emulated by Renaissance men such as ANDREA CAESALPINO, CHARLES DE L'ECLUSE, CONRAD GESNER, MATHIAS DE LOBEL, PROSPERO ALPINI, JEAN and GASPARD BAUHIN and JOHN RAY—most of whom succeeded better as botanists than as herbalists. The three real exceptions are HILDEGARD VON BINGEN's *Physica* (ca. 1150) and the herbals of PIERANDREA MATTIOLI (1611) and JOHANN VON BERGZABERN (1613); all three are significant materia medicas from the therapeutic standpoint. Although the majority are organized according to therapeutic categories, some Chinese pharmacopoeias (known as *ben cao*) are also

The Energetics of Western Herbs

arranged according to plant families. Examples include the famous Tang dynasty *ben cao* of LI ZE (ca. 670),[1] and the *Kai-bao ben cao* (ca. 974) of the Song dynasty.

An alternative botanical system sometimes is seen in which plants are classed according to the part used—root, leaf, flower, herb, fruit, seed, etc. This system often found favor in smaller works and catalogues such as WILLIAM SALMON's *Seplasium* (1693). It was sometimes combined with an alphabetical classification, as in JOHN QUINCY's *Complete English Dispensatory* (1736), and JOHANN SCHROEDER's *Pharmocopoeia Medico-Physica* (1641).

It is interesting to note that to our current knowledge, no classification comparable to the Chinese *Shennong ben cao* is found in the West—even though the modern view of herbal toxicity also falls into the same basic three categories (see p. 52). In this work, which may be considered the *Dioscorides* of Chinese medicine, 365 remedies are grouped according to three therapeutic grades, the first category consisting of *restoratives* or *tonics*, the second class consisting of herbs to be used with some care and discretion, and the third containing toxic herbs.

MODERN PHARMACOLOGIGAL

This is a more analytical type of natural scientific classification whereby plants are arranged according to the purported main "active principle"; in other words according to the main biochemical substance thought to be responsible for their effects. This approach began with the French school of biochemistry in the eighteenth century (BICHAT) and has grown exponentially with the development of Western science. Plant classifications according to biochemistry are the only ones officially accepted by Western medicine today. The considerations connected with these are discussed in Chapter 2.

TOPOLOGICAL

The second favorite Greek and Arabian way of grouping medicinal substances was *ton kata topous*, according to body part, also known as *a capite ad calcem* in the Renaissance. Texts aiming at a more therapeutic and practical mode tended to follow this method, and hence tended to be pharmacopoeias. Some of the significant works using this arrangement are GALEN's *Peri syntheseos pharmakon* ch. 1-10 (2nd century A.D.), IBN AL-BAITAR's *Kitab al-gami* (ca. 1225), AR-RAZI's *Aqrabadin al-kabir* (10th century), IBN SINA's materia medica in his *Al qanun* (11th century), PSEUDO-YUHANNA's materia medica in his *Aqrabadin* (13th century). Later on in Renaissance Europe the topological system was again taken up by writers such as WILLIAM COLE in *The Art of Simpling* (1656) and was a favorite for texts on therapeutics such as PHILLIP BARROUGH's *The Methode of Physicke* (1583) and VON BERGZABERN's *Arzneibuch* of 1582. In the late 1600's it eventually fused with the therapeutic classification, producing such herb classes as *pectorals* (treating the chest), *hepatics* (treating the liver), *cephalics* (treating the head), *cordials* (treating the heart).

ALPHABETICAL

Often the most practical arrangement, especially for students, this is not the modern invention it may seem to be: GALEN's *Peri kraseos kai dynameos ton haplon pharmakon*, for example, lists the remedies according to the letters of the Greek alphabet. Many later writers followed in ther master's steps, such as the humanist herbalists LEONHARDT FUCHS (1543) and EUCHARIUS RöSZLIN (1533). Official pharmacopoeias and dispensatories, following the examplary lead of the *Recettario Fiorentino* of 1498, also list simple or compound remedies alphabetically for ease of reference in the busy apothecaries where they were in constant use.

PERSONAL

Here the botanicals are arranged in an aleatory sequence, or one known only to the author himself! Like an alphabetical system of classification, it has no didactic or therapeutic intent whatsoever. Still, DIOSKURIDES in *Peri hyles iatrikes* (1st century A.D.), without which the Western herbal tradition is unthinkable, has his herbs listed in the most random order. This also seems to be a predilection of German writers, if important works on herbal medicine throughout the ages are anything to go by—witness those of OTTO BRUNFELS, WALTHER RYFF, BARTOLOMAEUS CARRICHTER, ALFRED DINAND and WERNER CHRISTIAN SIMONIS.

THERAPEUTIC

In this system, remedies are organized according to treatment methods or strategies, or "intentions of cure" as JOHN QUINCY nicely calls them. This classification was essentially introduced by GALEN who in his above-mentioned text gives synoptic lists of herbs according to their qualities, e.g. *heating herbs, cooling herbs, drying herbs* and so on. Even though CORNELIUS CELSUS and SERAPIO Junior followed up on this, it was left to the Neo-Galenic doctors of the seventeenth century, such as REMBERT DODOENS, MICHAEL ETTMUELLER, NICOLAS LEMERY and PITTON DE TOURNEFORT, to firmly establish therapeutic classifications. In developing and refining them, they originated the terms *diaphoretic, diuretic, calorific, refrigerant* and many others in order to indicate the treatment method that a botanical served. These short adjectives were chosen at the time in preference to long descriptive phrases such as *herbs that cause sweating* or *herbs that generate warmth*, simply for the sake of brevity.

Today also, most modern texts still use these adjectives to describe herbal remedies. **However, the treatment methods which they originally described were abandoned in medicine during the first half of the nineteenth century.** As a result, the vast array of herbs that had been used for two milleniums have since been bereft of the treatment methods which they had implemented and are now uselessly burdened with these outdated descriptions.

The treatment objectives that herbs were seen to implement, in continuous use since the days of HIPPOKRATES, were effectively abandoned due to the fact that Galenic medicine as a whole was jettisoned—not only its theoretical paradigm, but also its external methods such as phlebotomy and counterirritation. This was partly due to the rise of anatomical-clinical medicine, and partly due to the radical, shattering impact of the experimental physiology, pathology and pharmacology of one man, FRANCOIS MAGENDIE. Consequently, in spite of the mitigating influence on therapeutics of Eclectic medicine in later nineteenth century America, herbal remedies have since remained unorganized and isolated from any real therapeutic context. The pharmacopoeia itself is now reduced to a state where each herb is individually ticketed with a little string of qualifiers such as *sudorific, cathartic, hepatic*—worn-out labels meaningless to the modern practitioner untrained in Galenic medicine and oblivious to the meaning of its treatment strategies.

However, since the practice of Chinese herbal medicine has seriously begun in the West—an extremely recent event—the appreciation of a materia medica organized according to therapeutic methods based on energetic and vitalist principles, such as we find in Chinese herbal medicine, has grown considerably. We are now in a position to state that the Chinese system has certain advantages over the Galenic one, as well as certain disadvantages. (The significant differences were seen in Chapter 2.) Hence this attempt to reorganize the Western pharmacopoeia a very pertinent one, integrating as it does elements from Chinese and Galenic systems of therapeutic herbal classification.

Reclassifying the Materia Medica

A choice has to be made as regards both the type and style of an energetics-based classification of Western herbs. A completely new synthesis has been chosen, based on therapeutic principles from both Chinese and Galenic medicine.

Two elements have to be considered: the general structure of the Materia Medica, and its actual content. The overall **structure** or context is oriented to therapeutic intentions, i.e. methods of treatment. The classification used is not a theoretical but a pragmatic one, in which botanicals are classified according to their clinical use rather than their inherent properties. In this sense these herb classification belongs to the Chinese and ancient Greek style of classifying botanicals, namely the **clinical orientation** (seen in Chapter 2).

At the same time, the actual **content** and function of the classes belong essentially to the Western herbal tradition. As such, they are geared more to an understanding of the nature and dynamic of the herbs themselves and hence have a more theoretical emphasis. In content, therefore, this classification belongs to the more purely Western **remedy orientation** which relies heavily on pharmacology.

Where these two different orientations, the clinical and the remedy one, overlap is in the way they define the herb classes. It is the 25 herb classes therefore which weld the contextual structure and the individual content into a seamless unity. In other words, the herb classes lie precisely where treatment method and herbal property intersect, are one and the same. Moreover, to have them successfully serve both treatment intention and herbal property, clear definitions of the treatment methods must be made, clear to the point where they become more limited and precise than they usually are in the traditional systems. Paradoxically, however, they also become more malleable, for clearer and more precise definition of the herb classes creates the possibility of shifting or modulating from therapeutics to pharmacology without any break in logical continuity. It becomes possible to work with pharmacology, therapeutics and pathology as an **articulated chain** rather than as discontinuous units.

We can clarify this concept of **continuous articulation** by taking a particular example. Comfrey belongs to the class of herbs that *foster the Yin, provide moisture and lenify dryness*. In keeping with this it is a mucilage containing herb with *sweet moist* effective qualities and is used to treat conditions of **Yin deficiency** and **dryness** of various organs or parts. The pivot in the whole chain of Comfrey's nature, functions and indications is its effective qualities or energetics. Its *sweet moist* energetic qualities indicate its mucilage content on one hand and determine its Yin fostering, moisture providing therapeutic effects in Yin deficient and dry conditions on the other. All this together goes to secure Comfrey a place among botanicals that *provide moisture and lenify dryness*.

Besides attempting continuous articulation, this Materia Medica seeks to integrate the **systemic disharmony** orientation, so prevalent in traditional Chinese and Greek medicine, with the **specific disfunction** approach fostered in the later Western tradition. The overall structure of the herb classes naturally invites a form of therapy addressing systemic patterns of disharmony with their total symptom gestalt. Their detailed content, however, is also geared to the treatment of specific dysfunctions and symptom relief.

Taking Comfrey as an example once more, it is clear that since this plant is said to *foster the Yin*, we may expect it to be used for **Yin deficiency** syndromes of one type or another. (This systemic condition is characterized by dryness, sensations of heat, a thin pulse, etc.) In addition, Comfrey *provides moisture*, hence its use in **dry** conditions. As such, it can be used specifically to provide moisture locally in **dry, irritative, ulcerated, inflammatory** or **spasmodic** conditions.

Clearly, therefore, a definition such as Comfrey's of *fostering the Yin and providing moisture* in itself joins the systemic and the specific together like lacquer and glue, allowing us to draw on either modality at will.

To sum up, the articulated continuity between these aspects of herbal medicine—the clinical versus the remedy and the systemic disharmony versus the specific dysfunction approach—allows us in actual practice to modulate freely between the effect of an herb with reference to the systemic syndromes of disharmony it can treat and the effect of an herb with reference to the specific dysfunctions it addresses on the basis of its innate properties. Its energetic functional effects thus become a modular interface granting access to either pathology or pharmacognosy, syndrome treatment or symptom relief. With either Western or Chinese herbal systems alone this complete articulation is simply not possible. By aligning treatment methods (therapeutics) with herbal qualities and constituents (pharmacognosy) around the pivot of an herb's effects (pharmacology), it is then effectively possible to create a new system of classification which enjoys the benefits of both the Chinese and the Galenic styles of herbal therapy on one hand and the traditional and modern aproaches on the other.

The Twenty-Five Herb Classes

The aim of reclassifying Western herbs is to provide an accurate and practical materia medica usable to practitioners of both Chinese and Western botanical medicine alike.

While being only a first step in this direction, such a reclassification has the advantage of being both clear and useful in actual practice. It makes for easier memorization of the remedies in each category when being learnt, and is easier to use in a clinical situation. It avoids the unfortunate random sequence of herb classes as well as the blurring between different types of treatment methods prevalent in the current Chinese classification, while at the same time preventing the aleatory juxtaposition of therapeutically dissimilar remedies found in the Western one. The classification in this text is the result of many influences. They include HIPPOKRATES' idea of *eliminating* and *restoring* types of herbs, GALEN's classification of *eliminating, restoring* and *altering* type remedies, JOHN QUINCY's refinements of the Restoring methods, and the concept of Restoring and Draining types of treatment from Chinese medicine.

The Materia Medica is organized into 25 distinct classes of botanicals embodying treatment methods, and is divided into five parts.

1 **ELIMINATING:** Classes 1-6
   causing sweating
   promoting urination
   promoting bowel movement
   expelling phlegm
   promoting menstruation
   causing vomiting

2 **RESTORING:** Classes 7-11
   increasing the Qi and replenishing deficiency
   supporting the Yang and generating warmth
   restoring the blood and replenishing deficiency
   fostering the Yin and lenifying dryness
   causing astriction and drying mucous damp

The Energetics of Western Herbs

3   **DRAINING:** Classes 12-14
*circulating the Qi and loosening constraint
clearing heat and resolving fever
enlivening the blood and moderating the menses*

4   **ALTERING & REGULATING:** Classes 15-17
*promoting cleansing and resolving toxemia
regulating the Yin & the Yang
regulating hormones*

5   **SYMPTOM TREATMENT:** Classes 18-25
*enhancing pregnancy and childbirth
relieving indigestion
calming the spirit
lifting the spirit
relieving pain
promoting tissue repair
activating immunity and clearing toxins
killing and expelling parasites*

Concerning the placement of individual remedies in the herb classes, it is clear that many herbs could equally well have been put in several different classes. The real criterion was to find those botanicals which characterize a treatment strategy most accurately and completely. Obviously, we shall never know how the Chinese themselves would have classed Western herbs, had they been able to use them. JOHN QUINCY's comment of 1736 comes to mind in this connection:

> As to the general Denominations [of the classes] a Mean is here endeavoured, between the Obscurity of too great a Conciseness, and the perplexity of too many Subdivisions: so that, though a Simple in many places might, upon some account or other, be reckoned in another section or class; yet it is expected, it will be commonly found, that where it stands it has the most right, by reason of its most predominant Quality.

5 THE INTEGRAL PRESENTATION

The study of Simple Drugs is a study so agreeable, and so exalted in its own Nature, that it has been the pursuit of the first Geniuses of all Ages.

Pierre Pomet, *Histoire générale des drogues*, 1694

The individual presentation of each herb, as much as the overall classification of herbs, aims to integrate the phenomenological and the analytical paradigms. It therefore draws equally from elements of traditional energetics based Chinese and Greek herbal medicine and modern herbal therapy. The final advantage of incorporating various elements is to give a richer, more complex picture of each herb—a picture deep, all-encompassing in scope and precise in detail.

An integration of the two paradigms clearly implies some measure of balance between them. For this reason in the presentation of each herb the focus is first on its nature or character and second on its clinical functions, uses and preparations. To emphasize either paradigm would be one-sided; by presenting each in turn we are able to see the connections between them. This allows us to use the two treatment approaches together, modulating between one and the other at will.

The Herb's Definition and Nomenclature

The only aspect of nomenclature that requires some attention is the designation of the herbal remedy itself, i.e. its **pharmaceutical name**. Two basic issues are involved. First, Western pharmacy does not have a botanically consistent naming for the botanical parts used in its materia medica. Old name forms linger on in the pharmacopoeias of various countries, in spite of the universal acceptance of the Linnean designations and classifications by botanists. Second, there are two accepted styles of naming herbs: in the singular and in the plural. The Galenic tradition has always and invariably named parts of plants in the plural, and herbal pharmacy may continue to do so in spite of the singular form adopted, e.g., in 1979 by the *Pharmacopoeia Europaeana*, and the *Deutsches Arzneibuch*. Camomile flower tenaciously remains *flores Chamomillae*, Bittersweet twig is still *stipites Dulcamarae*, and so forth. At the same time, the Chinese pharmacopoeias have in modern times also consistently used the singular form—a practice now confirmed in Europe, as noted. Considering for a moment which logic is more compelling, we are bound to concede that if naming were taken as a literal description, then all plants and plant parts would have to be in the plural, a practice never adopted anywhere. Actually used in pharmacy are *rhizomae Calami, pericarpii Citri, cortices Xanthoxili*, and so on. We use the cut, crushed or powdered parts of many roots, rinds, barks, leaves, etc., not just a particular single one. On the other hand, if the description is not literal but a botanical description of the generic plant part, then the singular form may be used throughout. This is the choice made for the present Materia Medica.

The Energetics of Western Herbs

The following botanical terms have been adopted in this Materia Medica:

bulbus	=	bulb
cacumen	=	tree top
caulis	=	stalk, stem
cortex	=	bark
flos	=	flower, blossom
folium	=	leaf
fructus	=	fruit
gemma	=	bud
herba	=	herb
lichen	=	lichen
lignum	=	wood
pericarpium	=	rind, peel
radix	=	root
ramulus	=	twig
rhizoma	=	rhizome
semen	=	seed
thallus	=	thallus
tuber	=	tuber
turio	=	shoot, sprout

Terms such as *stipes, bacca, oculus,* and *summitas*, popular in the past, have been avoided since they are botanically redundant, e.g. *bacca* of *fructus*, *stipes* of *caulis*.

Ancient and folk names of the herb have been recorded in major Western languages, as they usually throw some light on the practical use of the plant, whether as food or remedy for human or beast. They may also point to its many other cultural, religious and mythical associations.

The Herb's Nature

The characterization of each remedy includes both current scientific information on the herb's biochemical constituents and information on its sense-perceptible composition.

CATEGORY: This defines the herb as **mild, medium-strong** or **strong** from the therapeutic viewpoint. Most remedies in this Materia Medica fall into the mild category, since they have minimal chronic toxicity. Since this factor is of basic importance, yet usually overlooked, the three therapeutic categories are discussed at the end of this chapter (see p. 52).

BIOENERGETICS: This concept defines the **bioenergies** which go to create and sustain a living plant. They originate in the four cosmic ethers and leave their imprint in the chemical constituents found through analysis. Although not sense perceptible, they are verifiable in various ways through inductive thinking. Since this aspect of plant remedies has not yet been adequately researched, it is omitted from the general presentation, although it may be mentioned in the notes. (Compare also p. 73).

CONSTITUENTS: Only the most important known **chemical constituents** are given here. However, the constituents found in a plant reflect research emphasis as much as anything else. (Compare p. 52).

EFFECTIVE QUALITIES: They describe an herb's nature in terms of certain **sensory**

The Integral Presentation

characteristics. Far from being passive or abstract qualities, they are **effective, energetic** or **dynamic,** because when the herb is ingested they produce effects that are therapeutically significant and usable. In Greek medicine they were known as *dynameis*, or *facultates* in Latin. The Chinese translation is *Qi*. (see p. 18 for further discussion).

There are primary and secondary effective qualities. The **primary qualities** of a botanical are taste, warmth and moisture. The **secondary qualities** are derivatives of both its primary qualities and its bioenergetic forces. The movement of an herb is also considered a secondary quality (see definition below).

Primary Qualities
TASTE: This refers to the Oriental six tastes—sweet, pungent, salty, sour, bitter, bland, plus the Aristotelian/Ayurvedic tastes astringent and oily: a total of **eight tastes**. Each taste has very specific effects in the body and all are exhaustively described in Greek, Chinese and Ayurvedic pharmacology manuals. In brief, *sweet* harmonizes, calms and restores; *pungent* activates, warms and causes sweating; *salty* softens and moistens; *sour* tightens and cools; *bitter* strengthens and cools; *bland* seeps water downwards; *astringent* strengthens and tightens; *oily* slows down and makes heavy.

WARMTH: An herbal remedy is said to have *warming* or *cooling* **effects** on the basis of both the person's subjective reaction to the plant, and the herb's ability to cause alterations of signs or symptoms of heat or cold. A five-step gradation is used—hot, warm, neutral, cool, cold—which may be qualified by "a bit" or "very". In cases where there is a difference between the initial warmth effect of an herb when taken and its subsequent warming or cooling effect, or if it shows both warming and cooling properties, this is noted. Discrepancies among these various aspects are explained in terms such as warming or cooling potential.

MOISTURE: This refers to the **degree of** *moisture* or *dryness* of an herb as it affects tissue. It is considered more important in Greek medicine than in Chinese, since dry and moist belong to the four effective qualities, together with hot and cold. In addition, they belong diagnostically to a modified eight principles set (see p. 29).

Secondary qualities: These describe an herb's general and global effects when taken internally or externally. They apply to solid and fluid body tissues as well as to energetic movements, to structure as well as to function. They are: *stimulating, calming, restoring, relaxing, nourishing, decongesting, astringing, softening, solidifying, dissolving, thickening, diluting.*

The **four movements** of an herb, which are described primarily in Chinese and Japanese texts, reflect the directions in which a remedy tends to move signs and symptoms. These are: *rising* (causing upward movement), *sinking* (causing downward movement), *dispersing* (causing outward movement), *stabilizing* (causing inward movement).

TROPISM: This term designates the organs, systems or other parts for which the remedy has an affinity or bias. (This phenomenon has been verified experimentally with essential oils.) In the Galenic tradition an herb was said to "appropriate" to certain body parts, while in the Chinese medicine it "enters" certain meridians. The tropicity of the five tastes in Chinese pharmacology (e.g. *saltiness* travels to the bones, *sweetness* to the flesh) also comes to mind in this connection. Tropism is the rationale behind traditional classifications such as *cordials* (going to the heart and circulation), *pectorals* (going to the chest and lungs), *hepatics* (going to the liver), *cephalics* (going to the head and brain), *nervines* (going to the nerves), *hysterics* (going to the uterus).

Organisms: These describe whole body systems which are governed by an organ function. There are **four organisms**, corresponding to the Greek four elements. These are the **Warmth** organism which deals with warmth and cold in every aspect and is housed in the blood; the **Air** organism dealing with movement and rest, with its substrate the nervous system; the **Fluid** organism which

The Energetics of Western Herbs

deals with transformation and change and is housed in the body fluids; and the **Physical** organism, dealing with structive tissue effects only and supported by the physical body. (See also appendix C.)

Meridians: These are the channels of Qi or life force as defined by Chinese medicine. Every herb is tropic for certain meridians and helps regulate an imbalance in these.

Tri Dosas: These are the fundamental **three forces** of Ayurvedic physiology, Vayu, Pitta and Kapha. They are dynamic principles governing all of life, like the diadic principle Yin/Yang. Herbs are said to increase or decrease one or more of the Tri Dosas, thus assisting in re-establishing a delicate balance in order to restore health. Succinctly, **Pitta** is active warmth and transformation, **Vayu** is movement and sensitivity, **Kapha** is structive substance and limitation.

GROUND: Also known as terrain, the ground is the arena where illness takes place and where herbal medicines unfold their therapeutic actions: this is the individual him/herself. For clarity of overview, ground is here presented according to three systems: *krasis* or **temperament**, **biotype**, and **constitution**. Herbs have a selective affinity for ground, as well as for conditions and syndromes, and may be used for constitutional, preventive treatment for general health maintenance in addition to short-term remedial treatment. They can successfully tackle an entire cluster of syndromes or conditions that the individual, as *krasis*, biotype or constitution, is prone to, and are often able to treat the typical ground on a systematic nervous and endocrine level.

Krases/**temperaments**: Treatment according to *krasis* (HIPPOKRATES) or *temperamentum* (GALEN) goes back to the Hippokratic writers in Greek medicine who sought to re-establish the particular *mesotes* or balance within the individual according to his/her *physis* or inherent natural constitution. GALEN later went on to define his *temperamenta*, i.e. temperaments, in terms of a *dyskrasia* of the *dynameis*, i.e. a poor mixture or imbalance of the four effective qualities. The four *krases* are the Sanguine, Choleric, Phlegmatic and Melancholic. (See also appendix D.)

Biotypes: Based on the preceding fourfold *krasis* system, the eight biotypes result from a correlation of the Bioenergetic psychosomatic types as developed by PIERRAKOS and KURTZ (founder of Hakomi body-centered psychotherapy) and the Chinese biotypes as interpreted by REQUENA. As a result, the eight biotypes are described by both their Hakomi and Chinese name, e.g. Expressive/Jue Yin. (For partial descriptions and studies of the eight biotypes, see the works of KURTZ, PIERRAKOS and REQUENA. See also appendix D).

Constitutions: The three constitutions also have their root in the vitalistic Western medical tradition and represent a more modern version of the four *krases*. Although they have been called by different names by various medical pioneers, they can be assimilated to three basic constitutional types, as evinced by the work of STAHL (1957), KRACK (1980) and others. HAHNEMANN, the founder of Homeopathy, spoke of the Sycotic, Syphilitic and Psoric constitutions; later, the pioneering homeopath VON GRAUVOGEL in the 1860's described the Hydrogenoid, Oxygenoid and Carbonitrogenic constitutions; more recently, developing the foundations of SHELDON's three constitutions, STAHL (1957) discusses the Carbonic, Sulphuric and Phosphoric constitutional types; while HENSE (date unknown) calls these the Lymphatic, Hematic and Mixed types. Finally, modern iris diagnosis pragmatically also refers to these as the Blue Iris, Brown Iris and Grey-Green Iris types. The summary chart of the three constitutions depicted in appendix E is limited for brevity's sake to three names, e.g. the Lymphatic/Carbonic/Blue Iris constitution, whenever it appears in the Materia Medica.

The Integral Presentation

The Herb's Functions and Uses

In this section of the herb's presentation, as in the preceding one, the aim is to integrate clinically derived uses with more theoretically derived ones. This has been achieved by creating an overall context of energetic functions and uses. These are conveyed, first, in the headings describing in phrase form the remedy's functions and, second, by describing the syndromes for which it is typically used. The phrases specifying an herb's functions do more than replace inadequate adjectives such as *diuretic* and *emmenagogue*: they spell out its functions in plain, nonspecialzed language, building up a precise picture, yet not shying from sensory descriptions.

Certain terms chosen, such as *astriction* (as in "creates astriction") and *lenify* (as in "lenifies dryness") are unusual, and may seem archaic. In every instance, however, the aim is to express a concept in as original and simple a form as possible. Thus to *astrict, astriction* are from the same root as the adjective *astringent*, which historically only found later usage. Similarly, the verb *lenify* has the origin as the adjective *lenitive*.

Throughout the text, all indications, whether symptoms or conditions, are expressed in the simplest way possible. I have tried to make the material as easily accessible as possible by reducing the number of technical terms and by spelling out the indication in full instead of using an abbreviation. It is for this reason that, for example, "high blood pressure" was chosen instead of "hypertension"; "painful or irregular periods" instead of "dysmenorrhea"; "ringing in the ears" rather than "tinnitus"; "high blood cholesterool" instead of "hypercholesterolemia".

Beneath the functions, the typical indications calling for the use of an herb are given. These indications consist of Chinese and Greek medical **syndromes, symptomatic indications** and **modern disease entities.** All three types of remedy uses are often listed, unless they so obviously overlap as to make repetition tedious. It is often the case that an indication will belong to two or more functions. Ribwort plantain, for example, treats blood heat; both its first function of *clearing heat, resolving fever and reducing inflammation* and its third function of *creating astriction, relieving congestion and staunching bleeding* contribute equally to resolving this syndrome. This overlap is inevitable and expected, seeing that herb functions are all interconnected.

Since the Chinese and the Greek approach are functional and energetic, and because they form a context for the modern analytical approach, it is an herb's typical syndrome uses which have been emphasized throughout. There is correspondingly less weight on Western disease terminology, although nothing essential or typical has been left out; in any case, the modern medical conditions implied will usually be obvious to the Western practitioner and will not need to be restated every time. Note that some remedies will be found less suited to syndrome uses than others. Blackberry leaf, for example, has no syndrome indications at all, only symptomatic ones.

All syndromes are in italics for easy recognition, while symptoms and conditions are not. Often an alternative designation for a syndrome is given, for the sake of clarity. The signs and symptoms given with each syndrome are only the main symptoms and not a list of all possible symptoms covered by that herb. They are the distinctive, typical, and specific symptoms which may be treated by that herb, as far as this has been possible to establish, hence the varying symptoms found under the same syndrome with different herbs.

Whenever the action of an herb is biased towards relieving a specific symptom, this is always listed separately in full capitals, implying that the symptom is treatable irrespective of the underlying condition or syndrome. This is the case with COUGH and Coltsfoot, or VOICE LOSS and Agrimony, for example. Some herbs are clearly oriented towards relieving specific symptoms, regardless of the origin and energetic context in which the symptoms are found. Elder flower, for

The Energetics of Western Herbs

instance, will relieve most types of swelling, e.g. whether due to water retention, a swollen lymph gland or simply a boil. Other remedies, by contrast, are definitely more syndrome or condition oriented, treating a whole configuration of symptoms.

The advantage of this kind of presentation is that it differentiates clearly among syndrome, symptom and condition, while also indicating which is paramount. Tormentil, for example, will treat leucorrhea of any kind on a symptomatic basis. Cinnamon, on the other hand, will address *genitourinary damp cold* specifically, the signs and symptoms of which include leucorrhea. The clear implication here is that Cinnamon, unlike Tormentil, is suited to treat the entire pattern of disharmony, not only the symptom of leucorrhea itself. Cinnamon therefore will treat leucorrhea in the context of symptoms such as fatigue, chilliness, poor appetite, etc.—symtoms of *genitourinary damp cold*.

Concerning terminology, the verb *strengthens* refers to physical tissue, as in *strengthens the lungs*, while the verbs *restores* and *stimulates* refer primarily to function, as in *restores the Spleen* and *stimulates the liver*.

When an organ or function is italicized in the main sentences describing an herb's function, as in RESTORES THE *SPLEEN*, this indicates that the Chinese functional organ is being referred to, not the anatomical organ itself.

The Herb's Preparation

In this section the main preparation forms suitable or available for use are given, together with their therapeutic applications, dosages and cautions. Dosages and cautions should always be heeded not only for reasons of safety, but also for the sake of maximum therapeutic effectiveness. General descriptions and details of preparations are found in the next chapter.

The Three Categories of Herbs

The classification of botanicals according to their intrinsic nature is not a new one. Hippokratic texts distinguish between three types: **restoring nutritive substances** (i.e. foods), **remedies** and **poisons.** These broad categories have served as the basis for works on pharmacology and therapeutics for over twenty-two centuries.

The classification in the *Shen nong ben cao jing*, used in Chinese medicine for almost the same number of years, is also relevant today. It is interesting that this classification turns out to be a prototype of a more modern version given by RUDOLF WEISS (1982), which forms the basis of the therapeutic categories presented here and used throughout the text.

The relevance of this threefold classification is not merely a theoretical one. It is essentially a therapeutic one, defining the therapeutic nature of botanicals. Since the category that an herb belongs to directly affects herb selection and usage in all aspects, its aim is to provide a comprehensive and safe framework for the user. The practical implications for herb selection, dosage, length of time it should be taken, etc., are discussed in Chapter 7.

Herbal remedies are divided into the following three categories:

1 **MILD HERBS** with very **structive** or **Yin** effects.

The therapeutic effect of these botanicals is gentle, slow-working and cumulative. They may and should be taken over long periods of time for their full healing potential to unfold. Side effects or negative reactions are minimal or nonexistent, and so theses herbs are said to posess **minimal or no chronic toxicity**. They consist of *restorative* or *tonic* remedies above all, and are used primarily for Restoring methods of treatment. Mild herbs are excellent used preventively as well as curatively. They are particularly suited to the treatment of chronic and systemic conditions where the vital forces, or Righteous Qi, need bolstering. Children and elderly people often rely exclusively on herbs in this category.

Mild remedies in this category include Elecampane, Camomile, Nettle, Flower pollen and Gentian. In fact, the majority of herbs in this Materia Medica are mild ones. It must be emphasized that mild means they have **structive** effects as opposed to active ones; it does not mean that they are ineffective. This is the mistake of scientific pharmacognosy when it labels an herb "inert" if it does not contain approved "active principles" such as alkaloids.[1]

2 **STRONG HERBS** with very **active** or **Yang** effects.

The effect of these botanicals is strong, rapid and immediate. They should be taken once only, or only occasionally. They provoke immediate side effects and negative reactions, and therefore are defined as possessing **acute toxicity**. These are mostly *draining* remedies, often used for symptom treatment. They are more appropriate in acute or local conditions where the principle is to deal with the pathogenic element directly; as a result, the vital force has to be strong enough to cope with the negative effects in the process. Strong herbs should be avoided where the vital force is weak, as well as in younger and older people.

Examples of herbs in this category are Aconite, Bryony, Digitalis, Poison hemlock, the sort of remedies one would not want to use without knowing precisely what the exact conditions are that call for their use, why they are excel at dealing with a problem, what the safe dosage is, and what side effects to look out for. Remedies in this category are not presented fully in this text, as they are not often used. This is not to say they are unsuitable when used in the right context: on the contrary.

3 **MEDIUM STRENGTH HERBS** with both **structive** or **Yin**, and **active** or **Yang**, effects.

These botanicals possess effects intermediate between the first and second types, combining as they do both structive and active properties. Since they have characteristics of both, they may have some negative side effects, and are defined as possessing **some chronic toxicity,** i.e. a toxicity which accumulates over time if the herb is ingested every day. For this reason they are typically used for one to three weeks, then discontinued. Their slow, cumulative low-level toxicity is obviously mitigated when used in small amounts in compound formulas or medications; it may even be annulled by using certain herbs in combination with them. Medium-strength herbs are found in all classes and are used in every variety of treatment method in both acute and chronic conditions.

Examples of these intermediary remedies are Fumitory, Arnica, Valerian and Bilberry. They should never be confused with outright toxic herbs of the strong, active type, as unfortunately they often are. Cereus and Lily of the valley, for example, still suffer from this confusion.

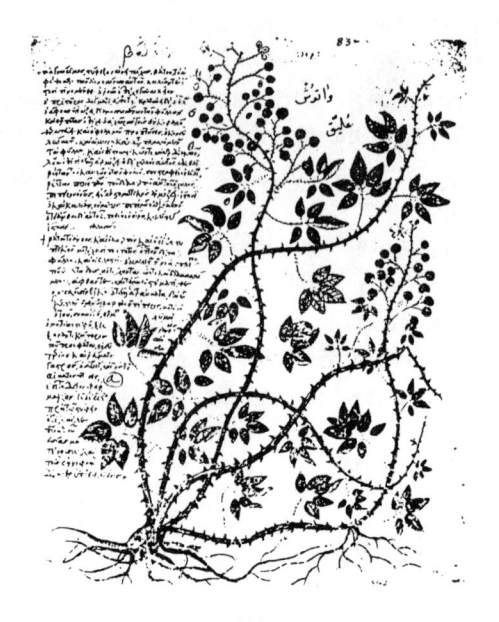

Blackberry, from Peri hyles iatrikes, *Pedanios Dioskurides, ca. 77 A.D.*

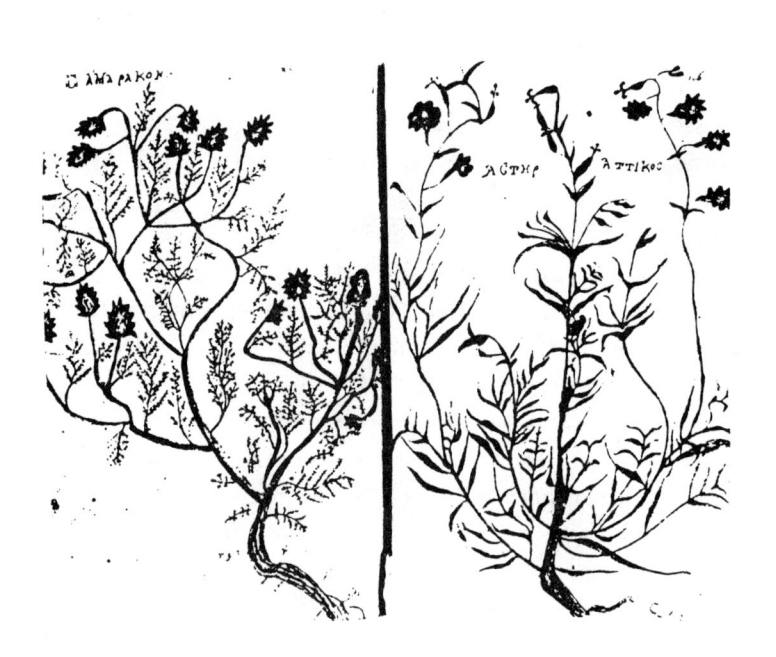

Left: Marjoram
Right: Starflower
From a 15th century manuscript.

6   Historical Antecedents

When obscurities and legends are removed in the light of modern methods, the treatment with simples so dear to our ancestors is still capable of rendering services. It can still fully justify the words of Oswald Crollius over three hundred years ago: We can see that those using simples in healing have more relevance and success in their enterprise than others.
                                           Henri Leclerc, *Précis de phytothérapie*, 1935

Of all the aspects of a new style Materia Medica, perhaps the most controversial, and certainly the most problematic, is the question of source material and its interpretation. Some idea of the considerable problems involved may be had if one considers two things.

First, by far the largest portion of herbal medicine practiced in the last 2,000 years was not actually written down in any way. It was practiced by lay healers, most of them women, who belonged mostly to the peasant classes.[1] Since they were denied literacy by the ruling Church, this knowledge was purely oral and practical, and handed down from mother to daughter or from one woman to another. This means that we have to rely on our imagination to conceive of what was probably a large number of botanicals used between Greek days and the eighteenth century.

Some oral traditions survived, however, despite the rigors of over 400 years of witch-hunts, and some were even written down. If these traditions are accurate, as they probably are, then plants such as Rye ergot, Foxglove and Deadly nightshade were used extensively, long before the modern clinic was invented. Moreover the large body of herbal folk knowledge that is found in Europe today is virtually a legacy, albeit in a highly diluted form, of the traditions of wise women, midwives and witches.

Second, where written sources exist, the variables inherent in them must be considered. The general variables concern the reliability of witnesses and accounts and the reliability of transmission from other authors, which may have been hindered by linguistic difficulties such as terminology and translation. More specifically, there are a variety of differing herbal descriptions in these written sources, which may be due to differences in nationality or personality of the writers, as well due to differences of the all-important therapeutic context they were describing. Differences of social, cultural and religious conditions, as well as of medical terminology and theory, can all result in specific variables affecting every aspect of a materia medica, including plant identification and the interpretation of described qualities, functions and uses.

While there is no space here for further inquiry into these problems, it is well to keep them in mind. They were vividly present as source information was selected from roughly four cultures on two continents using six languages over a span of two milleniums. The aim was to access the most reputable, accurate and original sources available for use as raw material for the Materia Medica to be presented here. Clearly, considering the issues involved, a very circumspect, cautious approach is needed in interpreting and integrating this mass of information. This approach is described later in this chapter in the methodology section.

In conclusion, it should be remembered that, while the approach using enquiring logic and analysis is useful, it must be balanced by striving to recreate a botanical healing art that is grounded

The Energetics of Western Herbs

and harmonious in every respect. In this respect, intuitive judgements inevitably came into play in shaping this Materia Medica. Since this pursuit of a more balanced herbal medicine is continually evolving, there will always be much that cannot yet be put into words, let alone explained and rationalized.

Historical and Modern Sources

Despite the severe limitations caused by a broken and depleted oral tradition of European medicine among women healers, a wealth of information on the use of plants in healing still exists from the Greek, Roman, Arab-Persian, Amerindian and American cultures. It covers the entire spectrum from simple, practical folk uses to medical theses by established physicians. The bulk of this information is a sunken Atlantis of knowledge and wisdom, accumulated by centuries of practical and theoretical development. The uses of remedies change as their various functions and purposes are discovered, utilized, forgotten and once again discovered over the centuries. Like changes in fashion, herb uses follow the tug of cultural, social and religious changes and upheavals, as well as the resulting changes in therapeutic contexts. Original records of medicine in transformation and its involvement with mythology, magic, farming, horticulture, botany, astrology, pharmacology, to name but a few contextual pursuits, sit for the most part in modest libraries the world over, bedecked in hoary dust.

Referring to historical and modern sources is simply one way of accessing plant remedies. Although not the only valid method, it still remains the basic way of obtaining a detailed picture. This method is all the more necessary today as the knowledge of the nature and effect of herbs has been drastically reduced, not only because of the dominance of experimental pharmacology since the 1850's, but also because of the availability of synthetic medicines on a mass scale. When the countless uses, past and present, of a single plant remedy are collected, the final overall view can only be described as iriscopic! This is not surprising, considering that the people contributing to herbalism represent a wide variety of trades: root-pickers and wildcrafters, barbers and bone-setters, midwives and housewives, wise women and witches, monks and mystics, classics professors and botanists, apothecaries and experimental chemists. The variety and richness of a remedy's uses, like mineral strata layered in rock, reflect every contextual variable imaginable and completely shatter any preconceptions one may have had.

Moreover, it is not enough to simply collect data on herb uses through the ages. More to the point is to understand that only the distilled balance of the whole can give us a true picture, one that we can realistically work with today. From the wide variety of cultural, medical and linguistic influences, it is necessary to extract a deeper, fuller picture of each herb. This can only be done through a process of distillation, involving elimination, acceptance, and sometimes transformation of raw information. It is here that right brain, intuitive elements come into play as logical information is systematically processed. The final comprehensive picture of a remedy should be such that all written sources may be seen to point to it, however faintly. This is the test of its universality, and this has been our aim in going to sources past and present.

The advantages of such a comprehensive approach go beyond the information in itself. One main advantage is the establishment of specific links with Chinese medicine. Since the underlying paradigms of traditional Greek and Chinese medicine allow such links to be made, as we saw in Chapters 1 and 2, they can greatly enhance our understanding of Western herbs. The most sympathetic texts in this respect are early Greek texts (1st-4th century B.C.), Persian texts up to the time of IBN SINA (5th century A.D.) and Renaissance texts between about 1480 and 1600. These texts require closer study if we are to fully appreciate what they can bring us in our attempt to create a more balanced, energetics-based herbal medicine.

How is one to view source material from a critical perspective, in order to extract reliable and useable information? Two factors are at play here, regardless of the modernity or age of the text: its originality and its integrity. A source is original if it was written or stated by its author. Secondhand or third hand sources automatically entail a multiplication of errors. The greater the number of subsequent copies or repetitions, the more mistakes in judgement not only increase, but actually gain credibility.[2] This happens with suprising ease, in spite of good intentions by all concerned, due to any of the variables noted. The writings of DIOSKURIDES during the Middle Ages, for example, when literacy was rare and poor scholarship rife, were to be found in an astonishing number of variations.

The advantages of returning to original sources are evident: by reading an author's own words rather than secondhand or tenth hand versions, one not only obtains more accurate information, but also maximizes the chances of gaining a correct understanding. However, one often meets with problems in reading original texts, not only the Greek, Latin, Persian or Arabic ones, but most texts well into the 1800's, the time of Galenic medicine's demise. There are a host of linguistic, semantic and terminological problems too formidable for anyone but the trained specialist to understand, making comprehension, let alone translation, almost impossible.[3]

On the other hand, reading later compilations does have some advantages. They tend to contain more information, giving us a fuller, more rounded picture of the remedies. The well ornamented masterpieces of Islamic Persian doctors such as AR-RAZI (Rhazes), IBN SINA (Avicenna) and AL-ABBAS, which are mainly texts on simples (single herbs) and prescriptions, all amply attest to this fact. By the same token, however, they are more liable to contain errors than the earlier texts—errors arising from poor interpretation as well as fanciful embellishment. In general, one has to strike a balance between the accuracy of original source material and the comprehensiveness of later works. Skepticism and an open mind together are the gateways which lead to a successful critical evaluation of any text.

The integrity of authors is another problematic issue directly affecting the quality and pedigree of herbal texts. It raises the issue of plagiary as well as of inaccurate texts, problems which are very hard to resolve. Certainly the character, personality and social status of an author plays a large part in determining the quality of his writings. The problem here is that plagiarism often goes unrecognized, while sincere work is unappreciated, due to some opinion about the author's character (which in turn is often based on his social standing). ADAM LONICER's Swiss *Kreutterbuch* of 1557, for example, was discovered by the author to be for the most part an unacknowledged rewrite of EUCHARIUS RöSZLIN's herbal of 1533—old wine revintaged by the most respected Basel town physician of the day!

But RöSZLIN had other plagiarists, too. His *Der Schwangerer Frauen und Hebammen Rosengarten* (ca. 1525), an outstanding Galenic medical text on pregnancy, birth and midwifery written in vernacular Swiss German, was copied and embellished by the Strasbourg citizen WALTHER RYFF in *Der Schwangerer Frauen Rosengarten* of 1580, long after the original text was out of print. RYFF at least did the work of reformulating the material in a more modern, imaginative, popular and attractive way. In RYFF's case the problem of plagiarism is severely compounded by the fact that the bulk of his work seems indeed to be originals, or at least completely reworked compilations. Like WILLIAM SALMON a century later, for reasons difficult to identify, he aroused the hostility of certain doctors who tried to discredit him and his works—and succeeded. His contribution to herbalism was considerable. He wrote a variety of works aimed at the average educated person, stylishly expressing the simple healing marvels that

The Energetics of Western Herbs

may be created in the kitchen, the still-room, the clinic and the pharmacy, using mainly native plants in a profusion of preparations both culinary and medicinal. His titles include *Practicierbüchlein Bewarter Leibartzeney* (1583), *New Kochbuch für die Krancken* (1545), *Lustgarten der Gesundheit* (1546), as well as the compendious *Reformierte Deutsche Apotheck* discussed below. Certainly the dividing line beween plagiary and reformulation in the natural sciences was, in those days, virtually nonexistent or, at best, extremely thin. The large output of both SALMON and RYFF at times belongs to this ambiguous area where compilation ends and plagiary begins. Today their works are of significant value in terms of their content and are prime examples of wrongly underrated literature.[4]

The example of NICHOLAS CULPEPER's *Herball* throws up problems of an entirely different kind. Here one simply questions whether a part of his assertions are the true result of his actual experience or whether they are the dictates of fancy. It is certain that his book contains between 20% and 30% material not found anywhere else in Galenic writings. Knowing his character and his avowed predilection for iatromathematics[5] (in RYFF's wake), one is inclined to consider the work a blend of sanguine conceit and astromedical conjecture.

Similar problems in an entirely different setting are raised when we look at early settlers' reports on the medical practices of the native American Indians. They contain very unrealistic or superficial descriptions at best, severely colored by fear, ignorance and prejudice. These descriptions must be understood in the context of severe culture shock on the part of the Spanish and French missionaries, with their dogmatic Christian ethics, and on the part of the English colonists, convinced of their superior civilization. In this connection, the doctors' blind use of complex pharmaceutical compounds from the Old World must be compared to the highly advanced preventive and remedial treatment with simple botanical remedies carried out by Native Americans.

Personal practical experience on the present writer's part represents another source of information for this Materia Medica. While it remains of limited influence, it does tend to shape and emphasize certain aspects more than others. Moreover, it is the personal experience of practitioners over a longer time which will validate or invalidate the syndrome uses presented here.

Primary Historical Sources

While herbal texts from Greek, Roman and Persian/Arabian times in a sense are the most authentic for Greek medicine, they are also the most inaccessible. The exception are the works of GALEN, AR-RAZI and IBN-SINA, which are more approachable to anyone schooled in a system of traditional medicine. The language used in these works is essentially similar to that of Chinese medicine and is still in use in the present day version of Greek medicine called Unani medicine *(Unani* means Ionian, i.e. Greek in Arabic). The Greek/Unani system is distinguished by a phenomenological paradigm using qualitative and dialectic terminology (compare p. 11). In most early texts, including those of GALEN, the functions and uses of a botanical are intimately linked to pathology, as in the Chinese system. However, as time went by, the approach became a more pharmacognosical one, i.e. based on an understanding of the plants themselves (their texture, taste, effective qualities, and so on). This bottomed out into sophistry in late medieval Arab literature with its 32 grades of warmth, for example, and directly led to biochemical scientific analysis which began in the eighteenth century.

Out of the plethora of herbals, dispensatories, toxicology manuals, etc., written between the fourth century B.C. and 1500 A.D., we have chosen to review in detail the following three outstanding volumes:

Peri hyles iatrikes, PEDANIOS DIOSKURIDES, Greece, ca. 77 A.D.

On Therapeutic Substances is a text which could be called the *Shennong ben cao* of Western/Greek herbal medicine and is also known under its Latin name *De materia medica*. It offers the most extensive and reliable source of information on the simples used in Greek medicine. The *Dioscorides*, as it was later called, was prized up to the seventeenth century, and longer still in India and the Middle East. It has been more studied, translated, discussed and commented on than any other Western herbal.

On Therapeutic Substances discusses in great detail 950 medicinal substances, of which almost 500 are botanical. It is laid out in five books covering:
1 aromatics, oils, salves, trees, resins & fruits
2 animal products, cereals & vegetables
3 herbs, roots & seeds
4 spores & fungi
5 wines, minerals & clays

In addition to presenting the uses, preparation and cautions of each remedy, DIOSKURIDES lists synonyms and possible fraudulent substitutes. This is the first Western work on herbal medicine freed of magical, ritualistic or talismanic uses from older times.

DIOSKURIDES' *On Therapeutic Substances* is distinct from THEOPHRASTUS's and later PLINIUS's writings on herbs, which are primarily botanical and historical compilations, however brilliant. Its value lies largely in the empirical approach of its author, who was a well travelled and experienced army doctor. It can actually be seen simply as a compendium of high quality empirical practice. It consists of two elements in very uncertain proportions: first, the empirical natural medicine as practiced mainly by women healers of the time; second, the author's own considerable experience.

Nevertheless, the *Dioscorides* has shortcomings. Understandably, being empirical material, it does not describe the remedies with reference to either the four fluids or the four qualities theory. Consequently, it fails to give the **specific conditions** for which an herb should be used. As a result, it reads like a manual of good symptomatic treatment—which in fact it is. Certainly it fails to present a clear picture of the more sophisticated medical practices found in various medical schools in those days. In the next generation GALEN is already pointing out examples of this in a critique of this herbal! He specifically complains, for example, that "Dioskurides writes that Polygonum provokes urination, and that it is useful for those with painful urination; however he fails to note exactly for what type of painful urination this plant is appropriate."[6]

Peri kraseos kai dynameos ton haplon pharmakon, CLAUDIOS GALENOS, Rome, ca. 165 A.D.

This is the main text in GALEN's vast output dealing with simple, not compound, remedies, i.e. with single herbs rather than formulas. Its title translates to English as *On the Mixture and Effective Qualities of Simple Remedies*. It has a companion text, *Peri trophon dynameos (On the Effective Qualities of Foods)* which presents culinary items alone.

Both books describe the nature, functions and uses of herbs and foods in a way that has become the hallmark of the Galenic approach; namely, in terms of their *dynameis* or effective qualities. These are functional, energetic descriptions of both their nature and effects based on the primary qualities hot/cold, dry/damp. As a result, GALEN's pharmacognosy and pharmacology are most similar to those of both the Chinese and Ayurvedic systems which are still widely used today. Nevertheless his work is distinct in showing a bias for therapy based on a profound, detailed understanding of the herbal remedy itself as opposed to an understanding of the clinical situation. It is the key text in Western medicine for the remedy approach (discussed in Chapter 2) which also underpins modern analytical pharmacognosy.

GALEN's *Peri kraseos* consists of eleven books, or what we would call chapters today. Books 1 to 4 present the basic principles of energetic pharmacognosy and pharmacology in fair detail, exhaustively describing various concepts involved, such as the four categories of *pharmakon* or remedies, their four types of effect (natural, accidental, potential and actual), their three kinds of *dynameis* or effective qualities (primary, secondary, tertiary), and their warmth grade or intensity (*taxis* or *apostasis*). Book 4, for instance, deals with the energetic or effective qualities of the six tastes, referring to many plant remedies as examples. Common, much-used substances such as water, vegetable oils, milk and vinegar are drawn upon as examples as GALEN develops his theories. Book 5 discusses the various uses of herbs, and classifies them into different types according to their therapeutic uses. Books 6 to 11 present a total of 216 remedies in terms of their main energetic properties, both primary (hot, cold, dry, moist), and secondary (astringing, softening, restoring, etc.). Books 6, 7 and 8 deal with botanical remedies in which the specific grade (*taxis*) of warmth is given in the case of 141 herbs. Book 9 covers earths, metals, minerals and stones; books 10 and 11 animal products, including blood, bile, sweat, milk, urine and stool.

GALEN's writing, which consists of over 500 works (including those that perished when his clinic burnt down in Rome), covers every branch of the medical arts. He established the foundation of a medical system which was developed and refined for fifteen centuries thereafter. His impact on the development of Western medicine was enormous for three reasons. First, he was a brilliant systematizer who, using integrative thinking, started from broad principles, then focused on particular facts; secondly, his approach managed to strike a nice, judicious balance between the analytical and the phenomenological methods; and thirdly, he was a compiler of a vast amount of medical knowledge who was able to reconcile conflicting schools such as the Dogmatists and Empiricists. Seen in this broad perspective, the importance of his *Peri kraseos* becomes clear.

Kitab al-Gami' li-mufradat al-adwiya wa-l-agdiya, IBN AL-BAITAR, Seville ca. A.D. 1225

IBN AL-BAITAR was a doctor, naturalist and botanist, who lived at the height of Greek medicine as practiced by Arabian physicians in Spain, when Islamic Arabic civilization was at its peak. Both his botanical and medicinal knowledge of plants was phenomenal, and he communicated widely with other naturalists. His travels led him via Egypt to the borders of Afghanistan.

IBN AL-BAITAR's gigantic text, whose title translates literally as *Collection of Simple Remedies*, contends for being the most serious, accurate, comprehensive and critical herbal ever written in the West. The author is exceptional in explaining his methodology at the outset. The text consists of the most relevant verbatim quotes from a total of about 150 authors, including HIPPOKRATES, ARISTOTLE, DIOSKURIDES, AR-RAZI, IBN SINA and the anonymous author(s) of *The Book of Experiences*. To these the author's commentaries are added to complete the picture. Using this technique, he compromises neither accuracy nor comprehensiveness. Morphology, nature, uses, side effects and their corrections, preparation methods and substitutions of the herbs are described. Remedies are arranged alphabetically and include many mineral and animal medicines.

The *Collection of Simple Remedies* is the unsurpassed compendium of the Greek materia medica, the culmination of about sixteen centuries of herbal experience in Mediterranean countries and beyond.

In contrast to the herbals in Greek, Latin, and Arabic that had been written up to that time, pharmacopoeias of Renaissance times (1400-1650), represent an ideal summary of Galenic pharmacognosy in languages more accessible to us. Here, as in all Galenic texts, we learn about a remedy's "temperature", moisture, qualities and specific effects on the four fluids and the three spirits, as well as syndrome and symptom indications for its use. There is little new in terms of form, although the content has been increased to cover many European plants that were not mentioned in the classics. Just as today there is a movement to exploring the energetics of local plants in addition to using the well-established Chinese herbs, so in those days the impulse arose to discover the energetic properties of European herbs to complement the Arabian remedies of the town pharmacies representing mainstream Galenic medicine. Many practitioners, such as BRUNFELS and BOCK, actively sought out the healers in the country, the women practitioners, and tried to salvage local plant uses for posterity. This must have been a compromising task, since a large number of these women were being burnt at the stake as witches. Many wise women practitioners practiced the ancient Wicca craft; and indeed, many were induced to reveal their therapeutic secrets under the appalling tortures during the mass psychosis of the witch-hunts.

At any rate, for the first time since DIOSKURIDES, the marvellous woodblock illustrations in these materia medicas illustrate recognizable plants—no medieval caricatures here: they are neither stylized nor symbolic. The best ones, found in the herbals of FUCHS and BRUNFELS, combine botanical precision with a fine rendering of the archetypal nature of each plant—a feat never bettered in that medium.

There are several materia medicas from this period that we deem valuable sources. Each satisfactorily resolves the problems arising from the difference between Greek and Central European flora, problems of plant identification, geographical variations, and qualities. Outstanding examples are:

De Historia Stirpium, LEONHARDT FUCHS, Basel, 1542

This book, which is simply a herbal, is without a doubt the most critical, erudite and reliable materia medica of the time. FUCHS was a superlative scholar as well as a highly competent and successful practitioner. Although relying extensively on PLINIUS, GALEN and DIOSKURIDES, FUCHS supplements the *Historia* with the results of his own extensive clinical experience. Every word is carefully considered, making this an extremely accurate text. Today we might criticize its humanistic bias and talk about a fossilized dependence on the classics. While this is justified, it does not detract from the intrinsic value of the material.

The plant descriptions are surpassed only by those of CHARLES DE L'ECLUSE and HIERONYMUS BOCK for their keen observation. The large folio contains over 500 breathtakingly beautiful full-page illustrations, the results of three artists working together.

Reformierte Deutsche Apotheck, WALTHER HERMANN RYFF, Strassburg, 1573

This is the major herbal from the Reformation period, for two reasons: first, because it is an original German text, instead of being a translation from Latin; and second, because it deals almost entirely with indigenous Central European medicinal plants (at a time when many authors were still clinging to their *Dioscorides*). The *Deutsche Apotheck*, or *German Pharmacy*, is a people's herbal. Written in the most engaging Swabian idiom of the day, it gets across the author's authentic feeling for his local herbs. RYFF's sympathetic and generous descriptions of their functions and uses do more to enthuse and inspire us to actually try them than the cool, pithy statements of a FUCHS or a RöSZLIN.

The Energetics of Western Herbs

The *Apotheck* is in two parts, *Materia Medica* and *Therapeutics*. Intended primarily as a reference work, the materia medica is replete with typical herb uses for syndromes and conditions and indicates herbal combinations and preparations of varying degrees of complexity.

New Kreuterbuch, JOHANN JAKOB THEODOR VON BERGZABERN, Frankfurt am Main, 1588

The *New Kreuterbuch* is the most encyclopedic herbal ever written in the West. Its two tomes of 1,600 folio pages contain over 3,000 entries of plant medicines arranged according to herbs, flowers, trees, shrubs, etc. It includes over 2,500 small woodcut illustrations, eleven separate indexes in ten different languages, and source references from 111 authors past and present. Its most recent edition, that of 1731, was edited by the botanist GASPARD BAUHIN. Each herb is typically presented in the following way: Introduction, Names, Nature/Faculty/Effect and Properties, Internal use, External use, Fresh juice internal use, Fresh juice external use, Distilled water, Wine extract, Conserve, Syrup, and Distilled oil.

The value of this apothecary's work lies in its sheer exhaustiveness. As in JOHN PARKINSON's *Theatrum Botanicum*, of about fifty years later which is closely modelled on this work, almost every statement is referenced, the opinions of past authors from KRATEVAS to FUCHS cross-referenced, and the whole distilled into definitive statements. This was the final Renaissance work on simples.

The nineteenth century also saw an extremely interesting and creative phase of botanical medicine, which consisted of Eclectic medicine on one hand and Homeopathy on the other. It is no coincidence that these appeared on the scene almost simultaneously; they are quite closely related in their methods and prescribing habits, their main difference being in the preparation method of remedial substances. While Homeopathy began in Europe and the Eclectic school grew out of the popular Thomsonian therapeutic movement in America (itself part of the Popular Health Movement), they continued to influence each other throughout the nineteenth century and well into the twentieth.

The scene had changed radically since the days of RYFF and FUCHS. Every aspect of human life had become different, healing and medicine included, as a result of social, technological and cultural upheavals. The already waning influence of GALEN had ceased entirely. The four fluids and the four qualities were myths from the past. A plethora of medical theories and systems had come and gone in their wake since the sixteenth century. Two movements had irrevocably shattered Galenic medicine: **clinical medicine** from France, with its sole reliance on signs and symptoms, and FRANCOIS MAGENDIE's **experimental physiology** and **pharmacology.**

Clinical medicine influenced medical practice in both Europe and America throughout the nineteenth century, and only waned as a result of the acceptance of cellular pathology in its latter years. Experimental physiology and pharmacology only became accepted at large when CLAUDE BERNARD continued and further developed the trend in the 1840's; since then it has been unstoppable.

Homeopathic medicine developed on its own, independent of the above trends—truly a unique event. Eclectic medicine, on the other hand, as seen in the writings of JOHN KING, JOHN SCUDDER, HERBERT WEBSTER, FINLEY ELLINGWOOD, JOHN URI LLOYD and HARVEY FELTER, is appropriately enough a fusion of several influences. The first is the botanical medicine of Native Americans and Black slaves as practiced in its watered down form by the Thomsonian practitioners. This influence provided the raw material and specific uses for well over two hundred indigenous botanicals.[7] It passed from the natives and Blacks over to the early

Historical Antecedents

pioneers and settlers, later to the Thomsonians, from the Thomsonians to the turn-of-the-century Philadelphia botanists, and from them over to the Eclectics. The second impulse originated in Homeopathic medicine which arrived from Europe with CONSTANTINE HERRING in the mid 1820's. It provided the general approach to botanicals, influencing not only the actual symptomatology of herbal remedies, but also therapeutics itself, emphasizing treatment aimed at rebalancing systemic disharmony rather than relieving isolated symptoms.

The third impulse came from both European clinical medicine and bacteriology as taught in the regular medical schools of the Eastern U.S.; this in turn provided the substratum of semiological, diagnostic and therapeutic methods for Eclectic medicine.

In view of the wide variety of influences that went into the shaping of Eclectic medicine, the reason why its instigator JOHN KING called himself an *Eclectic* becomes quite clear.

The works of Eclectic physicians are all hallmarked, first, by the more **analytical**, quantitative paradigm, which characterizes all medicine of the time; secondly, by the more empirical, **phenomenological** paradigm derived from both clinical medicine and Homeopathy, and, thirdly, by the **vitalist** paradigm which was inherent in herbal medical traditions. Moreover, their writings represent a perfect balance between the remedy based orientation, as emphasized by JOHN LLOYD (one of the most brilliant biochemists who ever worked with plants), and the clinical approach. A dynamic new whole resulted from the synthesis of the three methods. Eclectic practice represents an interesting example for the present Materia Medica, which integrates several therapeutic paradigms with ensuing benefits.

American Materia Medica, Therapeutics and Pharmacognoscy, FINLEY ELLINGWOOD, Evanston, 1898 (revised edition 1919)

The *American Materia Medica* is organized by topography (nervous system, heart, stomach, etc.) into ten groups of remedies, each divided therapeutically into several classes. A total of 389 substances are discussed, three-quarters of them botanical and the rest inorganic.

In his preface, ELLINGWOOD states that "This is a one-man work only in very small part. This book contains the results of the observations of perhaps 25,000 practising physicians. The statements are made from comparisons and from conclusions drawn from the bedside observations of all. With these the author has endeavoured to make severe and accurate adjustments of his own observations and experiences during forty years of family, hospital and out-consultation practice. Our earnest effort has been made to make the work widely cosmopolitan; as far as possible unprejudiced, scientific, strictly practical, and rational."

With these words, ELLINGWOOD clearly reveals himself as the clinician that he is. His Materia Medica is the most significant text of observation based herbal medicine in modern times and is therefore comparable to Homeopathy and Chinese medicine. The compilatory aspect is only bettered by medieval Arab writers, and in every sense the *American Materia Medica* is the *Collection of Simple Remedies* of modern times.

Each remedy is presented according to Physiological Action, Specific Symptomatology and Therapy, the first being the influence of experimental pharmacology, the second that of Homeopathy, the third that of clinical medicine. Here the three main influences mingling in a single text are seamlessly woven together, as Ellingwood stroke by stroke paints a picture that is as vivid in detail as it is breathtaking in scope. As a result, not only is much insight into the intrinsic nature of each plant obtained, but a clinical understanding of the specific conditions calling for each is generated—one that we can learn much from.

The entries are given varying attention, with typically six pages for important remedies such as Echinacea and Aconite. The detail of description and perspicacity of judgement found in the more

The Energetics of Western Herbs

modest accounts exceed anything else written by other Eclectics. Information on specific signs and symptoms, including tongue and pulse indications, is invaluable for differential diagnosis, whether of the Western or the Chinese kind.

It is interesting to note that the most recent edition of *King's American Dispensatory*, the one other important Eclectic pharmacopoeia, was also released in 1898. Updated and partially rewritten by JOHN URI LLOYD and HARVEY FELTER, it reads like a precise, summary account of the *American Materia Medica*. Published in two three inch tomes, its larger size than ELLINGWOOD's work is due to the inclusion of considerably more inorganic compounds as well as botanicals, on one hand, and, on the other, due to the greater amount of botanical, pharmacognosical and pharmaceutical information on each entry. Standard U.S.P. preparation forms are also given separate entries, appropriately enough for a dispensatory. *King's American Dispensatory* is a good complement from the field of pharmacy to the *American Materia Medica*, which is unquestionably richer and more elaborate where therapeutics is concerned.

Methodology

In order to make a balanced and integrated presentation of a botanical remedy, a working method had to be found which would allow the type of presentation based on the qualitative dialectic standards of Chinese and Greek medicine to be combined with the type of presentation based on the quantitative linear standards of modern Western herbal medicine. With this in mind, the following working procedure was developed.

First, all possible information on the herb's nature, functions, symptomatology and uses was gathered. Only sources of the highest pedigree were chosen, according to the criteria and considerations outlined above.

Secondly, since this mass of information was in a chaotic, or as it were liquid state, it was reorganized, sorted out and reworded in standard terms. This part of the process was extremely delicate, since it is here that jewels may be thrown out with the bathwater, in a mistaken if well meant attempt to separate reliable from imaginary uses of an herb. In general, any material that seemed dubious at first sight was retained if it made inductive sense or if it appeared in reliable sources from different periods or cultures. (It is this type of symptomatology which modern pharmacology often vindicates, as in the case of Cowslip for rheumatism; or which modern usage has reaffirmed, as with Mistletoe for tumors.)

Thirdly, this reorganized and distilled information was now scanned through the Chinese and Greek medical "viewfinder" in order to see what energetic, qualitative aspects (such as effective qualities, biotypes and syndromes) would crystallize. As the information on each remedy began clearly to take definite shape, its nature in terms of taste, warmth, secondary qualities and so on suddenly became evident. Moreover, a clear distinction among the types of uses of an herb emerged: symptom use, tissue condition use and syndrome use. At this point it was interesting to see how the overall character of the remedies became clearer and their therapeutic effects more understandable. Some remedies turned out to be simply syndrome naturals, like Angelica and Goldenseal, just as others, like Comfrey and Echinacea, stubbornly resisted attempts to manifest their syndrome uses, being symptom oriented. Others seemed tailor-made for overall tissue conditions. The bulk of botanicals, however, showed some balance of all three styles of usage.

Clearly, this third stage of the process has nothing in common with intuiting, theorizing or wishful thinking in regard to any aspect of a remedy. Speculation on symptomatology and uses of remedies, was rife in the past: it was at its peak with iatromathematics and the Neoplatonic revival during the Renaissance, and the example of NICHOLAS CULPEPER was given earlier on. Here, on the other hand, the method chosen is absolutely empirical: either syndrome uses were evinced in the symptomatology of an herb by a certain configuration of signs and symptoms, or they were not. This rescanning by pure observation is then the opposite of rationalizing about or analyzing its uses (in the Aristotelian-Arabian vein, as with modern pharmacology, for example). Any such pitfall is further corrected in the final step, where the remedy is tested.

In this fourth and last step of the process, the herb was reviewed in general and seen as a whole image or gestalt. This involved making systematic inductive links between its various aspects, in order to reach a larger, coherent whole. This procedure provides a test of findings in that it tends to either support or weaken the suggested presentation. At its best, an integrated herb profile revealed a meaningful, unified remedy picture, as opposed to a string of disconnected, inconsequential facts (which frequently is the case with contemporary presentations of herbs). As a result, the relations between an herb's nature, functions and uses became increasingly clear, forming a comprehensible whole. This allows us to see the links, for example, between an herb's *pungent taste,* its *sweat inducing* activity, and its usefulness in **external wind** conditions with fevers, colds or flus and related symptoms. In other words, we are able to articulate correspondences between the nature, functions and symptomatology of a remedy—a hallmark of integrative thinking.

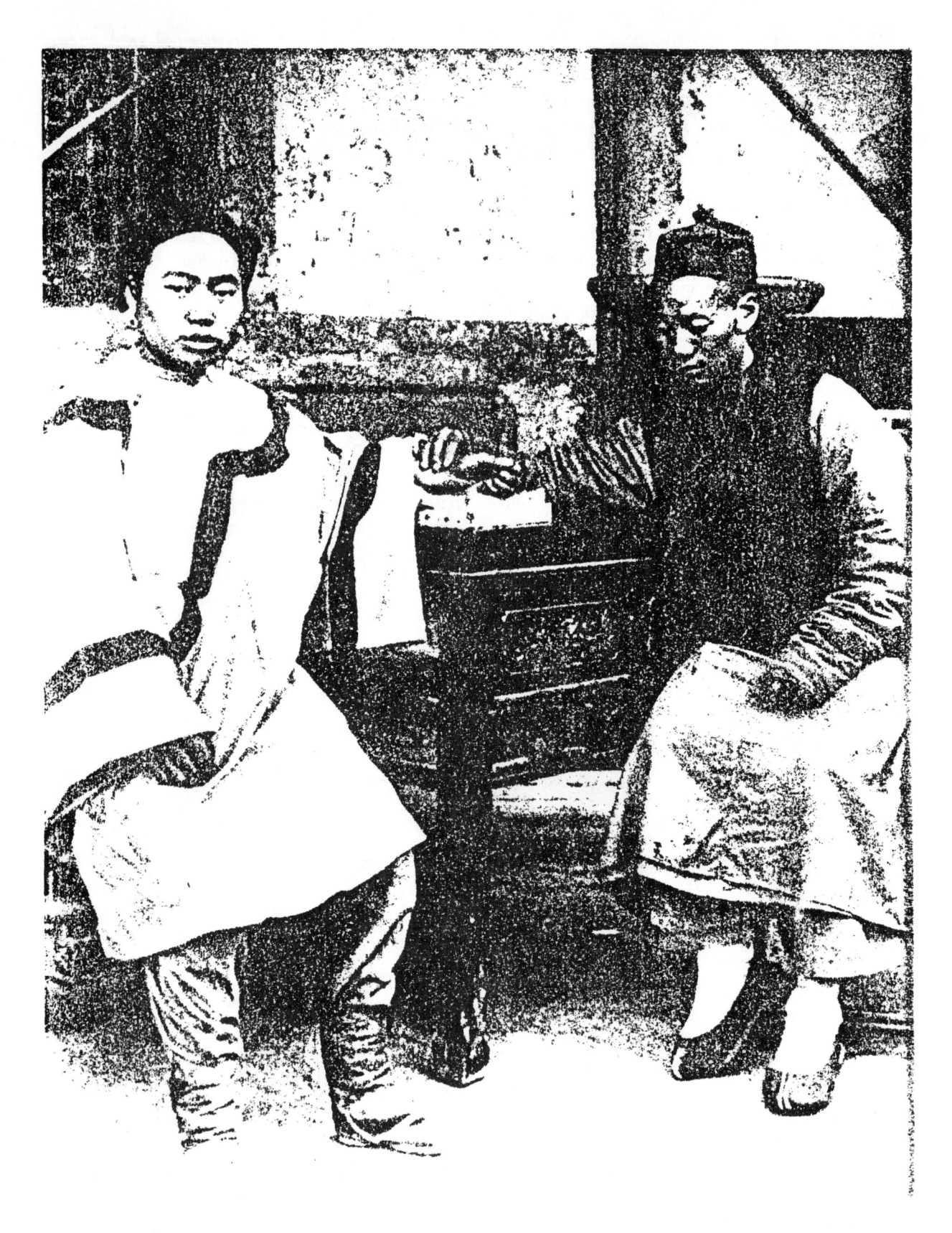

Pulse taking in Imperial China.

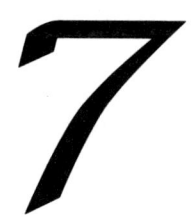

7 Guidelines to Prescribing

If those of these times would but be, by a joynt Concurrence, as industrious to search into the secrets of the Nature of Herbs, as some of the former, and make tryall of them as they did, they should no doubt find the force of Simples many times no lesse effectuall, than that of Compounds, to which this present age is too too much addicted.

William Cole, *Adam in Eden*, 1657

A variety of factors enter into play when we consider how best to use botanical remedies. The exact herb chosen, how long and how often it is taken, how it is prepared, what dosage is used, and what climate prevails are all factors which influence therapeutic effect and outcome. These factors are simply a part of the overall therapeutic context. Clearly, our aim is to find the right combination of prescribing factors for each particular condition being treated.

The following guidelines are just that—indications, not hard and fast rules. In any event, experience is the best teacher in prescribing.

The best way of working with these guidelines in any given condition is simply to decide which of the above-mentioned factors is the most important. Moreover, from both a theoretical and practical point of view it is usually impossible to take all factors into account. Elements such as the weather and season usually have low priority and in practice cause only slight if any modification of the preparation being prescribed.

In acute conditions, for example, **dosage** and **timing** of administration is likely to be the most crucial. In chronic conditions however, using the right **preparation form** may well be the foremost consideration. As another example, the different types of hot conditions all require different prescribing approaches. Full heat usually requires **large** doses of a **water preparation;** empty heat **smaller** doses of either **water** or **tincture** preparation; damp heat may need **repeated smaller** doses, as may blood heat.

The following variable factors are presented to help determine the type of herbal medication that should be prescribed. They are presented in order of importance.

Herb Selection

The selection of an appropriate remedy, or combination of remedies, is the core of herbal prescribing, regardless of the case under treatment. All other considerations follow from and depend on the herb selected.

It must be stressed that all the following factors governing herb selection only become effective when considered in the light of a **differential diagnosis** of the problem in question. Such a diagnosis includes an assessment of the nature, location, origin, etiology and progression of a disease condition. This holds true no matter whether a more analytical Western style diagnosis is done (based on tissue conditions, for example), or whether a more observational Chinese, Greek or Ayurvedic method is used. The principle of differentiating among various conditions giving rise to symptoms is the critical element of both types of diagnosis.

The Energetics of Western Herbs

When the various parameters of a condition are assessed, whether according to the eight principles in Chinese medicine or according to the *astringe/relax, stimulate/sedate* principles sometimes used in Western herbalism, herb selection is directly affected. The choice of a remedy affects all aspects of prescribing, right up to the dosage used.

The main factors to consider when choosing an herb are the following:

1) The **treatment principle**, i.e. whether treating
   - the constitutional individual ground preventively
   - the condition of disharmony remedially
   - the specific symptoms remedially

If treatment is geared to treating individual biotypes on a constitutional level, then mild (non-toxic) botanicals represent the ideal first choice. Medium-strength herbs may be used, but only in small quantities as part of an overall herbal formula.

If specific symptoms are being addressed, remedies from any category may be suitable. The same is true of treating syndromes or conditions.

2) The **treatment method**, i.e. whether the herb is to
   - eliminate
   - restore
   - drain
   - alter and regulate
   - treat symptoms

Within each of the above categories, the **specific** method must be chosen. For example, for the Restoring method, should the herb
   - increase the Qi, restore and strengthen (Class 7)
   - support the Yang, generate warmth and dispel cold (Class 8)
   - restore the blood, nourish and supplement (Class 9)
   - provide moisture and lenify dryness (Class 10)
   - cause astriction, dry damp and arrest discharge (Class 11)

If an Eliminating method such as promoting bowel movement is chosen, then remedies from that class, i.e. Class 3 should be selected. Botanicals in this Materia Medica are organized according to the treatment methods precisely to facilitate this selection. A full listing of possible herbs in each class may be found in the synopsis lists at the end of the Materia Medica.

3) The **type of conditions being treated,** i.e. whether
   - chronic or acute
   - global or local
   - internal or external
   - deficient or excessive
   - cold or hot

   ...as well as whether any injuries are present, such as
   - infection
   - toxemia
   - congestion (of blood, fluids, phlegm)
   - fever
   - internal wind
   - spirit disharmony

Guidelines to Prescribing

Chronic conditions demand mild remedies that can safely be taken over months at a time if necessary, whereas **acute** conditions may require stronger herbs.

Some remedies have more systemic, global effects, whereas others have more specific and local uses.

Most botanicals will treat internal conditions when taken internally. In addition, some can treat external conditions such as wind cold and wind heat, wind/damp/cold obstruction, etc. (Classes 1 and 8).

Deficient conditions require Restoring treatment methods using *restoring, stimulating, nutritive, astringing* or *moistening* herbs (Classes 7-11). Excess conditions need either Draining treatment methods using *relaxing, heat-clearing* or *decongesting remedies* (Classes 12-14), or Eliminating treatment methods using *diaphoretics, diuretics, laxatives, expectorants, emmenagogues* or *emetics* (Classes 1-6).

Cold conditions need herbs that generate warmth and dispel cold (Class 7), while **hot** conditions should be treated with those that clear heat and resolve fever and inflammation (Class 13).

Conditions accompanied by specific injuries such as congestion, infection (mentioned above) and causing acute symptoms require appropriate herbs primarily from the Symptom treatment section. For example, in conditions with **infection**, botanicals from Class 24 that activate immunity, restrain infection and clear toxin should be chosen. In conditions with **excess spirit** problems, or **internal wind**, botanicals from Class 20 should be selected. In conditions with **toxemia**, Class 15 remedies that *promote cleansing and clear toxemia* should be chosen.

4) The **individual ground** being treated, especially the condition of the vital force or righteous Qi.

For example, where the vital force is weak, all Eliminating strategies, i.e. herbs from Classes 1-6, should either be avoided or combined with Restoring herbs from Classes 7-11. The clearing heat method (Class 13) should also be used with circumspection in this case. Conversely, Restoring methods should be used most often, when this is possible.

Every individual biotype has herbs which represent *tonics* for that person, whether for deficiency or excess conditions. For the Expressive/Jue Yin type, for example, Yarrow, Camomile, Nettles and Dandelion are *ground tonics*. Each biotype has specific remedies which will benefit the individual by correcting the constitutional tendencies towards disharmony (diathesis) that the person is prone to.

5) The **intensity of effect** desired

Some herbs are stronger than others. Looking again at the remedies that *promote bowel movement*, we have a choice of intensity ranging from Aloes (the strongest) to Prune or Rhineberry (the mildest). The same is true of every class of herb. For example, some promote cleansing more strongly than others, while some calm the spirit more effectively.

6) The **season, climate and environment** (natural and man-made)

These factors can affect herb selection especially in regard to the herb's qualitative-energetic properties of taste, warmth, moisture.

In summer or hot weather, for example, people can warm up and cool down more easily. Therefore using treatment methods such as generating warmth, causing sweat, and clearing heat are much more effective. The converse is true in winter where cold and stagnation is more prevalent. The permutations of climate and how they affect treatment strategies and the selection of appropriate herbs is a subject well developed in both Chinese and Greek medicine. Whole textbooks on seasonal diseases and their treatment were written, some of which are available in translation.

The Energetics of Western Herbs

Environmental factors, especially in today's cities, should always be considered, in particular chemical pollution and psychical or mental stress. This in itself calls for remedies from Classes 15 and 12 respectively. Here again it is a matter of deciding on treatment priorities.

7) The **practical availability** of botanicals
This purely practical question needs no elaboration.

Duration

The length of time in hours, days, weeks or months for which a remedy should be taken can vary a great deal. The main considerations are:

1) The **nature of the botanical(s)** used, i.e. whether
   - mild with minimal chronic toxicity
   - medium strength with some chronic toxicity
   - strong with acute toxicity

If **mild** botanicals are used, they should be taken over a longer period of time, 7 days or more, to allow their accumulative effect to gather momentum. Taking Yellow dock root tea for only two days, for example, is a waste of time. It should be taken for at least 10 days, and then in tincture form if possible.

If **strong**, toxic herbs are used, they should be taken only once or twice, with an interval of several days, if repeated.

Medium-strength herbs fall in between these two. They are typically taken for 10-14 days, then stopped altogether, or a different herb may then be taken for 8 days. They have some toxicity which accumulates over time, a fact which must be respected. Examples of medium strength botanicals are Bilberry, Arnica, Fumitory and Valerian. (See p. 52 for a discussion of the three categories of herbs).

2) The **principle of treatment** used, whether the herb
   - treats the constitutional ground preventively
   - rebalances the condition of disharmony, or
   - relieves symptoms

If herbs are used **preventively** for the individual ground, extended or intermittent treatment is neccessary over a longer period of time. Treatment during the four seasonal changes is recommended.

If used to treat **actual conditions**, either short or long term treatment may be required.

If used for **symptom relief** (not symptom supression), short term medication is enough.

3) The **nature of the condition** being treated, whether
   - acute, subacute, chronic or degenerative
   - local or global
   - endogenous or exogenous
   - internal or external
   - deficient or excessive
   - cold or hot

With **chronic** or **degenerative** conditions (e.g. M.S., rheumatoid arthritis, heart conditions)

Guidelines to Prescribing

medication might be ongoing and permanent. With **acute** and **subacute** conditions, short-term treatment may be sufficient, and is typified by smaller regular doses at more frequent intervals. Examples of this type of condition and dosage include:
- at the onset of a cold, a hot infusion every 1/2 hr.
- with stalled labor, 1/4-1/2 tsp every 30 minutes up to a maximum of three times
- to stop hemorrhage or diarrhea, 1/2-2 tsps of tincture every 15 minutes

CAUTION: The imbalance resulting in acute symptoms often needs further attention and longer-term treatment!

Systemic conditions, such as those usually underlying skin eruptions, for example, are more likely to require longer treatment than purely local conditions such as an injury or local infection.

CAUTION: Local conditions of internal origin are always merely a part of a systemic condition!

Excess conditions, on the whole, are easier and quicker to treat through Eliminating or Draining treatment methods than **deficiency** cases. The latter may need longer Restoring work.

Hot conditions are more rapidly corrected than are cold ones.

External conditions such as wind cold/heat are treated more quickly than internal ones.

4) The **type of preparation** used, whether
- external (e.g. plaster, compress, liniment, enema) or
- internal (e.g. decoction, tincture, essential oil)

Some **external** applications are kept on for days (e.g. plasters), others for only a few minutes.

Water preparations may be taken over longer periods of time than alcoholic ones, since alcohol also has some chronic toxicity.

If **essential oils** are used, the duration of treatment varies. Again, the only guide is the category to which they belong.

5) The **individual ground** being treated

Some biotypes are more sensitive and responsive to herbal medication than others, requiring less extensive treatment. At present, the most effective treatment method will be a matter of individual experience.

6) The **season and climate** present at the time

In cold climates and seasons treatment may take longer than in warm ones.

Preparation

How a medicinal plant is prepared, whether by an infusion, tincture, essential oil or any other method, is not merely a haphazard choice. Each preparation method produces certain effects and is more suited to certain conditions than others. Each also has certain advantages, as well as disadvantages, which should be considered when an herb or group of herbs is selected. Because of these facts, a tremendous range of medicinal effects is actually possible, often with a single plant remedy.

A preparation method should be chosen which best meets the demands of the condition being treated. The following factors should be kept in mind when deciding on the optimal preparation to use for any given case:

1) The **nature of the herb(s)** being used:
- the part of the plant used (root, herb, flower, seed, etc.)

The Energetics of Western Herbs

- the category it belongs to (mild, medium strength or strong)
- its energetics, or effective qualities, (taste, warmth, moisture, secondary qualities)
- its main constituents (saponins, alkaloids, tannins, essential oils, mucilages, etc.)

In general, all parts of plants may be **tinctured** with good therapeutic effects. As water based preparations go, roots, which are denser and harder, should be **decocted** or **macerated**; softer flowers, herbs or leaves should be **infused**; seeds should be crushed and **infused**.

Mild, non-toxic herbs often come out equally well in either an infusion, decoction or tincture. **Medium** and **toxic** herbs on the whole are more effective if a tincture or fluid extract is made.

On the whole, the energetic qualities of remedies are clearer and stronger with **decoctions, infusions or macerations**, which is why Chinese medicine uses water based preparations rather than anything else. In **tincture** form, however, the taste, warmth and moisture of a botanical become more diffuse and compound as the plant's substantial constituents are enhanced.

Plant remedies with a **wide range** of constituents are best used in tincture form, whereas those with one or two outstanding ingredients such as essential oils or alkaloids are best prepared according to the optimum preparation for that constituent.

Herbs from the Labiate family such as Rosemary, Sage, Basil and Savory are best used in **essential oil** form if their full strength or range of effects is needed. The same is true with many tropical spices, barks, resins and flowers (Black pepper, Sassafras, Cajeput, Camphor, Jasmin, Orange...). Alternately, they may be tinctured, infused or macerated, being kept well covered while steeping.

Alkaloidal plants such as Lobelia, Motherwort and Fumitory may be decocted or tinctured equally well.

Herbs with a high **tannin** content such as Tormentil, Oak bark and Walnut are soluble in both water and alcoholic preparations.

Herbs containing **organic acids** such as Sorrel, Wood sorrel, Yellow dock and Grapevine leaf do well in either decoction or tincture form.

Herbs with **saponins** such as Wild yam, Sarsaparilla, Cowslip root and Heartsease are often better prepared as decoctions rather than tinctures, since saponins are more soluble in water.

Plants with much **mucilage** such as Marshmallow, Slippery elm and Irish moss are best either decocted or made into a glycerine extract. This preparation will enhance their *demulcent* and *emollient* effect.

2) The **therapeutic effect intended**:
- Eliminating
- Restoring
- Draining
- Altering

There is a basic difference between water preparations, such as decoctions and infusions, and alcoholic ones. **Water preparations** produce an effect which is almost entirely due to the physiological aspects of plant constituents, both on a quantitative-substantial and qualitative-energetic level. A **simple infusion** of a botanical that contains volatile oils and has a pungent taste can be relied upon to cause sweating and release external conditions.

This is not the case if a **tincture** or **fluid extract** of the same herb is used. Alcoholic preparations produce effects which are not always entirely explicable in terms of pharmacology alone. This is true for both energetic pharmacology (based on taste, warmth etc.), and substantial pharmacology (based on main constituents). **Alcoholic preparations** have both a physiological and a bioenergetic effect. Whereas the physiological effect is an allopathic one (treating something with its opposite), the bioenergetic effect is a homeopathic one (treating something with a similar thing). In pragmatic terms this means that alcoholic preparations have a homeopathic as well as an allopathic effect. In other words, they not only treat via opposites, as when cold remedies are used for hot conditions, and vice versa, but also by similars. Many warm or hot herbs, for example, are also anti-inflammatory, effectively clearing heat, when used in alcoholic form. The reasons for this are complex, and to do them justice would require lengthy explanations that unfortunately exceed the boundaries of the present work.

Alcoholic preparations represent a half-way stage between allopathic preparations (infusions, decoctions) and homeopathic ones. They share characteristics of both.[1] Alcohol-based tinctures and fluid extracts therefore will have a wider range of effects, and a more complex symptomatology, than decoctions and infusions. This also explains why many remedies have indications actually incongruent with their effective qualities; and why the functions and uses of many herbs are so much more extensive than what is described in the Chinese materia medica. It is not that Western herbs are more versatile, or that Western usage is more fanciful, or even that Chinese herbology likes to keep to the broad basics. The reason for the greater range of functions and indications of Western botanicals lies largely with the **preparation form used**.

With water preparations, for example, a hot herb will simply treat cold conditions, and vice versa, according to the law of allopathy. In tincture form a hot herb may *in addition* be used to treat certain hot conditions such as fever or inflammation, with Aconite being a good example. This is true because the *bioenergetics* released in a tincture effectively brings another dimension of activity into play—one which can either override the simple physiological effect or act in concert with it. Aconite for this reason can be used both as as a *warmth generating* remedy when decocted, where its *hot, pungent* and *penetrating* qualities exert their effects, and as a *heat clearing* remedy in tincture form, where its bioenergies are actively effective. Since Chinese herbalists have always preferred decoctions as a preparation form, they use Aconite allopathically to generate warmth and dispel cold. Eclectic and Homeopathic physicians, on the other hand, by choice used alcoholic preparations, and therefore employed Aconite in a homeopathic as well as allopathic way to clear heat and resolve fever.

Clearly, the difference in therapeutic effect between the two preparation forms is an important one. The main concept to remember is that water preparations are more limited in their functions and uses, while tinctures have a wider scope, being allopathic and homeopathic at the same time. Some individuals will respond better with one or the other preparation.

If an Eliminating treatment method is used (such as causing sweat, bowel movement, etc.), decoctions and infusions are preferable over tinctures.

If a Restoring, Draining or Altering method is chosen, all preparation forms may be suitable, depending on the case at hand. For example, if the loosening constraint method is used, an essential oil may be chosen since it is often strongly *relaxant* or *sedative*. Examples include Marjoram, Parsley seed, Bergamot, Angelica, and Aniseed. If the treatment objective is to clear full internal heat, it would be better to use decoctions in large doses.

3) The **intensity and type of effect** required

Generally speaking, **tinctures and fluid extracts** are stronger than water preparations. In milder conditions, therefore, or with children and older people, a decoction or infusion is often just right. Alternately, a smaller dosage of tincture may be used.

Essential oils are particularly strong when used internally, especially in acute conditions. In chronic conditions it is often preferable to massage them into the skin with a carrier oil.

Tinctures and **essential oils** are more *stimulating, mobilising penetrating* and *relaxing* than

The Energetics of Western Herbs

water preparations, hence are more appropriate to conditions of stagnancy, obstruction and cold.

Water preparations are better for *restoring, nourishing* and *heat clearing* purposes in deficient conditions of all kinds, as well as in hot conditions.

There are exceptions to these general guidelines, however. For example at the onset of a cold or flu when sweating is needed, a hot herbal infusion is better than a tincture dropped into hot water.

The most intense and appropriate effect is achieved when the preparation used is exactly matched to the condition being treated.

4) The **individual ground and condition** under treatment

Deficiency conditions or biotypes are better treated with water preparations, while conditions of **stagnancy** should be treated with alcoholic or essential oil mixtures.

5) The **season, climate and environment** present

In colder weather, more *active* preparations such as essential oils and tinctures are suitable; in warmer weather infusions and decoctions may be more appropriate.

Dosage

Dosage is another variable, and can range from fractions of a gram in the case of strong (toxic) herbs to several grams for mild (nontoxic) ones. It should be pointed out that very low dosages do not automatically put an herb in the homeopathic range. To qualify as a homeopathic remedy, an herb must be succussed (rhythmically shaken) as well as diluted.

Dosage selection should ideally match the condition being treated according to the following considerations:

1) The **nature of the botanical(s)** used:
   - mild with minimal chronic toxicity
   - medium with some chronic toxicity
   - strong with acute toxicity

For example, **mild** remedies work best in full doses. With nutritive and demulcent agents, there is usually no upper limit, e.g. in the case of Nettle, Kelp, Alfalfa, Microalgae, Dandelion, Couch grass.

Strong/toxic botanicals usually only need to be taken in very small doses to exert their effect. The exact dosage should be carefully established.

Herbs with **some chronic toxicity** (i.e. of the **medium strength** category) allow the greatest variation and freedom of dosage. Again, as with acutely toxic remedies, dosage should be ascertained individually.

2) The **therapeutic effect intended:**
   - eliminating
   - restoring
   - draining
   - altering
   - warming
   - cooling
   - restoring
   - relaxing

Many if not most herbs have different effects depending on the dosage level used. As a general rule, **low dosages** tend to have a *restoring* effect, **medium dosages** a *stimulating* one, and **high dosages** a more *draining* effect. At the same time, it is important to determine exactly what small, medium and large represents for each herb, since this too varies.

Guidelines to Prescribing

For example, in small quantities Dandelion root is *restoring* as a *bitter tonic* for liver and stomach Qi deficiency, or general weakness. In medium doses it works best as a *cleansing* remedy for toxemic conditions; while in larger doses it can act as a *draining, detoxifying* remedy in hot conditions. The same is true for most herbs with a *bitter* taste.

Botanicals with a ***pungent*** taste due to essential oils, such as Thyme, Peppermint, Rosemary, Sassafras bark and Ginger, have a *gastric stimulant* effect when taken in small doses for *intestines damp cold*, or simple indigestion. These herbs have a *circulatory stimulant* effect when taken in *medium doses* and a *diaphoretic* effect in *large doses*.

Remedies with a ***sweet*** taste such as Licorice, Red clover and Cornsilk, tend to be more *restoring* in small doses, and *calming* and *pain relieving* in large ones.

Herbs with a ***sour*** taste due to organic acids such as Wood sorrel, Grapevine, Lemon and Purslane are *digestive stimulants* in smaller doses and *heat clearing* and *resolvent* in larger ones.

Herbs with **anthraquinone glycosides** which promote bowel movement (Class 3) have an *intestinal stimulant* effect in small doses, a *laxative* effect in medium ones, and a *purgative* effect in larger doses.

Many Class 12 herbs with **alkaloids** or **essential oils** that loosen Qi constraint, and some Class 1 herbs for wind heat, such as Lobelia, Cowslip, Parsley seed, Sage, Catnip and Marjoram, have a *stimulant* effect in lower doses and a *relaxing* effect in larger ones.

3) The preparation method used

If the **essential oil** of an herb is used, for example, only a few drops are necessary, typically 3 drops three times a day. If a **tincture** is used, 2-4 ml or 50-100 drops is the dosage range. With **water based** preparations such as decoctions and macerations, 10 g are typically needed for a single dose.

External applications such as compresses and plasters need double or triple strength preparations.

4) The individual ground being treated:

Larger people require larger doses; smaller or thinner ones need smaller ones.

Infants' and children's dosages can be calculated as follows:

Method 1 (Young's rule)

child's dosage = adult dose x $\underline{\text{age}}$
  age + 12

Method 2 (Cowling's rule)

child's dosage = adult dose x $\underline{\text{age}}$
  24

Method 3

child's dose = adult dose x $\underline{\text{weight}}$
  150 lb.

The Energetics of Western Herbs

Herb Combining

This Materia Medica describes the nature, functions and uses of simple rather than compound botanical remedies. Its emphasis is on how to make best use of single herbs as opposed to combinations. Nevertheless, some guidelines on combining herbal remedies should be given. The point of mixing herbs together is to produce a more effective, healing medicine. It should never become an end in itself, however enjoyable the process may be. Simple combinations of just a few botanicals can greatly increase the suitability and efficacy of a remedy. This is true for a quick preparation of an emergency formula for bleeding, as well as for a formula used to treat an ongoing condition. In the first case, Shepherd's purse will definitely be enhanced by adding Lady's mantle for the treatment of uterine hemorrhage, for example, or Ribwort plantain in the case of coughing up blood.

OTTO BRUNFELS' words from the introduction to his herbal of 1532 are appropriate in this context: "…there are many useless formulas which are not to be recommended, and which can be replaced by simples. Moderation should be exercised in all things. In the old formulas also there are not more than four or five ingredients—hence their names *tetra pharmakon, diatessera* and such like."

When herbs are combined, specific therapeutic effects can be enhanced, altered or modified in a number of ways, so that complex conditions can be addressed on a variety of levels.

Conversely, those instances should also be singled out where combining herbs is **unnecessary**.

It is actually often the case that a single botanical can deal with a condition very adequately. These conditions tend to be mild, straightforward imbalances without any complications. A wind heat onset of flu, for example, is often competently dealt with by using Boneset or Linden flowers alone. A child's simple diarrhea can be relieved by Agrimony or Raspberry tea alone.

More importantly, if an herb is used in tincture form, its homeopathically effective bioenergetic qualities are brought out (see p. 72). As a result, its range of indications and depth of effective action is increased. Often the herb's effectiveness is enhanced to the point where no other remedy is really necessary. For example, a person with a condition characterized by cold extremities, palpitations, grief and despondency, worry, insomnia, night sweats and hot sensations could be treated in one of two ways. Either a complex formula can be made up to simultaneously treat both a heart Yang deficiency and a Kidney Yin deficiency, or a single remedy in tincture form may be given which matches this symptom pattern perfectly: Valerian.

Leaving these preliminary considerations behind, ways of combining botanicals may be looked at in more detail.

The easiest approach to herb combining is to examine the principles of traditional formulas as they exist in both Greek and Chinese medicine. The similarities here also far exceed the differences.

The following are the components that a formula may have, each represented by one or more herbs:
- the principal herb, which adresses the main entity being treated (whether condition or symptom)
- the secondary herb, which reinforces the effect of the principal herb
- the assistant herb, which assists and balances the principle nd secondary herbs by dealing with other aspects of the condition
- the envoy herb, which increases the tropism of the herbs to a certain organ, part or meridian.

This format is a flexible framework when combining botanicals, not a rigid structure to be adhered to. Good combinations can be made simply with a principle and a secondary herb, or with a principle and an assistant herb. The needs of every condition are different and require different types of combinations. It is the need to meet clinical cases in all their permutations of factors that led countless practitioners in both China and the West to formulate the vast body of prescriptions in existance today.

وقهوا الرصاص نغسل مكنى بغما يصلايه لها بدمن رصاص وتب
فيهاماوندلكها بيدها الى ان يسوداالما وتخرن بصفا خرقه ويعمل ذلك
ثانيه واكثرذا احتج الذلك ونغسل كما يغسل الاقلميا ويعمل ذلك

صنع الرصاص

الى ان يصير في السواد ويعمل منه اقراصا ويرفع

صفة اخرى

من الحكماء اخذ رصاصا نقيا فبرده واخذ لك لبن راد ن هل في صلايه
حجر ثم اصفا الاول فالاول تم رقن بحلس وينزع ذلك الما ويجعل

Preparing remedies—miniature from a medical treatise, Bhagdad, 13th century.

8 PREPARATION FORMS AND USES

It would not go against pharmacists, nor against doctors, if common, effective and easily available remedies were used—on the contrary, this would be an advantage. For what reason should our herbs not be as good as those from Asia and Africa?

Otto Brunfels, *Kreuterbuch*, 1532

The ways and methods of preparing herbal remedies for internal or external use, called pharmacy for short, are an integral part of botanical therapeutics. They reflect not only the treatment intention and medicinal effect, but on a deeper level the overall cultural bias of a system of herbal medicine. Both Chinese and Greek medicine as they were practiced up to the time of GALEN, for example, almost always use **dried roots** as medicines, while modern herbalism, especially since Renaissance days, has relied more on the **leafy** parts of plants. In this Materia Medica, the balance between the two is somewhat restored, but there are still half as many roots and rhizomes as there are herbs and leaves.

More specifically, herbal preparation forms should reflect the nature of the plant being used on one hand, and the type of use it is put to on the other.

Every herb as therapeutic agent has its own optimum preparation method. Plants whose effect depends largely on mucilage, for example, will do better as glycerine extract or decoction than in tincture form. Plants with much essential oil are better used in tincture or in pure essential oil form. These variations were fully discussed in the last chapter.

At the same time, in any given situation, there is always one preparation method which will bring out a certain property or characteristic in an herb most fully. It all depends on the treatment intention and effect desired. Rosemary in essential oil form, for example, is more *stimulating, warming* and *relaxing* than when taken as infusion, when it is possibly more *damp clearing* and *restoring*. This is the reason for the often lengthy notes on preparations found under each remedy.

Both the nature of the herb and the treatment method chosen will determine the choice of preparation.

It becomes clearer why traditional herbalism in general has devoted much thought to the preparation methods of plant remedies. Pharmacy was particularly developed during the Arabian phase of Greek medicine (ninth to fifteenth centuries) when compendiums of pharmaceutics such as the *Aqrabadin* (*Antidotarium*) by AR-RAZI (RHAZES) were written. Chinese medicine to this day makes extensive use of its traditional pharmaceutical skills. They are evident not only in the production of such traditional preparations as syrups, medicated wines, plasters, liniments, etc., but more particularly in the great care with which each plant is prepared before entering commerce and distribution and in the sheer variety of preparation methods themselves. Some examples are soaking the herb in wine or vinegar, roasting, honey-frying, baking with salt and steaming. Today, when the preparation of Western plant remedies is at a bare minimum and relies as much on the efforts of individuals as it does on commercial concerns, we would do well to take a fresh look at the functions and uses of a number of interesting preparation forms. This section is intended as a stimulus for experimentation with preparing remedies.

The Energetics of Western Herbs

In the following descriptions of various preparations, certain botanicals are given as examples. Those in italics indicate that they may be used in *essential oil* form, a stronger preparation on the whole. Those listed are meant as examples only and are not exhaustive.

The standard dosage range determines the quantity of the plant parts that should be used.

Preparations for Internal Use

DECOCTION

A decoction is the standard method used to prepare hard plant parts such as dried roots, barks and twigs, which need prolonged hot water application for their full extraction. Roots should be sliced diagonally for maximum extractability. Place in an earthenware, enamel or glass pan with cold water and bring to a boil, lower the flame, cover and simmer for 20-30 minutes, depending on the thickness of the root or bark.

The standard dose is the amount needed for one day's supply, which is three cups. The proportions used are 30 g (1 oz) of the chopped or sliced root to 600 ml (1 1/3 pints) of water. The actual amount of dried root used may vary, however, and the **standard dosage range** is between 20 g and 45 g (2/3 oz-1 1/2 oz.).

The decoction should be strained and one cup drunk unsweetened on an empty stomach, about 1/2 hour before eating, three times a day. When not in use, the decoction should be refrigerated; reheat before use. Not more than a three day supply may be made at one time.

Plant parts such as fruits, seeds and tough leaves may require a **short decoction**. This means they are decocted as described above, using a little less water, but for about 10 minutes only. They are then allowed to steep, covered, for another 10 minutes.

Decoctions are particularly good for extracting roots containing saponins such as Wild yam and Cowslip and tougher constituents such as resins and tannins.

INFUSION

An infusion is the usual method for preparing dried leaves, stems, flowers and other light plant parts, which need only short exposure to warm water to extract their essential oils. Heat water in a pan, and just after it begins to boil, pour over the plants, cover immediately and steep, or infuse, the herbs for 15-20 minutes.

Again the **standard dosage** is given for a one day's supply, i.e. three cups. The average proportions used are 30 g per 1/2 l (1 oz of herb per pint) of water. In actual practice, however, there may be dosage variations, as for the decoction method. One cup of the infused tea is drunk on an empty stomach, three times a day.

The **sun tea** preparation method is a useful variation on the infusion. Herbs are placed in cold water in a jar and set in the sun for 2-8 hours. This method is especially recommended for essential oil bearing plants such as Rosemary, Thyme, Mint and Sage.

ESSENTIAL OIL DISTILLATION

Essential oils are commercially available distillations of plants. They are the concentrated and potent constituents of many Mediterranean and tropical plants. The Mint family has many essential oil laden plants such as *Sage, Thyme, Peppermint* and *Rosemary*. The same is true for the seeds of such Parsley family plants as *Wild carrot, Angelica, Parsley, Cumin* and *Fennel*; for tropical barks such as *Sassafras, Cinnamon* and *Camphor*; and for flowers such as *Jasmin, Ylang ylang* and *Orange*.

It is possible to make one's own steam distillations with the right equipment, but requires

Preparation Forms and Uses

considerably more expense and time than preparations like tinctures and ointments.

Essential oils are used both externally and internally and should be carefully dosed. When used externally they need a fatty base or carrier oil to facilitate massaging them into the skin and to ensure an even penetration over the affected area. The quantity of essential oil used is 1-5%, i.e. 10-50 drops per 30 ml (or 1 oz) of base oil. The **standard dose** is a 2-3% preparation, i.e. 10-20 drops per oz. The higher doses are neccessary for infectious conditions only.

With local, acute, infectious or external conditions such as spasms, pain, skin conditions, injuries, etc., only the local area needs covering, using preparations such as a swab or compress, or applying the essential oil directly. When treating a more general, chronic, internal, emotional or mental condition, on the other hand, it is usually better to cover the whole body. Here essential oils are used in conjunction with massage therapy. Their scent is an integral part of the overall effect of the treatment and provide an additional healing factor.

In order to be taken **internally**, essential oils should be added to some warm water or herbal tea and drunk. The "tea" may be sweetened with half a teaspoon of honey or barley malt, especially for children. Some essential oils such as Cinnamon, Thyme and Oregano, however, are irritant to the skin and mucosa and should therefore be given in a gelatin capsule. After dropping the exact number of drops into the capsule, a little olive oil may be added to smooth absorption.

The **standard dose** is 2-4 drops in warm water or mild herbal tea twice or three times a day on an empty stomach. This may vary, however, depending on the oil. Due to the varying degree of toxicity of certain oils, the recommended dosages should never be exceeded.

The functions and uses of essential oils are very wide, but they all share most of the following characteristics: *stimulating, relaxing, restoring, antiseptic*. In addition to these, every oil exhibits a variety of other effects.

The reason for choosing essential oils over other preparations is that they are highly effective for the conditions they treat, have specific and rapid effects, and are easy and for the most part pleasant to use.

TINCTURE

A tincture is an alcoholic preparation suitable for almost any type of botanical, whether root, herb or fruit. The fresh (or sometimes dried) plant is finely cut or crushed and put into a glass jar and covered with alcohol. 25% strength grain alcohol (or stronger) should be used. Ethyl alcohol or a good grain alcohol such as vodka or brandy are ideal. If the **fresh** root or herb is used, 2 parts of alcohol are used to 1 part of the root/herb; if it is **dry** then 5 parts of alcohol are needed. (It is possible to use 1/2 alcohol and 1/2 spring water if the alcohol is at least 50%). This preparation is allowed to stand for two to four weeks, and should be briefly shaken once or twice a day. Once ready, the tincture is then strained and if possible the remaining tincture expressed using a small press or cheesecloth.

The **standard dosage range** for tinctures made from just alcohol is 2-4 ml (50-100 drops or 1/4-1 tsp or 25-75 min) in a little warm water or herb tea, three times a day. The **standard dose** is likely to be 3-4 ml, i.e. about 35-50 drops.

The advantages of tinctures definitely outweigh the disadvantages. They can extract substances which are unsoluble in water such as essential oils, alkaloids and resins; they are easily absorbed and act rapidly; they have a **bioenergetic** effect in the organism in addition to the purely **physiological** effect of non-alcoholic preparations (see p. 72); they are convenient to use, may also be used to make external preparations and do not deteriorate over time. Tinctures should be stored away from direct sunlight.

On the other hand, tinctures are not suited to treating everyone's condition nor are they suitable

The Energetics of Western Herbs

for those with an alcohol intolerance. Neither should they be used for preparing herbs with much mucilage such as Mallow or Comfrey root or with constituents only partially or completely unsoluble in alcohol, such as saponins, tannins and proteins.

A variation on the tincture is the **medicated wine**. This is prepared as a tincture, using pure wine instead of grain alcohol. Red wine has a more stimulating effect than white. This method is used especially for aromatic plants such as Rosemary and Sage, for bitter herbs such as Wormwood or Gentian (drunk in small *apéritif* doses) and for spices such as Fennel or Cumin. Here the benefits of wine (which should be organic if possible) in small quantities are combined with those of herbs.

FLUID EXTRACT OR CONCENTRATE

Fluid extracts or concentrates are alcohol or water-based preparations prepared using 1 part weight of dried herb to 2 parts volume of water or alcohol. They are between two and three times as strong as tinctures.

They can be prepared in one of three ways: first, using the percolation method in which alcohol is poured over the crushed or powdered herbal material about four times; second, using a tincture and heating it until all alcohol is evaporated; and third, making a decoction and then continuing to simmer uncovered until only a little liquid is left.

The **standard dosage** for a fluid extract/concentrate is between 1/2 and 1/3 that of the tincture. The advantage of using this type of preparation is that it involves less alcohol intake than the tincture. However, it is not suitable for all botanicals. *Nutritive* and *restorative* remedies such as Oats and Licorice make good fluid extracts. If heating is involved then a few constituents are lost, resulting in a medicine of a different quality.

MEDICATED GHEE

Medicated ghee is an Ayurvedic preparation made from clarified butter with the addition of herbs. Ghee has medicinal properties even when used alone; when used with herbs it facilitates their reaching their destination.

Ghee is first prepared by heating a pound of unsalted butter on a low flame for 10-15 minutes. As the butter begins to boil, the heat should be turned to low. Soon after the butter will turn a golden yellow and will begin to smell like popcorn. The ghee is ready when a drop or two of water dropped into it produces a crackling sound signifying that all water has evaporated. Allow to cool somewhat and strain, then pour into a container. Ghee will not go rancid at room temperature and may be kept for up to six months ready for use.

To make the ghee **medicated**, prepare a double strength herbal decoction; add this to half the amount of ghee, pouring and mixing slowly and thoroughly.

The **standard dosage** is 1 tsp.

Medicated ghee is used as follows:
- *to soothe irritated or inflamed eyes* (Rose petals, Eyebright, Camomile)
- *to clear excess mucous in the nose and sinuses* (Marjoram, Calamus, Camphor)
- *to relieve bronchitis and asthma* (Mullein, Hyssop, Rosemary)
- *to promote tissue healing* (Comfrey, Marigold, Selfheal)
- *to increase memory and intelligence* (Rosemary, Basil, Gotu kola)
- *to treat digestive atony or fevers* (bitters such as Wormwood or Gentian)
- *to treat peptic ulcers* (Licorice and Camomile 1/2-1 tsp twice or three times a day)
- Simple, unmedicated ghee also stimulates liver & stomach Qi, increases gastric secretions, and has a mild *laxative* effect, especially when drunk warm with goat's milk.

Preparation Forms and Uses

SYRUP

A syrup is a thick, sweet liquid used for conditions of the throat, lungs, stomach and intestines where continuous *soothing* effects are needed. It coats the digestive passages as it is taken in, maintaining direct and prolonged contact. Because of this, Class 10 *demulcent* or *Yin fostering* remedies make for excellent syrups. The gradual and gentle absoption of syrups is ideal for children and elderly people, as well as for chronic, Yin deficient, dry or inflamed conditions in general (e.g., with dry coughs, constipation, etc.). The herbs chosen for the syrup should reflect the therapeutic effect desired.

There are several ways of preparing syrups. In all of them the sugar content should be no less than 65% to prevent spoiling. A **simple** or **unmedicated syrup** is made by adding 1 lb. of sugar, molasses or honey to 1 pint of hot water. This mixture should be stirred continuously for a few minutes to avoid burning. Remove from heat and keep stirring constantly until cool. When cool, decant into clean bottles.

A **cordial syrup** is made by adding one part of a tincture to three parts of a simple syrup, or 2% of an essential oil may be used.

A **true syrup** may be prepared by making a decoction or tincture (using distilled water for longer storage), and adding 1 lb of honey or sugar to one pint of the water mixture. Bring to a boil, turn heat off and stir while the syrup cools. For a more viscous syrup the decoction may be reduced further by simmering down to 1/3 volume and then adding the same amount of honey or sugar. The true syrup far exceeds the other types in therapeutic efficacy.

A **cold syrup** is made by soaking fresh herbs in a simple syrup for one or two weeks, then straining and decanting it. The cold syrup is best suited to *sweet moist mucilaginous* herbs such as Comfrey, Coltsfoot and Licorice, and is used mainly to treat dry and Yin deficient conditions of the lungs and stomach. It is best prepared fresh each time, as it may not keep well.

A **glycerine syrup** is prepared by making a strong decoction/infusion, then adding 6 parts glycerine to 4 parts decoction (i.e. a 60% solution). This syrup is better for *nutritive* and *demulcent* remedies such as Irish moss or Slippery elm, and is used to treat the same conditions as the cold syrup. It will keep well and tastes sweeter than tinctures.

CAPSULE

In this preparation form, powdered herbal material, either dried or freeze-dried, is taken inside a gelatin capsule. It allows the remedy to be assimilated slowly in the small intestine rather than in the stomach. Although it can be used advantageously in chronic metabolic conditions, it will only have a maximum effect if **freeze-dried** rather than powdered dry herbs are used. Not only does the powdering process cause loss of herb quality, but the quantity absorbed—especially in the inimical conditions the remedy is supposed to address—is often minimal. Herbal constituents are simply not that absorbable when presented to the small intestine in bulk form. **Pills** have the same overriding disadvantages as capsules containing powdered herbs.

Convenience is the only advantage of taking capsules. In view of the above considerations, they should only be taken over another preparation when metabolic conditions require *nourishing* or *cleansing,* with Microalgae, Iceland moss, Kelp or Alfalfa, for example.

With properly fresh freeze-dried herbs, these considerations do not apply, however. On the contrary: they have virtually the same quality as the freshly expressed plant juice itself.

MOUTHWASH & GARGLE

A gargle is a double-strength herbal infusion used to wash out the mouth and back of the throat with a tea preparation (infusion, decoction) or, alternatively, with some tincture or essential oil dropped into hot water.

Gargling is used to provide *astringent* and *antiseptic* effects with conditions such as loose teeth, spongy, bleeding or inflamed gums, tongue and mouth sores and ulcers, mouth infections, chronic nasal drip, tonsilitis and laryngitis. The herbs commonly used therefore have an *astringent* and *antiseptic* quality, and are mostly found in Classes 11 and 13: Blackberry and Raspberry leaf, Agrimony, *Sage* and *Myrrh,* for example.

In addition, mouthwashes and gargles may be *stimulating* and *warming* with atonic, congested upper mucosal conditions such as chronic laryngitis, where Cayenne, Mustard or Bayberry may be used; or *lenitive* and *cooling* in the case of acute irritative or inflammatory conditions, where Mallow, Ribwort, *Lemon, Camomile*, for example, are more suitable.

DOUCHE

A douche is a vaginal wash using herbal tea preparations, diluted tinctures, or water with essential oils. Like the mouthwash, it treats the mucous lining in catarrhal or infectious conditions, here involving the external genitalia.

Again, *disinfectant* and *astringent* remedies are used for conditions such as intermenstrual bleeding, leucorrhea and cervical erosion (e.g. Cranesbill, Ribwort, Stoneroot, White deadnettle, *Lavender* or *Eucalyptus*); and yeast infections and cervicitis (Goldenseal, *Myrrh*, acidophilus powder in water, *Tea tree, Savory* or *Cinnamon*. 20 drops of the essential oils to 1 pint of water should be used). One tablespoon of cider vinegar is a good addition to help keep an acid PH.

It is best to use a douche bag for this purpose since sprays and syringes tend to damage the vaginal lining. An alternative is to pour in the liquid using a cardboard tampax cartridge as a funnel. The best position is lying on the back (to avoid spreading the infection to the womb), and the douche should be retained for 10-20 minutes. Douches should be done every day for up to a week when symptoms are acute; once a month is sufficient for maintenance thereafter.

It should be kept in mind that douching should not be done on a regular basis, as it disrupts the normal, healthy bacterial balance.

INHALATION

Taking in the vapors of an herbal infusion by inhalation is a good way to treat all the respiratory passages which are otherwise difficult to reach. The *stimulating, disinfectant* and *expectorant* herbs and oils *clear the airways of congestion and relieve wheezing and coughing* in catarrhal conditions. They also provide good symptom relief as local backup treatment to more systemic internal medication.

Typical symptoms relieved are sinus or eustachian congestion in the head, where *Thyme, Lavender, Camomile, Sage, Peppermint* or *Eucalyptus* essential oils may be used; and wheezing and asthmatic breathing, where Oshá, Angelica, *Hyssop* and *Thyme* are appropriate. In chronic lung and chest inflammations, *Benzoin, Camphor* and *Thyme* are excellent.

An infusion is made with the required herbs, or 6-12 drops of the essential oil is dropped into a small bowl of hot water. The head should be covered with a heavy towel, and inhaling should be carried out for 5-15 minutes three times a day. Alternately an inhaler may be used, available from some pharmacies and drugstores (these were very popular up to the middle of this century).

SQUATTING INHALATION

A squatting inhalation is to an inhalation what a douche is to a mouthwash. Here the benefits of a **medicated steam** are transferred through the vagina to the cervix for the relief of *spasmodic* conditions such as premenstrual cramping. The best remedies to use are *relaxant* essential oils such as *Pennyroyal, Juniper* and *Sage*, or herbs such as Yarrow, Tansy, Wormwood and Vervain. Urinary spasms due to stones or nervous tension are also relieved in this way.

The preparation method is simple: an herbal infusion is made, or the essential oil is dropped into a bowl of hot water (4 drops is enough), which is then set on the floor. Squatting over it allows the steam to permeate upwards and exert its *soothing, relaxing* effects. Dry off with a towel after 5-10 minutes.

Greek medical textbooks describe the benefits of **vaginal fumigations**, benefits identical to those described above. In fumigations the smoke of the smouldering ignited herbs is used rather than steam.

SMOKE

Smoking is used for the immediate temporary relief of lung problems such as coughs, bronchial congestion, asthma and bronchitis, as well as for general relaxation. The herbs used in this type of preparation may be blended from lung remedies such as Coltsfoot, Mullein, Nettle and Lavender. Good *relaxant* herbs for wheezing are Lobelia, Catnip and Calamint. For bronchitis, Rosemary, Thyme or Lavender should be included in the blend.

A good blend should include at least 10% Coltsfoot herb to ensure that the mixture burns well. For an optimum smoke the dried chopped herbs should be mixed with some honey and water, laid out to dry and then stored in an airtight tin or jar.

A single smoke consists of 6-10 inhalations. Note: Daily smoking of any plant is somewhat injurious to the lungs.

ENEMA

An enema (also called **clyster** in the past) is an injection of a medicated liquid by way of the rectum.

An enema may treat a purely local condition such as constipation. If **warm water** is used, it will *soften, dissolve* and *carry away waste;* if **cold** it will *stimulate peristalsis*. Where there is congealed fecal matter in bowel pockets, 2 cups of olive oil to 1 quart of warm water should be injected and retained 15-30 minutes in supine position with the hips raised. The upper abdomen (along the path of the colon) should also be massaged. In spastic conditions of the bowels, *relaxant* essential oils such as *Camomile, Sage* or *Carrot seed* should be used.

Enemas can also help *stop bleeding, diarrhea and dysentery* with the use of *astringent* remedies such as Agrimony, Oak bark or Bayberry, and *demulcent* ones such as Comfrey and chlorophyll if there is inflammation. The same *astringents,* used with cool water, will help treat hemorrhoids or prolapse by *strengthening tissue tone.* Moreover all colon diseases can be improved with the judicious selection of remedies used in enemas.

Systemic conditions such as Spleen Qi deficiency with poor nutrients assimilation are also amenable to treatment with enemas. In this case, Chlorophyll, Wheat grass juice, Kelp, Nettle, etc., should be injected and retained as long as possible. Enemas can also assist in *clearing injurious heat* in high fevers, especially with constipation present, and are an alternative to using internal *laxatives.*

Similar to but more effective than enemas are **colonic irrigations**. Here the entire colon is treated with water, with the possible addition of herb tea or essential oils. Being a specialized treatment form which needs a practitioner to be carried out, it will not be discussed in the present context.

Preparations for External Use

PLASTER

A plaster is an oil or wax based medication applied locally in cases where long-term effects are required. Its advantage over other methods is that healing effects unfold on a certain area over a longer period of time. They are produced by allowing continuous, slow absorption through the skin. In serious injuries and organic internal conditions, therefore, a plaster is the perfect complement to internal medication. Its functions are the following:

- *to relieve pain and swelling*, especially serious pain (*Lavender*, Arnica, Black cohosh, Lobelia, Hops), and to reduce liver or spleen swelling (Horseradish, Mustard)
- *to promote tissue repair* in fractures, wounds and related injuries (Comfrey, Marigold, Arnica, Tansy mustard, Selfheal, Ribwort)
- *to disinfect* as in chest and lung infections (Garlic, *Thyme*) or pelvic infections (Goldenseal, *Thyme*, Echinacea)
- *to relax organs* as in asthma and pleurisy (Lobelia, *Benzoin, Eucalyptus, Lavender*)
- *to stimulate and produce counterirritation*, as in bronchitis (Cayenne, Horseradish, Mustard) and phlegm congestion (*Pine, Myrrh, Turpentine*)

Preparation: For the plaster base, simple beeswax or other cerate bases such as lanolin, turpentine or wool alcohols may be used. Alternately, a simple ointment such as Arnica or Chickweed, thickened with wax and/or powdered herbs can be used as a starter. The final consistency should be thick, waxy and soft, easily adhering to the skin, to ensure penetration of the remedies. If skin irritating herbs are used, then the skin should be oiled before the plaster is applied, and its effects on the skin should be watched carefully.

A typical plaster base may be made from

100 g or 4 oz wax
50 g or 2 oz anhydrous lanolin
50 ml or 2 oz castor oil
200 g or 8 oz soft paraffin

Melt the wax in the top of a double boiler, add the lanolin, castor oil and paraffin. Remove from heat and stir constantly until cool. To this cooled mixture, add either the powdered herbs or essential oils (2-5%) in a 1:4 ratio.

POULTICE

A poultice (also known as a **cataplasm,** from the Greek *kataplasma*) is a water, tincture or fresh herb-based external medication applied topically for a short time. Since it can be changed and renewed often, it is more versatile than a plaster, both from a practical and therapeutic viewpoint. It is rapidly absorbed into the skin and has the following functions:

- *to stimulate circulation, generate warmth, relieve spasms, cramps and pain* in *cold* conditions with pain, spasms, griping or colic, which frequently occur in cold backaches, cold neuralgias or muscular cramps, and cold dysmenorrhea (Cayenne, Ginger, *Juniper, Marjoram, Camphor*); in Qi Constraint conditions with spasms, tension and internal pain (Lobelia, Black cohosh, Cramp bark, *Camomile*). When applied topically for a short time, the poultice is called a *rubefacient*; if it is left on, it becomes a *vesicant* poultice which promotes the formation of blisters causing derivation; in wind/damp/cold obstruction syndromes, including general fluids dyskrasia
- *to restrain infection, resolve inflammation and soothe irritation* locally or internally

(Selfheal, *Camomile, Lavender*, Marigold, Echinacea, Propolis, Barley flour)
- *to heal sprains, bruises* and related *wounds*, etc. (Arnica, Comfrey, Selfheal, Ribwort, Marigold, *Lavender*)
- *to draw out toxins such as pus or poison* in boils, furuncles, carbuncles and insect stings (Slippery elm, Marsh mallow, Onion, Cabbage, Comfrey)

Preparation: If a **fresh** herb is used it should be crushed, grated or chewed; applied locally without moistening; and wrapped in coarse muslin, cheesecloth or wool to keep it in place. If **dried** herbs are used, they should be mixed with a binder such as ground Comfrey, Slippery elm, Iceland moss, gum arabic, clay, pastry flour, flax flour or eggwhites. Once moistened with warm water they can be wrapped in a coarse cloth and applied. The poultice is always applied warm unless a specific cooling effect is intended. Should it become too dry it can be sprinkled with more water.

NOTE: Linen should be avoided due to its tight weave. Wool is best to create and retain warmth locally. Barley flour is the ideal binder when a *cooling* poultice is needed; barley flakes ground in a coffee grinder may also be used.

Variations: Some essential oils, tinctures or herb tea may be added to a poultice to enhance its effects. Lard or olive oil may be added to the mixture if a soothing, softening effect is required. This also prevents it from hardening too soon.

COMPRESS

A compress (also known as a **fomentation**) is simply water applied externally with a cloth. A simple compress uses cold or hot water to achieve its effects; if herbal tea or a tincture is also used, it is called a medicated compress.

A compress offers several advantages: heating and cooling effects can be obtained by simply applying cold or hot water at strategic places. It is the ideal method for *cooling*, in fact. Also, herbs too strong or too toxic for internal use such as Deadly nightshade may be used without harm. Like the poultice, a compress is very versatile. Its functions vary depending on the type used, as follows:

Cold Compress
- *to stimulate and decongest in full cold conditions*, as in edema, amenorrhea, constipation and scanty urination. Apply topically, especially on the lower abdomen
- *to clear heat, fever and inflammation, and decongest in hot conditions*, as in hot congested head, liver area, pelvis and feet. Apply locally, and also at a distance (calves, feet, nape of neck) for a greater effect
- *to relieve tiredness* due to overwork or stress when in good health. Placed on the feet, legs or hands it is very reviving. The cold water compress is definitely more *stimulating* and *decongesting* than the cold footbath

Warm Compress
- *to restore and strengthen in empty cold conditions*, as in weakness, fatigue, asthenia, shallow breathing. Apply locally.
- *to relax and loosen in Qi constraint and full cold conditions* as in spasms, cramps, pain and tension. Apply locally.

Alternating Warm and Cold Compress
- *to circulate Qi and blood and relieve stagnation in conditions of congealed blood, fluid congestion*, and *physical lumps and tumors*. Use in cases of bruising, injuries, sprains, edema, pelvic congestion, sore/lumpy/engorged breasts, lipomas, tumors, etc.

Medicated Compress
Herbs can reinforce the action of cold and hot compresses. The exact herb selected will depend on the condition under treatment.

The Energetics of Western Herbs

Preparation: A piece of towelling, flannel or other cloth is folded and immersed in cold or warm water or in a cold or warm herb tea, tincture or essential oil preparation (1 % dilution). It is applied over the affected part and may be covered with a dry towel or a waxed cloth, a hot or cold pad, water bottle, etc. It should be left on for 2-4 hours and changed if neccessary. A cold compress should always be kept moist.

WASH

A wash is a medicated water prepared by infusion, by decoction or with a diluted essential oil and applied with some cotton wool or soft cloth. In practice it is synonymous with a **swab**. Its function is to *cleanse, disinfect, soothe, cool* and *promote tissue healing*; it is used primarily in superficial conditions such as wounds, cuts, ulcers, skin eruptions and the like. Double-strength doses are used if the wash is prepared from an infusion or a decoction. If essential oils are used, a 1% dilution (i.e. 10 drops per 30 ml of water) is sufficient.

Marigold, *Lavender, Camomile, Bergamot, Geranium, Rosemary* and Echinacea are effective herbs to use in washes for cuts, wounds and ulcers

Red clover, Linden, Mallow, Camomile, Vinegar are used to *soothe and lenify* in dry or itchy (pruritic) skin conditions

Rosemary, Nettle and Birch are excellent for all scalp conditions.

OINTMENT

An ointment is an herbal oil or fat extraction applied to the skin by rubbing. It is also known as a *salve* or *unguent*. It has topical *protective, healing, soothing, moistening* and *cooling* properties and provides a long-term effect when continuously applied. It is also useful because of the large range of external conditions amenable to its influence. Its functions may be summarized as follows:

- *to cool and soothe* in hot, inflamed skin conditions, e.g. those due to *skin damp heat or fire toxin* with boils, sores, infected cuts, fungal skin infections, erysipelas, etc., (Marsh mallow, Slippery elm, Selfheal, Chickweed)
- *to warm and stimulate* in cold conditions and inactive skin conditions, e.g. broken veins and capillaries, cold arthritis, etc. (Cayenne, *Turpentine, Cinnamon*). This *rubefacient* method, if prolonged, and if stronger *pustulants* such as Cantharides, Tartar emetic, Croton or Laurel oil are used, will become a *pustulant* one for derivation purposes (see p. 666)
- *to moisten and protect* in dry, irritative, pruritic skin conditions, e.g. eczema, dermatosis, dry, chapped skin or lips (Marigold, Ribwort, Chickweed, Comfrey); psoriasis (Nettle, Cleavers, *Benzoin*)
- *to protect and heal* wounds, cuts, sprains and contusions (Marigold, Arnica, Self heal, Tansy mustard, Lady's mantle, *Lavender*). It is also used for varicose veins and indolent varicose ulcers (Marigold, Witch hazel, Horse chestnut). For ulcers the salve should be pasted around the affected part, and used in conjunction with an *antiseptic* wash.

Preparation: For an ointment base, various types of fat may be used to extract an herb's properties and afford continuous protection. Although animal greases such as pig and goose lard have rightly been favored as the best (their high protein content ensures rapid absorption), vegetable oils such as safflower, soybean, corn and almond, are still acceptable. The first three all the more so as they are high in linoleic acid which is nourishing to the skin. If these are preferred, wax or lanolin or both should be added towards the end of preparation to obtain the right consistency. Lanolin alone may even be used as an ointment base. It does not go rancid like vegetable oils and is ideal when a more protective type of salve is required. (Note: Some people are allergic to lanolin.) There are two basic preparation methods:

Preparation Forms and Uses

1) 1 part of finely powdered herb is thoroughly mixed with 4 parts of lard or oil base.
2) Into a slow cooker, i.e. a crock pot, 200 g or 1/2 lb of dried herbs (or 400 g or 1 lb of fresh herbs) should be placed with 600 g (1 1/2 lb) lard and 100 g (3 oz) lanolin or beeswax. This mixture is gently warmed (digested) in the oven at about 180°F for 4-8 hours. A hardened **medicated oil** is produced by this method (see liniment below) which is easier to spread.

If essential oils are used instead of herbs (with a 2-3% dilution), the base should be heated, the essential oils added and stirred, and then the whole mixture poured into a container and allowed to cool. NOTE: To better preserve a salve, only small amounts should be made at a time and stored in sealed containers. Preserving agents are also useful, such as a pellet of Benzoin or Balm of Gilead resin, or their essential oil or tincture, vitamin E oil (2 drops per 30 ml. or 1 oz.) or glycerine.

Variations: If a double-strength ointment is required, a second extraction of the same herbal material can be made, using the same oil, before adding the hardener.

Where *protective* qualities are required of an ointment above all, non-penetrating paraffins such as vaseline may be included in the base.

If *penetration* of the remedies is important, animal grease should be used alone.

CREAM AND LOTION

A cream is a light oil preparation emulsified with a medicated liquid. While similar to an ointment, it has the advantage of *penetrating faster* and *promoting healing*. Moreover it allows the skin to breathe by not clogging the pores. Creams should be used sparingly and often. They quickly *moisten, soothe* or *cool the skin* in all dry, irritative or hot skin conditions. The herbs used are generally the same as those for ointments.

A lotion is simply a thinner, more liquid cream, watered down with herb tea, tincture or vinegar. Good for treating more delicate, sensitive skin conditions (as in children and babies), it also soaks in more easily and interferes less with clothing. Again, it should be applied often. Lotions may be *cleansing, softening and soothing, astringing and toning*, or *pain relieving*.

Preparation: A simple cream may be prepared from an oil and water medication using an emulsifying agent to bind them. A better cream can be made using a medicated oil instead of plain oil (see liniment below). The best emulsifiers are Tragacanth or Acacia gum, lecithin, eggyolk, Almond flour or mucilagenous herbs such as Irish moss, Agar-agar, Marsh mallow, Comfrey, Purslane, Cannabis or Poppy seeds. Alternately, a ready-made emulsifying agent may be used. If an herbal tincture is used rather than a water preparation, the cream's storage life will be prolonged; the use of gums will decrease it. Lanolin will hold several times its weight in water and obviates the need to use an emulsifier. (Note: Some people are allergic to lanolin). Here are two sample ways of preparing a skin cream:

1) 400 g or 16 oz medicated oil
   100 g or 4 oz beeswax
   100 g or 4 oz anhydrous lanolin
   200 g or 8 oz tincture
   7 g or 1/4 oz borax

Both the medicated oil and the tincture can be made from herbs such as Rose petal, Ribwort plantain, Chickweed or Elder flower. The beeswax and the lanolin should be melted together on low heat. When melted, the pre-warmed medicated oil is added. Borax is dissolved into the tincture, heated to the same temperature and added to the other oils. The mixture is then removed from the heat and stirred until cool.

2) The medicated water (i.e. herb tea) is added to the lanolin drop by drop while beating constantly, similar to the way in which mayonnaise is made.

LINIMENT

A liniment is an oil based medication which is rubbed into the skin and muscles. It is also known as an **embrocation** or a ***medicated oil***. It can be applied by rubbing or massage, and has superlative *warming* effects. Its functions are as follows:

- *to stimulate, warm and relax the skin and muscles* in external damp/cold obstruction conditions such as myalgia, neuralgia, muscular atrophy and cold arthritis, with numbness, soreness and static pains. It may also be used for local paralysis and spasms (*Wintergreen, Marjoram*, Cayenne, Prickly ash, Ginger). If a *rubefacient* liniment made with Cantharides powder, Laurel or Croton oil is retained until blisters form, a drawing *vesicant* effect will be obtained. It is used to treat damp obstruction type sciatica, neuritis and other similar conditions (compare p. 667).
- *to relieve local injuries and swelling* in sprains, contusions, stings, and all injuries with unbroken skin (Arnica, St.John's wort, Tansy, Marigold)
- *to relieve burns and inflammation* (*Lavender*, St. John's wort, Camomile)
- *to treat an internal organ, bone or tissue* through a surface reflex area or point, i.e. a dermatome (nerve insertions along the spine, dorsal or abdominal reflex areas, acupuncture points etc.); in deep pains of the organs, bones, etc.
- *to repel insects* (*Pennyroyal, Citronella*)

Preparation: A simple liniment may be prepared with a 2-5% dilution of essential oil(s) in a good vegetable oil. If herbs are used, they are heated in lard or oil over a very low heat for 4-8 hours, then strained. 500 ml or 1 pint of lard or oil are used for 30 g (2 oz) of dried herbs. Alternately, the plant material can simply soak over two to three weeks, being shaken twice daily. After this period it is strained and stored in a dark jar.

Another way to prepare a liniment is with sun oil, weather permitting. Ingredients are placed in a glass jar and simply set in the sun for one or two weeks.

BATH

Therapeutic baths[1] may be taken using plain water or water to which herbs have been added (medicated water). There are various types, including foot baths, hip baths (or sitzbaths) and full baths. They all depend on one or more factors to be effective: the water itself, the water temperature, the type of herbs used and the aroma of the herbs or oils given off through the steam. The general functions of a bath are:

- *to restore, strengthen and revive* in deficient, atrophic and wasting conditions due to overwork and stress, in convalescence and after childbirth (seaweed or mineral extracts, *Thyme, Sage, Rosemary*)
- *to relax, calm and release tension* in excess conditions as in Qi constraint, spasms, irritability and general pain *(Camomile, Lavender*, Hops, Black cohosh)
- *to stimulate and warm* in cold conditions such as cramps, chilliness (Juniper, Black pepper, Prickly ash) and colds (Ginger, Horseradish, Mustard seed)
- *to clear heat and resolve fever* in feverish conditions (e.g. a cool bath for high fever; a warm bath with *stimulants* such as Cayenne, Ginger or Horseradish to cause sweating, with a cold towel over the forehead at the beginning of a fever); or simply when feeling hot (*Lemon*, seaweed, liquid trace minerals)
- *to draw out toxins* in toxemic conditions, especially general fluids dyskrasia due to poor diet and poor elimination (liquid trace minerals, seaweed, epsom salts), radiation, etc. (salt & soda)

Hand and Foot Bath

Ankles or wrists are immersed in water, either hot or cold, usually enhanced with herbs or essential oils. Hand and foot baths may be taken **cold** for 1-3 minutes to *stimulate, revive or cool* and to *increase vitality and resistance* in cases of chilliness, insomnia, fatigue, agitation and fevers. They may also be taken **warm** (25-26°C) for 12-15 minutes to *relax, calm, stimulate and warm* in cases of spasms, cramps, pain, internal congestion and painful periods, as well as weak vitality in general.

Alternating hot and warm baths are used *to move stagnant Qi and blood* where congealed blood, ecchymosis, contusions and blue marks are present.

Hip Bath

Also known as a **sitzbath**. A bowl may be used or a normal bathtub, filled with enough water to cover the hips up to the waist only. Add 1/4 l or 1/2 pint of the herbal preparation or 5-10 drops of essential oil to the water and mix well. A hip bath is very effective in urinary, genital and lower digestive conditions.

A **cold hip bath** should last only 1/2-3 minutes, depending on the person's strength. Cold hip baths have *stimulating, decongesting and regulating* effects and are ideal for treating blood congestion and most conditions with general plethora. They are unsurpassed for copious menstruation or intermenstrual bleeding. They can prevent colds and flus, and promote sound sleep.

A **hot hip bath** of about 15 minutes at 26°C will *stimulate, relax, soften, warm* and *relieve pain*, and is therefore used in conditions of cold, Yang deficiency and Qi constraint. It is typically used for gynecological conditions such as delayed or painful periods; for lumbar pain, urinary ailments including stones and dysuria, gout, hemorrhoids and constipation.

Full Bath

A **cold full bath** is taken for 1-2 minutes (never longer) and for those in good health is *reviving and stimulating*. For serious febrile conditions, a **tepid** bath may be used to cool slightly, after which the fever should be allowed to go down on its own.

A **warm full bath** has an undesirable tiring effect, which can only be avoided by taking it at the lower temperature of 20-25°C for no longer than 20 minutes. It is mildly *relaxing, warming* and *softening*.

Preparation: For medicated baths of any kind, either herbs or essential oils may be used. The choice of these depends on the type of effect required. If herbs are used, 1 liter or 2 pints of water is brought to a boil. The heat is turned off and the crushed or chopped herbs (up to 100 g or 4 oz) are immersed and allowed to steep, covered for 4 or 5 hours. This basic tea preparation should be stored in a non-metallic container and is used for several baths. Use 1/3-1/2 liter or 2/3-1 pint of the herb water for each bath.

If essential oils are used, place 5-10 drops in 1-5 pints of water. For a full bath, 5-20 drops are added directly to the water which should be swished just before entering.

Alternately, and for an occasional bath, an herb mix may be bound up in a muslin bag; this is called a **nodulus.** It is steeped in the hot water for the duration of the entire bath.

EYE PREPARATIONS

The basic preparations used in eye care are baths (or washes), compresses, ointments and creams.

Eye baths are made with *cooling, anti-inflammatory, disinfectant* herbs such as Camomile, Eyebright, Fennel, Meadowsweet, Melilot, Rose, Lavender, Elder flower, Corn flower, Barberry and Goldenseal. A weak infusion is made, strained thoroughly and poured into an eye cup, and the

The Energetics of Western Herbs

whole eye is washed. Alternately, a well-diluted tincture (1 part to 20 parts of tepid water) or distilled water may be used. A few grains of sea salt should always be dissolved into eye baths.

Eyebright is the best all-round eye remedy. It may be used for all eye disharmonies except for dryness.

Small compresses or **swabs** may be made using Camomile, Fennel or Apple pulp, and applied on resting, closed lids for 10 minutes.

Creams or **ointments** with any of the same herbs as above may be spread onto the upper lid and reapplied frequently.

All of the above three preparations may be used interchangeably for the following conditions:
- *tired, aching eyes*, often with low headache
- *dry, irritated eyes* caused by wind, strain or hay fever
- *mucosal inflammations* such as conjunctivitis and blepharitis, both simple and infective
- *eye catarrh* in head damp cold conditions
- *excessive weeping*

Eye baths may also be used to *strengthen eyesight*, using herbs such as Eyebright, Fennel or Valerian.

ENDNOTES

Chapter 1—Herbal Medicine East & West: Medical Philosophy

1   Interestingly, the Western life cycle of knowledge may be compared to typical biological phenomena such as the life cycle of the endometrium or the ovum. They also have long build-up phases and a sudden stage of collapse and change before making way for a new phase of build-up. The biological metaphor for Western thought can be further extended in that any new theory or system, in all scientific and artistic areas, is only accepted if it represents an **organic development** of an existing theory. In other words, the new theory must have a direct **parentage** and **derivation** from, a currently accepted, valid theory. Modern medicine has taken this approach to a logical conclusion in basing its method mainly on biochemistry.

2   This was acknowledged by Western commentators of Chinese medicine such as JOHN FLOYER as far back as the eighteenth century. His opinion was that "the want of Anatomy does make their Art very obscure, and gives occasion to phantastical Notions, but their absurd Notions are **adjusted to the real Phenomena, and their Art is grounded upon curious Experience, examined and approved for 4,000 years** [emphasis added]" (*The Physician's Pulse-Watch* p. 353). Another example of a pure phenomenon oriented healing system is, of course, Native American botanical medicine. This is very well summed up by the traveller JONATHAN CARVER, who, at the end of the eighteenth century, spent some time among the native tribes of Wisconsin and Minnesota: "They exercise their art by principles which are founded on the knowledge of simples, and on **experience which they acquire by an indefatigable attention to their operations** [emphasis added]" (*Travels through the Interior Parts of North America*, cited in *American Indian Medicine* by VIRGIL VOGEL, p.95).

3   Again the biological comparison which springs to mind is the self-regulating homeostatic endocrine system. Like Eastern thought, it is an ongoing, dynamic system in which continuous slight changes occur and all various parts are in constant dialogue yet never disturb the inherent stability of the governing pituitary gland.

4   Here the difference between *qi*, or soul spirits, and *shen*, or vital spirits, becomes clear. Qi is probably the key concept of Chinese medicine and is a significant emblem for the Oriental way of thinking with its pool of knowledge, a continuous flowing and eddying of ideas. Qi also has more of the nature of the soul or psyche and the realm of feelings, as well as the nature of stars and planets with their continuous, seemingly never ending, timeless cycles. The key concept of Greek medicine, on the other hand, is the vital spirit or *shen*. (It is a term as ubiquitous in Greek as Qi is in Chinese medicine.) It is a prime emblem for the more biological character of Western thought with its definite phases of growth and fall and especially its similarity to the realm of plants and their growth, maturity and decay.

5   The translation of Qi as "breaths" not only is a more correct rendering of its meaning, but is also in keeping both with the image of steam and clouds in the Chinese ideogram and with the actual sound of this word when pronounced. The plural form emphasizes the active, functional and effective nature of Qi. For a full discussion see *Survey of Traditional Chinese Medicine* by JEAN SCHATZ, CLAUDE LARRE and ELISABETH ROCHAT DE LA VALÉE (1985).

6   *The Touchstone of Complexions* is unusual for reasons other than a presentation of a Western

The Energetics of Western Herbs

version of the three treasures. On the face of it, it seems yet another popular book on health care, written at a time when the market was flooded with titles such as *The Jewell of Health* (1567), *The Castle of Health* (1539) and *Delights for Ladies* (1594). Closer inspection, however, reveals a very earnest, serious presentation of the meaning of preventive medicine, describing aspects such as lifestyle and spiritual attitude, in addition to giving dietary recommendations, undoubtedly based on readings of Arab texts.

7   The celebrated medical historian, CURT SPRENGEL, in his *Geschichte der Medizin* of 1795, in fact speculates on whether students of the Greek physician HEROPHILOS had not reached Samarkand and Baktria in their travels, thus to influence the "subtle pulse classification" of the Chinese. It is also interesting to note that as early as 1707 practitioners like JOHN FLOYER were complaining that "the Chinese have corrupted their art of feeling the Pulse by mixing their Philosophy of the Five Elements with it" (*The Physician's Pulse-Watch* p. 353). FLOYER was basing his observation on *Le secret du pouls,* written a few years earlier by the Jesuit missionary Father PLACIDE HERVIEU, in which WANG SHU HO's system of pulse diagnostics is fully presented.

8   RUFUS OF EPHESOS, *Synopsis peri sphygmon*, translated by Charles Daremberg as *Traité sur le pouls*, Paris, 1846.

9   It is not that Chinese medicine remained uninfluenced by alchemy; on the contrary, the history of Tang dynasty medicine is a record of a growing fascination with Indian alchemy, Indian medicinal plants, Indian mysticism and Indian Buddhism. All of these were copiously imported and assimilated into Chinese culture in a way only paralleled at the present time. (See *The Golden Peaches of Samarkand* by EDWARD H. SCHAFER, Berkeley, 1984.)

Chapter 2—Herbal Medicine East and West: Medical Theories

1   Pharmacognosy means the science of understanding a *pharmakon* or remedy; pharmacology denotes the study of its physiological effects. Both these may be energetic, as in Chinese and Greek medicine, or biochemic, as in modern medicine.

2   Therapeutics defines principles and methods of treatment.

3   Volume I of *The Touchstone of Medicine* goes into his theory of taste and smell in considerable detail, covering their nature, functions and therapeutic uses. Volume II gives exhaustive synoptic catalogues of the tastes and their effects and of the herb classes, followed by a detailed presentation of the latter, divided into three parts—*Evacuators, Hot or Cold Alterers, External Medicines*. Although, like Chinese medicine, FLOYER's method is phenomenon oriented, FLOYER himself is a remedy oriented person, like all good physicians of Greek medicine. In this sense he greatly resembles IBN AL-SINA, who was nicknamed the Arabian Galen. FLOYER's other significant works include a *Treatise on the Asthma* (1698) and several books on hydrotherapy.

4   In trying to isolate the mechanical cause of a problem and correct it with one or more suitable active constituents, contemporary herbalism does a better job than biochemistry itself. In using synthetic drugs, biochemistry actually violates its own rule of isolating the specific cause: the majority of drugs and other methods such as radiation therapy merely represent a blanket approach in which microorganisms and malignant cells are destroyed one and all. This is in contrast to the elegant **selectivity** and **tropic specificity** of organic plant compounds which invariably kill only injurious elements (e.g. bacteria) and moreover boost beneficial ones: the action of Garlic and Microalgae in the gut, of Poke root or Echinacea in the blood or of all *disinfectant* **essential oils** are a few examples out of countless possible ones.

Endnotes

5   There are also differences, however, between earlier alchemical chemists and later scientific ones. Whereas Persian and European iatrochemists could only induce chemical processes through the evidence of their senses, later European biochemists were able to look at the constituents of plants in microscopic, cellular detail. Similarly, whereas Arabian and Scholastic authors had to be content to determine a plant's nature to hair-splitting degrees through speculation, later organic chemists were working with plant material itself.

6   Thus, to give but one crude example, herbs that *extinguish wind and relieve spasms* from the Chinese pharmacopoeia, all *spasmolytic* and *nerve sedative* in action, are often labelled *carminatives*!

7   These are the definitions of MANFRED PORKERT, whose text, *The Theoretical Foundations of Chinese Medicine*, should be consulted for an in-depth presentation of Yin/Yang in Chinese medicine.

Chapter 3—The Meaning of Integration

1   Of course homeopathic medicine uses the same approach when comparing the sign and symptom gestalt of the patient with that of the remedies.

2   This procedure, which is identical to Hahnemannian homeopathic practice, extends to acupuncture points in addition to herbal remedies. Until recently, all Chinese texts on acupuncture points simply listed the symptoms, syndromes and illnesses indicated for their use. Like homeopathic remedies, they have no functions as such in terms of physiopathology. Both classical Chinese medicine and classical Homeopathy share a phenomenological approach enhanced by imagistic and comparative thinking.

3   It is no accident that Eclectic therapists, the largest group of practitioners of herbal medicine from about 1850 to the late 1940's, presented their remedies in a style similar to the homeopathic repertories of the day. Homeopathy was the dominant medical trend prevailing in the U.S. at the time. To chart the cross-influences between the Eclectics and the Homeopathists in terms of remedies used throughout this time would be a fascinating study.

4   For a very clear discussion of contradiction and its resolution through dialectic thinking, see MAO ZE DONG's *On Contradiction*. It is in this connection that as early as 1928 he already saw the need for combining traditional Chinese and Western medicine.

Chapter 4—The Materia Medica Reclassified

1   This *ben cao*, the most important prior to the Song dynasty, actually contains an entry on Roman Theriac, which must have been the complex antidote created by MITHRIDATES, king of Pontus, and still in use until the nineteenth century in Europe. A Byzantine embassy had brought this remedy—among a cornucopia of other gifts—to the Tang emperor in the year 667.

Chapter 5—The Integral Presentation

1   That this theory does not hold water is shown by the fact that many plants of the mild, i.e. non-toxic, category, such as Yarrow, do in fact contain "active" substances such as alkaloids, yet without the active and dramatic effect expected from them.

Chapter 6—Historical Antecedents

1   Very little has been written that documents the unofficial history of medicine in the West, and nothing at all about the healing practices it consisted of. *Old Wives' Tales* by MARY CHAMBERLAIN (Virago, London, 1981) is a good start, especially where the social context of this history is concerned. Chapter 2 of JEANNE ACHTERBERG's *Imagery and Healing* excells at placing women healers in the context of shamanism in general, while *Women Healers in Medieval Life and Literature* by MURIEL J. HUGHES (Books for Libraries Press, New York, 1943) specifically covers its medieval phase.

2   It is the sheer repetition of an opinion down the centuries by authority figures which often makes a statement attain the status of reliable, credible source material. The initial statement might have been merely a disparaging opinion or a caustic remark, the most obvious example being the beliefs held about the medical practices of the Native Americans, based as they were on the reports of early missionaries and explorers. For more detailed information, see in particular the works by VOGEL.

3   In a sense the problems become even more poignant with terminology closer to our era when many terms still in use are employed in a different way or carry different meanings and connotations than formerly. Familiar terms such as *astringent, cordial* and *alterative* meant far more in the seventeenth and eighteenth century than they do today, and many have been abandoned entirely. To understand them fully and realize their implications, one has to go first to their roots, which are found in none other than the writings of GALEN, and **then** try to understand their use in a certain period or a certain text or author. For example, how is one to be sure how syndromes such as *risings of the womb, windiness of the womb* or *strangulation of the womb*, were differentiated in those days?

4   Unfortunately, neither RYFF not SALMON were qualified M.D.s, which laid their character open to denigration and slander. Most biographers to the present day have the same opinion about them, disqualifying their work on the grounds that they were not doctors. RYFF, indeed, has almost been forgotten; none of the studies on herbals of this century even list his major work. This is yet another example of sheep-like repetition of opinion—which has nothing to do with proper research.

5   Like many of the continental trends, iatromathematics, also known as astromedicine or medical astrology, blossomed in England about a hundred years after its heyday on the continent. Like BARTHOLOMAEUS CARRICHTER in Germany, NICHOLAS CULPEPER was in fact one of the last exponents and popularizers of a branch of astrology that had its roots in the Italian Hermetic and Neoplatonic revival of about 1450 to 1510.

6   Cited in *Dictionnaire de la médecine ancienne*, OLIVIER DEZEIMERIS, p. 99.

7   That is to say that over 200 were accepted at one time or another by the *Pharmacopoeia of the United States of America* and the *National Formulary*. The actual number used by Native Americans (and Blacks, to a lesser extent) is closer to 500, according to research conducted by pharmaceutical historian HEBER YOUNGKEN (cited by VIRGIL VOGEL, *American Indian Medicine*, p.8); consequently, something nearer to this figure was also used at one time or another by early settlers, European immigrant servants, homesteaders, etc. In the above mentioned text VOGEL has written that "so complete, in fact, was the aboriginal knowledge of their native flora that Indian usage can be demonstrated for all but a bare half dozen, at most, of our indigenous vegetable drugs". (From *American Indian Medicine*, © 1970 University of Oklahoma Press).

Chapter 7—Guidelines to Prescribing

1   The implications of the homeopathic effect of tinctures, and especially of percolated ones, are far-reaching. It means that when using tinctures, for example, the whole symptom picture of an individual should be considered as much as the specific conditions and symptoms. His or her entire pattern of disharmony should be viewed as a whole as well as in fragments. The overall pattern or conformation can then be matched with the general pattern of indications of the botanical, to determine the best one to use. Getting exactly the right fit is, of course, ideal. However, it is not nearly as crucial with tinctures as with homeopathic remedies, since with tinctures the allopathic effect still accounts for at least half of the herb's effect.

This can be historically validated. Eclectic herbal medicine, for example, relied primarily on **specific medications** which were prepared by a percolation method, i.e. an alcoholic fluid extract. In harmony with this type of preparation, Eclectic practitioners also used homeopathic prescribing methods. They thought in terms of **specific symptomatology** (as seen in the texts of SCUDDER, KING, FELTER, ELLINGWOOD, etc.) as well as in terms of pharmacology.

Chapter 8—Preparation Forms and Uses

1   Therapeutic bathing, also known as hydrotherapy, has enjoyed varying popularity since Greek and Roman times, when it was a widely used method of treatment. Galenic medical textbooks such as IBN SINA's *Qanun* devote entire sections to it, and it has never been as popular as it was during the Arabian phase of Greek medicine. Even the nineteenth century manuals on hydrotherapy (e.g. KNEIPP) which discuss a whole range of water treatments do not go into as much therapeutic detail as these older texts. In Renaissance times, EUCHARIUS RÖSZLIN and WALTHER H. RYFF wrote delightful popularizations of these.

It is interesting to note that up to the sixteenth century, the late medieval bathhouse was an important locale of symptomatic and preventive treatment for both men and women. It was not only used for therapeutic bathing, but also for emetic therapy (causing vomiting) and for bloodletting. Writers of the period note with dry amusement that a trip to the bathouse usually involved the risk of getting sprinkled with blood through open windows, before having even set foot inside. Given hygienic habits as well as the narrowness of streets in those days, this must indeed have been a strong possibility.

Part Two
Materia Medica

MENTA
HORTENSIS TERTIA   Onser frawen müntz.

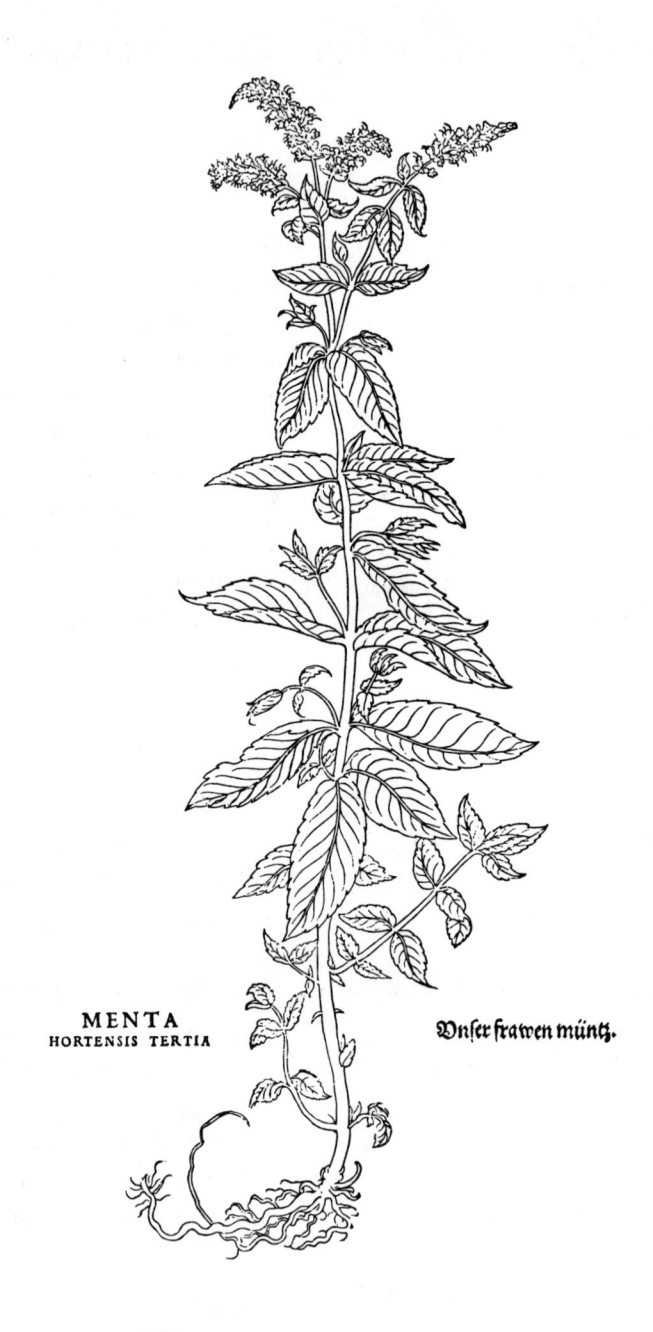

Mint

Guidelines to Using the Materia Medica

Conventions

The following conventions are adopted throughout this text.

All technical terms from Greek, Chinese and Ayurvedic medicine are kept in lower case when they are expressed in English. This is because concepts such as wind, cold, heat, damp, etc., although technical, are also words of common language describing everyday experience. In this sense, therefore, they are nontechnical, and allow us to understand energetic or vitalistic medicine as a non-technical healing art not separate from the realities of everyday life.

The names of the all-important organs are only capitalized when they refer to the functional Chinese organ or orb. Thus "Kidney Qi infirmity" refers to the Chinese Kidney, whereas "kidney Qi stagnation" refers to the anatomical kidneys; "Spleen Qi deficiency" evokes the Chinese Spleen functions, while "spleen weakness" refers to the anatomical spleen organ.

All words in italics denote a term in a foreign language, such as *tessara chumoi,* or the action and quality of an herb, such as *bitter cold febrifuge.*

All words in bold type signify either a pathological condition, such as **damp heat**, or a simple emphasis of meaning.

Layout

The Materia Medica is set out in five parts, according to the fundamental treatment principles of Eliminating, Restoring, Draining, Altering and Regulating, and Symptom Treatment. Each principle then comprises several specific treatment methods which corresponds to the basic herb classes.

Each class of herbs is introduced by a discussion of the treatment method that it serves, followed by the most important remedies for that class. Wherever possible these have been organized according to their taste qualities. Remedies in Class 12, for example, are grouped into *bitter pungent, bitter astringent, bitter sweet* and *pungent sweet* kinds.

Since every herb has more than one function (often several functions being equally important), it follows that it should actually be found in several classes. Therefore a listing of all possible remedies in each class is found in the synoptic list of treatment methods at the end of the Materia Medica.

Herb Presentation

Every botanical is presented according to its nature, functions and uses, preparation forms, dosages and cautions. The notes following each herb discusses the remedy in a more informal way, bringing out its main characteristics and clinical uses, useful combinations and significant similarities of usage with Chinese herbs. In addition, historical, botanical or taxonomic aspects of particular interest are also highlighted.

The sequence of functions for each herb begins with its use in the herb class where it is found—its most important use—and progresses with related uses. In this way a cumulative picture is built up and repetition of functions, since implicit, is avoided. The final function of each herb usually addresses external conditions such as injuries, skin conditions, etc. This implies that they

The Energetics of Western Herbs

should be treated not only with external preparations such as SWABS, WASHES, COMPRESSES, etc., but also by simultaneous internal use of that herb.

In the leading numbered sentences in capitals, describing the main functions of each herb, any word in italics, such as *SPLEEN*, refers to the Chinese functional organ or orb, not the anatomical organ.

Beneath the herb functions three types of indications are listed: Chinese syndromes, Western conditions and symptoms. They may be distinguished as follows: Chinese syndromes are always in italics, as in *blood deficiency*; symptoms and Western conditions are fully capitalized at the beginning and lower case thereafter, as in HIGH BLOOD PRESSURE, arteriosclerosis.

The **Preparation** section lists the most important ways of using the herb and the best preparation form for each. These applications are only limited by the imagination, however. Chapter 8 presents the possibilities inherent in each type of herbal preparation.

The **Dosages** given are the most common dosage ranges needed in practice. They are based on standard strength preparations (most often 1 : 5) using only alcohol. As a guideline, and if in doubt, the following dosage equivalents should be kept in mind for TINCTURES (as defined on p. [#]).

```
1 ml   = 15 min  =  25 drops  = 1/5 tsp
2.5 ml = 38 min  =  62 drops  = 1/2 tsp
5 ml   = 75 min  = 125 drops  = 1 tsp

ml  = milileter(s)
min = minim(s)
tsp = teaspoon
```

The dosages to be used will vary according to the parameters presented in Chapter 8. It should be noted that drops of pure alcoholic tincture are approximately half the weight and volume of drops of water. For this reason, if a TINCTURE is used made of, say, 66% alcohol and 34% water, then the dosage in drops would have to be reduced by 1/3 of that given in the text.

Cautions are not the same as contraindications. Cautions delineate areas where care should be taken when using the herb under certain conditions. Any contraindication, however, is absolute.

Detailed informartion on every aspect of the presentation of the herbs is given in Chapter 5.

ELIMINATING

Botanicals that eliminate are distributed among the following classes:

Class 1: **Herbs to cause sweating and release external conditions**
Class 2: **Herbs to promote urination and relieve fluid congestion**
Class 3: **Herbs to promote bowel movement and relieve constipation**
Class 4: **Herbs to expel phlegm and ease coughing**
Class 5: **Herbs to promote the menses and clear stagnation**
Class 6: **Herbs to cause vomiting**

All herbs in this section have in common the fact that they cause an active evacuation or elimination and as such are called *eliminant remedies*. They were called *contraries* by GALEN, since they go contrary to the condition being treated. They assist the natural eliminatory response in excretory functions such as sweating, urination, passing stool and menstruation. They include herbs that cause vomiting, because these too cause an active evacuation of injurious or toxic matter causing irritation.

The conditions treated by *eliminants* are all termed **full** or **excess** conditions (*plethora* or *mallon* in Greek medicine, *shi* or *yu* in Chinese medicine). Since these **excess conditions** involve an impairment of eliminative functions, *eliminants* uniquely address those types of excess conditions said to be characterized by **stagnation** and **obstruction**. This type of excess usually comes in the form of some undesirable redundancy of substance,[1] such as phlegm, feces, urine, menstrual blood, and the various types of toxins involved.

By removing an unwanted obstruction caused by an endogenous or exogenous irritant to an excretory channel, *eliminants* encourage the natural reflexes of the human organism's vital force, or *physis*, in its striving for homeostasis. They work directly to expel injurious waste matter and thereby support the natural response of an individual's vital force to stressful irritants.

The Class 1 herbs known as *diaphoretics*, for example, by causing sweating and releasing external conditions, assist the excretory functions of the skin, increase its ability to breathe as a membrane modulating the exterior and the interior, and remove surface obstruction in the form of stagnating metabolic wastes, including dead epithelial cells. In so doing they encourage the organism's vital natural response of righting itself to balance. The same principles of action are involved with botanicals that cause urination (*diuretics*), bowel movement (*laxatives*), that expel phlegm, (*expectorants*), that promote the periods (*emmenagogues*), and that cause vomiting (*emetics*).

Eliminant herbs are also used to sweep away exogenous irritants to both excretory organs and surface tissues, such as environmental pollutants (e.g. in the bronchi), poisons (e.g. in the stomach) and microorganisms such as bacteria and viruses.

Furthermore, *eliminants* are used to produce indirect or secondary effects beneficial in conditions not necessarily related to obstructed elimination. In this way sweating is used to resolve fever at the initial external stage. Causing bowel movement is often used to clear internal full heat conditions, to relieve blood or fluid congestion, and to promote cleansing.

However, although *eliminants* have some secondary cleansing effects, they should not be

The Energetics of Western Herbs

confused with *alterative cleansers* from Class 15. *Eliminants* remove a surface stasis and obstruction to excretory functions, whereas *cleansers* cause an alteration of internal toxemic conditions for the better. These are clearly different actions. It is precisely the confusion between eliminating and altering as herb actions and treatment methods that has led to the erroneous belief, still widely held, that cleansing can only be carried out by causing an elimination.[2]

Nor should *eliminants* be used interchangeably with *stimulants*. Although many of the Class 7 *stimulants* are *diaphoretic* and cause sweating, they serve rather different therapeutic aims. Whereas the point of using *stimulants* is to accelerate and improve the functioning of an internal organ or system, *eliminants* are used to promote elimination in an excretory organ suffering from stasis or obstruction. Since they disperse energy, *eliminants* are used to unblock channels of excretion towards the exterior to assist the elimination response, unlike *stimulants* which cause internal stimulation to support the Yang and generate warmth.

Equally important, *eliminants* are not *drainers*. Granted, both deal directly with excess conditions; both primarily treat acute manifestations of illness, either simple or with chronic underlay. But whereas *eliminants* evacuate a superfluity that has resulted from a substantial surface obstruction, *drainers* remove an excess due to an internal response of a more qualitative nature, such as heat (i.e. fever or inflammation) or Qi constraint. Moreover, *eliminants* owe their action to working in conjunction with the body's vital reflexes, whereas *drainers* do so in opposition to them.

In Hippokratic texts Eliminating is termed *kenosis*, meaning literally "emptying out". In spite of not addressing constitutional or long term disharmonies, Eliminating nevertheless treats an **overall condition** rather than a particular symptom or mechanism of disharmony. Since the very act of excreting sweat, urine, stool, phlegm or menstrual blood involves the vital force, or Qi, of the entire organism, not just the local parts concerned, Eliminating also qualifies as a **general treatment method**, as opposed to a local, cellular or molecular one. By engaging an individual's entire vital response to stressors or irritants, rather than correcting single symptoms, it achieves nothing less than the treatment of the entire field of disharmony, both in a vitalist and a mechanical sense. This is the *holon ton somatos* of the Greek physicians of the island Kos at the time of HIPPOKRATES, the *praemissum universalum* of the Renaissance therapists.

In rebalancing overall energetic conditions rather than arresting illness by physical symptom treatment, the Eliminating treatment method forms a sharp contrast to modern medicine. The latter, in the wake of MAGENDIE's experimental physiopathology, VIRCHOW's cellular pathology and PASTEUR's germ theory, concentrates on local treatment involving physical tissue or substance. In contrast, Greek/Galenic medicine for almost three thousand years has employed, like Chinese medicine, treatment methods that are general and vitalistic, engaging the individual *physis* and vital force. In China, the physician ZHANG ZI HE is seen as the main advocate of the "dispelling and purging" approach, which touted sweating, vomiting and purging as the three treatment methods for all illnesses.[3] The equivalent Chinese term for Eliminating is *tong*, as in the expression *tong wu yu* (eliminating the five obstructions), whose written character significantly contains the symbol for water. In Greek/Galenic medicine, imbalances were treated by utilizing the four fluids theory in which Eliminating played an important part. This integrative theory allowed inductive correspondences to be made, and treatment of whole patterns of disharmony to be carried out.

The use of *eliminants*, whether *diaphoretics, expectorants, laxatives, diuretics, emmenagogues* or *emetics*, is based on diagnostic findings as to the nature of the condition. Since these herbs engage the individual's vital response in their action, two concepts, the injurious Qi, or pathogenic

Eliminating

factors, and the righteous Qi, or benficient factors, need to be considered here. In Chinese medicine, these are called *fan zhi* and *zheng zhi* respectively, and in Greek medicine the righteous Qi is included in a term translated as *spiritus vitalis* or vital force. Both pathogenic and righteous factors have their own treatment principles.

Eliminating is used with **excess** conditions where the pathogenic factors (here in the form of stagnant waste) may be eliminated directly through one of the six methods. In **deficiency** conditions, on the other hand, Eliminating should not be used: rather the body's own righteous Qi, the vital force, should be tonified with *restoring* remedies in order to remove the excess. Where there is excess together with deficiency, eliminating methods may be used, but with care. Here an assessment must be made of the relative strengths of pathogenic factors and the organism's own vital forces and reserves. The choices here are either to address the pathogenic factors first and later support the righteous ones; or first to support the righteous facrtors and then deal with the pathogenic ones; or to do both at the same time.

Clearly, rather than being used in isolation, outside of any therapeutic context drawing in the individual's vital responses, *eliminants* are best used as agents that implement a treatment principle and method—in this case, to assist elimination responses to stressors. In this light, *eliminants* can be seen as therapeutic agents much like acupuncture needles, cupping glasses, phlebotomy needles, herbal moxa sticks, and so on. Their intention one and all is to carry out a certain energetic treatment method which, by encouraging a natural discharge, will promote a return to health.[4]

Equally important, it should be understood that there is no room here for causing the body to eliminate by force. In the context of the dialectic of the righteous factors versus the injurious ones there is always the choice of gently assisting the individual ground, of supporting an individual's *physis*, or innate, natural condition, in its striving for homeostasis. It is unfortunately all too common, even today, among practitioners of herbal medicine to randomly prescribe *eliminants* as a cure-all in the heroic manner of degenerate Galenic medicine, without understanding the need to assess and honor the body's own intrinsic ability to bring itself to balance—an ability respected in all medical traditions, and beautifully summed up in the concepts "righteous Qi" and "vital forces".

Clearly, it is the needs of a given situation that should determine the type and intensity of an Eliminating treatment method chosen; it is not a random choice. Admittedly, every era and every medical phase had its predilection for one or more method: nineteenth century medics, for example, saw bowel-cleansing and causing bowel movement as the radical solution to all disease, while Native American and its derived Thomsonian systems called for sweating with every conceivable ailment. The most judicious use of *eliminants,* however, entails drawing upon those appropriate to each case presenting.

Notes

1   The very substantial, material obstructions or accumulations involved in excess conditions requiring *eliminants* rather than *drainers* was often conveyed by the character *man* instead of or in addition to the term *shi* in traditional Chinese texts.

2   Responsible for today's widespread assumption that Eliminating is synonymous with Cleansing is the belief that causing any **alteration** in human physiology neccessarily entails a discharge of some kind. It is an idea that gained force from Renaissance times onwards, when, e.g., "injurious spirits" were "chased from the heart." The seventeenth to nineteenth century emphasis on attacking the disease through forceful Eliminating treatment tactics (consisting mainly of excessive bloodletting and purging with toxic South American botanicals or frightening disease away with concoctions of animal products—the so-called filth pharmacy) also prepared the stage for the equation **cleansing = eliminating.** The idea that cleansing can only be carried out by

The Energetics of Western Herbs

causing an active elimination of one of the impure fluids, however, was only properly formulated by the first Nature Cure practitioners in early nineteenth century Germany. It was strengthened by the Victorian Protestant revival with its Judaeo-Christian belief in original sin and its conviction that illness is punishment for sin and that the real remedy for it is suffering through purification. It was a revamping of the official Church moral attitude towards the poor during the Middle Ages, albeit a lenient one by comparison.

The Nature Cure school invariably treated any illness or disharmony by a cleansing of impurities and, therefore, by causing elimination at any cost. All disharmony was put down to a state of autotoxicosis, and all treatment consisted of promoting discharge or elimination. That this assumption is still widely held, however unconsciously, is not difficult to see; its influence even extends to seemingly unrelated theories such as OHSAWA's Macrobiotics, widely accepted today. (WILHELM HUFELAND, originator of Macrobiotics, was an extremely intelligent, creative and clinically successful physician; although a contemporary of PRIESSNITZ and later Nature Cure practitioners, his very Hippokratic outlook on health and illness has nothing in common with any of these or with Macrobiotics as practiced today.)

It is interesting to consider the origins of these beliefs. The autotoxicity or toxemia theory and the idea of **cleansing** originates in Greek religious-mythical-magical medicine before HIPPOKRATES, where *katharsis* meant a total spiritual, emotional and physical process of radical renewal (much as found in Native American healing ceremonies and rituals). This was later embodied in the Greek Asklepian temple cults of ritualistic soul, or psychic, healing, which survived into Byzantine days.

On the other hand, the idea of discharging and eliminating is a legacy from the Indian subcontinent, where sickness causing demons (the *balas* of Muslim psychotherapy and the *bhuta-preta* of the Hindu spirit pantheon) are **driven out** of the body in order to restore a pure, unpolluted body/soul/mind. The Indian caste system is a social expression of the same concern for internal purity. The parallel in chemical allopathic medicine today is the one dimensional attack on microörganisms and their expulsion from the body in an aspiration for antiseptic purity with no regard for PASTEUR's dying words, "BERNARD was right: the microbe is nothing, the **ground** is everything."

3   ZHANG ZI HE's ideas were subsequently modified by later physicians, each of whom placed emphasis on a different treatment method. So ZHU DAN XI recommended *watering the Yin* as of prime importance, while LI DONG YUAN promoted *strengthening the Spleen*, and LIU WAN SU advocated *cool and cold remedies*. Since the Qing dynasty Chinese medical treatment methods have coalesced into eight basic methods (*yi men ba fa*); these are the source of the expanded methods found in herbal textbooks today. Expressed succinctly, they are: sweating, vomiting, purging, harmonizing, warming, cooling, restoring, draining. In the terms of the present text, it will be seen that these consist of three Eliminating, two Restoring and two Draining methods and one Altering one.

4   It must be remembered that eliminative treatment methods go beyond the use of *eliminant botanicals*. In keeping with Galenic medicine, in a sense they include, in addition to the methods described above, bloodletting (see p. 479), cupping, and leeching, as well as derivative methods such as counterirritation, blistering, pustulation, fontanelles and cauterization (see p. 666). These are well described in ASCHNER's books on constitutional therapy.

CLASS 1

Herbs to Cause Sweating and Release External Conditions

The primary function of herbs that induce sweating is to "release" external conditions. By this is meant the resolution of conditions which take place on the external, superficial parts of the body and which Chinese medicine defines as the Tai Yang stage of illness. External conditions are acute conditions with rapid onset, are triggered by bacterial or viral invasion or flare-up, and are said to belong to the initial or alarm stage of general adaptation within the body's nonspecific response to stressors.[1] As such they represent an acute healing crisis in the organism's striving for homeostasis.

When environing pathogenic influences, simply called, e.g., wind, cold and heat in Chinese and Greek medicine begin to injure the functional integrity of the human organism, a conflict between the person's vital force (known as righteous Qi, *zheng qi*) and the pathogen is set up. The immune system engages, and symptoms such as chills, muscle aches, headache, stiff neck, fever and a floating, fast pulse begin to manifest. This is the symptom pattern which characterizes an external condition, typically found at the onset of colds, influenza, laryngitis and other acute upper respiratory infections.

The outcome of this initial struggle may assume different forms, depending on the exact interplay between certain factors. There is the person's own predisposing ground, i.e. his predisposition to infection in general, which is directly related to factors such as constitution, mental and emotional state, and levels of toxicity. However, more immediate factors must also be considered. These include not only the virulence of the environing influence or pathogen, but far more importantly, the vigor of the individual's own defense response. This vital response consists of both the internal struggle of the immune system and of the more manifest fever and sweating.

If defenses are weak, then no matter what the virulence of the offensive pathogen, the result will only be a slight fever, if any at all: a wind cold condition. If it continues over some time, it is liable to progress to the exhaustion stage of adaptation and produce a chronic condition in the Tai Yin stage of illness.

If on the other hand active defense response is good, then the strength of the fever will always accurately reflect the nature or virulence of the pathogen itself. If the pathogen is strong, then the response will be appropriately strong, resulting in a dynamic fever, with or without inflammation, i.e. a wind heat condition. If the pathogen is relatively mild, then the response will only be sufficient to overcome the pathogen—also a wind heat condition. In every case it is the **organism's own** immediate vital warmth response, as function of the warmth organism, which determines a wind cold or a wind heat condition, not the nature of the pathogen itself. The pathogen is merely the trigger in this dynamic situation; it is the integrity of the vital defensive forces that determines the outcome. It is known that a high temperature actually assists in the struggle against microorganisms, while the act of sweating itself not only keeps the temperature under control, but also speeds up the removal and elimination of toxic debris resulting from the conflict.

In either case, the person's vital force may either overcome or succumb to the pathogen. If its defense functions win out over the pathogen, the conflict is effectively resolved.

If pathogens endure, however, illness then enters the resistance phase of adaptation and becomes **chronic** by nature, going into the Yang Ming and any of the three Yin stages of disease

The Energetics of Western Herbs

described by Chinese medicine. In the case where the conflict continues with little variation, **subacute** conditions ensue, usually in the Shao Yang stage.

The overall treatment strategy for resolving external conditions hinges, therefore, around supporting the organism's own active defenses. Since these consist in first place of the warmth response called fever and sweating, it follows that the need is for botanicals that will encourage these functions: for *diaphoretics* or *sudorifics*, in short. In this supportive (not suppressive) approach the duration of defense response is shortened, and in the case of timely treatment the condition may be lenified or even prevented entirely. It is in this context that the Chinese expression *biao jie fa, exterior releasing method*, should be understood. Moreover, since the defense response may be a weak one (wind cold) or a strong one (wind heat), the treatment priority will be different in each.

Sweat inducing remedies, or *diaphoretics*, are *active, light, penetrating* and *dispersing* by nature, and invariably possess a *pungent, spicy taste* and a *warm* and *dry* nature. They are divided into *warming* and *cooling* kinds. Many contain volatile oils that account for these effective qualities.

1 HERBS TO CAUSE SWEATING, RELEASE THE EXTERIOR AND SCATTER WIND COLD

Remedies in this category are used for external conditions of acute onset characterized by sensations of chilliness, little or no sweating and fever, aches and pains, especially in the muscles, a stiff neck and a floating and tight pulse. If any inflammation with pain is present (as in angina), it tends to be mild. This is the typical **wind cold** condition occurring at the onset of infections involving the upper respiratory tract.

The treatment intention here is to support the body's defenses by stimulating a proper and adequate expression of fever and sweating, using *pungent warm circulatory stimulant diaphoretics* such as Cinnamon, Ginger, Oshá and Prickly ash. Their energetic tendency is to cause dispersion upwards and outwards, much like a water fountain. By pushing fluids towards the exterior and producing sweating, they effectively release the exterior and resolve the conflict. Many of these herbs are also to be found in Class 8 among the *circulatory stimulants* that support the Yang and generate warmth, since their nature is virtually identical.

2 HERBS TO CAUSE SWEATING, RELEASE THE EXTERIOR AND SCATTER WIND HEAT

Botanicals of this type are indicated when **wind heat** conditions arise, with few or no chills, a stronger fever and sweating than in wind cold, and a floating, fast pulse. They often involve more severe inflammation of the throat, eyes or head passages due to infection that causes additional soreness or pain.

The treatment priority here is to carefully control and resolve the warmth response. Fever should be steered to a resolution before the temperature becomes excessive (never above 105°F or 45°C). This is done by causing free perspiration, in this case to assist cooling the exterior as well as to cleanse and eliminate toxins. The remedies of choice in wind heat conditions are *pungent warm peripheral vasodilatory diaphoretics* such as Boneset, Linden, Catnip, Eucalyptus, Camomile and Elder flower. Should the temperature remain too high in spite of this, bitter cold herbs from Class 13, such as Wormwood and Gentian, are indicated in order to drain excessive heat and restore the person's strength.

It is interesting to consider the paradox that *pungent warm* herbs are often used for wind heat conditions. Clearly their intrinsic warmth in no way prevents them from resolving fever and clearing external heat. On the contrary: it is only through their affinity with our own warmth organism and their ability to induce sweating that they are able to help regulate and enhance our natural responses to pathogenic influences. Seen in this light, the possible additional use of hot remedies such as Eucalyptus, Camphor, Aconite, Garlic and Cayenne in wind heat conditions becomes more understandable[2].

Vasodilatory diaphoretics are also used in hot conditions affecting the upper trunk, or upper warmer, mainly infectious bronchial and lung conditions as seen in lung heat and lung phlegm Heat syndromes. Moreover, they represent the treatment of choice in all exanthemous (eruptive) conditions such as measles, mumps, chicken-pox and scarlet fever. Here as in all wind heat conditions sweating increases toxin elimination and fever resolution with special emphasis on promoting the eruption of rashes—the visible end result of a successful healing crisis on the exterior or skin level.

Causing sweat as an Eliminating method of treatment has two other applications of no less importance. The first is in chronic internal conditions of **toxemia** or **congestion** involving excretory functions; the second in chronic conditions of **constraint**.

Whereas, in the treatment of external conditions, causing sweat is produced as part of an overall strategy of managing the onset of external infectious conditions, when applied to internal conditions it effectively promotes cleansing by stimulating the elimination of toxins. WILHELM HUFELAND described the skin as "the organism's most general and powerful organ of secretion and cleansing," while PARACELSUS aptly named sweat an excrement of the blood. Clearly, in order to perform its functions as an eliminatory organ, as well as a nervous-sensory one, the entire skin surface needs to breathe freely. Like the lung to which it is closely connected it has to both receive and eliminate, hence it belongs to the rhythmical group of organs which includes the heart, lungs and stomach. When skin breathing is impaired for whatever reason, an important elimination pathway is also obstructed. Sweating is an effective treatment for reestablishing this breathing.

Traditional and modern methods abound for causing sweating, keeping the skin "open" and ensuring ongoing, unimpeded elimination. All traditional cultures use sweat cabins or types of hot baths for maintaining internal cleanliness. Native American sweatlodges, Finnish saunas and Turkish baths are typical examples of these peoples' hygiene. LAZARUS RIVIERE in sixteenth century France was perhaps the first European physician to use sweating as an eliminant method in its own right; he used diaphoresis where the other eliminative techniques were inappropiate.[3] Taking his cue from Native American practices, SAMUEL THOMSON in the second half of the nineteenth century turned sweating into the all-purpose treatment strategy *par excellence*. He thereby initiated an impulse in herbal therapeutics that lasted into the twentieth century, an impulse largely carried out through massive doses of Cayenne pepper. Hydrotherapy, or water treatments, including mineral baths from natural springs, has also been extensively used, especially since JOHN FLOYER's pioneering practice in the English West Country during the early 1700's; examples include the popularized work of VINZENZ PRIESSNITZ, KARL SCHROTH and SEBASTIAN KNEIPP in Germany a century later.

With its secondary cleansing effect, the *diaphoretic* method is important in treating a variety of toxemic and congestive conditions due to poor surface elimination, especially those of a chronic, intractable kind. Rheumatic conditions respond amenably to it, as world-wide empirical use has shown. This is true of both **wind obstruction** with its acute wandering pains and **damp obstruction** with its static chronic pains and neuralgias, as found in sciatica, lumbago, intercostal neuralgia etc. (see p. 665). Conditions of **general plethora** with adiposity, cellulitis, overweight,

The Energetics of Western Herbs

hypertension, etc., also respond well, as does **fluid congestion** with edema extending to the upper body. Any condition presenting rough, dry skin (either warm or cold) with an inability to sweat is improved by the diaphoretic method. Noninfectious, nonallergic skin conditions are typical results of hampered skin breathing: it causes itching, eruptions and, finally, inflammation. Moreover, dry skin is often found in chronic arthritic, rheumatic and diabetic conditions, as well as in Yang Ming Earth, Shao Yang and Yang Ming Metal biotypes. In all these conditions *cleansing stimulant diaphoretics* are used, such as Burdock, Celery seed, Cowslip root, Sassafras, Meadowsweet, Maidenhair fern, Birch, Heartsease and Sarsaparilla. In practice they are often combined with other Class 15 *cleansers*.

The act of perspiring involves not only vasodilation and increased sweat elimination, but relaxation besides. Both nerve and general tissue tone are lowered, creating a *relaxant* effect. Recognizing this, both Chinese and Galenic medicine use *diaphoretics* in conditions of **Qi constraint**. Their *relaxant* effect is ideal in excess Yang people where emotional or mental constraint and tension leads to irritability, unrest, internal spasms and so on. These botanicals are in fact *pungent warm relaxant diaphoretics* such as Inmortal, Linden, Camomile, Cowslip flower, Catnip, Calamint, Hyssop, Black cohosh, Angelica, Pleurisy root, Canada snakeroot and the related European Hazelwort.

Caution: Remedies in this class should not be used with copious sweating, with fluids depletion, blood loss, venereal infections, colitis and bleeding ulcers, or with chronic deficiency conditions such as cancer, TB and diabetes.

A summary listing of all herbs in this class is found on page 691.

Notes

1   HANS SELYE, *The Stress of Life*, Toronto 1976.
2   The mechanism of the righteous Qi as a **warmth** response versus the pathogens, i.e. as a mobilization of the Yang Qi or Wei Qi, is never considered in any Chinese text, yet clearly should be appreciated for a full understanding. As a result, even though Chinese medicine only uses *pungent cool*, not *pungent hot*, remedies for wind heat conditions, this should not blind us to recognizing its time-tested therapeutic effectiveness.
3   Before RIVIERE, Greek medicine tended to have a rigid dependence on the four qualities theory (hot/cold, dry/moist), which explains the relative unimportance of the diaphoretic method in Hippokratic texts. RIVIERE, however, had access to exotic botanicals that the Greeks did not, strong *diaphoretics* such Guaiacum (*lignum Guaiaci*), Sassafras (*cortex radicis Sassafrae*), and China root (*radix Chinae*). These he successfully employed in clearing up chronic, stubborn illnesses, as he records in his *Institutiones Medicae*. In supplementing the inadequate four qualities theory through his own success using the sweating method, RIVIERE brought widespread recognition to it as an important adjunct to other treatment strategies.

Herbs to Cause Sweating and Scatter Wind Cold

PEPPERMINT

Pharmaceutical name: folium Menthae piperitae
Botanical name: Mentha x piperita L. (N.O. Labiatae)
Ancient names: Minthe, Edosmon (Gr)
    Balsamita, Sisimbrium (Lat)
Other names: Menthe poivrée/anglaise (Fr)
    Pfefferminze, Edelminze, Hausminze (Ge)
Part used: the leaf

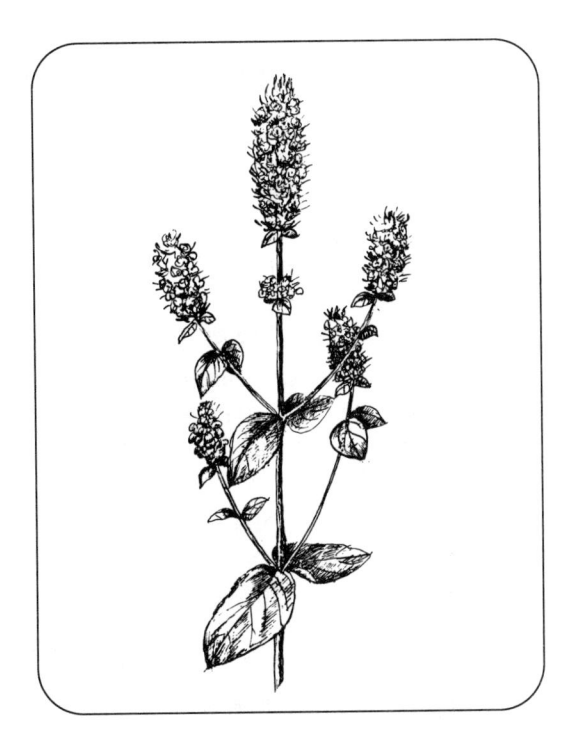

Nature

CATEGORY: medium-strength herb with mild chronic toxicity
CONSTITUENTS: ess. oil (incl. 30-70% menthol, terpenes, menthene, phellandrene, aldehydes), tannin, ketone (menthone), bitters, resins
EFFECTIVE QUALITIES
Primary: *Taste:* pungent, a bit sweet
    Warmth: warm with secondary cooling effects
    Moisture: dry
Secondary: stimulating, restoring, atringing, relaxing
    dispersing movement
TROPISM
Organs or parts: head, heart, lungs, stomach, intestines, gall bladder, liver, uterus, nerves
Organisms: Air & Warmth
Meridians: Lung, Spleen, Liver
Tri Dosas: increases Vayu and Pitta
GROUND
Krases/temperaments: Phlegmatic & Sanguine
Biotypes: Dependant/Tai Yin Earth & Expressive/Jue Yin
Constitutions: all three

Functions and Uses

1   CAUSES SWEATING, RELEASES THE EXTERIOR AND SCATTERS WIND COLD; DRIES DAMP AND CLEARS THE HEAD

external wind cold/heat: onset of cold or flu with fatigue, headache, chills and/or fever

Peppermint: Class 1

head damp cold & lung wind cold: stuffed head and sinuses, watery nasal discharge, chilliness

2. STIMULATES AND WARMS THE LUNGS, INTESTINES AND UTERUS; EXPELS PHLEGM AND PROMOTES THE MENSES; RESTRAINS INFECTION AND CLEARS PARASITES

lung phlegm cold: shortness of breath, full cough with thin white phlegm
CHRONIC BRONCHITIS, asthma, lung TB
intestines mucous damp: gurgling abdomen, lack of appetite, loose stool
ENTERITIS, cholera
ATONIC gastrointestinal ulcers
INTESTINAL PARASITES
uterus damp cold: delayed scanty menses with constant cramps before onset, leucorrhea
uterus Qi constraint: delayed painful menses with clots, moodiness before onset; PMS
SPASMODIC DYSMENORRHEA

3. STIMULATES AND DREDGES THE LIVER AND GALL BLADDER AND PROMOTES BILE FLOW; CLEARS FLATUS AND SETTLES THE STOMACH; RELAXES THE NERVE AND CALMS WIND

liver Qi stagnation: severe frontal or occipital headache, nausea, vomiting, abdominal & right flank pain
CHRONIC HEPATITIS
intestines Qi constraint: painful, difficult digestion with gas and cramps, worse with emotions and stress
Liver Yang rising (liver/endocrine dishramony): dizziness, headache, tremors
MIGRAINE, GALLSTONES, gall bladder spasms
NAUSEA or vomiting due to *stomach Qi reflux*

4. STIMULATES THE NERVES AND RESTORES STRENGTH; BENEFITS THE BRAIN

nerve deficiency: fatigue, weakness
VERTIGO, dizziness, headache, migraine, fainting

5. REDUCES INFLAMMATION AND BENEFITS THE SKIN, RELIEVES PAIN

SKIN INFLAMMATION, burns, scalds, acne, boils
SCABIES, ringworm
RHEUMATIC PAIN, toothache
MOSQUITO and gnat repellant

6. ARRESTS LACTATION AND REMOVES CONGESTION

EXCESSIVE breast milk; for weaning
CURDLED or congested breast milk

Preparations

USE: Peppermint ESSENTIAL OIL is the easiest and most convenient form in use today. It may be taken internally or massaged into the skin with a fatty base oil. An INFUSION is always reliable to fend **wind cold** or **wind heat** onsets of infections, especially with **head congestion**. INHALING is brilliant here, as well as for chest congestion. LINIMENTS can also

Class 1: Peppermint

be made for **painful rheumatic** and **neuralgic** states.

DOSAGE: Smaller doses *stimulate* and *warm*; **larger** ones cause sweating and tend to *relax* and *cool*. Standard doses are used.

ESSENTIAL OIL: 2-4 drops in some warm water

CAUTION: When using the essential oil especially, the doses should never be exceeded, as larger amounts may cause epilepsy. With children or sensitive people on a course of Peppermint (even with Peppermint tea!) it is adviseable to take a few days' break) after a week or so.

Peppermint is contraindicated in all dry conditions, in Yin deficiency, and with gastric hyperacidity.

Notes

Peppermint as a remedy often raises two contradictions: one concerning its warmth, the other its effect on sexual functions. The discussions on Peppermint's "temperature" predate even Renaissance times: we pick up the historical thread with ARISTOTLE who states that it cools the body. For GALEN it is a warm remedy in the third degee. Today's opinions range widely, from an intrinsically cool herb, which after a while creates warmth (or vice versa!), to both warm and cool simultaneously (from its taste), and so on. Contentions of this kind can only be resolved by clarifying the parameters of the debate. For a start, we should consider that the effect of an herb with regard to its warmth may vary according to the condition of the person, the climate and the preparation method. Even the experienced Bavarian doctor LEONHARDT FUCHS never really got close to the problem with his attempt to resolve ARISTOTLE's and GALEN's differences, his explanation being that excessive sexual indulgence caused by Peppermint's warm stimulation causes a cooling of the body. The simple differentiation between the exterior and the interior, one of the most basic diagnostic principles in Chinese medicine, is perhaps of greatest help here. On the whole, and even initially, in hot weather, Peppermint clearly generates warmth. This is **internal warmth** through *circulatory stimulation*. Traditional texts are full of quotes such as "warms a cold phlegmatic liver" (RYFF, 1548), and of indications for **damp cold** conditions of virtually all the organs, including the brain! However, in a hot climate or in feverish conditions, when taken in a larger dose, and especially if drunk hot, it will cause sweating, which effectively cools the exterior and lowers overall temperature if fever is present. In this sense Peppermint replaces *Bo he, herba Menthae,* from the Chinese materia medica. Moreover, since Peppermint, like Yarrow, is a systemic *relaxant* as well as as a *stimulant*, it does equally well with **wind heat** as with **wind cold** onsets, like *Jing jie, herba seu flos Schizonepetae tenuifoliae*. The point being made here is simply this. The final warmth effect of Peppermint will always depend on the precise combination of all these variables of the individual ground and the general environment.

A second contradiction lies in two beliefs held equally vehemently throughout herbal texts: One saying that Peppermint increases sexual drive, and the other, championed by ARNALD DE VILLANOVA, that it "takes away sexual desire, injures the sperm and in the long run causes impotence/infertility." It seems that Peppermint can act as a short term, mild sexual stimulant; and that its dry nature is liable to injure the fluids and the sperm (both being part of the Yin) if used continuously.

Peppermint should not be forgotten as one of the finest **liver** remedies available, with both *chologogue* and *antimigraine* effects, and probably stimulation of hormone metabolism. When thinking of its *stimulant, relaxant, anti-inflammatory* and *anodyne* effects on the **respiratory, nervous** and **reproductive** organs, we concur with OTTO BRUNFELS's conclusion in his 1532 entry on Peppermint: "*Summa summarum,* one could well write an entire book about the virtues of this precious herb."

Ginger: Class 1

GINGER

Pharmaceutical name: rhizoma Gingiberis
Botanical name: Gingiber officinalis Roscoe
    (N.O. Zingiberaceae)
Ancient name: Ziggiberis, Giggiberi (Gr)
    Zingiber (Lat)
Other names: Gingembre (Fr)
    Ingwer (Ge)
    Jiang (Ch)
Part used: the rhizome

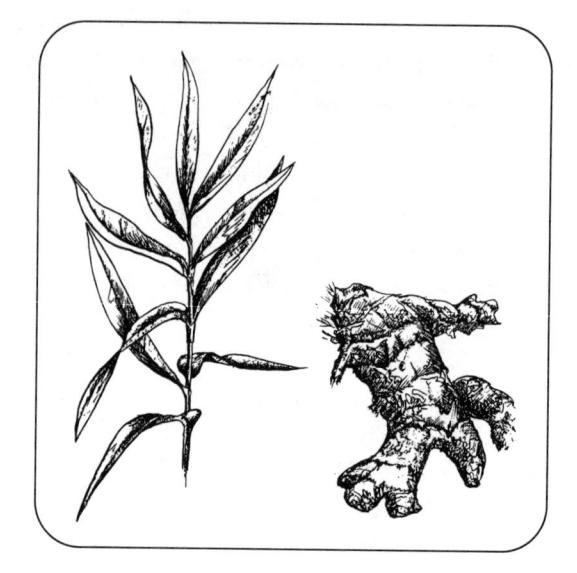

Nature

CATEGORY: mild herb with minimal chronic toxicity
CONSTITUENTS: oleoresin, ess. oil min. 1.5% (incl. phellandrene, camphene, zingiberene, sesquiterpenoid alcohols), gingerol & shogarol, acetic acid, asmazone, acetate of potash, sulphur, lignin
EFFECTIVE QUALITIES
Primary: very pungent, a bit sweet, hot, dry
Secondary: stimulating, relaxing, restoring
    dispersing movement
TROPISM: lungs, digestive system, uterus, immune system
    Warmth, Air organisms
    Lung, Spleen, Stomach meridians
GROUND: Phlegmatic & Melancholic krases
    Dependant/Tai Yin & Burdened/Shao Yin biotypes
    all three constitutions

Functions and Uses

1. **CAUSES SWEATING, RELEASES THE EXTERIOR AND SCATTERS WIND COLD; STIMULATES THE LUNGS AND EXPELS PHLEGM; RELIEVES PAIN**

   external wind cold: onset of cold or flu with dislike of cold, chilliness, fatigue
   wind/damp obstruction: with acute intermittent neuralgia
   CATARRHAL LUNG conditions with external cold

2. **WARMS AND INVIGORATES THE STOMACH AND INTESTINES AND DISPELS COLD; AWAKENS THE APPETITE, MOVES STAGNANCY, SETTLES THE STOMACH AND RELIEVES NAUSEA**

   intestines cold (Spleen Yang deficiency): no appetite, loose stool, chilliness
   ENTERITIS, dysentery
   stomach cold: dull epigastric pain better with massage or eating, vomiting clear sour liquid
   CHRONIC GASTRITIS
   stomach Qi stagnation: difficult painful digestion, flatulence, nausea, loose stool

Class 1: Ginger

NAUSEA or VOMITING in any condition, incl. travel sickness

3   STIMULATES AND WARMS THE UTERUS, PROMOTES THE MENSES AND FREES SPASMS

uterus cold: delayed, scanty or no menstruation with constant cramps, dull red clots, chilliness
MENSTRUAL CRAMPS, painful ovulation
IMPOTENCE due to cold or *Kidney Yang deficiency*

4   ACTIVATES IMMUNITY AND RESTRAINS INFECTION; ANTIDOTES POISON

PREVENTIVE IN EPIDEMICS
BACTERIAL & VIRAL INFECTIONS, scurvy
POISONING from herbs or food
TONSILITIS, laryngitis

Preparation

USE: Ginger may be used fresh or dried, or the ESSENTIAL OIL distilled thereof. The **dried** rhizome together with the TINCTURE, should be used for **internal** digestive or menstrual conditions for best effects, although the dried rhizome DECOCTED will also serve. In conditions affecting the **exterior,** the short DECOCTION of the **fresh** rhizome (with the lid on) has the most dispersing power, causing sweating as it does.

DOSAGE: ESSENTIAL OIL: 1-3 drops several times a day as required
TINCTURE: 2 ml or 50 drops
Other preparations: standard dose

CAUTION: Although Ginger is not contraindicated in patients with peptic ulcers, it should be avoided in stomach fire, as well as in hot lung syndromes. Use with care during early pregnancy, and only for nausea or vomiting.

Notes

Ginger has been as important in the Western pharmacopoeia as in the Far Eastern one, and for similar reasons. Not least of these is its ability to make other remedies in a herbal formula more acceptable to the digestive system through its *warming, carminative, stimulant, antiseptic* and *antitoxic* effects. HENRY BARHAM (1794) talks, for example, about "a corrective of many medecines...[which] taketh away their malice." In this regard also Ginger is an important **Spleen Yang** remedy since "it doth corroborate the naturall heate," also harmonizing menstrual problems due to cold.

As *diffusive circulatory stimulant* Ginger is a good **wind cold** remedy, especially when the lungs are involved; its anti-infective properties are an asset in all bacterial and viral conditions.

Recent research has verified that Ginger has a unique property of assisting other remedies in reaching their destination: it is a tropism enhancer, or an ideal *emissary herb,* that should be included in those combinations where its inclusion is appropriate from the energetic point of view.

Sassafras: Class 1

SASSAFRAS

Pharmaceutical name: cortex radicis Sassafrae
Botanical name: Sassafras officinalis Nees *et* Eberm. (N.O. Lauraceae)
Other names: Ague tree, Cinnamon wood (Am)
Bois de canelle, Laurier des Iroquois (Fr)
Sassafrasholz, Fieberbaum, Fenchelholz (Ge)
Part used: the root bark

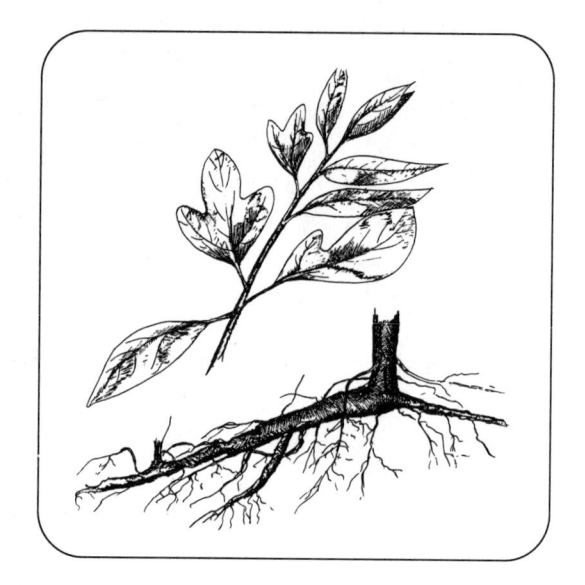

Nature

CATEGORY: mild herb with minimal chronic toxicity
CONSTITUENTS: ess. oil 1-2% (incl. 80% saffrol, pinene, phellandrene, eugenol, camphor), tannin, resin, sitosterol & other sterols, mucilage
QUALITIES
Primary: a bit pungent & sweet, hot, dry
Secondary: stimulating, decongesting, astringing, dissolving
TROPISM: lungs, skin, liver, bladder, kidneys
Air organism
Lung, Spleen, Kidney meridians
GROUND: Melancholic & Phlegmatic krases
Burdened/Shao Yin & Dependant/Tai Yin Earth biotypes
all three constitutions

Functions and Uses

1 CAUSES SWEATING, RELEASES THE EXTERIOR, SCATTERS WIND COLD AND RESOLVES FEVER

external wind cold onset of infections with fatigue, chills
head damp cold with sinus congestion & discharge
wind/damp obstruction with acute pains & neuralgias
REMITTENT FEVERS in Shao Yang stage

2 WARMS AND INVIGORATES THE INTESTINES, LIVER AND UTERUS; ABATES DISTENTION AND PROMOTES THE MENSES

intestines cold (Spleen Yang deficiency) with distention, painful flatus
liver cold stagnation with jaundice, headache
uterus cold with amenorrhea, cramps, infertility
WEIGHT LOSS

Class 1: Sassafras

3   CLEARS STASIS, SEEPS WATER, PROMOTES URINATION AND CLEANSING; STIMULATES AND DREDGES THE KIDNEYS, BENEFITS THE SKIN AND EXPELS STONES

kidney fluid congestion with leg edema
kidney Qi stagnation & *general toxemia* with cystitis, fatigue
CHRONIC RHEUMATISM, ARTHRITIS, GOUT
URINARY STONES
PAINFUL conditions of all types, incl. postpartum

4   RESTRAINS INFECTION AND DRIES DAMP; RESOLVES CONTUSION, RELIEVES PAIN AND BENEFITS THE SKIN

SKIN ERUPTIONS of all types
VENEREAL INFECTIONS with chronic *genitourinary damp cold*
SORES, bruises, chronic ulcers, animal bites

Preparation

USE: An overnight MACERATION in cold water is better than the DECOCTION for retaining all effects, and alcoholic preparations are good—all in standard dosages. The ESSENTIAL OIL if available may be taken in 1-3 drop doses in a little warm water (or hot if sweating is required).

Externally LINIMENTS, POULTICES and the like are used.

CAUTION: Avoid using in all acute inflammations.

Notes

To the progressive Seville physician NICOLAS MONARDES Sassafras was one of the wonders of the New Found World. His eulogies fill 22 pages (in the FRAMPTON translation) of the *Historia Medicinal* which he set down in 1574, and represent the first written record of this exotic wood. In a glowing style appropriate to his subject he narrates how the Native Americans helped the French deal with their infections and fevers with its use (infections engendered "by lying on the ground, and intemperate dyet" adds WILLIAM COLE a hundred years later). He devotes a whole paragraph to its virtues in "griefs of the stone," which it relieves by softening and eliminating them. He also emphasises that "the use of this [Sassafras] water doth make fatter... as those people who come from the Florida do praise it very much," indicating its use in wasting diseases, convalesence and exhaustion. (Chinese medicine would talk about a *Spleen tonic* at this point.) The Renaissance physician's presentation is completed with clinical case-histories, many from his own practice.

But it is only towards the end of his paean that the story-teller leaves off and the therapist really takes over. At long last MONARDES concludes that "it is to be considered, that principally it doth profit in long and cold diseases, and where there is windiness and other evils." He finally recognizes the true identity of this remedy as a *hot circulatory stimulant* and *diaphoretic,* as well as an *eliminant cleanser* in chronic toxemic conditions. And like all good Galenic practitioners of the time he was also aware of the temperaments and types for which is "convenient the use of this water". He leaves us with this warning: "And let them beware if they have much heate, or be of a hot complexion."

Oshá: Class 1

OSHA

Pharmaceutical name: radix Ligustici porterii
Botanical name: Ligusticum porteri Porter (N.O. Umbelliferae)
Other names: Porter's lovage, Indian parsley, Bear medicine, Colorado cough root, Chuchupate (Am)
Part used: the root

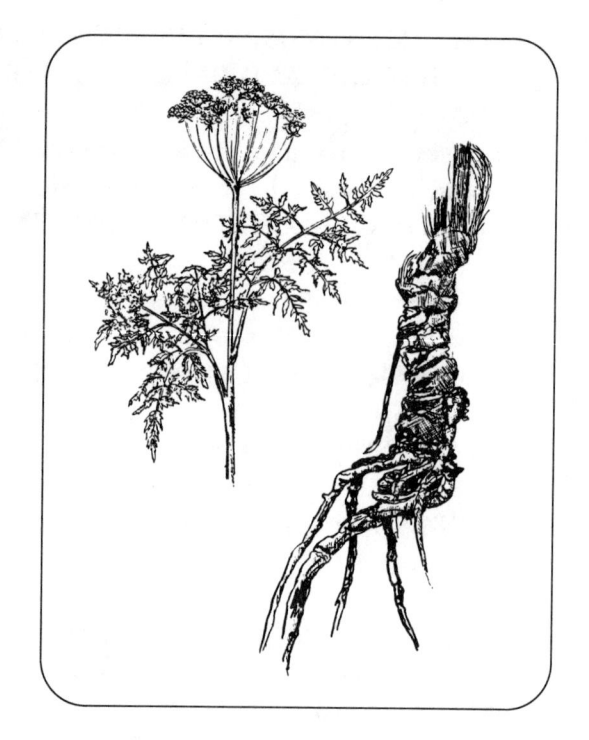

Nature

CATEGORY: mild herb with minimal chronic toxicity
CONSTITUENTS: ess. oil, resin (?), glycoside (?), silicon, bitters
EFFECTIVE QUALITIES
Primary: pungent, a bit bitter, warm, dry,
Secondary: stimuating, relaxing
TROPISM: lungs, stomach, intestines, uterus, kidneys, skin
  Air, Warmth organisms
  Lung, Stomach, Spleen meridians
GROUND: Phlegmatic & Melancholic krases
  Dependant/Tai Yin Earth & Sensitive/Tai Yin Metal biotypes
  Lymphatic/Carbonic/Blue Iris constitutions

Functions and Uses

1   CAUSES SWEATING, RELEASES THE EXTERIOR AND SCATTERS WIND COLD; PUSHES OUT ERUPTIONS

    external wind cold onset of infections with chills, fatigue, aches
    wind damp obstruction with acute neuralgic or rheumatic pains
    ERUPTIVE FEVERS

2   RESTORES AND STIMULATES THE LUNGS, EXPELS PHLEGM AND RELIEVES WHEEZING; RESTRAINS INFECTION AND CLEARS THE HEAD

    lung phlegm cold with coughing up white sputum, asthmatic breathing
    head damp cold (lung wind cold) with nasal congestion and discharge
    VIRAL INFECTIONS of SINUS, THROAT & LUNG with inflammation; minor skin infections
    EMPHYSEMA, silicosis, TB

Class 1: Oshá

3   WARMS AND INVIGORATES THE STOMACH AND INTESTINES; FREES SPASMS, RELIEVES PAIN AND FLATUS

stomach & intestines cold with epigastric pain, vomiting
Spleen Yang deficiency with weakness, loose stool
ENTERITIS, colitis
intestines Qi constraint with colic, distention & flatus
TOOTHACHE

4   STIMULATES THE UTERUS AND DREDGES THE KIDNEYS, PROMOTES MENSTRUATION AND URINATION; EXPELS THE AFTERBIRTH

uterus cold stagnation with delayed or stopped menses, constant lower abdominal pain
SPASMODIC DYSMENORRHEA
STALLED LABOR, RETAINED PLACENTA
kidney Qi stagnation with skin rashes, irregular urination, fetid stool

Preparation

USE: Oshá root is TINCTURED or DECOCTED for best results; equally good if not better is the overnight cold water MACERATION (heat up before serving). An ESSENTIAL OIL can be extracted from the **root** and **seed**, which probably has amplified *antiseptic, antispasmodic, diaphoretic* and *emmenagogue* properties.

DOSAGE: TINCTURE: 1-3 ml or 25-80 drops
                 DECOCTION: 1/2 oz per pint (or 1/2 l) of water

CAUTION: Oshá is contraindicated in deficient Yin and deficient blood patterns due to its *stimulating* nature, and during pregnancy as it is also a *uterine stimulant*.

NOTE: A European mountain plant of the same family, MASTERWORT, *Imperatoria ostruthia*, has virtually identical properties and may be used interchangeably with Oshá.

Notes

In many ways Oshá is the ideal *pungent warm* sweating herb if one happens to live in the regions where it grows. This is the mountain West of America, where it appears at 9,000 feet and increases in abundance with the altitude. Its spiciness is due to an essential oil with a particularly camphoraceous scent and taste, unforgettable once experienced. This makes for a large portion of its effects, although resins and glycosides most likely also contribute. These effects are largely *eliminating* ones, so that Oshá can be thought of as a multi-purpose *eliminant* remedy, where an obstruction or stasis in one of the waste channels exists. In practice it is used mainly to cause sweating, promote tardy obstructed menses and expel phlegm—where **cold** and **stagnation** has set in, as at the end of infections. Specifically, **viral infections** of the **upper airways** are most benefited by this plant, which has more affinity for the **lungs** than any other part. Its silica content helps explain its real *tonic* action on this organ, evident, for example, in the way it prevents scar tissue from forming in emphysema, silicosis, etc.

Very similar types of *Umbellifers* grow in mountain regions the world over. In Europe, for example, Masterwort has an impeccable reputation among Alpine inhabitants for precisely the same complaints treated by Oshá. In China, related *Ligusticum* types also grow aplenty and are similarly used: *Gao ben,* for example, like Oshá is also used to treat wind/damp obstruction and intestines cold with colic and diarrhea. However, Oshá does not relieve headaches caused by wind cold onsets as *Gao ben* has the reputation of doing.

Butterbur: Class 1

BUTTERBUR

Pharmaceutical name: radix Petasites
Botanical name: Petasites hybridus Gaertner,
    Meyer et Scherbius (N.O. Compositae)
Ancient names: Petasites (Gr)
    Bardana maior, Lappacium maius (Lat)
Other names: Langwort, Umbrella leaves, Bog
    rhubarb, Cleats, Eldin, Pestilence wort
    (Eng)
        Pétasite, Chapeau du diable (Fr)
        Pestwurz, Pestilenzenwurz, Grosser
            Huflattich, Schirme, Schweisswurz,
            Deutscher Kostus (Ge)
Part used: the root

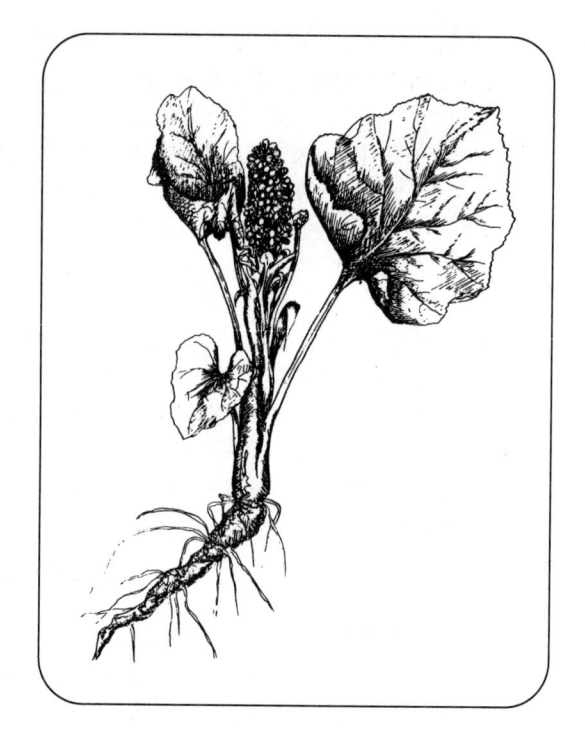

Nature

CATEGORY: mild herb with minimal chronic toxicity
CONSTITUENTS: ess. oil, alkaloid, potassium, helanthenin, inulin, tannins, mucilage
EFFECTIVE QUALITIES:
Primary: a bit pungent & bitter, warm, moist & dry
Secondary: stimulating, relaxing dispersing movement
TROPISM: lungs, skin, heart, kidneys, bladder, uterus, immune system
    Air organism
    Lung, Bladder, Kidney meridians
GROUND: Melancholic krasis
    Sensitive/Tai Yin Metal biotype
    all three constitutions for symptomatic use

Functions and Uses

1   CAUSES SWEATING, RELEASES THE EXTERIOR AND SCATTERS WIND COLD; PUSHES OUT ERUPTIONS; RESTORES THE HEART AND RELIEVES PAIN
    external wind cold onset of infections with head & neck pains, chilliness
    heart Qi deficincy with chest oppression
    wind/damp obstruction with acute neuralgias & rheumatic pains, esp. in lumbars & loins
    ERUPTIVE FEVERS

2   STIMULATES THE LUNGS AND EXPELS PHLEGM; OPENS THE CHEST AND RELIEVES WHEEZING; STIMULATES THE UTERUS AND PROMOTES THE MENSES
    lung phlegm damp with copious phlegm, wheezing, tight chest
    CHRONIC BRONCHITIS
    lung Qi constraint with asthmatic wheezing
    uterus cold with difficult or delayed menstruation

Class 1: Butterbur

uterus Qi constraint with painful menses, PMS
SPASMODIC DYSMENORRHEA

3 DREDGES THE KIDNEYS, HARMONIZES AND PROMOTES URINATION
kidney Qi stagnation with skin rashes, malaise
BLADDER IRRITATION
ANURIA

4 ACTIVATES IMMUNITY, RESTRAINS INFECTION, CLEARS TOXINS AND PROMOTES TISSUE REPAIR; BENEFITS THE SKIN
PREVENTIVE and remedial in epidemics
CHRONIC INFECTIONS, esp. of lungs, skin, bladder
CHRONIC WOUNDS, weeping or running ulcers, sores
SKIN ERUPTIONS and blemishes of all types

Preparation

USE: The TINCTURE or DECOCTION are used internally. A VINEGAR MACERATION was often recommended in the past. LINIMENTS, SALVES, COMPRESSES are used externally.
DOSAGE: standard doses throughout
CAUTION: Butterbur is contraindicated in pregnancy as it stimulates the uterus.

Notes

A new class of remedies should be created to oblige those herbs that could easily belong to any of the six Eliminating treatment methods. This elite of *super eliminants* would consist of botanicals such as Sassafras, Oshá, Wild ginger, the Snakeroots, Hazelwort, Pennyroyal—and Butterbur.

Specific to Butterbur in this connection is its *circulatory* and *cardiac stimulation*. It is ironic to see the Renaissance understanding of immune activation completely justified here (as it is with Lily of the valley, Cowslip, Valerian and many others). WHILHELM RYFF in his large herbal of 1583, for example, talks about its efficacy in "chasing from the body the poison in the heart through sweat." Today we have replaced this lively image, based on the Greek concept of the vital spirit housed in the heart (and corresponding to the Chinese *zheng, qi* righteous Qi), to the impoverished epithet *anti-infective*. We have thereby lost one of the guiding principles of all traditional systems, namely that of tonifying the individual's positive forces, as opposed to merely fending off invading pathogens. In this light Butterbur is as relevant a remedy today as it was in the Middle Ages.

In many ways Butterbur could serve as substitute for the Chinese *Qiang huo, rhizoma et radix Notopterigii*. Both share pungent *bitter warm* effective qualities, and are used in wind cold conditions with headache along the lines of acupuncture points LI 4, Lu 7, GV 14 & 16 and Gb 21, as well as wind damp type neuralgias and rheumatic pain.

With its large Coltsfoot-like leaves Butterbur was once used to wrap up dairy butter. However, women healers in the past knew other, more powerful ways of employing this plant. They used the root for bringing on menstruation obstructed by cold or shock and to relieve painful periods with tension, irritability and other PMS symptoms. They did not particularly need the linguistic refinement of a PITTON DE TOURNEFORT (1686) who later was to write "Les dames vaporeuses se trouvent bien de son usage," —which WILLIAM SALMON might have translated as "Ladies with rising hysterical vapours find it profitable to use."

Virginia Snakeroot

Pharmaceutical name: radix Aristolochiae serpentariae
Botanical name: Aristolochia serpentaria L., vel reticulata Nutt. (N.O. Aristolochiae)
Other names: a) Serpentaria, Snakeweed, Pelican flower, Snagrel, Sangree root (Am)
Couleuvrée/Serpentaire de Virginie (Fr)
Virginische Schlangen/Vipern-wurzel, Virginischer Baldrian (Ge)
b) Texas snakeroot/Ser-pentaria, Red River snakeroot (Am)
Part used: the root

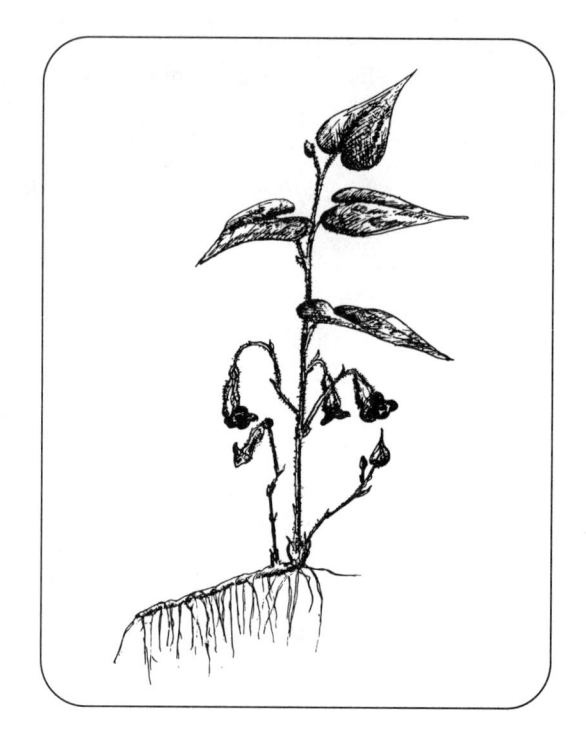

Nature

CATEGORY: mild herb with minimal chronic toxicity
CONSTITUENTS: ess. oil 1-2% (incl. borneol), aristolochic acid, tannins, aristolocampor, sesquiterpenoid (aristolactone), bitter, resin, gum, silica
EFFECTIVE QUALITIES
Primary: pungent, a bit bitter, warm with cooling potential, dry
Secondary: stimulating, decongesting, relaxing
　　　　dispersing movement
TROPISM: arterial circulation, uterus, lungs, intestines, liver
　　　Air, Warmth organisms
　　　Lung, Liver meridians

This remedy is virtually identical in its nature, functions, uses and preparations to WILD GINGER (p. 216) with the one difference that it is not used for promoting labor. It is very likely also to have some uterine stimulant effects, however.

All medicinal plants of the Aristolochia family, including BIRTHROOT, are very similar to, and stronger in effect than, WILD GINGER.

Therapeutically, the Snakeroots resemble *Wei ling xian, radix Clematidis,* from the Chinese repertory, in most of their functions and uses, so that substitution would be possible. Both botanicals treat patterns such as wind cold, wind & damp obstruction, uterus cold, fluid congestion, lung phlegm cold/damp, with lumbar pain, amenorrhea, acute neuralgias and rheumatic pains, and intestinal obstructions.

Herbs to Cause Sweating and Scatter Wind Heat

LINDEN

Pharmaceutical name: flos et folium Tiliae
Botanical name: Tilia cordata Miller, *seu platyphyllos* Scopoli (N.O. Tiliaceae)
Other names: Lime tree, Teil tree (Eng)
  Basswood, Bast tree, Spoonwood, Wycopy (Am)
  Tilleul, Tilleul à petites feuilles, Thé d'Europe (Fr)
  Linde, Steinlinde (Ge)
Part used: the flower and leaf

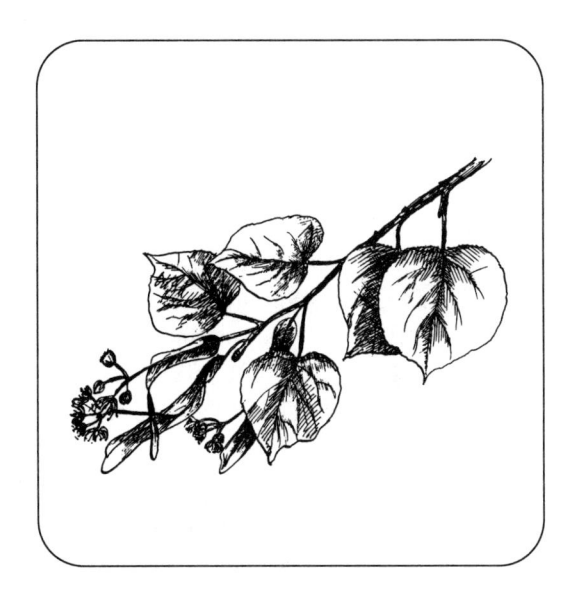

Nature

CATEGORY: mild herb with minimal chronic toxicity
CONSTITUENTS: ess. oil (inc. farnesol), flavonoid glycosides, saponins, quercitroside, protocatechic (condensed) tannins, mucilage, manganese, oxydase, sterols, vit. C, iodine, tartrates, malates, steroidal hormones
EFFECTIVE QUALITIES
Primary: *Taste:* a bit pungent & sweet & astringent
  Warmth: warm, with a secondary cooling effect
  Moisture: dry
Secondary: stimulating, relaxing, calming, dissolving, diluting
TROPISM
Organs or parts: lungs, heart, kidneys blood, central nervous system
Organisms: Air, Warmth
Meridians: Lung, Liver
Tri Dosas: decreases Pitta & Kapha, increases Vayu
GROUND
Krases/temperaments: Choleric
Biotypes: Tough/Shao Yang & Industrious/Tai Yang
Constitutions: Hematic/Sulphuric/Brown Iris

Functions and Uses

1. CAUSES SWEATING, RELEASES THE EXTERIOR, SCATTERS WIND HEAT AND RESOLVES FEVER

   external wind heat: onset of infections with fever, unrest, irritability, no sweating
   lung wind heat: swollen, red sore throat, coughing up yellow phlegm

2. CIRCULATES THE QI AND LOOSENS CONSTRAINT: RELAXES THE NERVE, FREES SPASMS AND CALMS WIND; CALMS THE SPIRIT AND INDUCES REST

Linden: Class 1

Qi constraint with nerve excess: emotional & mental nervous tension and restlessness
kidney Qi constraint: agitated depression, nervous unrest, abdominal cramps & flatulence
Liver Yang rising: headache, ringing in the ears, blurred vision
MIGRAINE
heart Qi constraint: palpitations, anxiety, shortness of breath, cardiac pains
internal wind: trembling, convulsions, stroke, epilepsy
HIGH BLOOD PRESSURE

3   DREDGES THE KIDNEYS, PROMOTES URINATION AND CLEANSING; THINS THE BLOOD AND SOFTENS DEPOSITS

kidney Qi stagnation with general toxemia: skin rashes or dryness, headache, nervousness, painful smelly urination
HIGH BLOOD CHOLESTEROL; uric acid diathesis
HARD DEPOSITS: arteriosclerosis, biliary & urinary stones

4   CREATES ASTRICTION AND ARRESTS DISCHARGE

BLEEDING, esp. from mouth & nose (hemoptysis, epistaxis)
DIARRHEA, dysentery

Preparation

USE: A warm INFUSION of Linden is ideal for children's conditions with constraint—like Camomile, but a bit stronger. Sipped hot it will fend off head and respiratory infections in adults as well as children. The TINCTURE or FLUID EXTRACT is stronger overall and, mixed with some hot water or herb tea, is also suitable for exterior conditions.
Past uses include WASHES on burns, boils and the like.
DOSAGE: standard doses throughout

Notes

There are two equally valid ways of looking at this remedy: as a *relaxing vasodilating diaphoretic,* and as a *diaphoretic cleansing relaxant.* From the first perspective Linden flower is an ideal **wind heat** type sweating agent when irritability, nervous tension and such prevail; it is better than Catnip, Boneset or Fieldmint in this respect. Here it excels with heavyset, excess type people with acute upper or lower respiratory infections where **heat** and **lack of sweat** (i.e. dry skin) predominate, corresponding to the classical Chinese *Ma huang* conformation, and to acupuncture points LI 4, TH 5, Bl 12 and GV 14. When the infection encroaches on the lungs, causing thick yellow phlegm, Linden is still a good remedy, like its Chinese similar *Sang ye, folium Mori albae*.

The second viewpoint, however, has a mirror-image perspective on this herb. Here **Qi Constraint** affecting the **heart, kidneys,** etc. is its field of operation, with spasms, palpitations, tremors, and excessive spirit manifestations such as insomnia and mania—especially with sluggish renal functioning and elimination. As a *relaxant,* therefore, Linden flower has much in common with *Chai hu, radix Bupleuri.* Both also combat high blood pressure and headache due to an excess of Liver Yang.

The overall profile of the Linden sympomatology is clear: it is one where **plethoric, excess** conditions with poor waste fluid elimination through skin and urine lead on one hand to **general toxemia**, with factors such as high blood pressure, sclerotic tendencies, skin and rheumatic conditions; and on the other hand to **excess spirit problems**, where Linden's mild *sedative* effects do well.

ELDER FLOWER

Pharmaceutical name: flos Sambuci
Botanical name: Sambucus nigra L. *seu*
  Canadensis L. (N.O. Caprifoliaceae)
Ancient names: Amantilla, Atrapasse (Lat)
Other names: a) Boretree, Scot tree, Pipe tree,
  Bottry, Devil's wood, Winlin berries
  (Eng)
  European/Common/Parsley elder (Am)
  Sureau noir, Seu, Sognon, Hautbois (Fr)
  Schwarzer Holunder, Holler, Holder, Flieder,
  Alhorn, Keilken, Kisseke, Schwitztee
  (Ge)
  b) American/Black/Common/Sweet elder
  (Am)
Part used: the flower; also the berry, *fructus Sambuci*

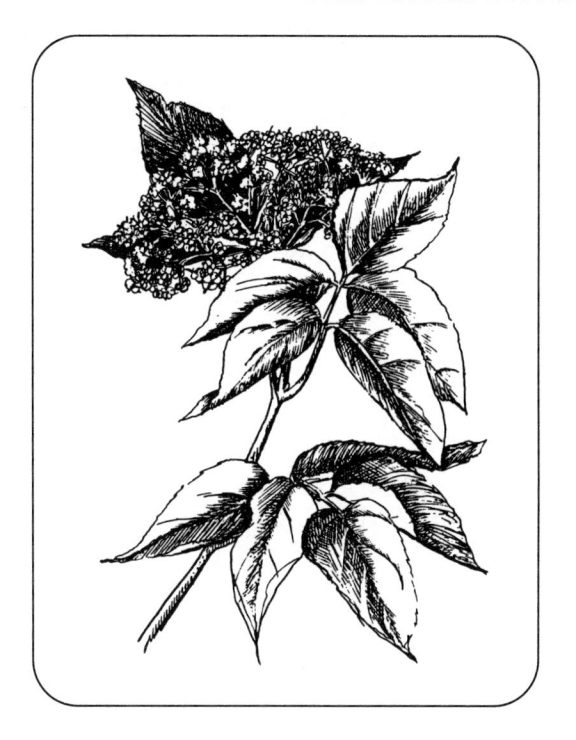

Nature

CATEGORY: mild herb with minimal chronic toxicity
CONSTITUENTS: flavonoids (incl. rutin & quercitin), tannins, mucilage, ess. oil (incl. terpenes), cyanogenic glycoside (sambunigrin, an isomer of prunasin), alkaloid (sambucine), potassium nitrate, resin
EFFECTIVE QUALITIES
Primary: *Taste:* a bit pungent & sweet & bitter
  Warmth: neutral with a secondary cooling effect
  Moisture: dry
Secondary: stimulating, decongesting, softening, dissolving
  dispersing movement
TROPISM
Organs or parts: lungs, skin, kidneys, bladder
Organisms: Warmth, Fluid
Meridians: Lung, Bladder
Tri Dosas: decreases Kapha, increases Vayu
GROUND
Krases/temperaments: Phlegmatic
Biotypes: Self-Reliant/Yang Ming Metal
Constitutions: all three

Functions and Uses

1 CAUSES SWEATING, RELEASES THE EXTERIOR AND SCATTERS WIND HEAT/COLD; PUSHES OUT ERUPTIONS AND RESOLVES FEVER; RESOLVES MUCUS AND DRIES DAMP, CLEARS THE HEAD AND RELIEVES IRRITABILITY

  external wind heat: onset of upper respiratory infections with aches, sore throat, chills and fever, anxiety, irritability

Elder Flower: Class 1

head damp heat (lung wind heat): thick purulent nasal discharge, red swollen sore throat, feverishness, slight chills

head damp cold (lung wind cold): nasal and sinus obstruction, watery nasal discharge, wheezing, chills & slight fever

TONSILITIS, LARYNGITIS, etc.

wind/damp obstruction: acute rheumatic joint & muscle pain

ERUPTIVE FEVERS: smallpox, measles, chickenpox

RHEUMATIC FEVER, HAYFEVER

2 STIMULATES AND RESTORES THE LUNGS, EXPELS PHLEGM AND RELIEVES WHEEZING

lung phlegm damp/heat: full cough with copious expectoration of white/yellow purulent phlegm

BRONCHIAL ASTHMA, bronchitis (acute or chronic)

PNEUMONIA, LUNG TB

3 SEEPS WATER, PROMOTES URINATION AND RELIEVES FLUID CONGESTION; DREDGES THE KIDNEYS, RESOLVES SWELLING, SOFTENS DEPOSITS AND EXPELS STONES

liver fluid congestion: local or general swelling or edema, fatigue, nausea

CARDIAC & renal dropsy

kidney Qi stagnation: headache, dry skin with rashes, abdominal distention, constipation

HARD DEPOSITS: arteriosclerosis, urinary sand or stone

SWOLLEN LYMPH GLANDS

4 CLEARS HEAT, REDUCES INFLAMMATION AND CLEARS TOXINS; SOFTENS BOILS AND DRAWS PUS; BENEFITS THE SKIN

bladder & kidney damp heat: frequent urgent urination, thirst, irritability

URINARY INFECTIONS

fire toxin: purulent sores, boils, furuncles, abscesses, ulcers, especially in the face, head, mouth, throat & lungs

MOUTH & THROAT INFLAMMATIONS, mouth ulcers, meningitis

EYE INFLAMMATION, sore tired eyes

LOW TIDAL FEVERS in Shao Yin stage with deficiency heat

SKIN ERUPTIONS and blemishes, chilblains

5 PROMOTES LACTATION

INSUFFICIENT breast milk

Preparation

USE: In most European countries herbalists, as well as country folk, make a distinction between the flowers, berries and bark of the Elder tree in therapy. While to a large extent all three share similar properties, for best results it is still worth keeping to the following guidelines:

the **flower**:
- for causing sweating and all other function 1 effects
- for restoring and stimulating the lungs, etc., function 2,
- for kidney Qi stagnation and other urinary conditions of function 3

Class 1: Elder Flower

  • for clearing empty heat and inflammation, etc., function 4

the **berry**:

  • for acute or chronic neuralgias, constipation, lung deficiency conditions of all kinds, food poisoning

the **inner bark** and **root**:

  • for **fluid congestion**, nephritis, obstinate constipation, rheumatism & gout

the **leaf**:

  • for skin damp heat (use an OINTMENT), skin cancer, and for support in diabetes

With external conditions, the INFUSION of the **flower** sipped hot is as good as the TINCTURE, while the latter wins out for other applications. EYE WASHES & BATHS, COMPRESSES, GARGLES and the like are useful in external conditions.

Traditional preparations of Elder flower &/or berry include the WINE, VINEGAR, OIL, SALVE, SYRUP, HONEY, PUREE (known as "false Theriac" in the past and made from the **berry**), the WATER, and SMOKE.

DOSAGE: standard doses throughout

Notes

No plant remedy has received more veneration in mythology, nor been put to greater practical use than the Elder tree. Its very name derives from a Greek musical instrument made of its wood, the *sambuke*. It is equally revered in the healing arts, from the ground level of folk use to the herbal physician's clinic. What is said here about it relates mainly to its **flower** and **berry.**

It is in treating **external** conditions involving the **skin, lungs** and **head** that Elder succeeds best. With its *sweet pungent* taste, its energy on the whole is *light* and gently *dispersing*. It also has a *dry* quality which is therapeutically important: all manner of **damp** conditions are helped through its use. These include **mucous damp** with mucosal weakness, congestion and catarrhal discharge (with or without infection) on one hand, and **water damp**, or fluid congestion with local or general edema on the other. Like Yarrow, Ribwort and Tansy, Elder is a *tonic astringent* that restores the mucosa to moderate its secretions. Its gentle stimulation is *vasodilatory diaphoretic,* which also assists in moving fluid congestion, and expectorant in conditions of congested phlegm damp. Truly an ideal remedy for relieving damp, of whatever type. It is used both in acute and chronic conditions of this kind, again testimony of its compassionate versatility.

Clearly, Elder flower could hold its own if asked to replace a Chinese herb for wind heat infectious conditions such as *Niu bang zi, fructus Arctii,* i.e. Burdock seed, or an acupuncture point formula such as LI 4, Lu 11, TH 5 and Bl 11 & 12. With lung conditions, on the other hand, it resembles *Sang bai pi, cortex radicis Mori albae,* or the acupuncture point combination Lu 5 & 10, P6, Bl 12 & 13 and St 40.

But Elder's moderate *bitterness,* moreover, makes for downward movement as well: fluid and waste are moved downwards through hepatic, intestinal and renal stimulation, with a net *cleansing* and *resolvant* effect. In the same vein, Elder flower is a good fever remedy, and any aspect of its energetics or constituents could be adduced in favor of this. The same goes for its *anti-inflammatory* and *antitoxic* property: like Ribwort, it has a solid reputation with symptoms of fire toxin.

Elder is a gentle, effective remedy when used with the right conditions and syndromes, and as **flower** a good ground tonic to the more heavy-set Yang Ming Metal biotype.

Catnip: Class 1

CATNIP

Pharmaceutical name: herba Nepetae
Botanical name: Nepeta cataria L. (N.O.Labiatae)
Ancient names: Kalaminthe (Gr)
  Mentha felina, Mentha gattaria, Herba felis,
    Calamentum maius (Lat)
Other names: Catmint, Catnep, Catswort, Field
    balm (Eng & Am)
  Cataire, Herbe-aux-chats, Chataire, Menthe
    des chats (Fr)
  Katzenminze, Nepten, Katzenraut,
    Nerventee, Bienenkraut, Mutterkraut (Ge)
Part used: the herb

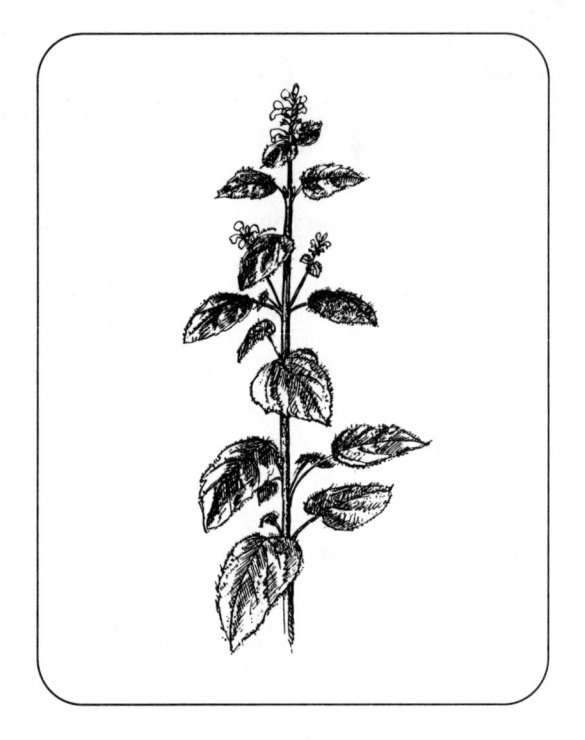

Nature

CATEGORY: mild herb with minimal chronic toxicity
CONSTITUENTS: ess. oil up to 0.7% (incl. nepetalactone 80-90%, camphor, cryophyllenes, dihydronepetalactone, humulene, nepetalacid, thymol, pulegone, aldehyde ester, hydroxylactone), tannin
EFFECTIVE QUALITIES
Primary: a bit pungent & bitter, cool, dry
Secondary: stimulating, relaxing
    dispersing movement
TROPISM: stomach & intestines, nervous system, uterus, skin
    Air organism
    Colon, Kidney meridians
GROUND: Choleric krasis
    Tough/Shao Yang biotype
    Hematic/Sulphuric/Brown Iris constitution

Functions and Uses

1   CAUSES SWEATING, RELEASES THE EXTERIOR AND SCATTERS WIND HEAT; RESOLVES FEVER AND CLEARS THE HEAD

    external wind heat: onset of cold & flu with headache, restlessness, chills & fever, sore throat
    head damp heat/cold: congested head & sinuses, watery nasal discharge, wheezing
    REMITTENT FEVERS in Shao Yang stage

2   CIRCULATES THE QI AND LOOSENS CONSTRAINT, RELAXES THE NERVE AND INDUCES REST

    Qi constraint with *nerve excess:* emotional, mental or nervous tension and unrest

Class 1: Catnip

intestines Qi constraint: abdominal colic, flatulence, indigestion, worse with emotions or stress
kidney Qi constraint with *internal wind:* kidney or sacral or flank pain, nausea, restlessness, agitated depression
TREMBLING, convulsions, hysteria
uterus Qi constraint: irregular or delayed painful menstruation, PMS

3   REDUCES INFLAMMATION AND BENEFITS THE SKIN
SKIN INFLAMMATION, dermatitis
GASTRITIS

Preparation

USES: Catnip should be sipped hot as herbal INFUSION, or the TINCTURE dropped into hot water, for feverish restless onset of infections. The TINCTURE or ESSENTIAL OIL is better for internal conditions of *constraint*. These also may be used for HIP BATHS in **menstrual** conditions or ENEMAS in **colonic** ones.

Catnip's cool quality may be used to advantage **externally** in **painful, hot lesions** or **swellings**, and **muscular pains or cramps**, in addition to **inflammatory stomach** conditions with internal use.

DOSAGE: standard doses throughout

Notes

This cat intoxicating plant is yet another ideal wind heat remedy where the fever is high and the skin still hot and dry. Being a mild herb of the Linden and Camomile type, it is ideal for children's fevers, and combines well with these.

Catnip has two special indications: first, congested head and sinuses with headache, i.e. **colds** in the **head** primarily; secondly, **restlessness** or **delirium**. In this case its nerve *relaxing* properties come nicely into play. As an *anti-inflammatory* and *anodyne relaxant diaphoretic,* Catnip is similar to *Sheng ma, rhizoma Cimicifugae,* from the Chinese materia medica.

Yet Catnip is surely more than a *pungent cool relaxant diaphoretic:* its high essential oil content, as well as traditional usage, points to an effective remedy for Qi constraint at its very root, the kidneys. Its relative CALAMINT, (*Calamintha officinalis* Moench), which was used interchangeably with Catmint in the past, is said to be stronger in this respect. Both are used for unrest of inner, psychic origin. If chronic, these can lead to sensations of internal trembling and finally visible trembling or spasm: internal wind in short.

Spearmint: Class 1

SPEARMINT

Pharmacological name: folium Menthae viridis
Botanical name: Mentha viridis L. (N.O. Labiatae)
Other names: Menthe verte, Nana, Menthe des
   Anglais (Fr)
   Grüne Minze (Ge)
Part used: the leaf

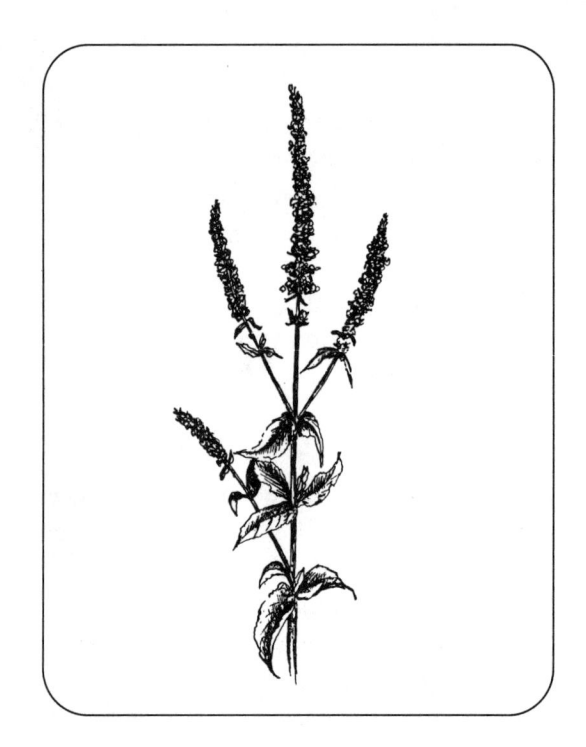

Nature

CATEGORY: mild herb with minimal chronic toxicity
CONSTITUENTS: ess oil (incl. camphor, menthol, menthone, thymol, cineol, limonene, isovalerate), minerals incl. iron, sodium, silicon, copper, chlorine, vit. A & C
EFFECTIVE QUALITIES
Primary: a bit pungent & sweet, cool, neutral
Secondary: stimulating, restoring, relaxing
TROPISM: lungs, upper respiratory system, stomach, bladder & kidneys
   Warmth, Air organisms
   Lung, Bladder meridians
GROUND: all krases, biotypes and constitutions for symptomatic use

Functions and Uses

1 CAUSES SWEATING, RELEASES THE EXTERIOR AND SCATTERS WIND HEAT; REDUCES FEVER

   external wind heat: onset of cold or flu with fever, some chills, headache, restlessness
   lung wind heat: sore throat, head congestion, coughing
   FEVERS in general

2 RESTRAINS INFECTION, REDUCES INFLAMMATION, CLEARS TOXINS AND RELIEVES PAIN

   INFECTIONS incl. upper respiratory, intestinal and urinary with damp heat
   DERMATITIS, burns, boils, wounds, sores
   fire toxin with purulent sores, abscesses
   RHEUMATIC PAIN, toothache
   EARACHE, pain in general

Class 1: Spearmint

3   STIMULATES THE LIVER AND ENDOCRINE SYSTEM; CLEARS FLATUS AND SETTLES THE STOMACH; RELAXES THE NERVE, INDUCES REST AND RELIEVES PAIN

liver Qi stagnation: headache, nausea, vomiting, malaise
INDIGESTION with flatulence
NAUSEA or vomiting due to *stomach Qi reflux*
ENDOCRINE DEFICIENCY in general
INSOMNIA, unrest

Preparation

USE: The ESSENTIAL OIL, TINCTURE and INFUSION of the leaves are used, in decreasing order of strenth. External WASHES, GARGLES, etc. can be prepared from any of these for *antiseptic* and *anti-inflammatory* effects. LEG BATHS or tepid COMPRESSES to the calves and nape of the neck would be good for unrelenting high fever.
DOSAGE: standard doses throughout

Notes

There are several reasons why Spearmint is a good wind heat herb, and comparisons with other *diaphoretic* herbs will define its exact role with more clarity.

First, Spearmint is a true *antipyretic* remedy, able, like Eucalyptus, to lower temperature no matter what else may be going on during a fever. It is also an unambiguously cool herb. This is in contrast to Peppermint which, being essentially *hot* and *stimulating,* resolves fever purely by causing sweating and accelerating all processes involved. Only in wind heat febrile conditions typified by an absence of chills is one liable to have to resort to lowering the temperature, and a wind cold *hot stimulant diaphoretic* like Peppermint might make matters worse if the temperature is high.

Secondly, Spearmint's *relaxant* properties are brought out merely because it does not also have the *stimulant* quality of Peppermint. Spearmint is a *relaxant diaphoretic* which gently opens the pores, thereby cooling the body and eliminating toxins as well as relaxing the nerves, calming and inducing rest, somewhat like Catnip (although definitely less strong in its *nerve relaxant* effect).

Thirdly, Spearmint has excellent *antiseptic* and *lymphatic stimulant* properties, both of which are very useful in wind heat conditions due to infections of any kind. As such, it resembles Marigold, and the two together should often be used for conditions such as tonsilitis, angina, laryngitis, etc. Fire toxin is systematically treated in this context.

Clearly, Spearmint is the closest thing in the West to the Chinese herb *Bo he, Mentha arvensis,* which is actually a type of Fieldmint. They may be used interchangeably, so close are their therapeutic uses, even down to lymhatic swelling. Both generally correspond to an acupuncture point selection such as LI 5, TH 5, Lu 6 & 10, and Bl 11 & 12.

Spearmint's secondary uses result from a tropism for the urinary tract. Here it is known to both decrease frequent dribbling urination and relieve supressed urination. It both *restores* the organs involved and *disinfects, cools* and *relaxes* in damp heat conditions. Clearly, it is invaluable support with stronger remedies or perfect for mild cases such as are found in pediatrics.

Eucalyptus: Class 1

EUCALYPTUS

Pharmaceutical name: folium Eucalypti
Botanical name: Eucalyptus globulus L.
   (N.O.Myrtaceae)
Other names: Australian fever tree, Blue gum tree
   (Eng)
   Eucaltyptus, Arbre à la fièvre (Fr)
   Eukalyptus, Blauer Gummibaum,
      Fieberbaum (Ge)
Part used: the leaf

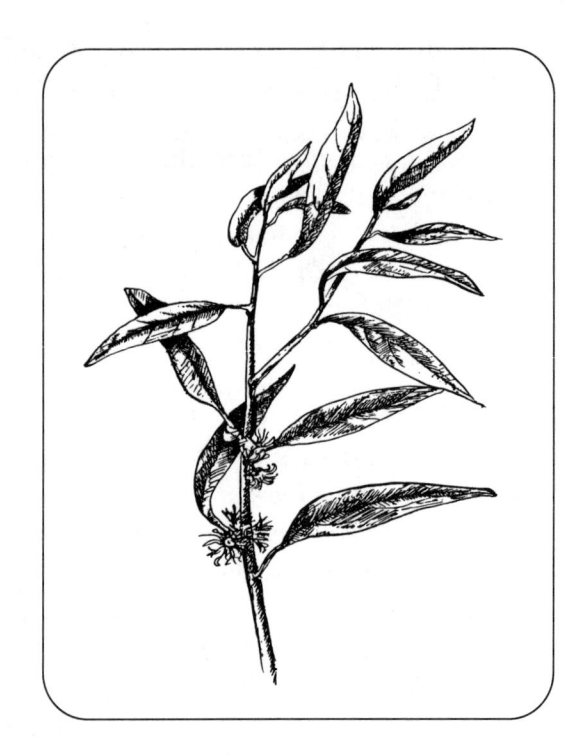

Nature

CATEGORY: mild herb with minimal chronic toxicity
CONSTITUENTS: ess. oil (incl. eucalyptol, phellandrene, aromadendrene, eudesmol, pinene, camphene, valeric aldehydes), tannin, bitter, flavonoid pigment, eucalyptine, bitter resin
EFFECTIVE QUALITIES
Primary: pungent, a bit bitter, cool, dry & moist
Secondary: stimulating, restoring, astringing
         dispersing movement
TROPISM: lower & upper respiratory system, head, pancreas, immune system, blood, stomach & intestines
         Air, Warmth organisms
         Lung, Colon, Bladder meridians
GROUND: Sanguine krasis Charming/Yang Ming Earth biotype
         all three constitutions for symptomatic use

Functions and Uses

1 CAUSES SWEATING, RELEASES THE EXTERIOR AND SCATTERS WIND HEAT; REDUCES FEVER, PUSHES OUT ERUPTIONS, CLEARS THE HEAD AND RELIEVES PAIN

external wind heat: onset of flu or fever with feverishness, sore throat, dislike of cold, aches and pains
head damp heat: nasal and head congestion, watery discharge
SINUSITIS, post-nasal catarrh, otitis
REMITTENT FEVERS in Shao Yang stage, incl. malaria, typhus, cholera
ERUPTIVE FEVERS: measles, chickenpox, scarlet fever
ACUTE RHEUMATISM, neuralgia due to *wind/damp obstruction*
HEADACHES, migraines

Class 1: Eucalyptus

2 STIMULATES AND SOOTHES THE LUNGS, LIQUIFIES AND EXPELS VISCOUS PHLEGM, RELIEVES COUGHING

lung phlegm heat/cold: full cough with copious purulent yellow-green phlegm or with fetid bloody pus, sore throat
ACUTE or CHRONIC BRONCHITIS, emphysema, pneumonia
lung phlegm dryness: coughing up plugs of phlegm, difficult coughing, asthmatic breathing
ALLERGIC ASTHMA (esp. after flu, TB, pneumonia, etc.)
lung Yin deficiency: low afternoon fever, dry mouth & throat, cough with sticky scanty sputum
LUNG TB

3 ACTIVATES IMMUNITY, RESTRAINS INFECTION AND CLEARS TOXINS; PROMOTES TISSUE REPAIR, REDUCES INFLAMMATION AND BENEFITS THE SKIN

LUNG INFECTIONS: whooping cough, pneumonia, dyphtheria, croup, lung abscess
THROAT INFECTIONS with mucous discharge
bladder & kidney damp heat: urgent burning urination, cloudy, mucusy urine, fever
genitourinary damp heat: purulent fetid yellow vaginal discharge, painful urination
UROGENITAL INFECTIONS incl. cervicitis, cystitis, pyelitis, nephritis
SKIN ERUPTIONS: herpes, parasitic skin infections, gangrene
SEPTICEMIA
CERVICAL EROSION
NEURALGIA, neuritis, muscular pain, rheumatoid arthritis
BURNS, WOUNDS, ulcers, abscesses
CHRONIC STOMACH ULCERS

4 EXPELS PARASITES, REPELS INSECTS

ROUNDWORM & pinworm, lice
TOPICAL insect repellant

5 SUPPORTS THE PANCREAS AND LOWERS BLOOD SUGAR

DIABETES (supportive), hyperglycemia

Preparation

USE: The ESSENTIAL OIL of Eucalyptus is used both internally or massaged into the body with a carrier oil. For external use WASHES, POULTICES, LINIMENTS, etc., are used on the skin, while *gynecological* conditions benefit additionally from DOUCHES, PESSARIES (eg. in postpartum care); and **ear, nose** and **throat** conditions from INHALATIONS.

DOSAGE: ESSENTIAL OIL: 2-5 drops three times daily in a little warm water
          All other preparations: standard doses

CAUTION: Because of its *pungent, penetrating* qualities Eucalyptus works best when acute inflammation has died down and become subacute or chronic.

Notes

This relatively recent addition to the materia medica has proved invaluable in three main areas: in **acute external** conditions, in **lung** syndromes and in **malarial** conditions.

As remedy for dealing with external conditions Eucalyptus is a major botanical where **wind**

Boneset: Class 1

heat is concerned—where the fever is high, the throat sore and swollen and the sinuses or head painful. As such it adequately replaces *Xin yin hua, flos Magnoliae liliflorae,* where necessary. In head colds with blocked sinuses with or without signs of heat it is ideal, and this is where inhalations come into their own. Since it causes sweat and alleviates pain, Eucalyptus is very useful in acute rheumatic and neuralgic complaints of the wind or damp type.

Closely connected is its action on the **lungs**, which span syndromes of **empty heat, phlegm heat/cold/dryness**. Here **congestive, spasmodic** and **infectious** conditions with purulence, fetor and secretions are relieved through its *stimulant, relaxant* and at the same time *lenifying* effects. The same applies to genitourinary conditions. As *antibacterial* agent Eucalyptus is fairly strong, belonging, as it does, to the aldehyde group. Like Ginger and several others, it also *stimulates immunity* systemically in the presence of infection.

The specific action of Eucalyptus on malaria is evinced in its transformation of malaria ridden areas wherever it is planted. It was called an *antiperiodic,* meaning that it resolves periodic, i.e. **remittent** and **hectic** or **tidal fevers**—the tertian and quartain agues of the past. Its combination of *spicy* and *bitter* qualities make Eucalyptus an important remedy for the Shao Yang stage, where chills and fever alternate, as well as for the Shao Yin stage, where the fever is recurrent every day or every second/third/ fourth day. Clearly, Eucalyptus is invaluable in a variety of febrile infections.

BONESET

Pharmaceutical name: herba Eupatorii perfoliati
Botanical name: Eupatorium perfoliatum L. (N.O. Compositae)
Other names: Feverwort, Thoroughwort, Indian sage, Crosswort, Agueweed, Teasel, Sweating weed (Am)
   Eupatoire perforée, Herbe à la fièvre, Herbe parfaite (Fr)
   Durchwachsdost, Virginischer Walddosten, Durchwachsurblättriger Wasserhanf (Ge)
Part used: the herb

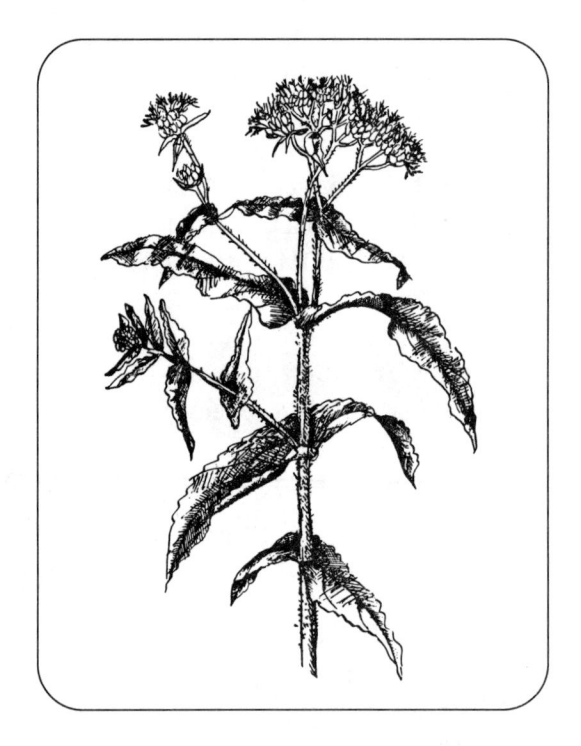

Nature

CATEGORY: mild herb with minimal chronic toxicity
CONSTITUENTS: ess. oil, bitter glycoside (eupatorin), wax, fatty resin (eupurpurin), resin, inulin, tannic acids, unsaturated alcohol (tremetrol), vit. D 1, sugar
EFFECTIVE QUALITIES
Primary: bitter, a bit pungent & astringent, cold, dry
Secondary: stimulating, restoring
TROPISM: lungs, throat, liver
   Warmth organism

Class 1: Boneset

        Lung, Liver, Spleen meridians
GROUND: Choleric *krasis*
        Industrious/Tai Yang biotype
        Hematic/Sulphuric/Brown Iris constitution

Functions and Uses

1   CAUSES SWEATING, RELEASES THE EXTERIOR AND SCATTERS WIND HEAT; RELIEVES COUGHING

external wind heat onset of infections with thirst, deep muscle pains as if in bones, backache, coughing
lung wind heat/dryness with dry irritating cough, hoarseness
COUGHING with measles, asthma in hot conditions

2   CLEARS HEAT AND RESOLVES FEVER; STIMULATES THE LIVER, PROMOTES BOWEL MOVEMENT AND MOVES STAGNANCY

liver fire with constipation, head congestion, feverishness
liver Qi stagnation with right side pain, constipation
JAUNDICE, acute or chronic
REMITTENT FEVER in Shao Yang stage; rheumatic fever

3   RESTORES THE STOMACH/*SPLEEN*, AWAKENS THE APPETITE AND GENERATES STRENGTH

Spleen Qi deficiency with fatigue, no appetite, diarrhea
CONVALESCENCE from acute or chronic fevers

Preparation

USE: The INFUSION and TINCTURE are the best preparations.
DOSAGE: Standard doses are used except for function 3 where **small** doses suffice, drunk warm or cool. **Larger** than normal doses make a safe *emetic*, especially used for conditions in function 2.

Notes

For millions of pioneering (and not so pioneering) Americans of the last century Boneset was **the** remedy for fevers, flus and colds. It was dreaded for its bitter taste by young and old alike, yet valued enough to be found hanging in country attic rafters throughout the year in readiness for use. Native Americans had very early shown white colonists the uses of this Indian sage, and it was apparently even introduced to England in 1699.

Although Boneset is essentially a very simple herb, to appreciate the means by which it achieves its simple results affords us a good insight into the interrelatedness of pharmacological energetics and functions. Bonesets's effects are fundamentally *stimulating* and *restoring*. In small doses it is a good *bitter astringent tonic* in **Spleen Qi deficiency** syndromes, relieving diarrhea, reviving the appetite and boosting energies. Next, it is a *bitter stimulant* suited to relieving **stagnant** and **hot** conditions of the the **liver/stomach/intestines** with constipation and feelings of heat, etc. Finally, its essential oil content assists in creating a *pungent diaphoretic* effect useful in **wind heat** situations with **deep aches and pains**.

It is in fever managment that Boneset's *bitter cold* and *pungent cold* qualities unite to create a superlative all-round *febrifuge* remedy. Its names Agueweed, Feverwort and Sweating weed witness the fact that it is one of the rare botanicals that for over 200 years achieved panacea status

Vervain: Class 1

with all three dominant cultures in America—Native American, African American and European American. Its *bitter cold* energies systemically clear heat by moving digestive stasis downwards; its *spicy vasodilation* causes sweating on the surface; both together rid toxins to shorten defense response. Both taste qualities together, then, conspire to deal with every aspect of fevers. Pleurisy root, Sassafras and Holy thistle are similar to Boneset in this respect.

VERVAIN

Pharmaceutical name: herba Verbenae
Botanical name: Verbena officinalis L., *vel* hastata L. (N.O. Verbenaceae)
Ancient names: Peristereon (Gr)
    Junonis lacrima, Ambrosia, Columbaria, Herba sacra, Verbenaca (Lat)
Other names: Herb of grace, Simpler's joy, Berbine, Ashthroat (Eng)
    Blue vervain, Wild hyssop, Simpler's joy (Am)
    Verveine, Herbe sacrée (Fr)
    Eisenkraut, Eisenreich, Taubenkraut, Segenkraut (Ge)
Part used: the herb

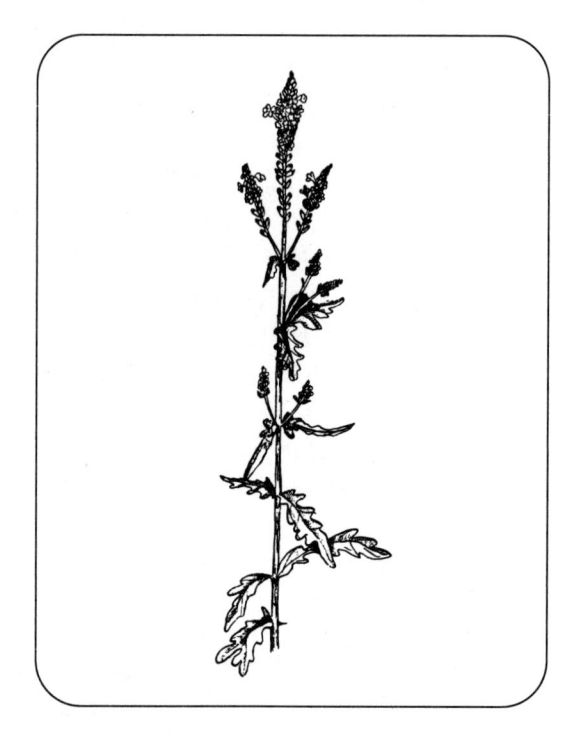

Nature

CATEGORY: mild herb with minimal chronic toxicity
CONSTITUENTS: ess. oil (incl. citral), glycosides (verbenaline & verbanine, bitter, tannins
EFFECTIVE QUALITIES
Primary: bitter, a bit pungent, cool, neutral
Secondary: stimulating, relaxing, restoring, dissolving
TROPISM: lungs, liver, kidneys, stomach, intestines, uterus, skin, nervous system, immune system
    Air, Fluid, Warmth organisms
    Lung, Liver, Kidney, Bladder, Chong & Ren meridians
GROUND: all *krases,* biotypes and constitutions

Functions and Uses

1 CAUSES SWEATING, RELEASES THE EXTRIOR AND SCATTERS WIND HEAT; RESOLVES FEVER AND RELIEVES COUGHING

external wind heat & lung wind heat: onset of infections with fever, weakness, restlessness, coughing
PNEUMONIA, WHOOPING COUGH in initial stages
REMITTENT FEVER in Shao Yang stage

Class 1: Vervain

2   CIRCULATES THE QI AND LOOSENS CONSTRAINT; FREES SPASMS AND RELIEVES PAIN

Qi constraint with deficiency with nervous tension, insomnia
Liver Yang rising (liver/endocrine disharmony) with vertigo, tinnitus, headache
MIGRAINE
intestines Qi constraint with colicky pains, indigestion
lung Qi constraint with asthmatic breathing
uterus Qi constraint with painful irregular menstruation (dysmenorrhea)
NEURALGIA, rheumatism, etc.

3   CLEARS STASIS, PROMOTES URINATION AND CLEANSING; STIMULATES THE LIVER, DREDGES THE KIDNEYS; EXPELS STONES AND BENEFITS VISION

liver & stomach Qi deficiency with no appetite, painful digestion
liver Qi stagnation with jaundice, edema
kidney Qi stagnation with skin rashes
URIC ACID DIATHESIS due to *general toxemia* with gout, rheumatism, skin eruptions
URINARY STONES
POOR VISION; cloud or film over eyes

4   STIMULATES THE UTERUS, PROMOTES MENSTRUATION AND LABOR; PROMOTES LACTATION

uterus Qi stagnation with delayed or stopped menses
AMENORRHEA
STALLED LABOR
SCANTY BREAST MILK
THREATENED MISCARRIAGE

5   RESTORES THE NERVE AND LUNGS, INCREASES THE QI AND CREATES STRENGTH; LIFTS THE SPIRIT AND RIDS DEPRESSION

nerve deficiency with weakness, depression
lung Qi deficiency with poor breathing, despondency, fatigue
CHRONIC NERVOUS DEPRESSION

6   ACTIVATES IMMUNITY AND ANTIDOTES POISON; PROMOTES TISSUE REPAIR, REDUCES INFLAMMATION AND SWELLING; EXPELS PARASITES AND BENEFITS THE SKIN

PROPHYLACTIC in epidemics
POISONOUS bites
INTESTINAL WORMS
WOUNDS, sprains, bruises
MOUTH & GENITAL sores or ulcers, spongy gums
ECZEMA, running sores

Vervain: Class 1

Preparation

USE: Internally the INFUSION or TINCTURE is used. Externally POULTICES, WASHES, OINTMENTS, etc., are appropriate not only for acute conditions but also **chronic painful** ones.
DOSAGE: standard doses throughout
CAUTION: Being a *uterine stimulant,* Vervain is contraindicated during pregnancy, and may only be used immediately before or during labor itself. Paradoxically, Blue vervain, like Wild yam root, has also been successfully used to prevent threatening miscarriage, and should apply to the above mentioned biotypes.
NOTE: There is no significant difference in the uses of the European and the Blue vervain: they may be used interchangeably.

Notes

Vervain is yet another example of a gentle remedy with a very wide field of applications. Unfortunately botanicals such as these lend themselves to erroneous ideas. They are often thought to be dispensable since there are many others more effective for each of the conditions they treat. This may be so, but misses the point that they can deal effectively with a **mixed** condition of disharmony, where both acute and chronic ailments compete for attention.

In complex situations of this kind Vervain excels at a multi-faceted managment approach—like Yarrow and Wood betony, for example. **Qi deficiency** with **constraint, Qi stagnation** and toxemia—common with untreated chronic conditions—would be typical of a Vervain conformation. Its functional profile as a whole should be taken into account if we are to make best use of it. Vervain is clearly not a collection of single effects: plant pharmacology is as mysteriously interrelated as is human physiology itself, of this we may rest assured. Given this, we are in a better position to apply a remedy such as this to a particular **ground**, such as uric acid diathesis and Shao Yang, Jue Yin and Lymphatic biotypes in the case of Vervain.

The mild, undramatic action of Vervain might be another reason for considering it dispensable, along with other gentle, wide-ranging herbs such as Speedwell, Elder, Meadowsweet and countless others. Again, there are sufficient conditions and individuals who actually need a treatment such as this, that is both low-intensity and yet efficacious. European herbals of the last eight centuries, as well as more recent American ones, are replete with testimonies of this.

Although Vervain is very similar to *Chai hu, radix Bupleuri,* it should only be used in the same way after careful consideration. Certainly this is possible with conditions such as wind heat with coughing and restlessness, Shao Yang stage fevers, and Qi constraint including Liver/Spleen disharmony and uterus Qi constraint. Both herbs basically share the same primary and secondary qualitative energetics and effects. Vervain, however, will not raise central Qi with proplapse, is not *relaxant* and *nerve sedative,* nor *liver-protective* like *Chai hu.*

CLASS 2

Herbs to Promote Urination and Relieve Fluid Congestion

Herbs in this class increase the elimination of fluids through urination, irrespective of the volume of water actually drunk. They are said to cause **diuresis**, and are used primarily to treat **fluid congestion**, or water retention. In second place, *diuretics* in this class provoke urination in cases of obstructed or difficult urination, assist in resolving urinary infections, and help promote cleansing for conditions of general toxemia.

Fluid congestion denotes any accumulation of intracellular or extracellular fluid, which are known as dropsy and edema respectively. Although the congestion may occur anywhere, it is liver and kidney functions which are the main regulators of the body's whole fluid organization. Liver Qi deficiency is usually at the bottom of conditions such as generalized edema or edema from the waist down, with possible symptoms such as poor appetite, somnolence, lethargy, withered complexion, a white smooth tongue coat and a deep, slow pulse. This condition is known to Greek medicine as liver fluid congestion.[1] Among the causative factors, allergies, infections and liver cirrhosis are prominent. Treatment aims to stimulate liver functioning and promote urination.

In the case of kidney fluid congestion however, whether due to the presence of kidney disease or not, the edema begins around the ankles and moves upwards, and may be attended by symptoms such as puffy eyes in the morning, lumbar pain, heavy knees, a pale thick tongue and a deep and thin or deep and slow pulse. In this case a stimulation of the kidneys, of the Kidney Yang in Chinese medicine, is neccessary. If the heart is involved causing heart fluid congestion, i.e. cardiac edema due to congestion of electrolytic fluid (chronic congestive heart failure), symptoms will present such as peripheral or central edema, watery stools, muscular weakness, fatigue. This is known as heart & Kidney Yang deficiency fluid congestion in Chinese medicine. Here the treatment is to strongly stimulate the heart and circulation and promote urination.

Fluid congestion is generally treated by causing excess fluid to "seep" downwards (as the Chinese expression goes) through increased absorption and excretion. This seeping process may be compared to water from melting snow percolating or seeping down a mountainside beneath a solid layer of surface snow. The manifest result of this process is an increase of water content in the urine and a reduction of fluid caused swelling. Botanicals that achieve this may be known as *seeping diuretics*: they are true *diuretics* in the original sense of the term.

Many liver herbs that open up liver Qi promote regular fluid metabolism and cause fluid seepage downwards and out. These *hepatic diuretics* tend to have a variety of tastes which are known to engage liver functioning. Some are *bitter cool* due to their bitter substances, such as Dandelion, Squills, Wormwood, Gentian and various thistles. Some are bland, like Asparagus, Sea holly, the Mallows and Couch grass;[2] some are *sour astringent cool* with plenty of organic acids such as Shepherd's purse, Wood sorrel, Herb Robert, Lemon, Grapevine, Blackberry and Lady's mantle. Others, *pungent warm* and *dry,* and belonging to the Umbellifers, which significantly contain essential oils, include Lovage, Parsley, Celery, Wild carrot, Fennel, Sea holly and Buplever. Others yet are *pungent hot,* such as Angelica, Buchu, Juniper, Black pepper, Onion and Garlic: these should be used when fluid congestion is associated with cold.

The Energetics of Western Herbs

Renal stimulant diuretics are also used to relieve fluid congestion, especially with a Kidney Yang deficiency. They include *osmotic diuretics* with their frequent mannitol or saponin content, such as Couch grass, Horsetail, Asparagus, Birch, Cowslip root, Goldenrod, Hydrangea, Restharrow, Rupturewort and Bittersweet.

Thirdly, *cardiac stimulant diuretics* are used, especially where fluid congestion is due to heart & Kidney Yang deficiency. These increase glomerular filtration by increased blood flow to the kidneys. *Diuretics* of this type include Sqills, Lily of the valley, Cereus, Digitalis, Strophanthus, Canadian hemp and Adonis, among others.[3]

Promoting urination is also used for acute conditions with **difficult** and **obstructed urination** (dysuria, anuria) and **urinary tract infections**. Obstructed urination, which may be due to blood congestion, acute fevers, acute or chronic glomerulonephritis or prostate enlargement, causes a dangerous retention of urine. The importance of keeping this excretory channel open at all times to avoid uremia and kidney damage is clear. In addition to those mentioned above, remedies used here include members of the *Cruciferae* family with their mustard oil glycosides; examples include Horseradish, Watercress, Cabbage and Mustard. With urinary infections such as cystitis, urethritis and pyelitis, causing urination is achieved not only by the *cool urinary antiseptics* of Class 13, but equally by the *seeping diuretics* in Class 2. In chronic infections, moreover, the Class 7 *urogenital tonics* (such as Gravel root and Buchu leaf) should also be adopted.

Finally, being an *eliminant* therapy, promoting urination also has a global *cleansing* effect. Causing diuresis is the method of choice when general toxemia, i.e. a general overload of metabolic wastes in the fluids, is caused by sluggish renal functioning due to stagnant kidney Qi. The *diuretics* of choice for this job, however, are the *cleansing diuretics* of Class 15, although most herbs in Class 2, such as Dandelion leaf and Couch grass, also have *cleansing* properties. The latter botanicals, by assisting in the removal of toxins, will speed up the resolution of general toxemia with symptoms such as skin eruptions and headaches, as well as prevent more chronic imbalances such as high blood pressure, the formation of hard deposits (sclerosis and calculi), rising uric acid levels and general bioelectrical imbalances denoting a general fluids dyskrasia. If these more advanced conditions have already set in, Class 15 *cleansing* remedies should be selected by preference.

Caution: The use of *seeping diuretics* should be avoided in conditions of Yin deficiency and fluids depletion.

A summary listing of all herbs in this class is found on page 692.

Notes
1   This syndrome is known in traditional Chinese medicine as Spleen Yang deficiency fluid congestion.
2   Compare the bland tasting remedies of the Chinese pharmacy, such as *Fu ling (Poria cocos), Tong cao (medulla Tetrapanacis), Zhu ling (Grifola),* and *Ze xie (rhizoma Alismatis).*
3   Certain alkaloidal plants are also known to cause urination, among which are Broom (sparteine), Canadian hemp, Dogbane, Adonis, and others.

LOVAGE

Pharmaceutical name: radix Levistici
Botanical name: Levisticum officinale Koch (syn. Ligusticum levisticum L.) (N.O. Umbelliferae)
Ancient names: Ligustikon (Gr)
    Libisticum, Ligusticum (Lat)
Other names: Old English/Cornish/Italian lovage (Eng)
    Livèche, Ache des montagnes, Céléri bâtard, Pavais (Fr)
    Liebstöckel, Grosser Eppich, Maggikraut, Badkraut (Ge)
Part used: the root; also the fruit, *fructus Levistici*

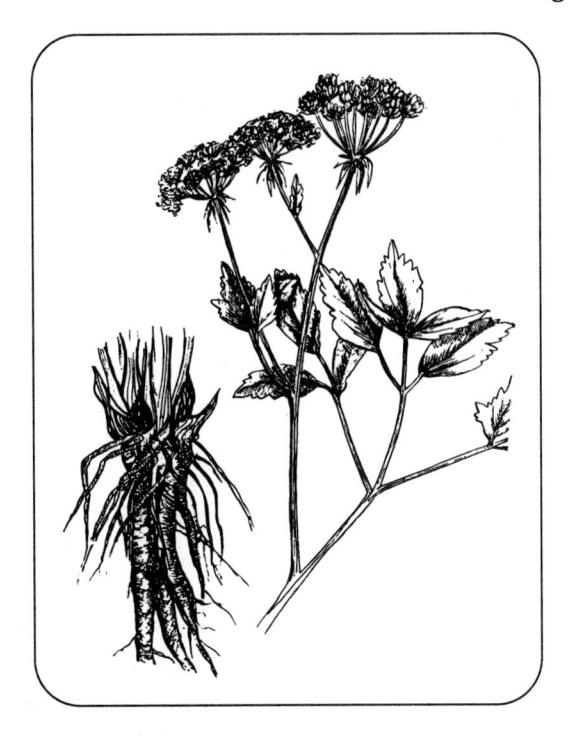

Nature

CATEGORY: mild herb with minimal chronic toxicity
CONSTITUENTS: essential oil (incl. ligustilide, bergapten, umbelliferone, butyl-phthalidin), resins, sugars, coumarin, gum, tannins, malic & angelic acid
EFFECTIVE QUALITIES
Primary: *Taste:* a bit bitter & sweet & pungent
    Warmth: warm
    Moisture: dry
Secondary: restoring, stimulating, decongesting, diluting, dissolving
    sinking movement
TROPISM
Organs or parts: stomach, intestines, liver, uterus, kidneys, bladder
Organisms: Fluid
Meridians: Spleen, Liver, Kidney
Tri Dosas: decreases Kapha, increases Vayu
GROUND
Krases/temperaments: Phlegmatic
Biotypes: Self-Reliant/Yang Ming Metal
Constitutions: Lymphatic/Carbonic/Blue Iris

Functions and Uses

1   SEEPS WATER, PROMOTES URINATION AND RELIEVES FLUID CONGESTION; STIMULATES AND DREDGES THE LIVER AND KIDNEYS; SOFTENS DEPOSITS AND EXPELS STONES

    liver & kidney fluid congestion: tiredness, nausea, water retention from waist or ankles down
    kidney Qi stagnation: headache, skin rashes, constipation
    CHRONIC CYSTITIS, rheumatism, gout

Lovage: Class 2

GENERAL TOXEMIA
HARD DEPOSITS: urinary stones, liver sclerosis, arteriosclerosis
NEPHROSIS
OBSTRUCTED URINATION in any condition

2 RESTORES THE UROGENITAL ORGANS, STIMULATES THE UTERUS, PROMOTES MENSTRATION AND CHILDBBIRTH

genitourinary Qi deficiency (Kidney Qi infirmity): lumbar pain, frequent scanty urination, bedwetting
uterus damp cold: delayed scanty menstruation with continuous lower abdominal pain, dizziness, leucorrhea
uterus Qi stagnation: delayed, short menstruation with pain at start, clotted flow
SLOW PAINFUL LABOR
RETAINED PLACENTA

3 RESTORES THE LIVER AND STOMACH AND AWAKENS THE APPETITE; MOVES STAGNANCY AND ABATES DISTENSION

intestines mucous damp (Spleen damp): gurgling swollen abdomen, fatigue
liver & stomach Qi deficiency: no appetite, abdominal pain & distension
stomach cold: constant dull epigastric pain better with food, nausea, colicky pains

4 RESOLVES SWELLING AND DISSIPATES TUMORS; RESOLVES CONTUSIONS, RESTRAINS INFECTION AND BENEFITS THE SKIN

SWELLINGS, lumps, tumors
SKIN CONDITIONS: acne, psoriasis, eczema, seborrhea
WOUNDS, boils, mouth sores & ulcers

Preparation

USE: The **seed,** not the root, was held to be the most effective by most practitioners in the past (e.g. DIOSKURIDES), probably due to its higher essential oil content. However, either one will make effective medicines in TINCTURE or DECOCTION form (the latter being the less strong). Lovage used externally makes good SALVES, WASHES, etc., for conditions on the skin. HIP BATHS are excellent in suitable menstrual complaints.

DOSAGE: Standard doses apply to all preparations of both root and seed unless the **fresh root** is used, when they should be slightly reduced.

CAUTION: Being *uterine stimulant,* Lovage should not be used during pregnancy. It comes ino its own, however, to promote or ease labor with hypotonic action.

Notes

Lovage root is a wrongly neglected plant both as a *diuretic* and as *digestive remedy.* These labels do little to help us understand its nature, however: so much more is gained by looking at its effective qualities. Lovage combines the *sweet, pungent* and *bitter* tastes, creating a gentle yet penetrating warmth which *restores, stimulates, cleanses* and *decongests.* Working mainly in the **metabolic region**, it addresses conditions of **excess cold** where **stagnation** has set in. Hence it treats accumulated mucous damp in the digestive system (the Spleen), fluid congestion or water damp anywhere due to either/both kidney and/or liver/Spleen Qi stagnation, and damp cold of the reproductive organs with white discharge. In other words, it treats syndromes involving **damp** as are treated by acupuncture points St 40 & 41, Sp 3 & 9, Gb 26 and CV 9 & 12.

A specific indication for Lovage is **painful digestion**, since it frees smooth muscle spasm (essential oil content) as well as promoting digestion through greater secretions. Its traditional use for bladder concretions, anuria and urinary weakness completes the picture of Lovage as an important *urinary remedy*.

One is struck by the similarity with *Bai zhu* and *Cang zhu* in the Chinese pharmacopoeia. One feels sure that Lovage's range of indications will match those of the Chinese *Atractylodes* types.

As **gynecological** agent Lovage has a very solid reputation. Women physicians during the Middle Ages such as TROTULA OF SALERNO and HILDEGARD OF BINGEN, not to mention the thousands of midwives throughout Europe at the time, held it in high regard. All valued Lovage both as a **menstrual** and **obstetrical** remedy. In finding it useful for late, painful menstruation and leucorrhea due to damp cold or Qi stasis in the pelvic or uterine area they were mirroring Chinese pratitioners using *Chuan xiong, radix Ligustici walichii,* and *Dang gui, radix Angelicae sinensis.* Pharmacognosy now supports this practice by finding a similar content of ligustilide and several of its components (giving them their characteristic celery-like scent) in both Lovage and *Dang gui*. Ligustilide, the major component of their essential oil fraction, is said to be responsible for their *uterine stimulant* effect.

In light of this it comes as no surprise to learn that past midwives also esteemed Lovage as a medium-strength *partus preparator* for its *stimulant* and *pain relieving* effects before and during labor. Unfortunately, since the entire legacy of women healers was first supressed and then almost eradicated in the later Middle Ages as a result of the patristic enterprises of church, legal system and medical establishment (including over 300 years of witch-hunts), hardly any records of its uses as a woman's remedy have come down to us. However, this does not prevent us from remembering the true nature of this remedy. We can once again use it properly and as it was used for centuries.

Goldenrod: Class 2

GOLDENROD

Pharmaceutical name: herba Solidaginis
Boptanical name: Solidago virgaurea L. (N.O. Asteraceae)
Ancient names: Virga aurea (Lat)
Other names: Woundwort, Aaron's rod, (Eng)
  Verge d'or, Solidage, Herbe aux Juifs (Fr)
  Goldrute, Heidnisch Wundkraut (Ge)
Part used: the herb; also the root, *radix Solidaginis*

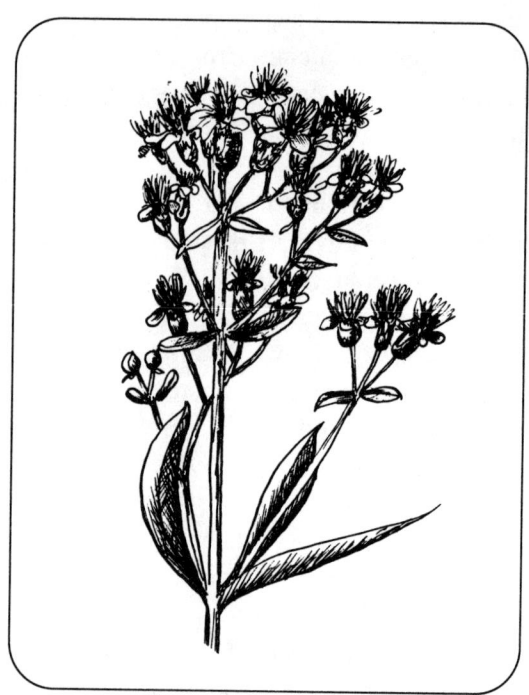

Nature

CATEGORY: mild herb with minimal chronic toxicity
CONSTITUENTS: ess. oil, salicylic acid, catechin tannins 8-15%, saponins, alkaloidal substance, flavonoids 1.4% (incl. quercetin, rutin, quercitrin, isoquercitrin, campherol, astragalin), anthrocyanidin, polyacetylenes, bitter, nicotinic & phenolcarbonic acids, amide, glycoside
EFFECTIVE QUALITIES
Primary: bitter & astringent, cool, dry
Secondary: astringing, restoring, stimulating, decongesting; sinking movement
TROPISM: kidneys, bladder, intestines upper respiratory tract, fluids, blood, skin
  Fluid organism
  Liver, Kidney, Triple Heater meridians
GROUND: Sanguine krasis
  Charming/Yang Ming Earth biotype
  Mixed/Phosphoric/Grey-Green Iris constitution

Functions and Uses

1 SEEPS WATER, PROMOTES URINATION AND RELIEVES FLUID CONGESTION; RESTORES, STIMULATES AND DREDGES THE KIDNEYS; PROMOTES CLEANSING AND BENEFITS THE SKIN

   kidney fluid congestion: swollen ankles and legs spreading upwards, puffy eyes mornings, lumbar pain
   ACUTE ANURIA, e.g. during acute nephritis
   kidney Qi stagnation with *general toxemia:* dry skin, rashes, painful urination, irritability
   ARTHRITIS, gout
   CHRONIC SKIN CONDITIONS: dermatitis, psoriasis, eczema, acne, herpes
   CHRONIC KIDNEY INSUFFICIENCY, chronic nephrosis
   HIGH URINE ACIDITY & CHOLESTEROL, albuminaria
   HIGH BLOOD PRESSURE

Class 2: Goldenrod

2 CREATES ASTRICTION AND PROMOTES TISSUE REPAIR; RESOLVES MUCUS, DRIES DAMP AND ARRESTS DISCHARGE

head damp cold/heat: head & nasal congestion, watery nasal discharge
HAYFEVER
intestines damp heat: loose mucoid stool, fatigue
CHRONIC ENTERITIS or diarrhea
MUCOUS CYSTITIS, white leucorrhea
MENORRHAGIA in all deficiency conditions
WOUNDS, sores, ulcers, ruptures, insect bites
LOOSE gums and teeth, mouth/throat/genital sores & ulcers

3 REDUCES INFLAMMATION AND RESTRAINS INFECTION

CHRONIC URINARY INFECTIONS with *genitourinary damp heat,* incl. cystitis, nephritis, colibacillosis
CHRONIC INTESTINAL INFECTIONS, Crohn's disease, rectocolitis diphtheria

Preparation

USE: Goldenrod may be used in INFUSION or TINCTURE form both for acute and chronic **urinary, respiratory** and **intestinal** conditions. Goldenrod is of good repute as a *vulnerary* with **injuries, ulcers** etc. and should therefore be found in SALVES, WASHES and similar preparations.
DOSAGE: standard doses throughout
NOTE: Two of the numerous American species, *Solidago canadensis* and *S. serotina* have been shown to contain a higher proportion of diuretic constituents than the European Goldenrod; these will therefore meet all the main reqirements above, to say the least.

Notes

Goldenrod is one of numerous remedies which has come down to us through Greek medicine, having been used extensively by healers and physicians of all sorts. In WILLIAM COLE's entry of 1657 we can read how the Oxford dean and herbalist is not above agreeing, for a change, with the infamous *bête noir* of the medical establishment, NICHOLAS CULPEPER, heartily endorsing his opinion that home grown remedies are superior to outlandish remedies "far fetch and dear bought". The same could be said for many botanicals, of course. The truth is that since every plant is unique in its own environment and therapeutic effect it is best suited for the conditions and people of the reguion where it grows: this has been shown experimentally.

Two areas benefit the most from Goldenrod: the **urinary system** and the **upper respiratory tract**. When afflicted by damp heat infections they respond gratefully to its *restoring, drying and anticatarrhal, cooling* and *anti-inflammatory* effects. The kidneys especially are rehabilitated functionally and structurally. Water elimination is increased so that **acute** urinary obstruction (in acute nephritis for example) is promptly relieved. On the other hand Goldenrod can be used for long-term treatment of **urinary** and **hepatic** conditions with **deficiency, stagnation** and **fluid congestion,** where its *antiseptic* properties are an added asset. Clearly, Goldenrod herb has much to recomend it for the replacement of *seeping diuretics* from the Chinese range such as *Yin chen, herba Artemisiae capillaris, Qu mai, herba Dianthi,* and *Mu tong, caulis Akebiae.*

On the other hand, Goldenrod's *tonic astringent* effects are most prominent in the **nasopharinx**. Radically restoring the mucosa in addition to drying up secretions, it is similar to Ribwort, Elder and several others. As a result, chronic, intractable damp cold conditions, or chronic catarrhal infections anywhere along the secreting membrane are treated in a systemic way.

Squills: Class 2

SQUILLS

Pharmaceutical name: bulbus Scillae
Botanical name: Scilla maritima L. (syn. *Urginea maritima* Baker)
Ancient names: Skilla (Gr)
    Squilla, Pancratium (Lat)
Other names: Sea onion, Maritime/red/white squill (Eng)
    Scille maritime, Charpentaire (Fr)
    Meerzwiebel, Mäusezwiebel (Ge)
Part used: the bulb

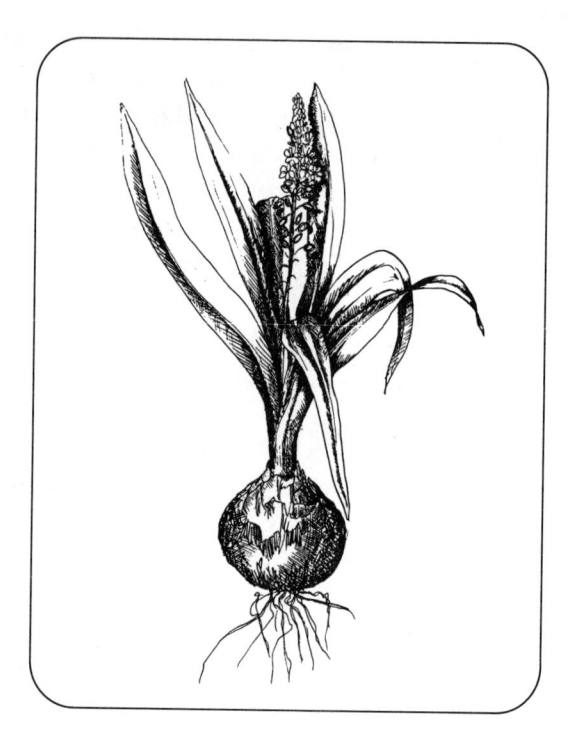

Nature

CATEGORY: medium-strength herb with some chronic toxicity
CONSTITUENTS: cardiac glycosides (bufadienolides: scilaren A & B), mucilage 4-11%, tannin, fixed oil, ess. oil
EFFECTIVE QUALITIES
Primary: a bit bitter & sweet & pungent, cool, moist
Secondary: stimulating, decongesting
TROPISM: kidneys, liver, heart, lungs, uterus
    Fluid organism
    Kidney, Bladder, Lung meridians
GROUND: all krases, biotypes and constitutions

Functions and Uses

1   SEEPS WATER, PROMOTES URINATION AND RELIEVES FLUID CONGESTION; STIMULATES THE HEART AND KIDNEYS AND LENIFIES IRRITATION
    PALPITATIONS, chest oppression due to cardiac insufficiency
    heart fluid congestion with central or peripheral edema
    kidney fluid congestion with leg edema
    ASCITES
    URINARY IRRITATION

2   FOSTERS THE YIN, MOISTENS, SOOTHES AND STIMULATES THE LUNGS; LIQUIFIES AND EXPELS VISCOUS PHLEGM AND RELIEVES COUGHING
    lung Yin deficiency with dry cough, afternoon fever
    lung wind dryness with dry unproductive cough, dry throat
    lung phlegm dryness with scanty viscous phlegm
    DRY, IRRITATING COUGH, hoarseness

Class 2: Squills

3   CLEARS STASIS AND DRAINS PLETHORA; STIMULATES THE LIVER AND UTERUS; DREDGES THE KIDNEYS AND PROMOTES THE MENSES

liver Qi stagnation with jaundice, flank pain
kidney Qi stagnation with high chloric & uric acid, scanty urine
GENERAL PLETHORA with overweight, abdominal distension
uterus Qi stagnation with delayed, painful menstruation

Preparation

USE: The DECOCTION, TINCTURE, FLUID EXTRACT and POWDER are all good. Traditional preparations of this highly regarded remedy include Squills WINE, VINEGAR, OXYMEL and SYRUP.

DOSAGE: Smaller dosages are used for its *demulcent* and *expectorant* effect in the lung and chest area, while larger dosages are more *diuretic* and *stimulating* to cardiac and renal functions.

DECOCTION: 2-7 g per pint of water for three doses
TINCTURE: 0.25-2 ml, i.e. 10-50 drops
POWDER: 0.05-0.10 g as *expectorant;* 0.10-0.50 g as *diuretic*

CAUTION: Avoid doses higher than these for safety, and take breaks of several days after ten days if using continuously to avoid Squills' low toxicity from building up.
Squills is forbidden during pregnancy, as it promotes uterine contractions, and in damp heat conditions with acute inflammation.

Notes

Squill bulb has always played an important part in Galenic medicine as a strong *diuretic*. As a *cardiac stimulant* useful in heart fluid congestion, or with general heart Yang deficiency symptoms, Squills increases the water in the urine, relieving edema due to both faulty renal and cardiac functioning. Its cardioactive glycosides are cause in this; they are nonaccumulative, like the glycosides in Lily of the valley and Cereus.

At the same time Sqills is used where physical accumulation of adipose tissue, mucus, etc. exists, causing toxemia and overweight. In this context PIERANDREA MATTIOLI in the sixteenth century praised Squills as "an egregious medicine for the maintenance of human health," claiming that its use was first discovered by PYTHAGORAS.

In correcting a variety of **lung** conditions with **dryness** Squills evinces important *cool moist demulcent* and *lenitive* as well as *secretolytic expectorant* effects. This puts in on a par with the equally moist Chinese *Yin tonics* such as *Mai men dong, radix Ophiopogonis,* and *Bai he, bulbus Lilii,* both used for the same dry lung conditions. Anyone who has a chance to compare the similar physical consistency and feel of these three plants will be in no doubt about this.

Wild Carrot: Class 2

WILD CARROT

Pharmaceutical name: radix seu fructus Dauci
Botanical name: Daucus carota L. (N.O. Umbelliferae)
Ancient names: Daukon (Gr)
Other names: Queen Anne's lace, Bird's nest (Eng & Am)
Carotte (Fr)
Karotte, Möhre, Gelbe Rübe (Ge)
Part used: the root or the fruit

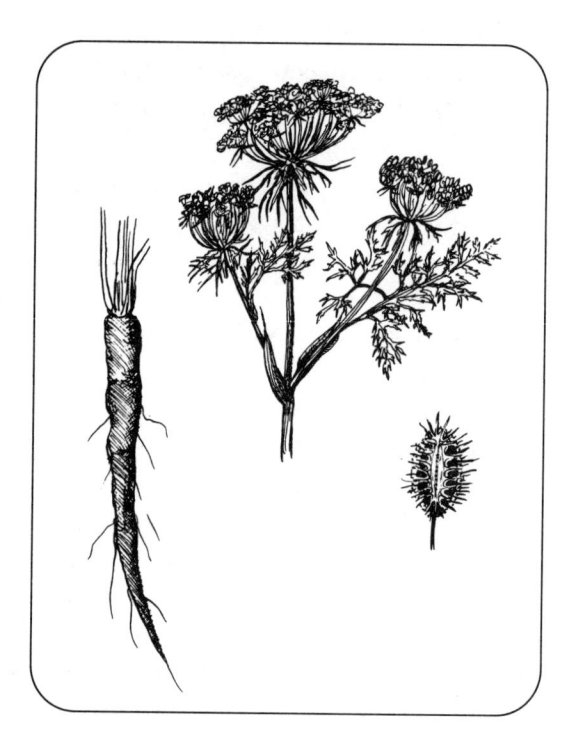

Nature

CATEGORY: mild herb with minimal chronic toxicity
CONSTITUENTS: ess. oil, carotene, vit C, B1, B2, B6, E, H, glucose, sucrose, pectin, malic acid, xantophyll, pentosane, asparagin
EFFECTIVE QUALITIES
Primary: a bit bitter & sweet & pungent, neutral, moist
Secondary: stimulating, relaxing, decongesting, dissolving
sinking movement
TROPISM: bladder, kidneys, uterus, intestines, stomach
Air, Fluid organisms
Bladder, Kidney meridians
GROUND: Sanguine krasis
Charming/Yang Ming Earth biotype
Lymphatic/Carbonic/Blue Iris constitution

Functions and uses

1   SEEPS WATER, PROMOTES URINATION AND RELIEVES FLUID CONGESTION; STIMULATES AND DREDGES THE KIDNEYS, PROMOTES CLEANSING AND SOFTENS STONES

kidney fluid congestion with leg edema, puffy eyes
kidney Qi stagnation with *general toxemia* with malaise, skin rashes, gout
URIC ACID diathesis
URINARY STONE or sand

2   STIMULATES AND RELAXES THE UTERUS AND INTESTINES; PROMOTES THE MENSES AND EXPELS THE AFTERBIRTH

uterus Qi stagnation with delayed, painful menstruation

Class 2: Wild Carrot

RETAINED PLACENTA
intestines Qi constraint with flatulent colic
CHRONIC COUGHS, hiccough

3 **RESTORES THE UROGENITAL ORGANS, HARMONIZES URINATION AND ENHANCES SEXUAL DESIRE**
genitourinary Qi deficiency (Kidney Qi infirmity) with impotence, frequent scanty urination
bladder Qi constraint with difficult, painful or obstructed urination
CHRONIC NEPHRITIS

4 **RESOLVES SWELLING AND DISSIPATES TUMORS; PROMOTES TISSUE REPAIR**
SWELLING, sores, abscesses, carbuncles
TUMORS, lipomas
WOUNDS, rodent or gangrenous ulcers
SKIN DRYNESS or pruritus

Preparation

USES: The short DECOCTION or TINCTURE of the **root** is used. POULTICES are used externally, or the root pulp applied **raw**. The ESSENTIAL OIL extracted from the **seed** is more strongly *antispasmodic* and *anodyne* as well as *diuretic* and *emmenagogue,* and may be used to enhance labor contractions and expel the placenta.
The fresh JUICE of domestic organically grown carrots, drunk regularly, goes quite some way in dealing with the symptomatology above if taken over a longer period.
DOSAGE: DECOCTION & TINCTURE: standard doses
                    ESSENTIAL OIL: 2-6 drops in some warm water
CAUTION: Carrot seed or its essential oil are forbidden during pregnancy as it may stimulate uterine contractions.

Notes

Wild carrot is a good remedy for all general purposes of *promoting urination* in kidney deficiency conditions. Its action unfolds almost entirely on the **urinary** and **genital** system and is primarily a *stimulant* one. Together with its *decongestant* effect on fluid congestion primarily in the lower limbs, Wild carrot has a *restoring* edge locally and a *cleansing* effect on all fluids and tissues, like all good *diuretics*. VAN HELMONT himself, in the sixteenth century, was full of praise for its stone dissolving effects.

GALEN classes Carrot seed as one of the **minor warming seeds.** It was subsequently much used in compound formulas by Persians such as AR-RAZI and PSEUDO-YUHANNA, and, in the words of eighteenth century Parisian pharmacist PIERRE POMET (1694) "expels Wind, and is good against pains of the Wombe and Bowels, vehement Colicks, Vapours and Hysterick Fits.".. ("Hysterick" here means *uterine,* from the Greek *hysteros,* womb.) Its ability to stir sluggish or lost menstruation and relieve attendant cramps, as well as to expel sticky placentas, was much used in the past. Today we have the convenience and advantage of using the extracted essential oil for more reliable effects in this area.

Dandelion leaf: Class 2

DANDELION LEAF

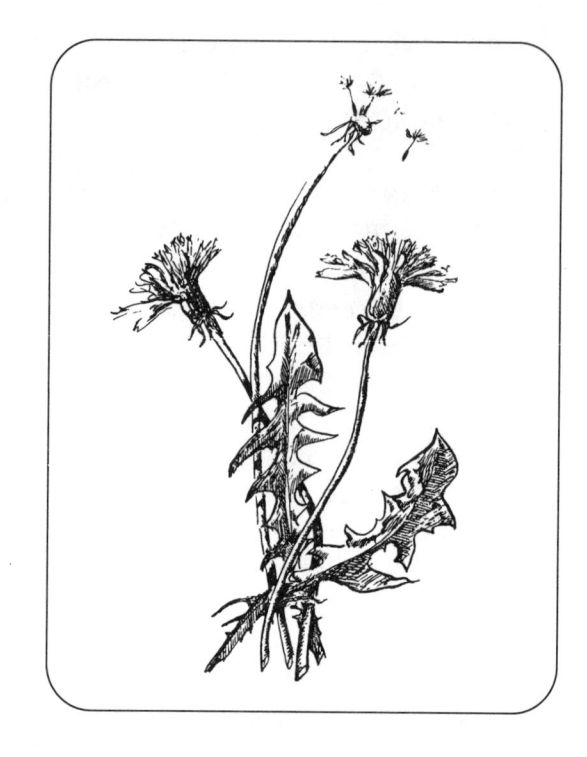

Pharmaceutical name: folium Taraxaci
Botanical name: Taraxacum officinale Weber
    (N.O. Compositae)
Part used: the leaf

Although Dandelion leaf is identical in its constituents, qualities, functions and uses to DANDELION ROOT (p. 580), its higher potassium content (among other things) makes it a powerful diuretic. Hence it is used in all types of fluid congestion, i.e. edema with swelling, as well as supportively in high blood pressure.

Preparation

USE: The fresh JUICE, INFUSION or TINCTURE of the **freshly dried** leaf is used. The FREEZE DRIED EXTRACT, if available, is the next best thing to the fresh JUICE itself. After several weeks some of the potency of the dried leaves is already lost. The young leaves are also EATEN in salads in spring, along with other *cleansing* greens such as Lamb's lettuce (Cornsalad) and Endive.
DOSAGE: JUICE: 10 to 20 ml three times a day; standard doses otherwise

ELDER BARK

Pharmaceutical name: cortex Sambuci
Botanical name: Sambucus nigra L. (N.O.
    Caprifoliaceae)
Ancient names: Amantilla, Atrapasse (Lat)
Other names: Boretree, Scot tree (Eng)
    European/Common/Parsley elder (Am)
    Sureau noir, Seü, Sognon, Hautbois (Fr)
    Schwarzer Holunder, Holler, Holder, Flieder,
        Alhorn, Keilken, Kisseke, Schwitztee
        (Ge)
Part used: the bark

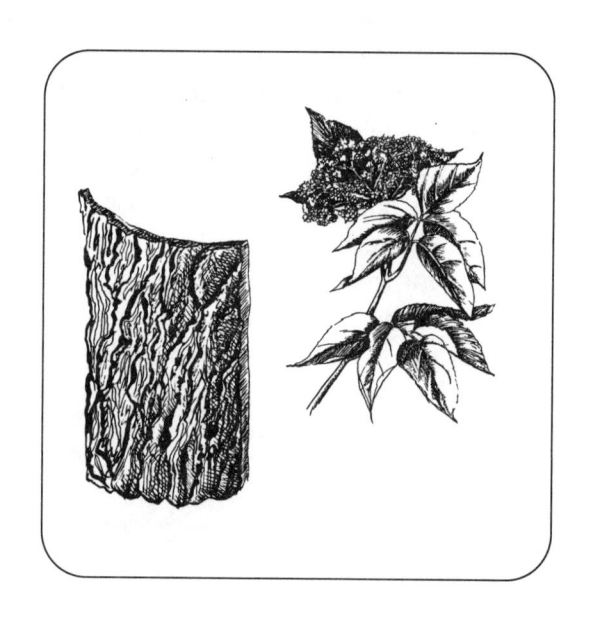

Class 2: Elder Bark

Nature

CATEGORY: mild herb with minimal chronic toxicity
CONSTITUENTS: (see Elder flower, p. 121)
EFFECTIVE QUALITIES
Primary: a bit bitter & pungent, dry, warm
Secondary: stimulating, decongesting, dissolving
sinking movement
TROPISM: liver, kidneys, intestines
Fluid organism
Liver, Kidney meridians
GROUND: all for symptomatic use

Functions and Uses

1 SEEPS WATER, PROMOTES URINATION AND RELIEVES FLUID CONGESTION; STIMULATES THE LIVER AND DREDGES THE KIDNEYS, PROVOKES BOWEL MOVEMENT AND PROMOTES CLEANSING

liver & kidney fluid congestion with local or general water retenion, nausea
GENERAL TOXEMIA
CHRONIC GOUT, arthritis, rheumatism
NEPHRITIS
OBSTINATE CONSTIPATION
EPILEPSY (as emetic in larger dose)

Preparation

USE: The DECOCTION and TINCTURE are both used.
DOSAGE: Standard doses, exceeded only if a safe emetic effect is needed.
CAUTION: Being highly *stimulant,* Elder bark is contraindicated in pregnancy as well as in Yin deficiency and in fluids depletion conditions.
NOTE: Besides the Eurtopean elder, two other types of Elder may be used for their *diuretic* and hence *cleansing* effect: first, the root of Dwarf elder, (Danewort, Blood elder, Walewort, Wild elder), *radix Sambuci ebuli* (of which the fruits are poisonous); secondly, the root bark of the Red elder, *cortex radicis Sambuci racemosae* (of which the seeds are poisonous). The bark of the American elder, *Sambucus canadensis,* should not be substituted for this herb as it contains much more toxic hydrocyanic acid and the alkaloid sambucine than the European elder.

Couch Grass: Class 2

COUCH GRASS

Pharmaceutical name: rhizoma Tritici
Botanical name: Triticum repens L. (syn.
    Agropyrum repens Beauv. (N.O.
    Gramineae)
Ancient names: Agrosis (Gr)
    Gramen dioscoridis/caninum (Lat)
Other names: Twitch grass, Dog grass, Quich
    grass, Wickens (Eng)
    Quack grass, Witch grass (Am)
    Chiendent (Fr)
    Quecke, Rechgrass, Quickengrass,
    Schliessgrass, Rebel (Ge)
Part used: the rhizome

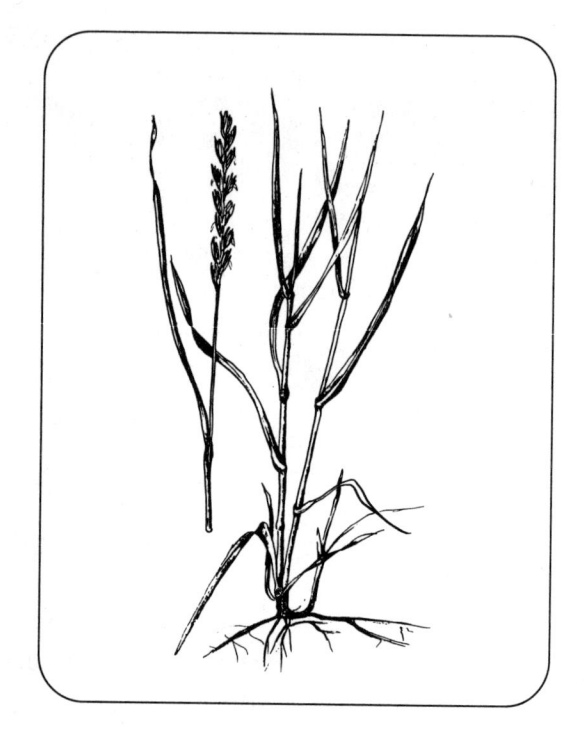

Nature

CATEGORY: mild herb with minimal chronic toxicity
CONSTITUENTS: mannitol, inositol, saponins, mucilage 8%, inulin-like triticin, silicic acid, organic acids, glycosides, iron, trace minerals, antibiotic substances, vit. A & B
EFFECTIVE QUALITIES
Primary: a bit sweet & bland, cold, moist
Secondary: nourishing, stimulating, decongesting, softening, dissolving
    sinking movement
TROPISM: bladder, kidneys, intestines, lymphatic system, skin
    Fluid organism
    Kidney, Bladder, Liver, Three Heater meridians
GROUND: all krases, biotypes and constitutions for symptomatic use

Functions and Uses

1. SEEPS WATER, PROMOTES URINATION AND RELIEVES FLUID CONGESTION, DREDGES AND STIMULATES THE KIDNEYS AND LIVER; PROMOTES CLEANSING, ENLIVENS THE LYMPH AND BENEFITS THE SKIN
    kidney & liver fluid congestion with leg or general edema
    kidney Qi stagnation with *general toxemia* with chronic skin eruptions, muscular rheumatism
    LYMPH CONGESTION, esp. chronic swollen glands

2. RELAXES AND MOISTENS THE UROGENITAL ORGANS, HARMONIZES URINATION, LENIFIES IRRITATION AND PAIN
    GENERAL BLADDER IRRITATION with difficult, urgent urination
    PAINFUL urination or stone passage
    DERMATOSIS

3 CLEARS HEAT, REDUCES INFLAMMATION AND RESOLVES FEVER; RESOLVES MUCUS AND DRIES DAMP; SOFTENS BOILS AND DRAWS PUS

bladder damp heat due to acute infections, with discharge
intestines damp heat due to acute infections with mucopurulent stools
INFECTIONS of urinary and intestinal tract
CATARRHAL conditions of intestines & bladder with white discharge
skin damp heat with boils, abscesses, furuncles

4 STRENGTHENS THE LUNGS AND REPLENISHES DEFICIENCY

ANEMIA, scrofulosis, rickets
LUNG conditions with deficiency, e.g. TB

Preparation

USE: The pressed JUICE, DECOCTION, TINCTURE or GLYCERINE EXTRACT are all good preparations.
DOSAGE: Larger than standard doses may be used in complete safety if required.

Notes

The rhizome of this common weed furnishes one of the more versatile urinary remedies used in herbal medicine. Unlike some *diuretics,* which do a specific job, Couch grass may be used successfully in a number of different urinary disharmonies. On one hand, Couch grass is a remedy *for* **chronic** conditions. Containing much mucilage, it is a *urinary demulcent* with a *sweet, moist* taste. Here it joins Cornsilk, the Mallows, Hydrangea and Licorice with its soothing, *lenitive* effect ideal for irritative conditions. At the same time, Couch grass is one of the strongest *seeping diuretics* of all (mannitol, saponins), goading the liver and triple warmer as it does into managing the fluid economy as a whole (its significant *choleretic* effect is a part of its liver tropism). As such, it closely resembles the *sweet bland diuretics* used in Chinese medicine such as *Yi yi ren (semen Coicis), Tong cao (medulla Tetrapanacis)* and *Dong gua ren (semen Benincasae),* some of which also contain saponins, and its actions correspond in the main to an acupuncture formulation such as CV 3 & 9, Sp 9, Li 8, and Bl 22 & 28.

In addition, Couch grass is more intense in its *cleansing* effect than all others in this class: this is ensured by a generous trace minerals content. These trace minerals also account for its secondary applications in blood deficiency conditions, consumption, etc. **Lymphatic congestion** with chronically swollen glands and **eczemas** both dry and suppurative come into its orb (as with Cleavers, Nettle and Figwort...).

On the other hand, **acute** conditions of **damp heat** with purulent discharge are also manageable with Couch grass, conditions where the *antiseptic* substances and the organic acids also play a large part. This herb goes quite some way in replacing *Ze xie (rhizoma Alismatis)* and *Di fu zi (fructus Kochiae scopariae)* from the Chinese herbal range. In severe cases, stronger *cold disinfectants* such as Birch, Celery and Uva ursi should be added, as well as others according to the whole symptom picture presented.

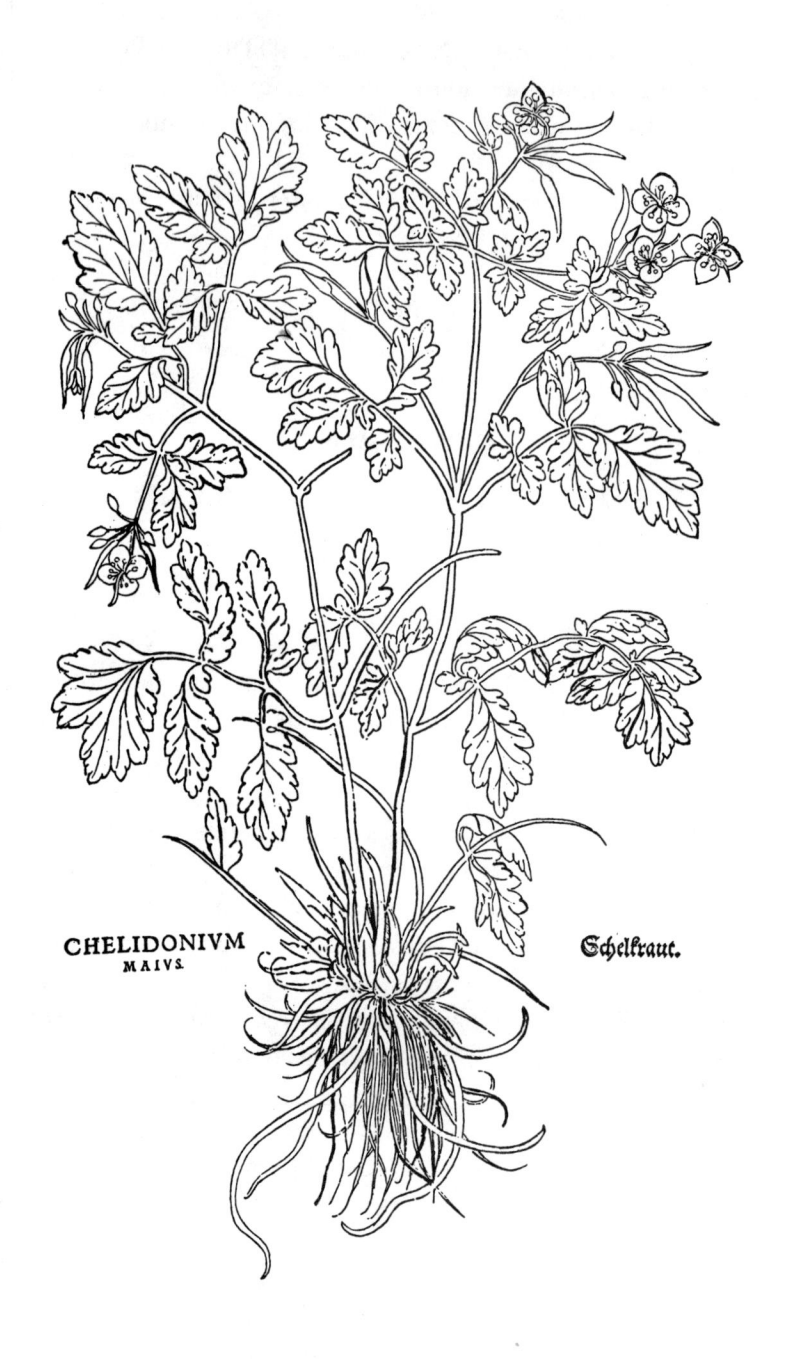

Celandine

CLASS 3

Herbs to Promote Bowel Movement and Relieve Constipation

Botanicals in this category in one way or another promote bowel movement, also known as purging. They are used primarily where bowel movement has become sluggish, causing a retention of feces. These herbs effectively break up an eliminatory obstruction and induce a natural elimination of waste by stimulating colonic peristalsis. Secondarily, they are also used to alter systemic conditions for purposes of rebalancing.

Constipation may have a variety of origins, all of which should be examined so that the right type of herb—one that will rebalance the overall syndrome in addition to relieving the symptom of constipation—may be selected. Shallow breathing, lack of exercise, inadequate dietary roughage, raw fruits and vegetables, excessive cheese consumption, insufficient water intake, nervous fatigue and emotional upsets are among the major causes of constipation.

When used for the local treatment of constipation, the aim of promoting bowel movement goes beyond just emptying bowel contents. The long-term objective is to create a regularity which assures a spontaneous and timely evacuation of colonic contents.[1] With the assistance of indicated lifestyle and dietary measures even the most rebellious colon can eventually be managed. Promoting bowel movement in this sense is as much **preventive** of toxic conditions as it is **remedial** of constipation. Its importance as a prophylactic cannot be overestimated.

The purging method not only deals symptomatically with various types of immediate constipation, but also radically treats the many conditions that bring constipation in their wake. These may be divided into two types, Qi stagnation and dryness. Typical syndromes include intestines Qi stagnation, liver Qi stagnation, intestines dryness and intestines dry heat.

Since constipation is found in a wide variety of conditions, it is important to distinguish between them and use the herbs appropriate to each.

1 HERBS TO REMOVE INTESTINAL STAGNANCY, ABATE DISTENTION AND PROMOTE BOWEL MOVEMENT

Botanicals in this class remove stagnation in the central and lower intestinal tract resulting from **intestines Qi stagnation** or **intestines damp cold**. Typical symptoms are abdominal distention, sensation of weight in the abdomen or pelvis, lack of appetite, stale taste on awakening in the morning, nausea, constipation with occasional watery stool, a dirty grey or brown tongue moss and a tight, slippery or full pulse. If left untreated the accumulation and stagnation of metabolic by-products causes increasing toxicity and toxic mucus accretion.

Remedies used for this condition are *stimulant laxatives* of the most general kind, which cause free bowel movement within eight hours. They are used either occasionally in otherwise healthy people, or regularly, on a more long-term basis, for chronic conditions—but then only in the context of rebalancing the overall disharmony. The main herbs used vary from gentle *laxatives* such as Yellow dock, Licorice, Rhineberry and Tamarind to active *laxatives* such as mineral salts (e.g. Glauber's and Epsom salts), Rhubarb, Buckthorn, Cascara sagrada and Senna seedpods, and to active *purgatives* such as Senna leaf and Aloes. Some of the more active ones may cause a certain degree of griping or cramping. They are made more bearable when combined with *spicy*

The Energetics of Western Herbs

carminatives, small fruits with much essential oil, such as the seeds of Anise, Fennel, Cumin, Coriander, etc. *Stimulant laxatives* all vary in their qualities of warmth and taste, due to the variety of constituents which stimulate peristalsis. It is important to choose the most appropriate herb according to the duration and type of condition, the ground of the individual person, his or her constitution and other conditions. For example, Senna leaf and Aloes are hot in quality and are therefore contraindicated in all *hot* and congestive conditions.

Another type of botanical used to relieve intestines Qi stagnation is the *bulk laxative*. These gentle, safe herbs are often found in commercial preparations and are more suitable for long-term use. They swell up when drunk with warm water and increase peristalsis through their sheer bulk in the colon. Psyllium husks and the bran of grains (e.g. rice or wheat bran) are the best *bulk laxatives*.

2 HERBS TO STIMULATE THE LIVER AND GALL BLADDER, BREAK UP OBSTRUCTION AND PROMOTE BOWEL MOVEMENT

These botanicals remove upper digestive tract stagnation and obstruction causing dull pain and distention while eating, acid regurgitation, nausea, constipation, fat intolerance, a swarthy complexion, right flank or midback pain, headache, moodiness, low will power, depression, and a tight, full pulse. These symptoms are typical of **liver Qi stagnation** involving as it does biliary insufficiency with chronic dyspepsia.

Remedies that open liver Qi, break up obstruction and move the bowels are known to stimulate the flow of bile and other digestive secretions. They stimulate the entire digestive tract to digest and assimilate normally, in the process helping to dredge and evacuate stagnant food, mucus and other toxins. Botanicals such as Blue flag, Fumitory, Celandine, Oregon grape and Milk thistle belong in this category. Known as *choleretic* or *cholagogue laxatives,* they have proven to have a particular affinity for Shao Yang, Yang Ming Metal and Tai Yin Earth biotypes. It is their *bitter* and *pungent* qualities which stimulate and deobstruct. These herbs also combine well in most conditions where they may be needed as back-ups. They may require extended use, depending on the severity of the condition and the tenacity of the constipation. The *warm* quality botanicals in this category, such as Culver's root, Celandine, Holy thistle and Rosemary may be used to treat constipation due to cold. This is typically found with liver Yang deficiency and liver cold stagnation. Both have symptoms of chilliness, cold limbs, nausea and occipital or frontal headache; with the former syndrome there is additional debility, a pale tongue with no moss and a slow, weak pulse; with the latter there is thick white tongue moss and a slow, tight, full pulse. Class 7 *warm Qi tonics* (all types) and Class 8 *hot circulatory stimulants* should be added as appropriate.

Cholagogue and *choleretic laxatives* are contraindicated with blood congestion in the pelvis (e.g. with hemorrhoids, with large gallstones and with blood in the stool.

3 HERBS TO CLEAR HEAT AND PROMOTE BOWEL MOVEMENT

Remedies in this category also treat internal excess conditions of the intestines, but only in hot conditions such as **liver fire** and **intestines dry heat** (in the Yang Ming stage). The heat of a fever may cause internal dryness through excessive fluid absorption, with constipation or small, dark, dry feces. Typical attendant symptoms are intense congestive headaches, sweating, thirst, feverishness, irritability, delirious speech, yellow dry tongue moss and a fast or slippery full pulse.

The botanicals used are *cold laxatives* and *purgatives*. There are two types. The first are saline *laxatives* that work by osmosis, including sea vegetables such as Kelp and Bladderwrack, sea trace mineral products and Epsom and Glauber's salts. Their *salty* quality naturally softens and moistens, enhancing digestion as well as breaking up stagnant waste and promoting bowel movement.

The second type is *cold anthraquinone purgatives* such as Rhubarb, Cascara sagrada and Alder buckthorn; their action is due to the alkaloid anthraquinone. Being *cold*, *bitter* and *downward-moving* by nature, they should be avoided during pregnancy. Since their action is only engaged in the presence of normal bile secretion, if the latter is insufficient, as in liver Qi stagnation, they should be combined with *choleretic laxatives* in the category above. They are often used in conjunction with Class 13 herbs in order to clear heat and resolve fever.

4 HERBS TO MOISTEN THE INTESTINES AND PROMOTE BOWEL MOVEMENT

Herbs in this category moisten or lubricate the intestinal wall to induce bowel movement when there is insufficient mucus. They are used in **dry** conditions of the **small** and **large intestine** with chronic constipation, in the context of patterns such as **Yin deficiency, blood deficiency** and **fluids depletion.** Intestinal dryness may arise acutely due to hemorrhage or fluid loss, or chronically during convalescence after fevers, following childbirth, from an overindulgence in physical exercise such as running, or simply from old age. These *laxatives* tend to have mildly *sweet*, *cool* and *moist* qualities. Because of their high mucilage content they are known as *demulcent laxatives*. Psyllum, Cannabis and Flax seeds, dried Tamarind fruit, and Prune, Peach, Apricot and Plum kernels all cause a slipping of bowel contents due to the lubricating effect of their fatty oil. They are particularly suitable for children, pregnant women and the elderly.

Demulcent laxatives should be used in combination with herbs that treat the main imbalance. In the case of Yin deficiency with internal dryness, for example, Class 10 herbs that foster the Yin and promote moisture are chosen to complement these *laxatives*.

Another, equally important aim of causing bowel movement is to generate changes in other parts of the body. Although constipation is usually present, here relieving it is not the primary consideration. Of real import is the **heat clearing** and **draining** effect of purging downwards, as well as its **decongesting** and **cleansing** one through the fluid organism. The recognition that purging, judiciously used, can generate deep and lasting systemic changes, thus producing a conversion in the entire organism, is as old as history itself. Egyptian, Indian Ayurvedic, Greek, Chinese and Tibetan medicines all used, or still use, purging as a treatment strategy. It is particularly well developed and articulated in the Ayurvedic medical canons, the Susruta and the Charak Samhita, written before the emergence of Greek medicine. HIPPOKRATIC texts as well as those of GALEN discuss purging as the treatment of choice in **plethora**, i.e. excess conditions, where one or several of the *four chumoi* (fluids) are in excess. Important and highly successful doctors such as LAZARUS RIVERIUS (Montpellier), THOMAS SYDENHAM (London), HERMANN BOERHAAVE (Leyden), WILHELM HUFELAND (Berlin) and JAMES HAMILTON (Edinburgh)[2] made regular use of this method for a wide variety of conditions, often with astonishing results. Causing bowel movement and bloodletting were the most extensively used (and often misused) treatment methods in Western Galenic medicine. Today we may in addition draw on colonic irrigation therapy for achieving the same results as those obtained by *laxative* herbal and mineral remedies. As HAMILTON points out, traditional enemas do not have the same effect since they cleanse only a part, not the whole, of the colon.

The *purgative* method can be used in conditions involving **full heat at the Qi level**, such as stomach fire, gall bladder fire, gall bladder damp heat, liver fire, heart fire, Spleen damp heat, intestines dry heat and fire toxin. Inflammatory diatheses of all kinds (especially **below the waist**) come under consideration here, and include conjunctivitis, iritis, otitis media, cholecystitis, bronchitis, enteritis, appendicitis, cellulitis, endometritis and chronic nephritis. For these, both *cold laxatives* such as Glauber's or Epsom salts, Rhubarb, Buckthorn, Cascara sagrada and Tamarind,

The Energetics of Western Herbs

and *hot laxatives* such as Senna and Aloes may be used.[3] The energetically draining effect of purging may be used in spirit excess cases of mental or emotional conditions such as manic-depressive syndrome, psychotic states and manic conditions in general.

Purging also addresses the two main forms of stagnation: **congestion** and **toxemia**. It relieves any type of fluid congestion by promoting the downward seepage and elimination of exudates and transudates. Uterus blood congestion, pelvic blood congestion, heart blood congestion, liver fluid congestion, abdominal plethora[4] and head congestion are the main congestive syndromes helped by this treatment method. With any kind of blood congestion only *cool* and *cold purgatives* are indicated, however: *hot, irritant* herbs such as Senna and Aloes are contraindicated.

In cases of severe **fluid congestion**, nevertheless, where fluid accumulation needs to be rapidly reduced, *hydragogue purgatives* should be adopted. This drastic method of treatment is indicated for acutely dangerous fluid congestion in the chest or abdomen (as in pleurisy and ascites), or whenever very strong purging is required. These herbs produce instant violent diarrhea which rapidly flushes out excess fluid. Since they irritate the bowels so strongly, to avoid injuring the Qi and the Yin they should be used with great care in children and the elderly, as well as in all deficient conditions. They include Jalap, Hedge hyssop, Mercury, Colocynth, White bryony and Poke root, and are fairly toxic. They should be avoided entirely wherever the vitality is low and should always be supplemented by herbs from Class 7 which increase the Qi and restore.

Since purging directly alters the entire fluid environment, any overload of wastes is eased and toxicity is gradually cleared with its use. Purgation was dubbed an *antidyskratic* treatment in the past for this very reason. As such it can also be used as supportive treatment in all **toxemic** conditions with **excess** and in general plethora as well as general fluids dyskrasia and the resulting scrofulitic, skin and uric acid diatheses, including eczema, herpes, erysipelas and inflammatory arthritis. Finally, and purely empirically, inducing bowel movement has been found eminently useful for the following other types of conditions; children's conditions such as jaundice of the new-born, cramps, fits and convulsions, hot conditions and skin complaints, as well as infectious conditions in general. In the case of infections, causing bowel movement may be used at the onset to mitigate the process and at the very end to remove toxins and avoid complications.

Caution: Causing bowel movement is best avoided in severe deficient conditions, with exhaustion, with chronic diarrhea, gastrointestinal bleeding and severe abdominal pain. During pregnancy, only a few herbs in this class are suitable.

A summary listing of all herbs in this class is found on page 692.

Notes

1   Its function in the short or long run is to reestablish the colon as a powerful rhythmical organ with spontaneous peristalsis; an organ where "radical change" *(bian hua)* can take place—in contrast to the slower rhythmical, more gradual transformation-assimilation processes which take place in the upper and middle digestive tract.

2   JAMES HAMILTON, director of the Royal Infirmary, Edinburgh, *Observations on the Utility of Purgative Medicines,* Edinburgh, 1805.

3   From the times of the Greek-Galenic practice up to the present century, clearing heat through purging was carried out not only with tartaric acid salts such as sodium bitartrate and cream of tartar, but also and especially with that old standby Calomel. Calomel, a highly toxic mercurous chloride, was very much a two-edged remedy: it produced spectacular results when specifically indicated and used according to precise dosage, condition and ground, and unfortunate effects

when not. Eclectic physicians such as SCUDDER and WEBSTER at the end of the nineteenth century gave exact indications, which include tongue, urine and other signs that they considered called for its possible use (see *King's American Dispensatory)*. Physiomedicalists, on the other hand, considered Calomel too unreliable and unpredictalble in its effects, since, unlike botanical remedies, it works directly against the vital force, not with it. Calomel's traditional reputation was stellar to the extent that it aquired such flattering titles as *Mercurius dulcis, Draco mitigatus* and *Panacea mercurialis.* It was used (the Eclectics and Physiomedicalists would say abused) for a wide range of stagnant congestive, inflammatory and febrile conditions, and had a special reputation with chronic articular rheumatism; Biliary and Choleric biotypes were said to respond best to it. However, JOHN KING was emphatic that "there is no single remedy known to man which has produced a greater amount of mischief by its *indiscriminate* use than mercury" (italics original). In contrast to the issue of bloodletting, therefore, the question of whether there is any condition for which nothing else will act as swiftly and effectively as Calomel is virtually overruled by considerations of its unpredictable, Russian roulette type action. Certainly, the possibility of using mercury in homeopathically potentized form clearly obviates the need to rely on larger physical doses of this important remedy.

4   Abdominal plethora is a Galenic syndrome which is actually the result of liver Qi stagnation combining with intestines Qi stagnation. Here the accumulation of toxic metabolites and portal congestion together create chronic abdominal distention, constipation, etc.

Celandine: Class 3
Herbs to Stimulate the Liver and Gall Bladder, Break up Obstruction and Promote Bowel Movement

CELANDINE

Pharmaceutical name: herba seu radix Chelidonii
Botanical name: Chelidonium majus L. (N.O. Ranunculaceae)
Ancient names: Chelidonion (Gr)
　　Erundina, Meliton (Lat)
Other names: Tetterwort, Greater celandine (Eng)
　　Chélidoine, Eclaire, Salogne, Herbe aux Hirondelles (Fr)
　　Schöllkraut, Schwulstkraut, Augenkraut, Schinnkraut (Ge)
　　Bai qu cai (Ch)
Part used: the herb or root

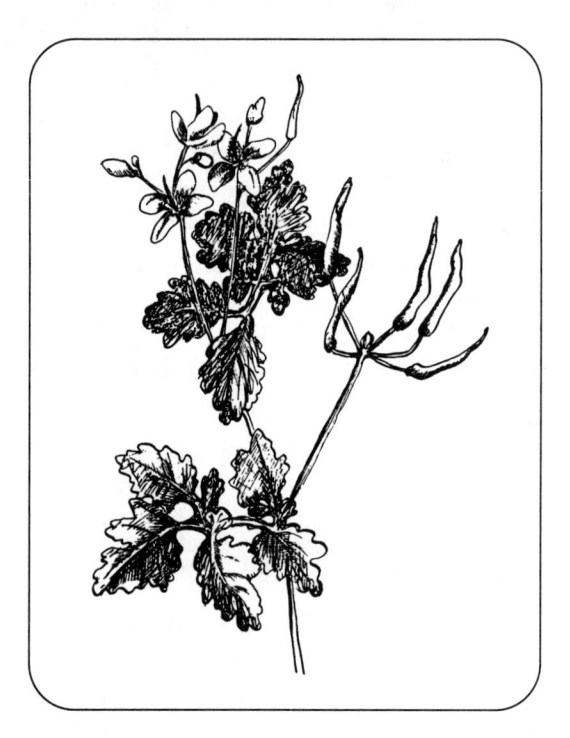

Nature

CATEGORY: medium-strength herb with some chronic toxicity
CONSTITUENTS: alkaloids (incl. chelidonin, chelerythrin, sanguinarin, glaucin), bitter, ess. oil, chelidonic/citric/nicotinic/malic/bernstein acids, proteolitic enzymes, resin, methylanin, histamine, sparteine, vit C, calcium, ammonium-magnesium phosphate
EFFECTIVE QUALITIES
Primary: *Taste:* a bit pungent & bitter
　　　Warmth: warm
　　　Moisture: dry
Secondary stimulating, relaxing, decongesting, dissolving
TROPISM
Organs or parts: liver, gall bladder, spleen, lungs, kidneys, blood, lymph, eyes
Organisms: Warmth, Air, Water
Meridians: Gall Bladder, Liver, Lung, Heart
Tri Dosas: increases Pitta, decreases Vayu
GROUND
Krases/temperaments: Phlegmatic & Melancholic
Biotypes: Dependant/Tai Yin Earth & Burdened/Shao Yin
Constitutions: Hematic/Sulphuric/Brown Iris

Class 3: Celandine

Functions and Uses

1. **BREAKS UP OBSTRUCTION, PROMOTES BOWEL MOVEMENT AND REMOVES STAGNANCY: STIMULATES, WARMS AND DREDGES THE LIVER AND GALL BLADDER, PROMOTES BILE FLOW AND CLEARS MUCOUS DAMP**

    liver Qi stagnation: constipation, light pasty stools, bilious headache, throbbing right hypochondriac pain radiating to shoulder
    liver & gall bladder damp cold: depression, chilliness, yellow skin, fatigue, nausea
    JAUNDICE due to damp or damp cold obstruction
    CHRONIC HEPATITIS
    GALLSTONE, cholecystitis, liver sclerosis

2. **STIMULATES THE HEART AND CIRCULATION AND GENERATES WARMTH; REMOVES BLOOD CONGESTION AND FREES SPASMS**

    liver cold stagnation: cold limbs, lack of will-power, fatigue, no appetite, frontal or occipital headache
    heart blood congestion: palpitations, shortness of breath, stabbing cardiac pain
    intestines Qi constraint: flatulence, colicky pain
    lung Qi constraint: wheezing, coughing
    SPASMODIC COUGHING, bronchitis

3. **CAUSES SWEATING, RELEASES THE EXTERIOR AND SCATTERS WIND COLD; RESOLVES FEVER AND RELIEVES PAIN**

    external wind cold: onset of cold or flu with fear of cold, aches and pains, fatigue
    REMITTENT FEVERS with alternating chills and fever
    wind damp/obstruction: with pain or neuralgia

4. **SEEPS WATER, PROMOTES URINATION AND RELIEVES FLUID CONGESTION; DREDGES THE KIDNEYS, CLEARS STASIS AND PROMOTES CLEANSING**

    liver fluid congestion: general and ankle swelling, heavy stiff swollen limbs, dizziness, heavy feeling head
    kidney Qi stagnation with *general toxemia:* fetid stools, irritability, skin rashes
    GOUT, arthritis, rheumatism

5. **RESOLVES CONTUSION AND PROMOTES TISSUE REPAIR; DISSIPATES TUMORS AND BENEFITS THE SKIN**

    SPRAINS, bruises, contusions
    RODENT ULCERS, running sores, warts
    TUMORS, lumps, lipomas, cancer
    CANCER, esp. of stomach and skin
    SKIN ERUPTIONS: nettle rash, eczema, tetters, ringworm
    TOOTHACHE

6. **STRENGTHENS AND CLEARS THE VISION**

    EYE INFLAMMATION
    POOR EYESIGHT
    FILMS & STAR in the eyes, cataract

Celandine: Class 3

Preparation

USE: The most effective use of this plant is the fresh JUICE or its FREEZE-DRIED EXTRACT. Good second choices are the TINCTURE and INFUSION (drink hot to bring on sweating). These **must** be made from plant material not older than 4 months if its antispasmodic properties are to be retained (WEISS, 1972). Celandine's external uses are many, notably EYE BATHS, WASHES, GARGLES, COMPRESSES and CREAM.

Chelidonium is also much used in Homeopathy for actions 1, 3 & 4, as well as for acute rheumatic pains and headaches in 3 x potency.

DOSAGE: TINCTURE: 1/2-2 ml or 12-50 drops
JUICE: 2 tsp (10 ml)
INFUSION: 5-10 g (1/6 - 1/3 oz)

CAUTION: Pregnancy is a contraindicaton due to Celandine's *uterine stimulant* property.

It is a safe herb as long as correct doses are maintained and, if taken on its own, breaks of several days are taken after every 14 days of use.

Notes

With its little glossy golden flowers, Celandine immediately strikes one as a typical liver remedy. This it certainly is, yet in order to understand it more fully it is more helpful to see it as much as a *warming, energizing cardiovascular stimulant* as a *hepatic stimulant*. By stimulating cardiac functions, Celandine is able to relieve heart blood congestion causing angina pectoris type complaints; drunk hot in flu like and feverish conditions it will bring on sweating and scatter wind cold as a *diaphoretic,* and is helpful with acute damp cold neuralgias due to its *analgesic* property. Its many alkaloids, the result of its typical Poppy family bioenergies, are active in these respects.

Still, the benefits accrued from goading a phlegmatic liver into activity for the circulation as a whole should not be underestimated. Celandine essentially treats conditions of a **Yang deficient** or **Yin excess**, **cold**, **stagnant**, and **damp** nature with fatigue, introversion and cold limbs and constipation foremost. Damp cold in the liver and gall bladder is perhaps its most telling condition, with Yin-type jaundice, hepatitis, etc., being eventual outcomes. Again, besides noting the fact that Celandine is a *choleretic laxative,* it is equally important to recognize that only constipation due to **cold** will fully respond to it. Of course, it is always possible to make symptomatic use of this herb for **any** type of liver congestion, jaundice, hepatitis, cholecystitis, and so on. Celandine has certainly proved its worth in these conditions, being reportedly able, for example, to either increase **or** decrease bile release, thin **or** thicken the bile, etc. Yet a purely symptomatic approach is a sad waste of therapeutic efficacy, since none of Celandine's contextual energetic qualities are put to use as they are in a vitalistic system—the only approach that has demonstrably endured, despite fashions.

It is really difficult, if not impossible, to find an equivalent to this plant in the Chinese pharmacopoeia—proof being that Chinese researchers and hospitals have been successfully using this unique plant for decades. Its action on the liver and gall bladder, however, roughly corresponds to an acupuncture point selection such as Li 3 & 13, St 40, Sp 5 & 9, Gb 24 & 25.

In the context of the above conditions, Celandine is also much used with vagal hypertonia and ensuing bronchial or intestinal spasms (alkaloid chelidonin at work), while its *spasmolytic* effect also favorably affect the bronchials and intestines as well as the gall bladder. Moreover, as liver remedy Celandine also operates within the water element, relieving edema, when generalized, and promoting *toxin elimination* from both the hepatic and renal end (alkaloid spartein).

Celandine is said by some practitioners to be superior even to Arnica or Witch hazel in treating bruises and sprains, and is equal to Eyebright in removing films from the eyes (whence its German name *Augenkraut*). Tumors benign and malignant are also asterisk symptoms, as Chinese research confirms.

Small wonder, then, that even Native Americans with their long empirical tradition and their abundant reserves of extremely reliable herbs considered Celandine a very useful remedy once they had been shown its uses by the Pennsylvanian Germans in the eigteenth century.

MILK THISTLE

Pharmaceutical name: fructus Cardui mariani
Botanical name: Carduus marianus L. (syn.
 Silybum marianum Gaertner (N.O.
 Compositae)
Ancient names: Sillybon (Gr)
 Cardus Sanctae Mariae, Eryngium (Lat)
Other names: Lady's thistle, Mary thistle, Marian
 thistle, Lady's milk (Eng)
 Chardon Marie (Fr)
 Mariendistel, Weisse Wegdistel, Frauendistel
 (Ge)
Part used: the fruit

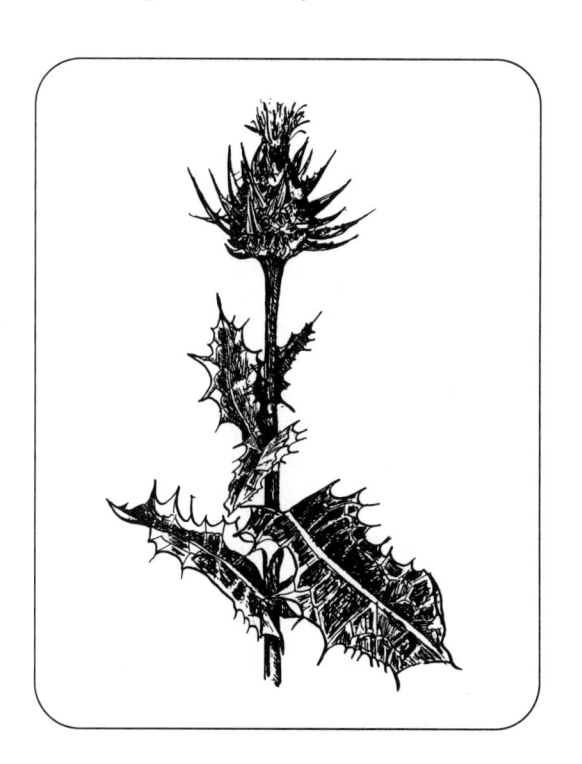

Nature

CATEGORY: mild herb with minimal chronic toxicity
CONSTITUENTS: flavonol sylimarin, (incl. sylibin, silydristin, silydianin), flavonoid, bitter, amines (tyramine, histamine, agmatine), tannin, polyacetylenes
EFFECTIVE QUALITIES
Primary: pungent & bitter, warm, dry
Secondary: stimulating, decongesting, astringing, restoring, dissolving, softening
TROPISM: liver, kidneys, heart, lungs, bladder, uterus
 Warmth, Fluid organism
 Liver, Heart, Chong & Ren meridians
GROUND: Melancholic & Phlegmatic krases
 Burdened/Shao Yin & Dependant/Tai Yin Earth biotypes
 Hematic/Sulphuric/Brown Iris constitution

Functions and Uses

1 PROMOTES BOWEL MOVEMENT AND REMOVES STAGNANCY; RESTORES AND STIMULATES THE LIVER AND GALL BLADDER AND PROMOTES BILE FLOW; DREDGES THE KIDNEYS, PROMOTES URINATION, SOFTENS STONES AND BENEFITS THE SKIN

liver Yang deficiency with *cold stagnation* with nausea, headache, jaundice, constipation

Milk Thistle: Class 3

PREVENTIVE & REMEDIAL in liver degeneration & toxicosis
LIVER CIRRHOSIS, hepato- & splenomegaly, gallstone colic
ACUTE & CHRONIC HEPATITIS
kidney Qi stagnation with skin rashes, fatigue
URINARY STONES, psoriasis

2   DRAINS THE YIN AND DISPELS COLD; STIMULATES THE HEART, CIRCULATION, LUNGS AND UTERUS AND PROMOTES URINATION; EXPELS PHLEGM AND PROMOTES THE MENSES

Yin Excess with heaviness, cold limbs
heart Yang deficiency with mental depression, dizziness
LOW BLOOD PRESSURE
heart fluid congestion with edema, no appetite
lung phlegm cold with thin white phlegm, coughing
uterus cold with delayed or absent menstration, cramps

3   CREATES ASTRICTION, ENLIVENS THE BLOOD AND RELIEVES CONGESTION; MODERATES THE MENSES, STOPS BLEEDING AND ARRESTS DISCHARGE

uterus blood congestion with early copious menstruation, hemorrhoids
MENORRHAGIA, hemorrhage in general
INTESTINAL & urogenital discharges due to damp cold

4   PROMOTES TISSUE REPAIR AND BENEFITS THE VEINS

VARICOSE ULCERS & veins
RODENT ULCERS

Prepartion

USE: The short DECOCTION and TINCTURE of Milk thistle seeds are good preparation forms. Both internal and external application is recommended for function 4.
DOSAGE: standard doses throughout

Notes

Although there are similarities of functions between all types of Thistles, Milk thistle stands out for several reasons. For one, it has a *systemic inhibiting* effect on the parasympathetic nervous system which, together with its *warming circulatory stimulant* effect, makes it an ideal remedy for draining **excess Yin**. Where heart, liver, intestines or genitourinary organs are involved in conditions of this type, it simply excells, addressing cold and damp conditions of these organs due to Yang deficiency. Greek medicine has been able to rely on the effects of this plant for over two thousand years.

Modern pharmacology, however, has uncovered a specific property of Milk thistle's constituent silymarin, which is highest in the fruit: by protecting the cell membranes of liver parenchyme, it prevents substances toxic to the liver, including viruses and drugs, from penetrating liver cells. This stalwart Galenic remedy has thus found a new paplication in preventing and treating virtually any liver damage. As such, it enjoys an even better reputation as other known *liver protective* botanicals such as Alfalfa and Licorice and several Chinese herbs, including Schizandra and Lycium fruit. Milk thistle's important preventive role in organic liver disease, and wherever liver poisoning is suspected, is therefore clear. Both acute and chronic hepatitis, for example, stand to benefit from its use.

Like several other herbs from the Composite family, Milk thistle stands out as a *restoring* as well as a *dredging* **liver** remedy. Its actions include *softening* and *dissolving* in hardening processes such as sclerosis and stone-formation. These properties are amply supported by an *astringent decongestant* effect on both veins and capillaries, which relieves stagnant congested blood as an integral part of metabolic stimulation. Since Milk thistle also has a marked tropism for the uterus, it emerges as a significant woman's ally for the treatment of functional heavy periods, and should be considered when **cold stagnation** or **excess Yin**, such as is typically found in the Shao Yin biotype, is uppermost in the symptomatology.

CULVER'S ROOT

Pharmaceutical name: radix Leptandrae
Botanical name: Leptandra virginica L. (syn. Veronica virginica L.)
(N.O. Scrophulariaceae)
Other names: Black root, Bowman's root, Brinton root, Leptandra (Am)
Part used: the root

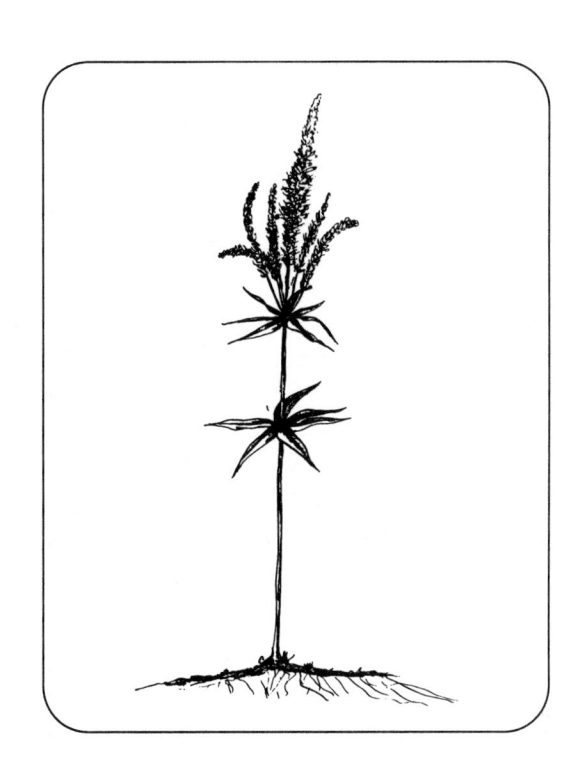

Nature

CATEGORY: mild herb with minimal chronic toxicity
CONSTITUENTS: bitter substance leptandrin, glycoside, saponin, mannitol, tannin, citric acid, phytosterols, ess. oil, gum, resin
EFFECTIVE QUALITIES
Primary: bitter, a bit astringent, warm, dry
Secondary: stimulating, restoring, cleansing, astringing
sinking movement
TROPISM: liver, intestines, stomach, kidneys, uterus
Fluid, Warmth organisms
Liver, Colon meridians
GROUND: Melancholic krasis
Burdened/Shao Yin biotype
Hematic/Sulphuric/Brown Iris constitution

Culver's root: Class 3

Functions and uses

1. **BREAKS UP OBSTRUCTION, PROMOTES BOWEL MOVEMENT AND REMOVES STAGNANCY: STIMULATES AND DREDGES THE LIVER AND GALL BLADDER AND PROMOTES BILE FLOW**

    liver Qi stagnation with yellow skin, flank pain, semi-digested stool, gloominess
    stomach & intestines Qi stagnation with constipation, swollen abdomen
    HEPATITIS, acute or chronic
    JAUNDICE due to cold & damp

2. **WARMS AND INVIGORATES THE STOMACH, INTESTINES AND LIVER; DISPELS COLD AND ARRESTS DISCHARGE**

    intestines cold (Spleen Yang deficiency) with no appetite, diarrhea
    CHRONIC ENTERITIS, dysentery, children's cholera
    liver Yang deficiency with chilliness, depression, inertia, dull frontal or occipital headache, vertigo

3. **DREDGES THE KIDNEYS AND PROMOTES CLEANSING, BENEFITS THE SKIN**

    kidney Qi stagnation with signs of *general toxemia*
    SKIN ERUPTIONS, rashes, scrofula, syphilis

4. **CAUSES SWEATING, RESOLVES FEVER AND PUSHES OUT ERUPTIONS**

    REMITTENT FEVERS of Shao Yang stage, incl. malaria, typhus
    ERUPTIVE FEVERS of all types

Preparation

USE: The **dried** root should be used in preference over the **fresh** always, to avoid nausea and griping. TINCTURES, FLUID EXTRACTS and DECOCTIONS are all used.
DOSAGE: Standard doses throughout. **Larger** doses are more *laxative*.
CAUTION: Culver's root should be avoided during pregnancy because of its *sinking* movement.

Notes

As a liver-centered herb Culver's root may usefully be compared to Celandine. Both have an essentially *warm* and *restoring* nature suited to **cold liver** syndromes with chilliness, cold extremities and the train of symptoms associated with liver congestion. Both remedies in addition have a cleansing effect particularly with a **skin** bias; both cause sweating and help resolve intermittent and eruptive fevers. To this extent they are identical.

However, their differences are significant, too. Whereas Celandine is essentially a *decongesting* and *relaxing stimulant,* Culver's root is a *restorative* and *stimulant*. Like Milk thistle, it should be used where Qi stasis is accompanied by **deficiency** and **cold**. This herb, which was considered "a sure tonic to intestinal glandular saction, improving the functions of all intestinal glands," was applied when the tongue was "pale, coated uniformly white, or greyish-white and moist" (ELLINGWOOD, 1898). Culver's root clearly treats deficiency cold in the stomach and intestines as much as in the liver & gall bladder. Spleen and liver Yang deficiency conditions are addressed here, and diarrhea and constipation are both regulated, in a similar way to that achieved by acupuncture points Bl 18, 20 & 25, St 25, Li 13 and CV 8 with moxa.

Another remedy originating in Native American uses, Culver's root is of medium-strength and combines well. In functions 1 & 2 it shows some similarity to *Qing pi, pericarpium Citri reticulatae viride,* from the Chinese pharmacy.

BLUE FLAG

Pharmaceutical name: rhizoma Iridis
Botanical name: Iris versicolor seu germanica L.
 (N.O. Liliaceae)
Ancient names: Ireus, Iris (Gr)
 Affrodisia, Gladiolus, Illiria (Lat)
Other names: Flower-de-luce (Eng)
 Flag lily, Liver lily, Snake lily, Wild iris (Am)
 Iris d'Allemagne, Glaieul bleu, Flambe, Lis (Fr)
 Schwertlilie, Blaue Schwertel, Lilgen, Veilchenwurzel, Himmelschwertel (Ge)
Part used: the root

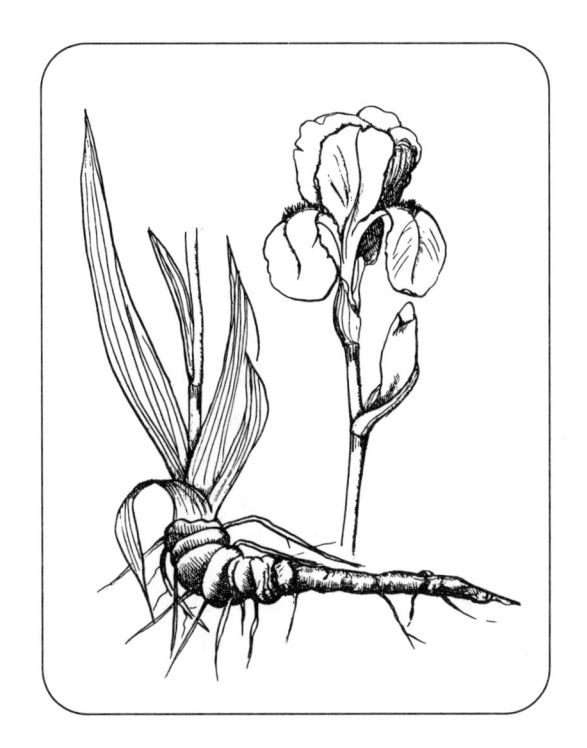

Nature

CATEGORY: medium-strength herb with some chronic toxicity
CONSTITUENTS: alkaloid, tannin, acids, ess. oil (incl. ketone, irone), glycoside (iridin), gum, resin, mucilage, starch, sugar
EFFECTIVE QUALITIES
Primary: *Taste:* pungent, a bit bitter & sweet
 Warmth: cool
 Moisture: dry
Secondary: stimulating, decongesting, dissolving, cleansing
TROPISM
Organs or parts: liver, stomach spleen, intestines, lungs, bladder, blood, lymph
Organisms: Warmth, Fluid
Meridians: Gall Bladder, Liver, Lung, Bladder
Tri Dosas: decreases Kapha & Pitta
GROUND
Krases/temperaments: Phlegmatic & Sanguine
Biotypes: Self-reliant/Yang Ming Metal & Expressive/Jue Yin
Constitutions: Hematic/Sulphuric/Brown Iris

Functions and Uses

1 BREAKS UP OBSTRUCTION, PROMOTES BOWEL MOVEMENT AND REMOVES STAGNANCY: STIMULATES THE LIVER AND GALL BLADDER AND PROMOTES BILE FLOW; STIMULATES THE UTERUS AND PROMOTES THE MENSES

 liver Qi stagnation: distended right flank with sharp pains mid-back pain, constipation, clay

Blue Flag: Class 3

    colored stools, scanty urine, jaundice
    stomach & intestines Qi stagnation: swollen, painful abdomen, acid belching, nausea, vomiting sour semidigested food, sick headache
    CHRONIC CONSTIPATION
    SPLEEN & LIVER ENLARGMENT
    uterus Qi stagnation: delayed painful menstruation with purple clots, sore breasts, fibroids

2. CLEARS HEAT, TRANSFORMS DAMP AND CLEARS TOXINS; DREDGES THE GALL BLADDER AND MOVES THE LYMPH
    liver/gall bladder damp heat: nauseating headache with bitter vomiting, swollen painful flanks and sides
    HEPATITIS, LYMPHOMA
    Spleen damp heat: exhaustion, distaste for rich foods, bitter taste in mouth, thirst
    ACUTE LIVER or GASTRIC INFECTIONS, cholecystitis
    bladder damp heat: urgent painful burning urination, thirst
    genitourinary damp heat: venereal infections with purulent discharge, incl. syphilis
    fire toxin: abscesses, sores

3. PROMOTES CLEANSING, CLEARS TOXINS, RESOLVES TOXEMIA AND DRAINS PLETHORA; PROMOTES URINATION AND BENEFITS THE SKIN
    general toxemia: fetid stools, skin rashes
    ARTHRITIS, gout, rheumatism
    CHRONIC ECZEMA, psoriasis, tetters, ringworm
    HERPES ZOSTER
    liver fluid congestion: generalized edema, heaviness of body, shortness of breath
    general plethora: cellulite, high blood pressure, obesity

4. STIMULATES THE LUNGS, EXPELS PHLEGM AND RELIEVES COUGHING
    lung phlegm heat: full cough with thick yellow phlegm, sore throat, hoarseness

5. RESOLVES SWELLING AND DISSIPATES TUMORS; STIMULATES THE PANCREAS AND THYROID
    UTERINE FIBROIDS & polyps, pelvic & uterine infections
    SOFT TUMORS and soft enlarged lymph glands, scrofula, goiter thyroid enlargment
    THYROID or PANCREATIC INSUFFICIENCY

Preparation

USE: Blue flag's actions come out best when used in the form of TINCTURE or FLUID EXTRACT, while the DECOCTION of the dried root is still serviceable. If the **fresh root** is used, its *purging* properties become stronger: use with care.

External preparations are appropriate mainly in **skin** conditions and **wounds**. **Venereal infections** should be dealt with by DOUCHES.

Historical preparations of Blue Flag include SYRUPS (it was much used for lung conditions with phlegm), PESSARIES, GARGLES and medicinal SNUFFS. SCHROEDER (1611), for example, gives a 15 ingredient SYRUP for "cold coughs and cold lung conditions," which also returns lost speech. MATTIOLI (1610) presents a *laxative* WINE of Blue Flag, Agrimony, Holy thistle, Centaury, Wormwood, Betony, Anise, Fennel, Tamarind, Senna, Rhubarb and Scabious, which "cleanses the body of all pernicious damp, assists those with phlegm in the lungs and chest, and with coughing and difficult breathing . . ."

DOSAGE: **Smaller** doses are sufficient for *stimulating* and *cleansing* effects (functions 1, 3, 4, 5). **Larger** doses have *purging, detoxifying, heat clearing, phlegm breaking* effects (function 2).

Smaller dose:
　　TINCTURE: up to 2 ml (50 drops)
　　DECOCTION: 4-8 g

Larger dose:
　　TINCTURE: up to 4 ml (100 drops)
　　DECOCTION: 8-16 g

CAUTION: As Blue flag is a strongly *stimulating* remedy, if used on its own, breaks of a few days are advised about every week, and the dosage should never be exceeded.

Blue flag should never be used in **deficiency** conditions of any kind, and, if used alone should be given cautiously during pregnancy.

Notes

Blue flag at one time was not only a standard remedy in the European pharmacy, but also the most widely used medicine of all among Native Americans, according to VIRGIL VOGEL (1970). Of course, it was also taken up by the medical profession during the nineteenth century.

Eclectic medical prescribing at that time, like that of contemporary Homeopathy, was very **specific** with respect to remedy symptomatology. This was only partly due to the bleed-through from homeopathic to other forms of allopathic medicine during this period. With Blue flag, for example, the type of liver congestion amenable to its influence is typified by clay colored stools, scanty urine, a thin, narrow red tongue with yellow moss in the middle, palpitations and inactive, jaundiced skin. These specific symptoms immediately paint a picture of the **general condition**. In the same vein we may say, using Chinese medical terminology, that its use in **liver/gall bladder damp heat** is characterized by "a neuralgic pain over one eye, or involving one side of the face, usually the right side" (ELLINGWOOD, 1898).

Blue flag is essentially used for clearing **damp heat** of various kinds, covering **congestive catarrhal** conditions with **infection** of the **chest, upper digestive** and **urogenital** areas. Its *stimulating, decongestant* (and *choleretic*) influence is centered on the liver, stomach gall, bladder and small intestines, where chronic Qi stagnation with acid belching, sick headache, jaundice and constipation is relieved. In this respect it addresses the therapeutic ground covered by a Chinese herb such as *Yin chen hao, herba Artemisia capillaris*, more than adequately, and corresponds to the use of acupuncture points such as Gb 34 & 44, Si 4, Bl 18 & 19, and Li 13. As a result, overall cleansing is also enhanced, with evident benefits in chronic **blood, lymph, fluids** and **skin** disharmonies resulting from high toxin levels. Gynecological tumors found in this context will benefit especially. Where thyroid insufficiency is at the bottom of this type of condition, it will also relieve it. Besides combining congenially with other *cold cholagogue laxatives* such as Cascara sagrada, Dandelion and Gentian, therefore, Blue flag is also complemented by a variety of Class 15 *cleansers*.

Inasmuch as Blue flag is a *bitter pungent* **lower warmer damp heat** *remover,* also treating fire toxin and fluid congestion, as well as being an *antirheumatic* herb, it shows therapeutic similarities with *Han fang ji, radix Stephaniae tetrandae,* from the Oriental pharmacopoeia.

May Apple: Class 3

MAY APPLE

Pharmaceutical name: rhizoma Podophylli
Botanical name: Podophyllum peltatum L. (N.O. Berberidaceae)
Other names: Mandrake, Racoonberry, Hog apple, Indian apple, Wild lemon, Duck's foot, Wild Jalap, American mandrake (Am)
Citron (Fr)
Part used: the rhizome

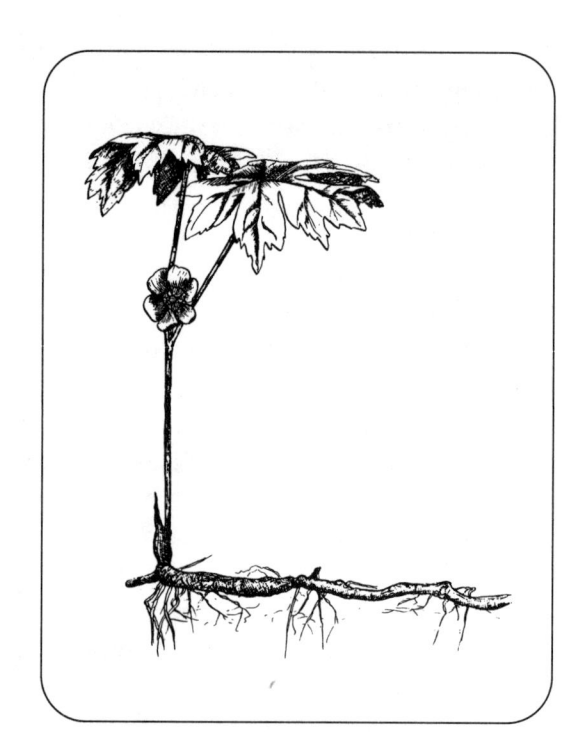

Nature

CATEGORY: medium-strength herb with some chronic toxicity
CONSTITUENTS: crystalline antitumor substance podophyllotoxin, tannin, resin, podophyllin, picropodophyllinic & gallic acid, podophylloquercitin, glycosides, calcium oxalate, ess. oil
EFFECTIVE QUALITIES
Primary: pungent, a bit bitter & sweet, cool, dry
Secondary: stimulating, decongesting
TROPISM: liver, gall bladder, intestines, uterus, kidneys
Fluid organism
Liver & Gall Bladder meridians
GROUND: Phlegmatic krasis
Self-reliant/Yang Ming Metal biotype
Hematic/Sulphuric/Brown Iris constitution

This remedy is virtually identical in its nature, functions and uses to BLUE FLAG, rhizoma Iridis, with the following differences.

1   Being stronger than Blue flag in dredging the liver and moving stagnancy, May apple is indicated when **chronic liver congestion** causes pain beneath the scapula, painful distention of the liver region and chronic constipation with hard, dry clay colored stools. Like Blue flag it is also used in *liver/gall bladder damp heat* with lymph stagnation (painful sides), vertigo, nausea, etc. ELLINGWOOD (1898) notes that the pulse is "full, large, sluggish and oppressed," and the tongue "heavily coated, uniformly yellowish, or yellow center, a thick dirty coat, especially atthe back."

2   May apple also treats **chronic skin eruptions** of most kinds due to liver Qi stagnation and general plethora, but not general fluids dyskrasia as Blue flag does.

3   In addition to being a *cholagogue hepatic decongestant,* May apple is also a *circulatory* and *cardiac stimulant* and may be used in wind heat onsets of flu or fever with hepatic congestion.

Class 3: May Apple

4   May apple will not treat intestines or bladder damp heat, liver fluid congestion or lung phlegm heat.

5   May apple, like Blue flag, also has *antitumoral* effects. It has no known effect on the thyroid, on the other hand.

Preparation

USE: DECOCTION, TINCTURE, etc. are all suitable.
DOSAGE: DECOCTION: 1 tsp per pint (1/2 l) of water
                 TINCTURE: 10-25 drops, or up to 1 ml

Small doses will restore Spleen Qi as a *bitter tonic,* while **medium to large** ones are more *stimulating, decongesting, detoxifying* and *cooling.*

CAUTION: If used alone May apple should be discontinued for a fea days from time to time, as its slight toxicity may accumulate. Use in pregnancy is also forbidden for this reason. Doses larger than those indicated will cause vomiting and severe diarrhea.

May apple is not a remedy for **deficiency** conditions. It should be kept to conditions of **Qi stagnation, damp heat** and **toxemia** with liver and gall bladder involvement.

Notes

With its fragrant, mawkish white flowers and lemon-like edible fruit, May apple was a common vegetable drug of the Native Americans; like many herbs, it only drew the attention of physicians when the work of Philadelphia botanist WILLIAM BARTON appeared in the early 1800's.

May apple, or American mandrake, as this botanical has become known overseas, demonstrates once again the influence on Eclectic practitioners of the **specific** symptomatology developed by the mid-nineteenth century homeopathists. In this way May apple acquired a core pattern of symptoms around which other symptoms or disharmonies may appear. This central pattern of disharmony is described in Note 1 above. It describes liver stagnation and liver damp heat from the Chinese syndromes fairly well—but not liver fire: May apple is simply not cold enough, unlike the bitter heat-clearing *liver dredgers* from Class 13. Its role is to disperse **longstanding** and **systemic stasis** and **obstruction**, typically causing chronic constipation, cool, dingy yellow skin, and dull headaches with vertigo. This it does better than any other remedy in this class. Indeed, early Eclectics nicknamed it vegetable Calomel for this very reason, a reminder of the late-Galenic legacy of the mineral remedies used to promote elimination.

Fringe tree: Class 3

FRINGE TREE

Pharmaceutical name: cortex radicis Chionanthi
Botanical name: Chionanthus virginicus L. (N.O. Oleaceae)
Other names: Snowdrop tree, Snow flower, Old man's beard, Poison ash (Am)
　Arbre de neige (Fr)
　Schneeflockenbaum, Schneeblume, Franzenblume (Ge)
Part used: the root bark

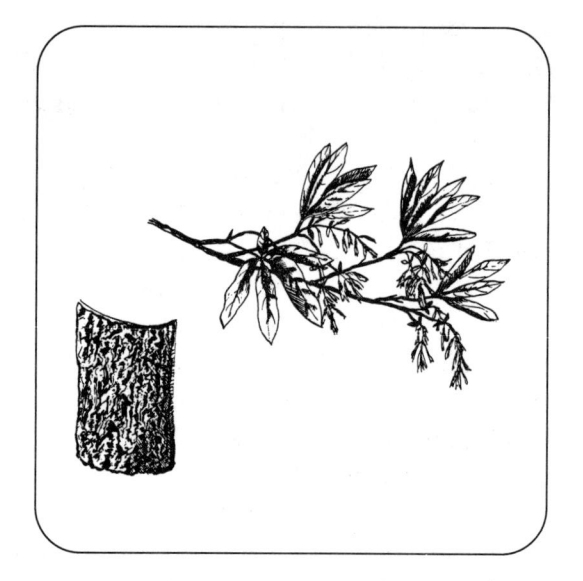

Nature

CATEGORY: mild herb with minimal chronic toxicity
CONSTITUENTS: saponins, phillyrin, chionanthin, forsythin, aglucone phyllogenin, phillyroside
EFFECTIVE QUALITIES
Primary: bitter, a bit astringent, cold, neutral
Secondary: stimulating, decongesting, restoring, dissolving, softening, diluting
　sinking movement
TROPISM: liver, gall bladder, stomach, spleen, pancreas, veins
　Warmth, Fluid organism
　Liver, Gall Bladder, Spleen meridians
GROUND: Sanguine & Choleric krases
　Expressive/Jue Yin & Tough/Shao Yang biotypes
　Hematic/Sulphuric/Brown Iris constitution

Functions and Uses

1　BREAKS UP OBSTRUCTION, PROMOTES BOWEL MOVEMENT AND REMOVES STAGNANCY: STIMULATES AND DREDGES THE LIVER AND GALL BLADDER, CLEARS HEAT, TRANSFORMS DAMP AND PROMOTES URINATION
　liver Qi stagnation with jaundice, flank fullness & dull pain, somnolence, fatigue, greyish dry stool, constipation
　liver & Spleen damp heat with vomiting, painful and swollen sides
　liver fire with feverishness, bilious headache, constipation
　JAUNDICE, portal congestion

2　RESOLVES FEVER AND REDUCES INFLAMMATION
　REMITTENT FEVERS in Shao Yang stage; malaria
　INFLAMMATIONS, wounds

3　RESTORES THE LIVER, STOMACH, PANCREAS AND SPLEEN
　liver & stomach Qi deficiency with epigastric pain, heartburn, slow heavy digestion
　EXHAUSTION due to chronic illness

DIABETES (supportive)
SPLEENIC & HEPATIC ENLARGEMENT

Preparation

USE: The TINCTURE and DECOCTION are the best preparation forms, used internally, or externally in WASHES or COMPRESSES (RAFINESQUE).
DOSAGE: standard doses throughout

Notes

In the eighteenth century the botanist LINNAEUS named this lovely white-flowered shrub from the southeastern American states *Chionanthus*, a fanciful rendering of *snowflower* in Greek. We may appreciate this healing herb even more if the specific energetic and tissue conditions meeting its use are understood.

Fringe tree is in first line a *cholagogue stimulant* addressing **stagnation** of all the organs directly involved in digestion, as well as **heat** and **damp heat** in the liver and spleen. Nineteenth century medical practice, which generously utilized botanical remedies, ascertained its symptomatology very precisely. Foremost among these were dull pain in the liver area, sleepiness, jaundiced skin, a thick, flabby tongue with greasy white or yellow moss, and dry, grey colored floating stool. Clearly, it addresses similar liver syndromes for which *Huang qin, radix Scutellariae*, from China is used, and for which acupuncture points such as Li 3 & 14, GV 9, Bl 18 & 19, Gb 34 and SI 4 are used. We also know that Fringe tree's *diluting, softening* action, partly due to its content in saponins, will thin the bile and prevent, if not help break up, biliary stones. Its *restoring* property extends to all the upper digestive organs, and includes hepatic and spleenic enlargement, as well local venous blood congestion. Its *cool, anti-inflammatory* nature is supported by the evidence of early travellers observing Native American practices, such as JOHN BRICKELL, who reported that it was "cooling and good in all Inflammations and soreness of the Eyes, Ulcers in the Mouth and Throat..."

If used as a simple *tonic* remedy in small doses after or during chronic conditions, Fringe tree will stimulate upper gastric secretions, enhance assimilation and improve elimination through the stool and urine - hence its net *cleansing* effect

Balmony: Class 3

BALMONY

Pharmaceutical name: herba Chelonis
Botanical name: Chelone glabra L (N.O. Scrophulariaceae)
Other names: Snakehead, Turtlebloom, Shell flower, Salt rheum weed, Bitter herb, Hummingbird tree, Glatte (Am)
Chélone, Galane (Fr)
Schildkrötenblume/staude, Kahler Fünffaden, Bartfaden, Brummvogelbaum (Ge)
Part used: the herb

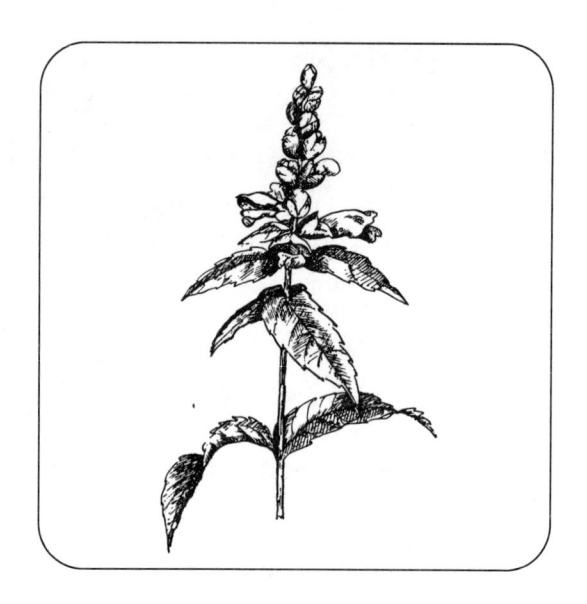

This herb is virtually identical in its nature, functions and uses to FRINGE TREE, cortex radicis Chionanthi, with the following exceptions.

1   Balmony is not used to treat diabetes or spleenic enlargement as Fringe tree is.
2   Balmony is excellent used externally in OINTMENTS for mastitis, hemorrhoids, painful ulcers, etc.

FUMITORY

Pharmaceutical name: herba Fumariae
Botanical name: Fumaria officinalis L. (N.O. Papaveraceae)
Ancient names: Kapnos, Phoumaria (Gk)
Fumus terrae (Lat)
Other names: Beggary, Wax dolls, Earth smoke, Snapdragon (Eng)
Fumeterre, Herbe à la jaunisse, Fiel de terre (Fr)
Erdrauch, Taubenkropf, Katzenkörbel (Ge)
Part used: the herb

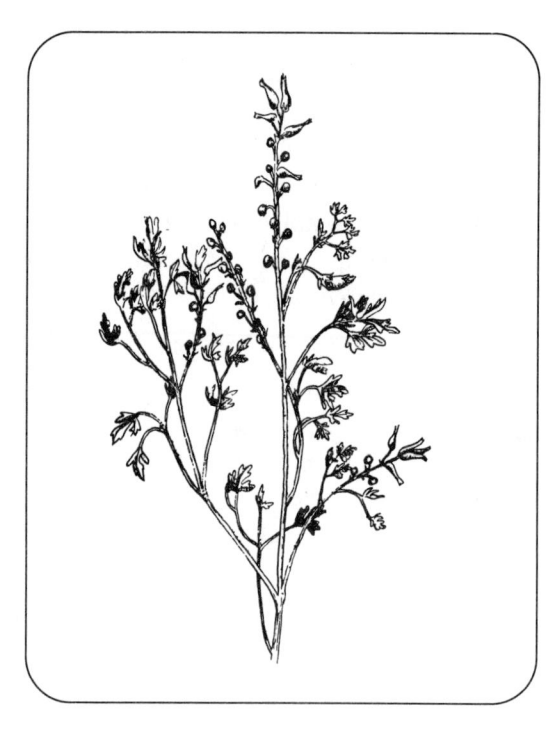

Nature

CATEGORY: medium-strength herb with some chronic toxicity
CONSTITUENTS: alkaloids (incl. fumarine, cryptocavin, corydalin, sinactin, aurotensin), fumaric acid, cholin, flavonoids (rutin, quercitin & other glycosides), mucilage, resin, bitter

Class 3: Fumitory

EFFECTIVE QUALITIES
Primary: bitter, a bit salty, a bit cool, dry
Secondary: stimulating, diluting
　　　　　　sinking movement
TROPISM: liver, gall bladder, intestines, uterus, blood, skin, nervous system
　　　　　Warmth, Fluid organism
　　　　　Liver, Gall Bladder meridians
GROUND: Choleric & Sanguine krases
　　　　　Tough/Shao Yang & Expressive/Jue Yin biotypes
　　　　　Hematic/Sulphuric/Brown Iris constitution

Functions and Uses

1 BREAKS UP OBSTRUCTION, PROMOTES BOWEL MOVEMENT AND REMOVES STAGNANCY: STIMULATES AND DREDGES THE LIVER AND GALL BLADDER, REGULATES BILE-FLOW AND ALLAYS IRRITABILITY
   liver Qi stagnation with right hypochondriac pain and swelling, jaundice, constipation
   liver & stomach Qi deficiency with slow painful digestion, poor appetite, timidity
   gall bladder damp heat with nausea, violent headache, irritability
   ANY DEFICIENCY or EXCESS of BILE FLOW, esp. if chronic

2 CLEARS STASIS: FLENZES MUCUS AND PROMOTES MENSTRUATION
   intestines mucous damp (Spleen damp) with alternating constipation and diarrhea, swollen gurgling painful abdomen
   uterus Qi stagnation with delayed painful menstruation, dark clots

3 PROMOTES CLEANSING, CLEARS TOXINS, RESOLVES TOXEMIA AND DRAINS PLETHORA; BENEFITS THE SKIN AND CLEARS CONTUSION
   general toxemia with foul stools, skin rashes; chronic gout and rheumatism
   GENERAL PLETHORA: obesity, hypertension, atherosclerosis
   SKIN CONDITIONS in general: eczema, psoriasis, dermatosis
   CONGEALED BLOOD due to bruising, contusions

Preparation

USE: The INFUSION, TINCTURE and FLUID EXTRACT are all used to represent Fumitory's actions, including those for external application.
DOSAGE: standard doses throughout
CAUTION: If used over about ten days Fumitory will show an increasing sedative effect on the CNS: use with discretion. Avoid during pregnancy because of its stimulant action in the lower warmer.

Notes

Fumitory, whose latin name means "earth smoke", is a special remedy among the many that both break up obstructions and cleanse. Belonging to the Poppy family, like Celandine and Blood root, it has an impressive array of seven alkaloids. Unlike its cousins, however, it has an amphoteric *regulating* action on bile production and release: it is unique among the gall bladder herbs in this respect. This effectively suggests its use in all conditions of **liver/gall bladder stagnation** in both **deficiency** or **excess** conditions. Similarly, being of a *mild, slightly cool* warmth

Fumitory: Class 3

grade, it is suitable for all gall bladder conditions, combining well with both *cool* or *warm* botanicals. Besides, it has been used successfully for both acute situations and chronic conditions since Greek days. Its alkaloids also provide a *relaxing* and *cooling* effect—becoming *sedating* with continuous use—which is ideal when stagnation turns into heat.

Fumitory excells in conditions of **general toxemia** with physical **toxin** and **mucos accumulation** on one hand, and actual **gall bladder** dysfunction on the other—where symptoms of tension, irritability, skin rashes and, for women, late, painful, clotted menstruation, in the case of women, predominate. Galen's summary statement that it "deobstructs the liver, evacuates burnt bile and cools the blood" cannot be bettered. The emerging profile suggests the disharmonies of the Shao Yang biotype which are basically those of the Gall Bladder and Triple Heater meridians. In moderate and occasional doses, Fumitory is a good preventive ground tonic for this type, with their constitutional sympathetic nervous excess.

Herbs to Clear Heat and Promote Bowel Movement

RHUBARB

Pharmaceutical name: rhizoma Rhei
Botanical name: Rheum palmatum L. (N.O. Polygonaceae)
Ancient names: Rheon, Rha (Gr)
Rhabarbarum, Radix pontia (Lat)
    Rewerd (Pers)
Other names: China/East Indian/Turkey rhubarb (Eng)
    Rhubarbe (Fr)
    Rhabarber (Ge)
    Da huang (Ch)
Part used: the root

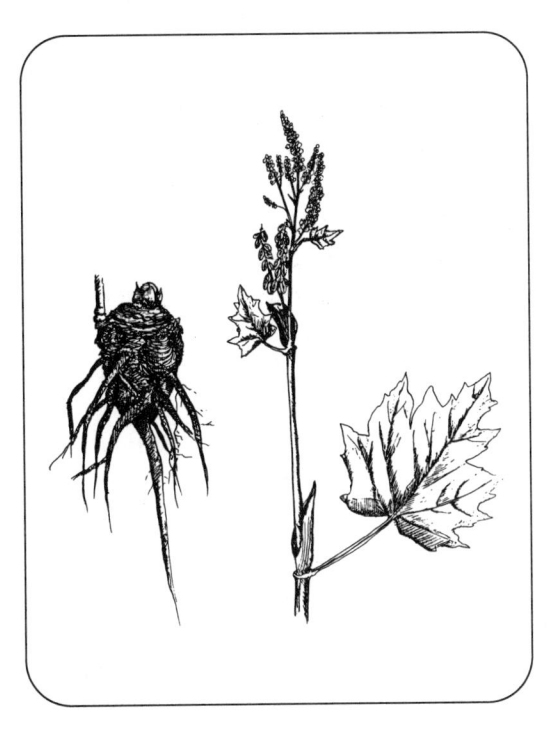

Nature

CATEGORY: mild herb with minimal chronic toxicity
CONSTITUENTS: anthraquinones and derivatives (incl. emodin, chrysophanic acid, rhein, rheochrysidin), tannins, oxalic, gallic & cinnamic acids, iron, magnesium, vits B & C
EFFECTIVE QUALITIES
Primary: *Taste:* bitter & astringent
        Warmth: cold
        Moisture: dry
Secondary: stimulating, restoring, astringing
        sinking movement
TROPISM
Organs or parts: stomach, small & large intestines, liver
Organisms: Air, Warmth
Meridians: Stomach, Spleen, Liver, Colon
Tri Dosas: increases Vayu, decreases Kapha & Pitta
GROUND
Krases/temperaments: Choleric
Biotypes: Industrious/Tai Yang & Tough/Shao Yang
Constitutions: Hematic/Sulphuric/Brown Iris

Rhubarb: Class 3

Functions and Uses

1 PROVOKES BOWEL MOVEMENT, REMOVES STAGNANCY, TRANSFORMS DAMP AND CLEARS HEAT: DREDGES AND CALMS THE LIVER, STIMULATES THE COLON AND ABATES DISTENSION

intestines dry heat: constipation, fever, hard abdomen
liver/gall bladder damp heat: nausea and vomiting, swollen tender sides and flanks, fever, irregular stool, jaundice
liver fire: irritability, congestive face with throbbing headache, constipation, dark scanty urine
stomach fire: great appetite, thirst and drinking cold water, fetid breath

2 RESTORES THE STOMACH AND LIVER, CLEARS STASIS AND AWAKENS THE APPETITE; STIMULATES THE LIVER AND GALL BLADDER AND PROMOTES BILE FLOW

stomach Qi stagnation: difficult slow digestion, sour eructations or regurgitation, swollen painful abdomen, poor appetite, weakness
liver Qi stagnation: nausea, tender swollen flank and abdomen, constipation or pasty light colored unformed stools, flatulence, jaundice
GALLSTONES, HEMORRHOIDS

3 CREATES ASTRICTION, DRIES DAMP AND ARRESTS DISCHARGE

intestines damp cold: indigestion, loose or copious watery stool, nausea, tender swollen abdomen, restlessness, chilliness
MUCOENTERITIS, chronic diarrhea, children's cholera, summer diarrhea
GASTROINTESTINAL IRRITATION

4 RESOLVES CONTUSION

CONGEALED BLOOD due to injuries and contusions; with sharp pain and delayed menstruation

Preparation

USE: With more than any other remedy, perhaps, Rhubarb's effects and uses are inextricably tied up with its **dosage**.

The DECOCTION is particularly suited to function 3, using small doses every 30 or 60 minutes, since the tannins are thereby brought out; the root may also be dry-toasted or roasted beforehand for better effect. Conversely, the TINCTURE or FLUID EXTRACT wins out for Rhubarb's other functions.

The days of the Eclectic practitioners saw splendid formulas such as Locke's Neutralising Cordial, Beach's Neutralizing Physic, and Glyconda, and we are the poorer for their abscence. Older traditional preparations include compound Rhubarb PILLS, SYRUPS, CONSERVES and HONEY BALLS. RYFF (1568) gives a 13 herb receipt for these.

DOSAGE: The **small dosage** has an *astringing* and *calming* effect, and is used for all gastric conditions with "enfeebled digestion and irritation" (FELTER) without severe inflammation, i.e. for damp cold intestinal syndromes (function 3).

The **medium dosage** has a *stimulating* and *laxative* effect, and is appropriate for gastrointestinal stasis due to gastric or hepatic insufficiency, i.e. in stomach/intestines/liver Qi stagnation (function 2).

Class 3: Rhubarb

The **high dosage** is effectively *purging* and *cooling,* and suited to stomach, intestines, liver and gall bladder heat syndromes (function 1).

The larger the dose, the more Rhubarb should be adjusted by combination with *carminatives*.

Small dose:
>   TINCTURE: 6-12 drops
>   DECOCTION & POWDER: 0.05-0.5 g; a few sips of the decoction every 30 or 60 minutes until improvement sets in.

Medium dose:
>   TINCTURE: 12-50 drops
>   DECOCTION & POWDER: 0.5-2 g

High dose:
>   TINCTURE: 50-100 drops (1/4-1/2 tsp)
>   DECOCTION & POWDER: 2-3 g

CAUTION: Rhubarb's *downward-moving* and *stimulating* qualities, largely due to its content in anthraquinone glycosides, in medium and high doses make it contraindicated during pregnancy and lactation and with hemorrhoids, gout and stones due to oxalic acid.

If, when using this herb, the urine turns red, this is simply an alkaline reaction and no cause for concern.

Rhubarb should never be combined with *emetics* to cause vomiting.

Notes

The history of Rhubarb's medicinal uses would fill many pages, as it spans its origins in China, its adoption into the Ayurvedic medical system on the Indian subcontinent, its uptake by Greek/Tibb Unani medicine throughout the Islamic empire, and finally its more modern European use. Rarely has any botanical been so widely used by mankind, and the art of causing bowel movement, the *purging* treatment method, would be inconceivable without it.

For all that, Galenic medical theory held the position that "Rhubarb is so effective for the Liver that it is called the Life, Soul and Treacle of the Liver, purging from thence Choler, Phlegme and Watery humours" (WILLIAM COLE). In other words, it was used to treat any kind of **liver excess** due to a *dyskrasia* of the three noted humors or fluids. Here we connect with functions 1 and 2 above characterized by **chronic liver** and **intestinal stagnation** and the generation of **internal heat** and **damp heat**. It is these conditions for which *Da huang* (the identical botanical) is mainly used in Chinese medicine today.

Galenic physicians had, on the whole, gone far beyond Rhubarb when needing to cause bowel evacuation: they had long graduated to more drastic purges such as Scammony, Colocynth and Jalap, not to mention the mineral cathartics of the "chymists". No, Rhubarb was a solid liver remedy, which "is likewise good against the Windinesse, Wambling and Weaknesse of the Stomach." Here WILLIAM COLE touches on its *restoring* effects, given as function 2, in language very evocative of the diarrhea and enteritis that it treats.

The Persian physicians' zealous page-long prescriptions based on Rhubarb were all avidly emulated up to Renaissance times, and they live on in transformed shape in the formulas of the Eclectic school. Rhubarb is hardly ever used alone: it is ususally assisted by a second herb or is used itself as a corrective addition to other remedies. The *laxative* effect of Rhubarb lies between the strength of Senna leaf and Cascara sagrada or Buckthorn. For many reasons, it is the best *laxative* for long-term use and perfectly safe for children, older people and those with deficiency of any kind.

Cascara sagrada: Class 3

CASCARA SAGRADA

Pharmaceutical name: cortex ramuli Rhamni
Botanical name: Rhamnus purshiana DC (N.O. Rhamnaceae)
Other names: Sacred bark, Chittem bark, Bearwood, Bearberry, Coffeeberry bark, Mountain cranberry bark (Am)
Amerikanische Faulbaumrinde (Ge)
Part used: the bark

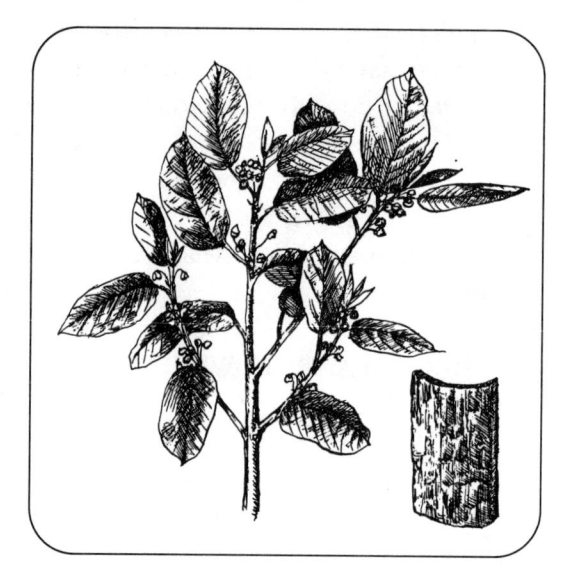

Nature

CATEGORY: mild herb with minimal chronic toxicity
CONSTITUENTS: anthraquinones (incl. emodin, chrysophanic acid, aloe-emodin, cascarosides A,B,C,D), ess. oil (rhamnol arachidate), glycosides, bitter, resins, lipids, methylhydrocotoin
EFFECTIVE QUALITIES
Primary: bitter, a bit astringent, cold, moist
Secondary: stimulating, restoring, dissolving, cleansing
sinking movement
TROPISM: liver, gall bladder, stomach, small intestine
Warmth organism
Liver, Gall Bladder, Small intestine, Colon meridians
GROUND: Sanguine krasis
Expressive/Jue Yin biotype
Hematic/Sulphuric/Brown Iris constitution

Functions and Uses

1 PROVOKES BOWEL MOVEMENT, REMOVES STAGNANCY AND CLEARS HEAT: STIMULATES AND DREDGES THE LIVER, GALL BLADDER AND COLON AND PROMOTES BILE FLOW

liver Qi stagnation: tender swollen right flank, constipation, nausea, headache, midback pain, hemorrhoids
CHRONIC CONSTIPATION, gallstones, liver cirrhosis, jaundice
intestines dry heat: hard swollen abdomen, constipation
liver fire: red face, constipation, bursting headache

2 RESTORES THE LIVER AND STOMACH AND PROMOTES DIGESTION

liver & stomach Qi deficiency: abdominal swelling and pain, flatulence, painful slow digestion, foul breath

3 DREDGES THE KIDNEYS, CLEARS TOXINS AND PROMOTES CLEANSING

kidney Qi stagnation: skin rashes, dry skin, poor appetite

Class 3: Cascara sagrada

general toxemia: chronic rheumatism, gout
URINARY STONES due to calcium (preventive)

Preparation

USE: Cascara sagrada may be used in DECOCTION, POWDER or TINCTURE form. The main consideration in its use, however, is the dosage.

DOSAGE: **Small** doses have a *restoring* effect (function 2), **medium** doses have a *laxative* and *cleansing* effect (function 1 & 3), **large** doses a *cathartic* and *cooling* effect (function 1).

Small dose:
  TINCTURE: 6-20 drops
  POWDER & DECOCTION: 1/4 to 1 g

Medium dose:
  TINCTURE: 20 to 50 drops
  POWDER & DECOCTION: 1-2 g

Large dose:
  TINCTURE: 50 to 100 drops given once only
  POWDER & DECOCTION: 2-4 g given once only

CAUTION: Cascara should be used with a little care during pregnancy, as it does have an active, downward-moving energy. If being used continuously, **small** doses are recommended for maintenance once the liver Qi stagnation or chronic constipation has cleared: continuous large doses are certainly liable to produce unpleasant side-effects. As with all strong *laxatives,* the large dose should not be used in deficiency conditions of any kind.

NOTE: Other Buckthorns such as California buckthorn, *Rhamnus californica,* may be used in the same way. The latter is said to tone the mucous membrane and reproductive organs, but is somewhat gentler in its *laxative* effects—often welcome in children and the elderly.

Notes

This bark from a tree of the Buckthorn family native to the American Northwest coast was used by Native Americans long before the present Spanish name of "sacred bark" was given it in praise of its efficacy. Therapeutically it is medium-strength, and somewhat weaker than Rhubarb root and Senna leaf.

Cascara sagrada forms a transition between the two main types of *laxatives* in his class, the *stimulant laxatives,* which cause evacuation by stimulation of the colon itself, and the *choleretic laxatives,* which cause bowel movement by increasing bile flow and quality. This botanical does some of both. While it may be used symptomatically in chronic conditions with intestines Qi stagnation, one is better served by treating it as a liver opening remedy with a special focus on the **constipation** so often present, as we do with acupuncture points Li 3 & 13 and St 25 & 37. Internal portal congestion with hemorrhoids, right flank pain and chronic constipation or irregular bowel movement are all relieved in the process. Its downward moving emphasis entails an increase of urine output and renal cleansing as well. Moreover, like Rhubarb root (*Da huang* in the Chinese pharmacopoeia), Cascara sagrada is effectively useful in **excess internal heat** conditions. In addition, Cascara exhibits *resolvent cleansing* effects which are only partly due to its *eliminant* activities. Overall metabolism in enhanced, and chronic low level symptoms such as skin rashes, fetid stools and tendency to stone formation are improved. It is clearly a good choice for treating symptoms due to **stagnant** conditions of **excess** and **general toxmia**, and specifically those involving the liver, stomach intestines.

Alder buckthorn: Class 3

ALDER BUCKTHORN

Pharmaceutical name: Cortex ramuli Rhamni frangulae
Botanical name: Rhamnus frangula L., syn. Frangula alnus Mill. (N.O. Rhamnaceae)
Ancient names: Alnus nigra, Avornus, Frangula (Lat)
Other names: Alder dogwood, Arrowood, European black alder, Persian berries (Eng & Am)
Bourdaine, Bourgène, Aune noir, Rhubarbe des paysans (Fr)
Faulbaum, Glatter Wegdorn, Pulverholz, Grindholz (Ge)
Part used: the branch bark

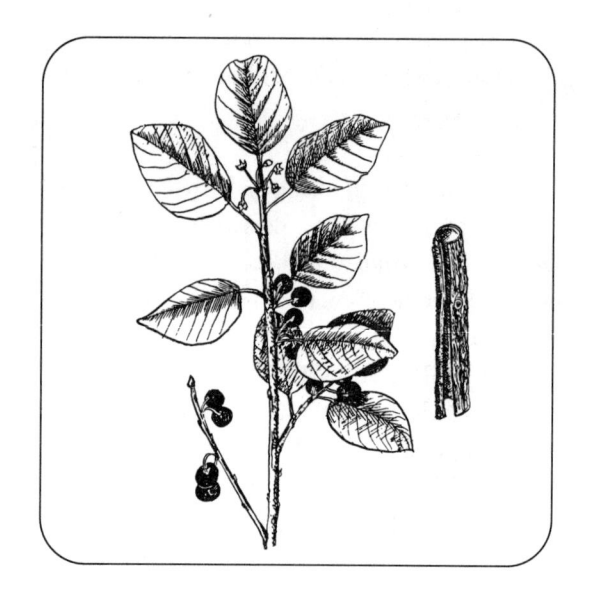

This herb is virtually identical in its constituents, qualities, functions and uses to CASCARA SAGRADA. Some practitioners, including R.F. WEISS, believe it to be less strong or reliable than the latter, but this is a matter of some dispute.

A closely related shrub is RHINEBERRY, also called Waythorn, Hartsthorn, Common buckthorn (Eng), Purging buckthorn (Am), Nerprun, Bourgépine (Fr), Wegdorn, Kreuzdorn (Ge), *fructus Rhamni,* from *Rhamnus catharticus* L. Its berries are also used in the same way as function 2 of Cascara sagrada. Its main active ingredients are also anthraquinones. One teaspoon of the dried berries are used to a 1/4 litre (1/2 pint) of water in INFUSION.

SENNA

Pharmaceutical name: folium Sennae
Botanical name: Senna acutifolia Del., *vel angustifolia* Vahl. (N.O. Leguminosae)
Other names: Alexandrian Senna, Tinnevelly Senna (Eng)
Fan xia ye (Ch)
Part used: the leaf; also the pod, *folliculum Sennae*

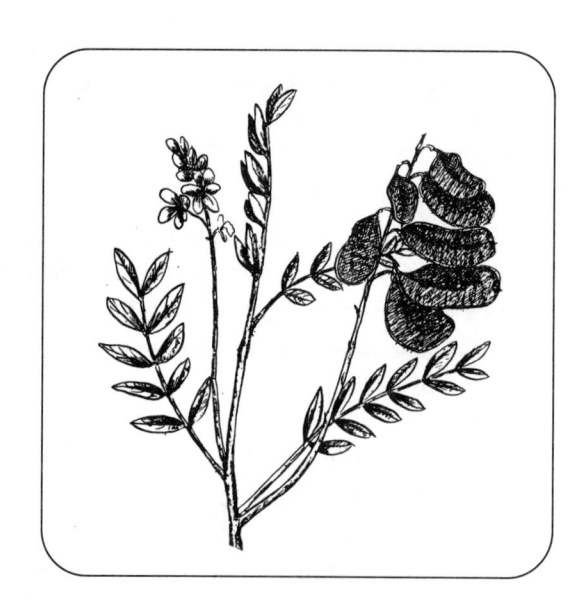

Nature

CATEGORY: mild herb with minimal chronic toxicity
CONSTITUENTS: anthraquinone glycosides (incl. rhein, aloe-emodin, sennosides A & B), chrysophanic acid, chrysophanol, mannitol, mucilage, acetic acid salts, resins, ess. oil (traces),

Class 3: Senna

EFFECTIVE QUALITIES
Primary: bitter, hot with a secondary cooling effect, dry
Secondary: stimulating
  sinking movement
TROPISM: intestines, uterus
  Warmth organism
  Small intestine meridian

Functions and Uses

1 PROVOKES BOWEL MOVEMENT, REMOVES STAGNANCY AND CLEARS HEAT; STIMULATES THE COLON AND ABATES DISTENTION; STIMULATES THE UTERUS AND PROVOKES MENSTRUATION

intestines Qi stagnation with temporary constipation due to any cause, abdominal distention
EXCESS HEAT CONDITIONS with constipation in general
uterus Qi stagnation with amenorrhea

Preparation

USE: The ideal preparation is a cold water MACERATION for 8-10 hours: this causes less extraction of the resins responsible for causing intestinal irritation and griping. The little loss of efficiency entailed is adequate compensation for the cramping it otherwise causes, especially for those average cases of temporary constipation where a stronger *laxative* is unnecessary.

The TINCTURE and INFUSION are useful, nevertheless, and should be combined with one or more *carminatives* such as Ginger, Cumin or Fennel in 1 part to 4 for most comfortable results.

Other pharmaceutical preparations existed in the past, and some are still available today.

Senna is commonly used in formulas treating syndromes other than those above, where a pronounced *laxative* effect is required.

Senna **pods** are only mildly *laxative* and are especially suited to children and pregnant women, taken in INFUSION of 3-8 g.

DOSAGE: MACERATION & INFUSION: 1-2 g per cup of water (1 g is usual)
  TINCTURE: 10-40 drops; 25 drops or 1 ml is usual

CAUTION: Senna leaf is used to relieve **temporary** constipation or amenorrhea only, since it is habit forming and should not be used for more than a few days at a time. The dosage should not be exceeded. Pregnancy is a contraindication as Senna is *uterine stimulant*. So are all **congestive inflammatory** and **catarrhal intestinal** conditions as found in intestines damp Heat, blood heat, uterus blood congestion and intestines damp cold. This is because Senna has a *hot, stimulant* and *irritant* quality which causes hyperemia in the pelvic organs.

Like Aloes, however, Senna leaf **can** be used for internal heat conditions in the absence of these contraindications. This can be called an internal *counterirritant* technique, since through derivation blood (and therefore heat) is effectively drawn downward.

NOTE: American senna, *Cassia marilandica,* has been said to be the therapeutic equivalent of the two species normally used. Bladder senna (*Colutea arborescens*) and Wild senna (*Globularia alypum*), on the other hand, are milder than any of these.

Notes

Since the classification of Senna and Aloes as *hot* herbs is likely to cause concern among practitioners of Chinese medicine, it is thought best to devote a little space to this theme. Senna leaf is known as *Fan xia ye* in Chinese medicine.

Senna: Class 3

It should be clear, first of all, that by definition all *irritant* substances have a **hot** nature. Tissue irritation causes increased activity, i.e. blood flow, and therefore heat. (*Rubefacients* take advantage of this in *counterirritation* therapy.) If continued, external irritation causes inflammation or blistering (as do *vesicants*). Garlic, Cayenne, Aloes and Senna, for example, are all *hot,* and all are contraindicated in local hot or inflammatory congestive conditions.

The reason that Chinese and Ayurvedic pharmacology calls Senna and Aloes **cold** is that by causing intestinal irritation and hence bowel movement they effectively clear heat. As *hot irritant purgatives* Aloes and Senna are heat clearing by **internal counter-irritation**. The definitive consideration from the Chinese point of view, then, is not the warmth quality of the herb itself, but its final effect in these particular conditions of heat. However, in conditions without heat, Senna and Aloes are definitely not cooling, increasing activity as they do and clearing stagnation in the lower warmer. These remedies have been used since prehistoric times for simple colonic and menstrual obstruction without heat. Moreover, since both are hardly ever used in acute full heat conditions on their own, but are combined, instead, with cold sustances such as minerals, defining their warmth solely by the pragmatic criterion of their final effect actually defeats its own purpose. Far better to understand the *derivative* effect of *hot irritant* herbs, which can clear heat of a noncongestive kind when required. Only in this way can Senna's use in simple obstructive conditions be differentiated from its use in hot conditions.

Galenic medical authors from Greek, Jewish, Persian, Arabic and European cultures were not ignorant of these problems when they classified Senna and Aloes as **hot** or **heating** substances, on the contrary. The Aristotle trained minds of Persian physicians spent much time ruminating over the intrinsic nature and actual effect of medicinal substances—as they did with every substance known: they were alchemists and philosophers, after all, who virtually founded modern pharmacy. These are the conclusions they drew, based on over a millenium of experience. Today, when energetic medicine is in its infancy once again, we can learn much from them.

ALOES

Pharmaceutical name: folium Aloidis
Botanical name: Aloe vulgaris L. *et* spp. (N.O. Liliaceae)
Other names: Aloès (Fr)
   Aloe (Ge)
   Lu hui (Ch)
Part used: the leaf

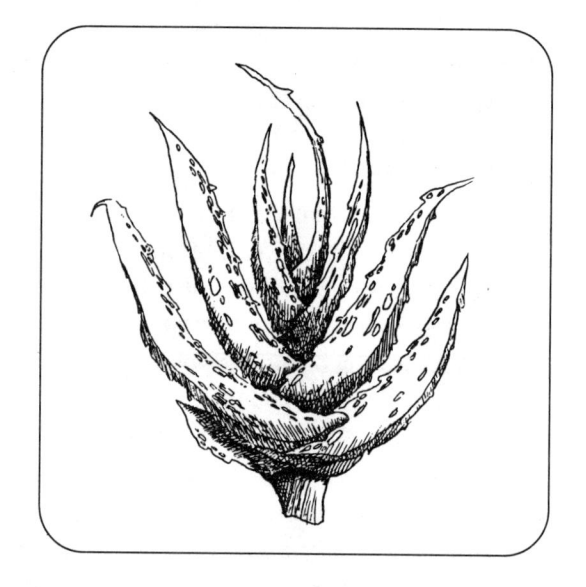

Nature

CATEGORY: mild herb with minimal chronic toxicity
CONSTITUENTS: crystalline glycosides aloin (incl. barbaloin, isobarbaloin), amorphous aloin (ß-barbaloin), aloe-emodin, capaloin, resin 16-63%, ess. oil, fructose, glucose, arrabinose & mannose, mucopolysaccharides, formic acids (asparagin, salin, serin, glutaminic acid), calcium,

Class 3: Aloes

potassium, magnesium, magnesium lactate, pradiciminase, glycoprotein aloctin-A
EFFECTIVE QUALITIES
Primary: bitter, hot with a secondary cooling effect, moist
Secondary: stimulating
sinking movement
TROPISM: liver, stomach, intestines, uterus
Warmth organism
Liver, Small Intestine meridians
GROUND: all krases, biotypes & constitutions for symptomatic use

Functions and Uses

1. PROVOKES BOWEL MOVEMENT, REMOVES STAGNANCY AND CLEARS HEAT; STIMULATES THE COLON AND ABATES DISTENSION; STIMULATES THE UTERUS AND PROVOKES MENSTRUATION

    intestines Qi stagnation with abdominal distension, chronic constipation
    uterus Qi stagnation with delayed, obstructed menses
    STUBBORN CHRONIC CONSTIPATION or OBSTRUCTED MENSES due to stagnation or heat
    liver fire with red face, headache, constipation

2. STIMULATES THE LIVER AND STOMACH AND AWAKENS THE APPETITE

    liver & stomach Qi stagnation with poor appetite and painful, slow digestion

Preparation

USE: Used is the golden brown **powdered concentrate** derived from the bitter tasting **juice** in the peripheral leaf cells of *Aloe ferox, Aloe vulgaris* and *Aloe soccotrina* mainly. This contains the active anthraquinone glycosides. A TINCTURE or FLUID EXTRACT of the **leaves** has similar functions.
DOSAGE: Dosage is critical, here as with other remedies of this class. **Smaller** doses have a *stimulating* effect on upper digestive activities (function 1), while **larger** doses function in *laxative, purgative, emmenagogue* and *cooling* ways (function 2).
Smaller dose:
   TINCTURE: 24 drops
   POWDER: 1 grain (0.07 g)
   JUICE: 1 ml (1/5 tsp)
Larger dose:
   TINCTURE: 2-6 ml (50-140 drops)
   POWDER: 2-6 grains (0.2-0.5 g)
   JUICE: 2-4 ml (a weak 1/2-1 tsp)
CAUTION: Since Aloes is very *irritant* and *heating* locally (due to its resin content), it is contraindicated in pregnancy and in congestive conditions of the urogenital organs and pelvis, especially with copious menstrual or any intermenstrual bleeding (e.g. uterus blood congestion or blood heat). Hemorrhoids therefore also forbid its use. Besides, Aloes should not be used continuously **for any condition.** In any case, it is best always combined with smaller amounts of, e.g. Tamarind, Fennel, magnesium carbonate, etc. to mitigate griping or cramping.

Aloes is only fully effective with normal bile secretions and alkaline chyme, since it depends on this environment to unfold its effects. Hence it is not fully effective where liver Qi stagnation, especially with jaundice, is present.

Aloes: Class 3

Notes

The Aloe plant is a succulent from the East and South African tropics and one of the few botanicals used worldwide today for which we have indigenous African medicine to thank. Greek medicine found use for it from its earliest days (DIOSKURIDES, CELSUS, PLINIUS), and the island Sokotra soon became its Mediterranean home base. Chinese medicine also found use in it and established trading routes with East Africa under the Tang dynasty in the sixth century. (At that time the silk road began in Canton and ended at Alexandria, and Chinese coins and porcelain have been found as far south as Zimbabwe in Rhodesia). More recently, the plant gained the West Indies with the slave trade, and then the Southern states of North America, where it was diligently cultivated by Spanish missionaries and their servants. Through runaway slaves Aloes then passed over to the Seminole, Creek and Choctaw Native Americans. With this, its journey around the world was completed.

Therapeutically speaking, two facts about this remedy are significant. First, Aloes is the strongest of all *anthraquinone laxatives*. A glance at its constituents (no tannins, free anthraquinones, volatile oil, etc.) evinces this. It is simply in a class apart from Rhubarb, Cascara sagrada and Buckthorn. For this reason, it should be used as a *purgative* only as a **last resort** and hardly ever as a *laxative*. Secondly, it must be reserved for really **chronic** intestines Qi stagnation or uterus Qi stagnation where it can act as a catalyst to break habitual colonic and uterine inertia.

Paradoxically, even though Aloes has a *hot, irritant* nature like Senna, it may still be used for clearing heat through its *purgative* effect, a use particularly well developed by Chinese physicians. The dynamics of this effect is simply a *derivative* one using counterirritation—no less! (see footnote to SENNA).

TAMARIND

Pharmaceutical name: fructus Tamarindi
Botanical name: Tamarindus indica L. (N.O. Leguminosae)
Other names: Indian dates, Sour-bean tree (Eng)
   Tamar hindi (Ar)
Part used: the fruit

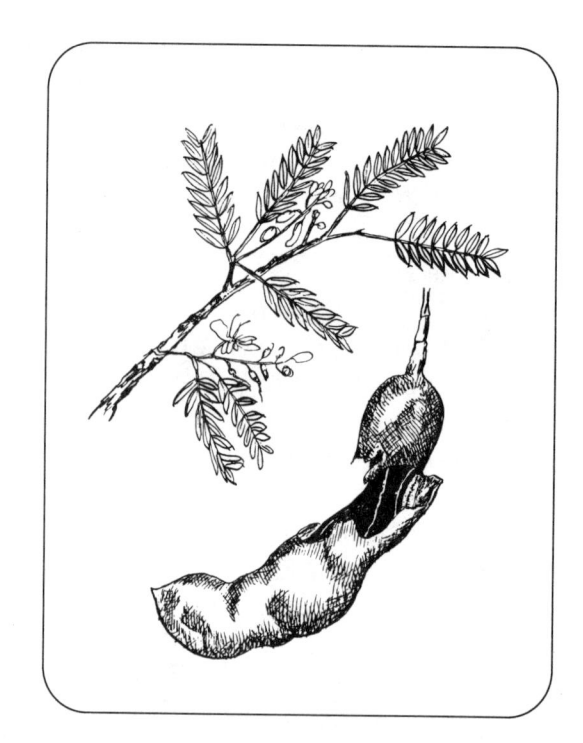

Nature

CATEGORY: mild herb with minimal chronic toxicity
CONSTITUENTS: 10-15% tartaric acid, acetic/malic/succinic acids, sugars, pectin

Class 3: Tamarind

EFFECTIVE QUALITIES
Primary: sour & oily & sweet, cool, moist
Secondary: softening
  sinking movement
TROPISM: stomach, intestines, urogenital organs
  Warmth, Fluid organisms
  Colon, Small Intestine meridians
GROUND: all krases, biotypes & constitutions for symptomatic use

Functions and Uses

1 CLEARS HEAT, RESOLVES FEVER AND REDUCES INFLAMMATION; MOISTENS AND SOOTHES THE INTESTINES, PROMOTES BOWEL MOVEMENT AND RELIEVES THIRST

intestines dry heat with constipation, dry throat & mouth
CONSTIPATION with dryness due to any condition
EXCESS HEAT conditions with hard scanty stools, fever, thirst FEVERS in general
INFLAMMATION of the intestines, kidneys, liver, gallbladder with heat or damp heat

2 RESTRAINS UROGENITAL DISCHARGE

DISCHARGES in venereal infections
PREMATURE EJACULATION, seminal discharges

Preparation

USE: A short DECOCTION of the fruit pulp is best; a TINCTURE is also possible.
USAGE: Generous standard doses are used whether Tamarind given on its own or combined with other *laxatives, demulcents* or *cooling remedies,* as is often the case.

Notes

The soft, dark, oily fruit of the Tamarind tree has always been used in Indian cooking as well as in medicine. Like Camphor, Myrrh and many others it has come to us via the Arabian pharmacy. In Ayurveda it balances the dosas by increasing Kapha and lowering Vata, whether taken as part of daily fare or as concentrated medicine. Its action unfolds primarily on the small and large intestines, where it has a *moistening, soothing, cooling, softening* effect. In Physiomedical terms Tamarind is a *relaxant*. Two main usages outline themselves once its qualities are understood. First, **dry intestinal** conditions of all kinds with constipation are relieved through its *demulcent laxative* effect; the stool is softened, and bowel movement follows. If the overall syndrome is a hot one, Tamarinds will tend to promote cooling and relieve thirst. "They purge moderately and temperately," stated the London apothecary JOHN QUINCY in 1736, and are milder than all others in this class. They were combined with others such as Rhubarb, Rose and Senna in Persian style preparations in electuaries, syrups, juleps, bolus, etc.

Secondly, **damp heat** conditions of the **intestines** are relieved with its *cooling, lenitive* and slightly *astringent* effect; fluid discharges are also lessened. Here its *sourness* acts in a similar way to that of *Wu wei zi, fructus Schizandrae*, and *Shan zhu yu, fructus Corni*, in the Chinese pharmacy. It remains to be seen whether this astrictive effect extends to restraining night sweat in lung Yin deficiency syndromes, for example.

TVSSILAGO Roßhůb.

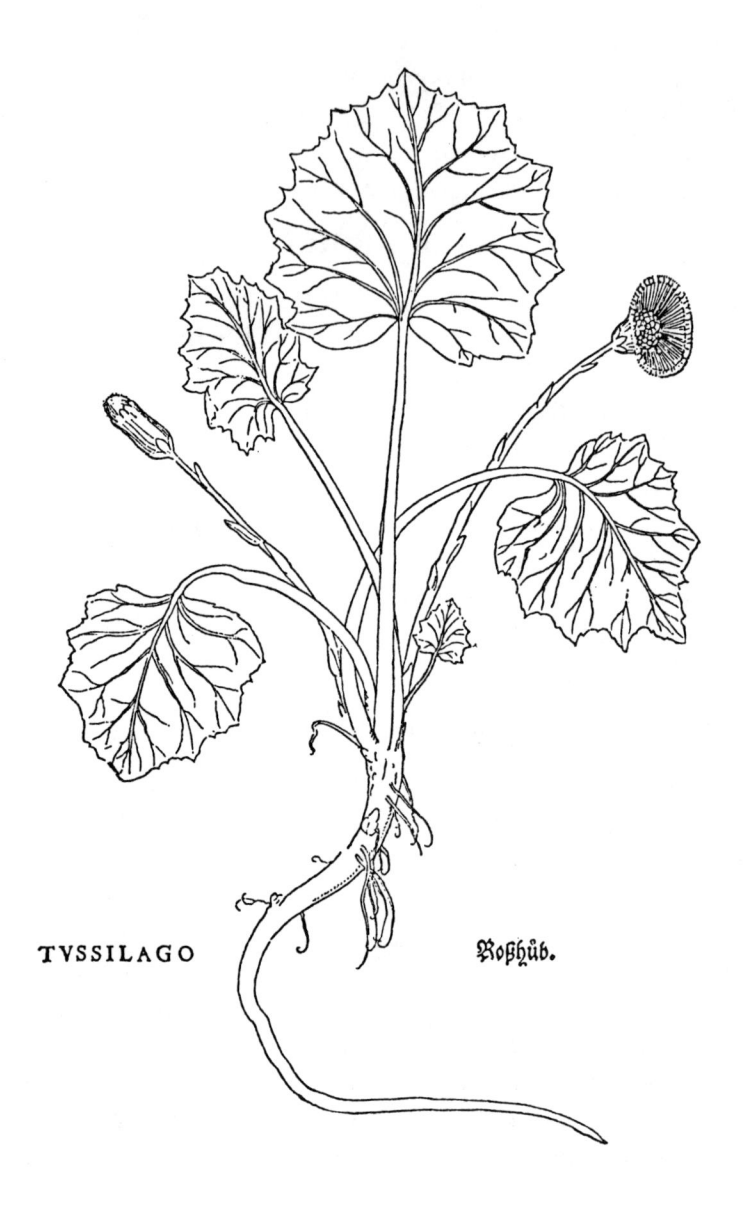

Coltsfoot

CLASS 4

Herbs to Expel Phlegm and Relieve Coughing

Herbs in this class treat conditions characterized by a stasis or obstruction of excessive phlegm and toxins in the bronchi, and thereby relieve coughing. Their stimulating action on the bronchi makes coughing an easier act of elimination, thus encouraging a natural response of the vital force to irritants.

Phlegm represents unmetabolized mucus secretions in the lungs. Since no longer serving a protecting and moistening function but stagnating and hardening instead, it is clearly an injurious substance. By hindering normal secretion it provides a hotbed for bacteria and therefore infection. Phlegm is treated by stimulating the cough reflex which will loosen and expel it.

Stagnant phlegm in the lungs is found in a variety of syndromes which vividly describe the state of the phlegm being eliminated: lung phlegm cold, lung phlegm heat, lung phlegm dryness. If phlegm accumulates over a long time causing chest fullness, asthmatic breathing, etc., (as found in, e.g., chronic bronchitis or bronchial asthma) then the *emetic* treatment method described in Class 6 should be used.

1 HERBS TO GENERATE WARMTH AND EXPEL PHLEGM

Botanicals in this category treat **lung phlegm cold/damp** conditions typified by a full cough, expectoration of profuse thin white phlegm, intermittent continuous coughing, wheezing or shortness of breath on exertion or when lying down, a slippery or wiry pulse and a greasy white tongue moss. These symptoms are usually found in conditions such as chronic bronchitis and chronic bronchial asthma.

Treatment aims to stimulate the lungs to expel phlegm by using herbs with *warm, pungent, dry, stimulating* qualities: *warm stimulant expectorants* in other words. These remedies, usually containing essential oil and/or saponins, include Angelica, Hyssop, Elecampane and Horehound among others. They increase elimination through the bronchial mucous membrane, promote the expectoration of phlegm, and generate warmth through increased circulation. They are contraindicated if there is any coughing up or vomiting of blood.

2 HERBS TO CLEAR HEAT, RESTRAIN INFECTION AND EXPEL PHLEGM

This group of remedies is directed at **lung phlegm heat**, a syndrome which includes more severe or acute lung infections such as acute bronchitis, bacterial pneumonia and pleurisy. Typical symptoms are some chills and slight fever; coughing, wheezing; chest pain, muscle aches; coughing up phlegm which may be thick, fetid, yellow-green or containing pus or blood; a fast and slippery pulse, and a yellow-coated tongue.

Here the treatment is to clear the infection and heat as well as to eliminate the offensive phlegm. The appropriate remedies have a *cool stimulant nature* as well as *disinfectant* properties. Ribwort plantain, Pleurisy root, Comfrey and Elder flower are prime examples. Some, being *anticatarrhal tonic astringents* like Ribwort and Elder flower, provide the bonus of inhibiting excessive mucus production.

The Energetics of Western Herbs

3 HERBS TO LIQUIFY AND EXPEL PHLEGM AND RELIEVE COUGHING

This group of remedies addresses **lung phlegm dryness**. This can follow exogenous conditions such as wind heat or wind dryness or endogenous ones such as lung Qi constraint. The latter typically involves spasmodic asthma, a nervous condition affecting the lungs over longer periods of time. In this case there may be mental tension or emotional holding, chest distention with pain, asthmatic breathing with wheezing, and a wiry pulse. Alternatively, lung Qi constraint may represent an allergy that has been driven inwards causing asthma (i.e. allergic asthma) and commonly found in the aftermath of influenza, pneumonia and tuberculosis, especially after antibiotic treatment. Whatever its origin, however, lung phlegm dryness always manifests coughing up hard plugs of sticky phlegm, with difficulty of coughing; this holds true even when an external pathogen such as dry wind is the immediate trigger.

The treatment of lung phlegm dryness with herbs is pitched at several levels, depending on the condition's context and etiology. If lung Qi constraint is at the root, remedies which circulate lung Qi, *respiratory relaxants,* are used. Botanicals such as Black cohosh, Wild cherry, Red clover, Lobelia and Inmortal will allay tension and anxiety, open the chest and ease breathing. If the context is an allergic diathesis, then this should be the priority of treatment. In all cases, however, it is viscous bronchial phlegm which needs softening, loosening and eliminating with *secretolytic expectorants*. These contain saponins, which help turn a dry cough into a more wet, productive one. Mullein, Cowslip, Soapwort and Grindelia are good examples of this type of expectorant.

All forms of lung dryness call for the additional support of Class 10 *demulcent expectorants*.

4 HERBS TO DRAIN HEAD PHLEGM AND CLEAR THE SINUSES

When phlegm blocks the **nasal** and **other passages** in the **head,** not only difficult breathing, but also giddiness, confused thinking and a heavy feeling head may follow. This is normally a follow-on from head damp cold or lung wind cold, and is treated by softening and draining the phlegm downwards. This is achieved using *pungent warm aromatic* herbs with a high essential oil content: Peppermint, Marjoram, Eucalyptus and Camomile. They are best applied using steam inhalations or medicated snuffs.

A summary listing of all herbs in this class is found on page 693.

Herbs to Generate Warmth and Expel Phlegm

HYSSOP

Pharmaceutical name: herba Hyssopi
Botanical name: Hyssopus officinalis L. (N.O. Labiatae)
Ancient names: Yssopon (Gr)
   Hyssopus (Lat)
Other names: Ezob, Isop (Eng)
   Hysope (Fr)
   Ysop, Essigkraut, Klosterhysop, Eiserichkraut (Ge)
Part used: the herb

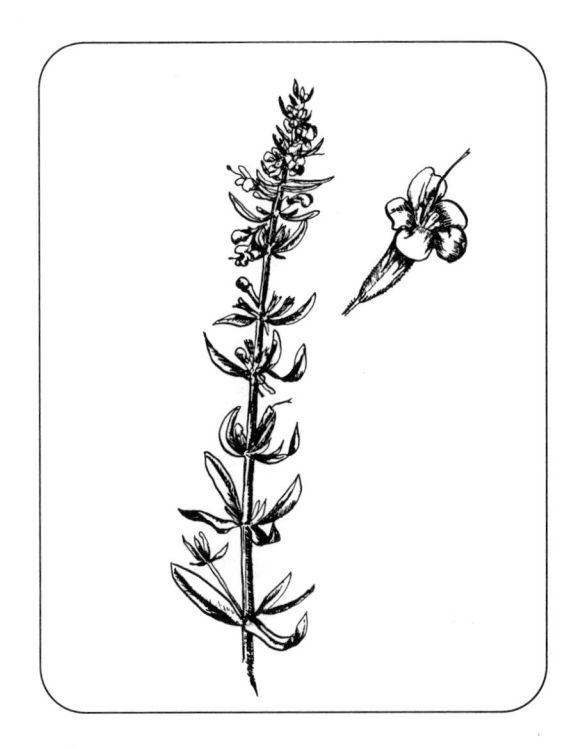

Nature

CATEGORY: mild herb with minimal chronic toxicity
CONSTITUENTS: ess. oil (incl. pinocamphone, phellandrene, borneol, thujone, limonene, geraniol), flavonoid glycoside (diosmin), tannins 8%, saponin, cholin, malic acid, silica, potassium nitrate, hyssopine
EFFECTIVE QUALITIES
Primary: a bit pungent & bitter, neutral, dry
Secondary: stimulating, restoring, relaxing
TROPISM: lungs, intestines, circulation, uterus, kidneys
   Air, Warmth organisms
   Lung, Spleen, Colon meridians
GROUND: Phlegmatic krasis
   Dependent/Tai Yin Earth biotype Lymphatic/Carbonic/Blue Iris constitution

Functions and Uses

1 STIMULATES AND WARMS THE LUNGS; LIQUIFIES AND EXPELS VISCOUS PHLEGM; RELAXES THE BRONCHI, OPENS THE CHEST AND RELIEVES WHEEZING

   lung phlegm cold: full cough with expectoration of thin white phlegm, chest fullness and distention
   CHRONIC BRONCHITIS or bronchial asthma
   lung Qi constraint: irritable, dry nervous cough, wheezing, coughing up plugs of hard phlegm
   SPASMODIC ASTHMA, whooping cough
   LUNG TB, HAYFEVER

Hyssop: Class 4

2. CAUSES SWEATING, RELEASES THE EXTERIOR AND SCATTERS WIND COLD; STIMULATES AND BALANCES THE CIRCULATION, RESOLVES FEVER AND PUSHES OUT ERUPTIONS

   external wind cold onset of flu or cold with chills, feverishness, dislike of cold, fatigue
   wind/damp obstruction: acute neuralgia worse in damp & cold
   LOW or HIGH BLOOD RESSURE
   REMITTENT & ERUPTIVE FEVERS

3. RESTORES THE LUNGS, INCREASES THE QI AND REPLENISHES DEFICIENCY; RESTORES THE NERVE, GENERATES STRENGTH AND RIDS DEPRESSION

   Qi deficiency: weakness, grief, melancholy
   lung Qi deficiency: shallow breathing, shortness of breath, poor resistance to colds
   NERVOUS EXHAUSTION due to stress, overwork, convalescence
   NERVOUS DEPRESSION, melancholy
   AUTOIMMUNE DISEASE of all types

4. WARMS AND INVIGORATES THE INTESTINES/*SPLEEN;* ABATES DISTENSION, REMOVES STAGNANCY AND EXPELS PARASITES

   intestines cold (Spleen Yang deficiency): lack of appetite, distended abdomen, abdominal colic, chilliness
   INTESTINAL PARASITES

5. STIMULATES THE UTERUS AND PROMOTES MENSTRUATION; DREDGES THE KIDNEYS, PROMOTES URINATION AND SOFTENS STONES

   uterus damp cold: missing or delayed, scanty menses with cramps, white leucorrhea
   kidney Qi stagnation: headaches, skin rashes, cystitis
   URINARY STONES & SAND (oxalic & phosphatic)

6. RESTRAINS INFECTION, RESOLVES CONTUSION, PROMOTES TISSUE REPAIR AND BENEFITS THE SKIN

   EAR, NOSE & THROAT INFECTIONS
   WOUNDS, CUTS
   BRUISES, contusions, wounds
   SKIN CONDITIONS incl. eczema, psoriasis, cancer
   TOOTHACHE

Preparation

USE: Like Class 7 *Qi tonics,* Hyssop can be used as a preventive over long periods of time; best suited to this is the INFUSION. This together with the TINCTURE and ESSENTIAL OIL are the main preparations of this remedy in therapy, in increasing grades of stimulation. The hot INFUSION is sipped mainly as a *stimulant diaphoretic* in **external wind cold** conditions affecting the **head** and **lungs**, while the other types of preparation open up Hyssop's full potential. The ESSENTIAL OIL may be applied externally with a base oil or taken internally (but see caution).

As a prime **lung** remedy Hyssop is, and was often, used in SYRUPS, as this recipe from RYFF's *Reformierte Deutsche Apotheck* testifies: Hyssop, Celery root, Fennel root, Liquorice, Gum tragacanth, Poplar seeds, Quince seeds, red and black Raisins, Rose petals (fresh), Squills, Figs and Dates—a typical *stimulating, warming* and *soothing* SYRUP from the traditional central European pharmacy. The CONSERVE of Hyssop flowers on the same page is unfortunately too long to reproduce; however we would recommend a simpler SYRUP or TINCTURE of Mullein and Hyssop flowers and tops (with a touch of Licorice) for stubborn asthmatic conditions due to Qi constraint.

GARGLES, WASHES, etc., are the most appropriate for external use.

DOSAGE: ESSENTIAL OIL: 2-3 drops in a little warm water
Others: standard doses

CAUTION: The recommended dose for the ESSENTIAL OIL should never be exceeded, as it contains the toxic cetone pinocamphene. For the same reason it should not be used continuously internally over 4 weeks, nor taken by individuals prone to epileptic fits.

During pregnancy Hyssop should be used with caution, if at all, being additionally *uterine stimulant*.

Notes

Hyssop is one of several remedies with an uplifting effect on the spirit and mind, being the only *nerve restorative* in this class. More specifically, it is an important herb for **chronic deficient** conditions with depression and low vitality, often of emotional origin, such as grief or suppressed feelings. **Qi deficiency** conditions specifically are here addressed: Hyssop is both a *Spleen* and *lung Qi tonic,* bolstering both ailing appetites and failing forces with its *bitter* taste. Deficiency cold conditions of the Spleen, lungs and uterus are all replenished and warmed through, especially those with an element of catarrhal damp and consequent discharge or of painful spasm. In addition, being a *sympathetic nervous stimulant,* Hyssop is a *systemic Yang tonic,* deeply *warming* and *stimulating,* like its fellow Mint Basil. Its use in these types of deficiency onditions must have been widespread in the Middle Ages during which, following Charles I's edict, Hyssop was much cultivated in the polynia-like physick gardens next to cloisters and walks.

Hyssop is a foremost remedy for **chronic cold** and **phlegmatic bronchial conditions**, especially those accompanied with above-mentioned symptoms. Clearly, there are some resemblances with *Jie geng, radix Platycodi,* used in Chinese herbalism, as seen mainly in functions 1 and 2 above, although, curiously enough, high blood pressure is another indication common to both botanicals. Among *stimulant expectorant* and *secretolytic* herbs in this class, Hyssop is typically *diaphoretic* and *relaxant:* wind cold with Yang deficiency and its accompanying symptoms due to poor arterial circulartion is its specific application here.

Pine: Class 4

PINE

Pharmaceutical name: folium Pini
Botanical name: Pinus sylvestris L. et spp. (N.O. Coniferae)
Ancient names: Poune, Pitous (Gr)
Other names: Pin sylvestre, Mantel (Fr)
    Waldkiefer, Föhre, Hartzbaum, Kinholz (Ge)
Part used: the needle

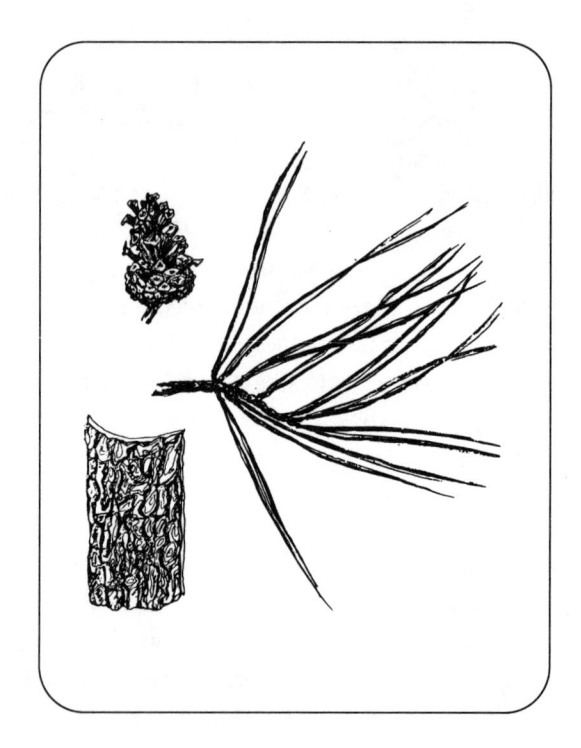

Nature

CATEGORY: mild herb with minimal chronic toxicity
CONSTITUENTS: turpentine resin, mallol, ess. oil (incl. sylvestrene, pinenes, bornyl acetate, cardimene, pumilone, phellandrenes, pinicrin), tannin, vit. C, glucose, galactose
EFFECTIVE QUALITIES
Primary: a bit pungent & bitter, neutral with both warming & cooling potential, both dry & moist
Secondary: stimulating, restoring, solidifying
    stabilizing movement
TROPISM: lungs, liver, stomach, urogenital organs
    Warmth, Air, Fluid organisms
    Lung, Kidney meridians
GROUND: Melancholic krasis
    Burdenned/Shao Yin & Sensitive/Tai Yin Metal biotypes
    Lymphatic/Carbonic/Blue Iris constitution

Functions and Uses

1   RESTORES AND STIMULATES THE LUNGS, LIQUIFIES AND EXPELS VISCOUS PHLEGM AND CLEARS THE HEAD; OPENS THE CHEST AND RELIEVES WHEEZING; LENIFIES IRRITATION
    lung & Kidney Yang deficiency with fatigue, chilliness, asthmatic breathing
    lung Yin deficiency with dry coughs, weakness; lung TB
    lung phlegm dryness with scanty hard phlegm
    lung phlegm damp with copious white phlegm
    ASTHMA, pneumonia, bronchitis, TB
    head damp cold with head congestion, colds

Class 4: Pine

2   SUPPORTS THE YANG AND RESTORES STRENGTH; STIMULATES THE ADRENALS
Spleen & Kidney Yang deficiency with mental, physical and sexual fatigue, chilliness, poor appetite, impotence
ADRENAL INSUFFICIENCY

3   RESTORES THE LIVER AND STOMACH, REMOVES STAGNANCY AND QUELLS NAUSEA
liver & stomach Qi deficiency with stagnation with swollen, painful distended abdomen, sour regurgitation, nausea

4   RESTRAINS INFECTION AND REDUCES INFLAMMATION; PROMOTES TISSUE REPAIR AND RELIEVES PAIN
INFECTIONS of the lungs, upper respiratory, urinary & genital organs (incl. flu, sinusitis, prostatitis, pyelitis)
CHOLECYSTITIS, gallstones
RHEUMATIC & gouty conditions, toothache, backache
SCABIES, lice
WOUNDS
EXCESSIVE PERSPIRATION of feet

Preparation

USE: The most efficient preparation of Pine needles is the distilled ESSENTIAL OIL: this can be used both externally with a base oil (RUBS, LINIMENTS, etc.), and internally (incl. in SYRUPS). Strengthening BATHS can be prepared, and INHALATIONS are excellent for sinus and bronchial infections. Alternately the needles may be shortly DECOCTED or TINCTURED. To some extent the **inner bark** may be used, as also the **buds** and **cones**.
DOSAGE: ESSENTIAL OIL: 3-5 drops in some warm water

Notes

Most parts of the Pine tree served as internal and external remedies for a variety of Native American tribes. Although a variety of Pines were used, White pine (*Pinus strobus*), Yellow pine (*Pinus echinata*) and the Long leaved pine (*Pinus palustris*) were the main ones. In Europe, *Pinus sylvestris* has played the same role for thousands of years.

Pine is one of the major **lung** remedies and, as such, similar to Balm of Gilead, Coltsfoot and Thyme in its great versatility. It will both *soften* and *stimulate* bronchial secretions, as well as *lenify* and *relax* the tissues involved, hence is applicable in a range of **cold, damp, dry** and **constrained** conditions of these weather-sensitive organs of the Earth element. Infections both acute and chronic are equally well treated by this herb which has the potential of either warming or cooling, thanks to its excellent *antiseptic, anodyne* and *anti-inflammatory properties*. When used for its more systemic functions, Pine has a good *Yang supporting* effect appropriate for Spleen and Kidney Yang deficiency syndromes where **fatigue, coldness** and **sexual exhaustion** are prominent. This is partly explicable through its *adrenal stimulation* (on both the medulla and cortex), which also ensures good results with forms of asthma due to lung and Kidney Yang deficiency.

Bloodroot: Class 4

BLOODROOT

Pharmaceutical name: rhizoma Sanguinariae
Botanical name: Sanguinaria canadensis L. (N.O. Papaveraceae)
Other names: Red puccoon, Indian paint, Tetterwort, Pauson (Am)
    Sanguinaire (Fr)
    Kanadisches Blutkraut, Blutwurzel (Ge)
Part used: the rhizome

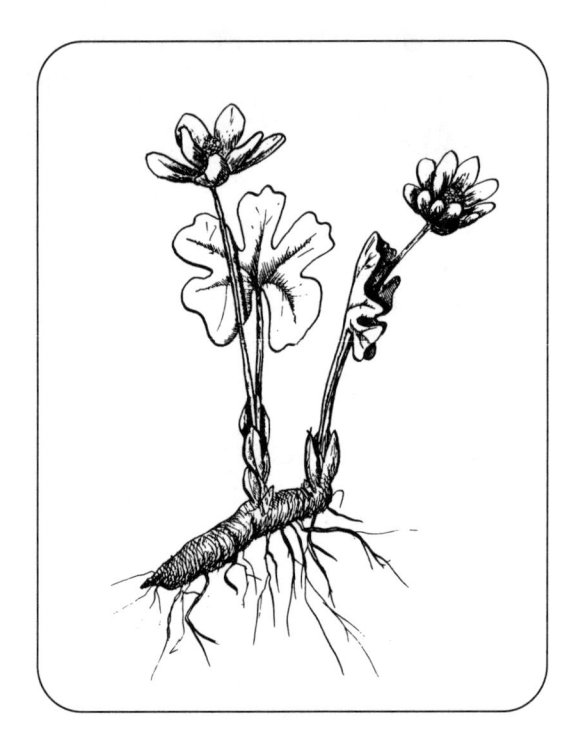

Nature

CATEGORY: medium-strength herb with some chronic toxicity
CONSTITUENTS: alkaloids (chelerythrin, sanguinarine, homochelidonin, protopin), resin, sanguinaric acid, citric & malic acids, starch
EFFECTIVE QUALITIES
Primary: pungent & bitter, hot, dry
Secondary: stimulating, restoring
TROPISM: lungs, heart, liver, stomach, intestines, uteus, urinary organs
    Air, Warmth organisms
    Lung, Heart, Liver
GROUND: Phlegmatic & Melancholic krases
    Dependant/Tai Yin Earth & Burdened/Shao Yin biotypes
    Lymphatic/Carbonic/Blue Iris constitutions

Functions and Uses

1   STIMULATES AND WARMS THE LUNGS, EXPELS VISCOUS PHLEGM, RELIEVES COUGHING AND CLEARS THE HEAD; RESTORES THE HEART AND LUNGS
lung phlegm cold with chilliness, full cough with white sputum
CHRONIC BRONCHITIS
lung dryness with harsh dry cough, irritation/tickle in throat
LUNG hepatization
head damp cold with nasal catarrh
heart & lung Qi deficiency with palpitations, chest oppression

Class 4: Bloodroot

2   PROMOTES BOWEL MOVEMENT AND REMOVES STAGNANCY: STIMULATES AND DREDGES THE LIVER, WARMS AND INVIGORATES THE INTESTINES AND PROMOTES BILE FLOW

liver cold stagnation with nauseaous headache, cold limbs, catarrhal jaundice
stomach & intestines cold with gurgling abdomen, epigastric pain

3   STIMULATES AND WARMS THE UTERUS, RESTORES THE UROGENITAL ORGANS AND PROMOTES THE MENSES

uterus cold with delayed, cramping menstruation
genitourinary cold (Kidney Yang deficiency) with scanty or frequent urination, chilliness

4   BENEFITS THE SKIN

SKIN ERUPTIONS, sores, ulcers, scrofula
Fungal growths, tumors

Preparation

USE: The TINCTURE and DECOCTION are good all round preparations. A simple or compound SYRUP may be used in lung conditions, while external uses include a SALVE and WASH for skin conditions.

DOSAGE: TINCTURE: 10-40 drops (i.e. max. 1.5 ml)
                 DECOCTION: 2-10 g per pint or 1/2 l of water for a day's supply

Smaller doses relieve lung irritation by a *lenitive* action, while **larger** ones irritate and cause *stimulation* and *expectoration.*

CAUTION: Blood root has some chronic toxicity due to its alkaloids: dosages should not be exceeded, nor should Blood root be taken continuously without breaks, especially if used as a simple. Its *pungent hot stimulant* energetic property also makes it contraindicated during pregnancy and with acute inflammations; it is also best avoided in young children.

Notes

The root of this valuable Native American remedy becomes red when broken, whence its name. Botanists like JOHN BARTRAM and JAMES BIGELOW around the turn of the last century helped to make this cousin of the Celandine known to Western science, and it became an important agent in Eclectic medicine for most of the nineteenth century.

Bloodroot's *stimulating* and *warming* influence is felt equally in the rhythmical organs above the diaphragm as in the metabolic ones below. Containing some similar and some identical biochemical constituents, such as alkaloids and acids, to those of Celandine, it has many uses in common with it. Both are used as *diaphoretics* in fevers and to stimulate and mobilize the liver Yang in liver cold type syndromes with stuck or insufficient bile-flow. But here their ways do part. Blood root is *restorative* to both heart and lung Qi, as well as a *stimulant expectorant.* In severe or chronic bronchial, hepatic and urogenital conditions presenting with **deficiency, cold, phlegm** and **weakness** due to deficient Yang, Blood root can play an important role. It addresses the same lung conditions as *Xuan fu hua, flos Inulae,* in the Chinese pharmacy, i.e. those which acupuncture would treat with points Bl 13, Lu 7, St 40, Gb 34 and CV 6 & 12 with moxa. While combining well with other types of *expectorant* remedies in this class, it may also be used, for example, for convalescence from pneumonia with exhaustion and coughing together with Wild cherry, Mullein and Coltsfoot.

Yerba Santa: Class 4

YERBA SANTA

Pharmaceutical name: folium Eriodictyonis
Botanical name: Eriodictyon californicum Greene, *vel E. tomentosum* Benth., *vel E. angustifolium* L. (N.O. Hydrophyllaceae)
Other names: Mountain balm, Bear plant, Holy herb, Consumptive's weed (Am)
Part used: the leaf

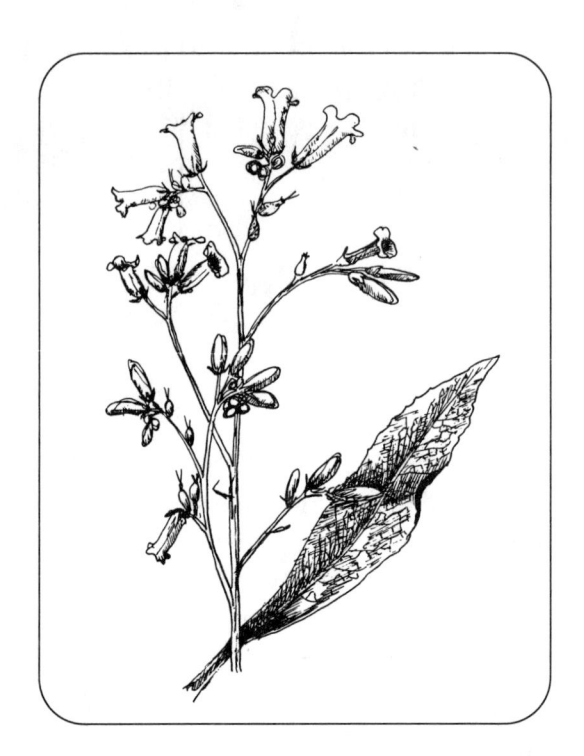

Nature

CATEGORY: mild herb with minimal chronic toxicity
CONSTITUENTS: resins, phenols, ess. oil, ericolin, eriodictyonic acid, tannin, gum
EFFECTIVE QUALITIES
Primary: a bit pungent & bitter & sweet & astringent, warm, dry
Secondary: stimulating, relaxing
TROPISM: lungs, liver, stomach, head, sinuses
　　　　　Air organism
　　　　　Lung, Colon meridians
GROUND: all krases, biotypes and constitutions for symptomatic use

Functions and Uses

1   STIMULATES THE LUNGS AND EXPELS PHLEGM; RELAXES THE BRONCHI, OPENS THE CHEST AND RELIEVES WHEEZING
    lung phlegm cold with copious white phlegm, wheezing
    CHRONIC BRONCHITIS, consumption
    lung Qi constraint with dry harsh cough, asthmatic beathing
    CHRONIC ASTHMA with weakness

2   RESTORES THE LIVER AND STOMACH, AWAKENS THE APPETITE
    liver & stomach Qi deficiency with no appetite, slow painful digestion, fatigue

3   RESTRAINS INFECTION, CREATES ASTRICTION AND CLEARS THE HEAD
    BLADDER & urethra INFECTIONS, esp. mild or chronic
    head damp cold with head congestion
    HAYFEVER
    LEUCORRHEA

Class 4: Yerba santa

Preparation

USE: Standard doses of the TINCTURE are used for a full-strength remedy; the DECOCTION is still useful however. The SYRUP, simple or compound, is an excellent way of using Yerba santa for lung conditions. For skin and bronchial congestion the STEAM INHALATION may work wonders, while a DOUCHE wil help stop discharges.

DOSAGE: TINCTURE: O.5-2 ml, or 15-50 drops
　　　　　　DECOCTION: 3-10 g

Notes

The long, slender, Rosemary-like green leaves of this low shrub from the mountain West of the U.S. and northern Mexico are called Yerba santa, Holy herb, in the Spanish culture. They have a distinctive, gently bittersweet taste with a spicy top note reminiscent of Echinacea.

The value of Yerba santa is mainly as a *stimulating expectorant* and *bronchial* and *urinary disinfectant*. It is equally good with chronic **phlegm cold and asthmatic lung** conditions, both infectious and non infectious. Its somewhat *bitter* taste also serves *restoring* functions to the upper digestive tract, which are not marked enough, however, for any heat clearing results. In the **urinary tract** Yerba santa also proves an *antiseptic diuretic* due to its phenol, resin and essential oil content and serves mild bladder conditions of the damp heat or damp cold type well. In congestive head conditions, with or without chest involvment, Yerba santa has also proved very effective. Hayfever is often prevented or relieved, in this connection.

Since having four taste qualities, and hence four eneregetic directions, Yerba santa combines well with other remedies. It could even be seen as a possible substitute for a Chinese herb such as *Xuan fu hua, flos Inulae*.

Inmortal: Class 4

INMORTAL

Pharmaceutical name: radix Asclepiadis
Botanical name: Asclepias asperula Gray, *vel capricorna* L., *vel syriaca* L., *vel decumbens* L. (N.O. Asclepiadaceae)
Other names: Antelope horns, Milkweed, Silk-weed, Wild cotton, Swallow-wort (Am)
   Herbe à la ouate, Asclépiade du Canada (Fr)
   Echte Seidenpflanze, Egyptischer Hundskohl (Ge)
Part used: the root

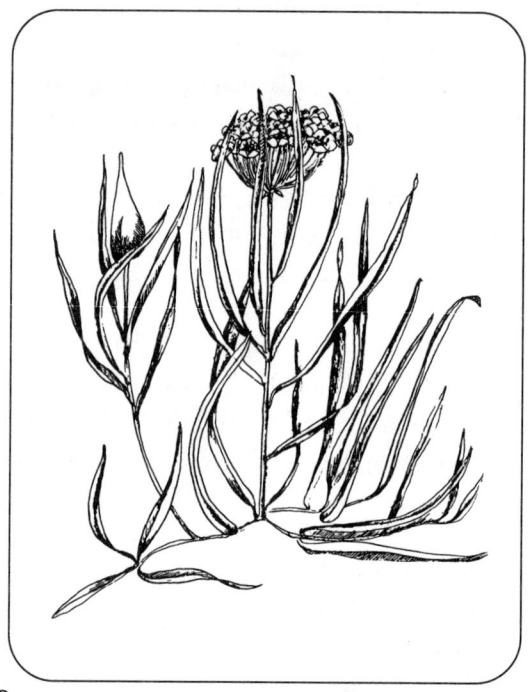

Nature

CATEGORY: mild herb with minimal chronic toxicity
CONSTITUENTS: glycosides (incl. cardiac glycosides & asclepiadin), bitters
EFFECTIVE QUALITIES
Primary: bitter, neutral with both warming & cooling potential
Secondary: stimulating, decongesting, restoring, relaxing
TROPISM: lungs, heart, circulation, stomach, liver
   Warmth & Air organisms
   Lung, Heart, Chong & Ren meridians
GROUND: Melancholic krasis
   Sensitive/Tai Yin Metal biotype
   Lymphatic/Carbonic/Blue Iris constitution

Functions and Uses

1. STIMULATES THE LUNGS AND EXPELS PHLEGM; RELAXES THE BRONCHI, OPENS THE CHEST AND LEVELS ASTHMA
   lung phlegm damp with coughing, some expectoration, wheezing
   CHRONIC BRONCHITIS, bronchial asthma
   lung Qi constraint with asthmatic breathing, tight chest
   SPASMODIC ASTHMA
   PMEUMONIA, pleurisy, chest & side pains

2. CAUSES SWEATING, RELEASES THE EXTERIOR AND SCATTERS WIND COLD; STIMULATES THE LYMPH AND BENEFITS THE SKIN
   external wind cold onset of infections with fatigue, chills, low vitality
   REMITTENT FEVERS in Shao Yang stage
   LYMPH CONGESTION
   SKIN conditions in general

Class 4: Inmortal

3 STIMULATES THE CIRCULATION, STIMULATES AND SUPPORTS THE HEART, RELIEVES BLOOD CONGESTION

heart Yang deficiency with mental depression, palpitations
heart blood congestion with shortness of breath, cardiac pain

4 STIMULATES THE UTERUS, PROMOTES THE MENSES AND EXPELS THE AFTERBIRTH

uterus Qi stagnation with delayed, painful menstruation
RETAINED PLACENTA

5 RESTORES THE LIVER AND STOMACH, AWAKENS THE APPETITE AND PROMOTES BOWEL MOVEMENT

liver & stomach Qi deficiency with poor appetite, slow painful digestion, constipation

Preparation

USE: The DECOCTION, TINCTURE and FLUID EXTRACT are taken for internal use. Either makes a fair INHALANT for clogged sinuses.
DOSAGE: half the standard doses throughout
CAUTION: Being a *uterine stimulant*, Inmortal is forbidden during pregnancy.

Notes

Inmortal is an effective plant remedy from the Native American and Spanish traditions of New Mexico. Its thin, spiky horn-like leaves have earned it the name *Antelope horns,* and it belongs to the Milkweed family, named *Asclepias* after the celebrated early Greek physician. There are several species which may be used to produce the remedy Inmortal (pronounced with the accent on the final syllable, as in "recall").

Inmortal's effect is essentially *stimulating,* unfolding mainly in the rhythmic sphere of **circulation, heart** and **lungs**. Heart and lung Yang are activated, and congestions (whether of blood or phlegm) cleared. A good *relaxant* effect on the bronchi is also obtained, evident from the improvement of bronchitic and asthmatic conditions of both the phlegm damp and the Qi constraint type. Lymphatic drainage from the lungs is also enhanced in chronic conditions. Moreover, drunk hot, Inmortal initiates sweating and relieves the surface with onsets of flu or other infections where low vitality and chills are present. Inmortal's action here roughly equates to those of acupuncture points LI 4, Lu 7 & 5, Bl 13 and Ht 9.

With a definite tropism for the **reproductive** organs, Inmortal's *stimulating* effects extend down to the uterus where stagnant Qi type menstrual conditions are mobilized; in childbirth, labor pains are eased, and sticking placentas eliminated.

The suitability of this botanical for **chronic** conditions is underscored by a *bitter restoring* effect acting on the liver and stomach, as well as by its effectiveness in skin conditions generally, the dual result of *diaphoresis* and increased *lymph drainage* in general.

Herbs to Clear Heat, Restrain Infection and Expel Phlegm

PLEURISY ROOT

Pharmaceutical name: radix Asclepiadis tuberosae
Botanical nanme: Asclepias tuberosa L. (N.O. Asclepiadaceae)
Other names: Butterfly weed, Yellow milkweed, Archangel, Canada root, Tuber root, Orange swallow-wort, Wind root, Flux root, Chiggerflower (Am)
Asclépiade tubereuse (Fr)
Seidenpflanze, Knollige Schwalbenwurz (Ge)
Part used: the root

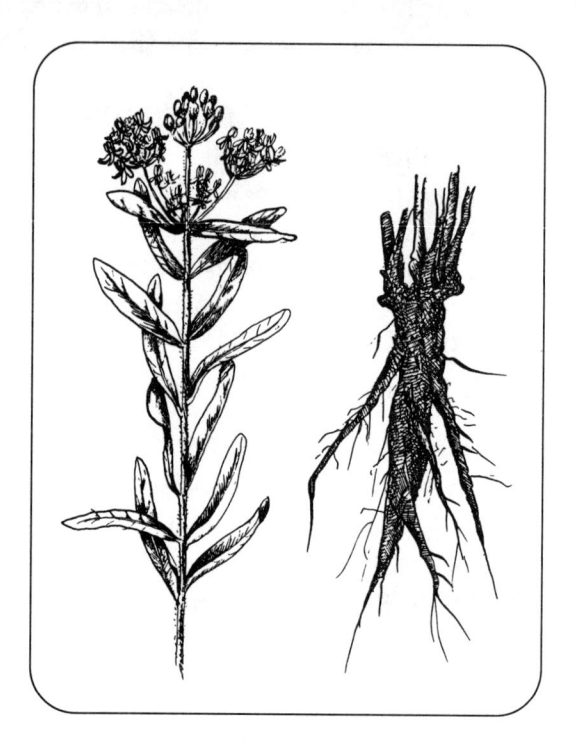

Nature

CATEGORY: medium-strength herb with some chronic toxicity
CONSTITUENTS: glycosides (incl. asclepiadin & cardioactive glycosides), alkaloid, tannic & gallic acids, resin, bitters, ess. oil, fixed oil, resins
EFFECTIVE QUALITIES
Primary: *Taste:* bitter, a bit pungent
Warmth: cool
Moisture: dry
Secondary: restoring stimulating, relaxing, decongesting
TROPISM
Organs or parts: lungs, heart, stomach, intestines, kidneys, uterus
Organisms: Air
Meridians: Lung, Spleen, Colon
Tri Dosas: regulates Vayu, decreases Kapha
GROUND
Krases/Temperaments: Choleric
Biotypes: Tough/Shao Yang
Constitutions: all three

Functions and Uses

1 STIMULATES THE LUNGS AND EXPELS PHLEGM; CLEARS HEAT AND REDUCES INFLAMMATION; RELIEVES WHEEZING AND COUGHING

lung (wind) heat: headache, fever, tight dry cough with scanty sticky phlegm, sore throat
PLEURISY, CROUP

Class 4: Pleurisy Root

lung phlegm heat: asthmatic breathing, coughing up fetid blood-streaked phlegm, full cough
ACUTE PLEURITIS, pneumonia, bronchitis, peritonitis
heart/lung fluid congestion: difficult breathing from exertion or lying down, irritability, chilliness, coughing up blood
ACUTE LUNG EDEMA

2   CIRCULATES THE QI, LOOSENS CONSTRAINT AND FREES SPASMS: RELAXES THE BRONCHI, INTESTINES AND UTERUS; OPENS THE CHEST, RELIEVES PAIN AND LEVELS ASTHMA

lung Qi constraint: asthmatic breathing, dry irritating cough, tight chest
SPASMODIC ASTHMA
CHEST PAINS, acute or intermittent
PLEURITIC CHEST PAINS, acute or chronic
intestines Qi constraint: colicky pains, flatulence
ACUTE GASTRITIS
uterus Qi constraint: delayed, scanty menstruation with cramps

3   CAUSES SWEATING, RELEASES THE EXTERIOR AND SCATTERS WIND HEAT; RESOLVES FEVER, PUSHES OUT ERUPTIONS AND RELIEVES IRRITABILITY

external wind heat: onset of INFECTIONS with aches and pains, irritability, fever
ACUTE RHEUMATIC FEVER
ERUPTIVE FEVERS: chickenpox, measles, scarlet fever
wind/damp obstruction: acute neuralgias or rheumatism

4   RESTORES THE LIVER, STOMACH AND INTESTINES/*SPLEEN*

liver & stomach Qi deficiency: painful slow digestion
Spleen Qi deficiency: weakness, poor appetite, diarrhea

5   DREDGES THE KIDNEYS, PROMOTES URINATION AND CLEANSING; PROMOTES TISSUE REPAIR AND BENEFITS THE SKIN

kidney Qi stagnation with general toxemia: skin rashes, dry skin, fatigue, mucous cystitis, abdominal bloating
WOUNDS, ulcers
SCROFULA, syphilis

Preparation

USE: The DECOCTION, drunk hot to *promote sweating,* is used in beginnings of colds and flus. This and the TINCTURE and FLUID EXTRACT (both made from the **dried** root) are all used for all functions above, with the TINCTURE being the most *stimulating* and *dispersing* in action.

DOSAGE: TINCTURE: 1-3 ml, or 25-75 drops
                DECOCTION: standard doses

Small doses only are needed for *restoring* and *cleansing* (functions 4 & 5)

CAUTION: Pleurisy root is contraindicated in pregnancy as it is a *uterine stimulant.*

Notes

Pleurisy root was one of the "finds" of early medical botanists in the US around the turn of the last century. Already the German medic JOHANN DAVID SCHOEPF had catalogued it in 1787,

Scabious: Class 4

probably based on SAMUEL STEARN's *American Herbal* of 1772. Affirmations about its "great certainty and permanency of operation" (CHAPMAN) were freely bandied about, and it rapidly became recognized as "powerfully promoting suppressed expectoration, and thereby relieving the breathing of pleuritic patients in the most advanced stage of the disease" (GRIFFITH). Of course, by that time little thought was given to the fact that Native Americans had been using this remedy for the same complaints for over a thousand years. Such is the fate of a remedy projected into the bright lights of Western medical publicity.

Pleurisy root is without doubt one of the best *expectorants* there is. But it is also a *cool relaxant stimulant,* like Elder flower, White horehound and Coltsfoot, and more: a *pungent bitter cool stimulant* like its Oriental similar, *Qian hu, radix Peucedani* from the same class of herbs. This makes all the difference in **wind heat** conditions with fever, coughing and wheezing, as also in inflammatory chest conditions of all types—as the Chinese know from their experience with *Qian hu.* Clearly, Pleurisy root is in harmony with an acupuncture point selection such as Lu 5 & 10, TH5, LI 4 and Bl 12.

Its *bitter* component, like the points Bl 38 and CV 12, here provides useful *tonifying* support where needed by working on the liver and stomach/*Spleen,* in harmony with its other qualities. Since Pleurisy root is equally effective in all its functions, it has a good combining potential with other herbs in this class.

SCABIOUS

Pharmaceutical name: planta tota Scabiosae
Botanical name: Scabiosae columbaria L. (N.O. Dipsaceae)
Ancient names: Psora (Gk)
　　Gallinacea, Columbaria (Lat)
Other names: Devil's bit scabious, Blue ball, Blue buttons, Devil's bit, Lamb's ears, Hardhead, Forebit (Eng)
　　Scabieuse, Bonnet bleu, Herbe de St. Joseph, Mors/Morsure du diable (Fr)
　　Taubenskabiose, Skabiosenkraut, Teufelsabbiss, Apostemenkraut, Grindkraut (Ge)
Part used: the whole plant

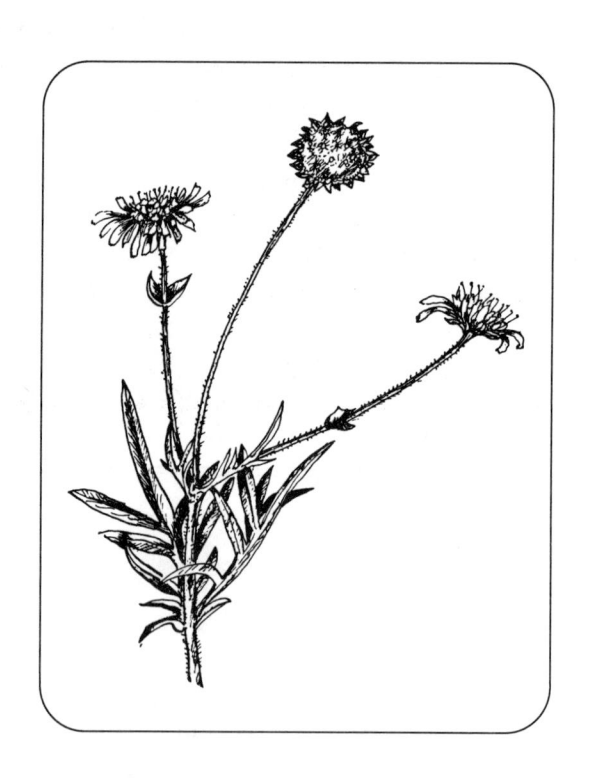

This plant is virtually identical in its nature, functions and uses to PLEURISY ROOT, with the following differences:

1　Unlike Pleurisy root, Scabious is not used as a *relaxant expectorant* in asthmatic and Qi constraint conditions of the lungs and intestines (function 2).
2　Scabious' additional functions and uses are:

CLEARS HEAT AND TOXINS AND REDUCES INFLAMMATION; RESTRAINS INFECTION AND RESOLVES CONTUSION; PROMOTES TISSUE REPAIR AND BENEFITS AND SOOTHES THE SKIN

WOUNDS, sores, ulcers, abscesses (esp. of lungs & mouth)
fire toxin: with boils, carbuncles
THROAT & MOUTH INFECTIONS
DRY SKIN ERUPTIONS with itching (incl. scurf, scabies, tetters, ringworm, vaginal pruritus)
SKIN BLEMISHES incl. freckles, sunburn

Preparation

USE: The DECOCTION and TINCTURE are the most viable. Scabious excells at external use with SWABS, COMPRESSES, OINTMENTS, etc.
DOSAGE: standard doses throughout
NOTE: To some extent *Scabiosa arvensis,* (Field scabious, Clodweed, Cardies, Pincushion) and *Scabiosa atropurpurea* (Lady's pincushion, Gypsy rose) are used instead of this species, with some loss of therapeutic efficacy.

Notes

This valuable medicinal plant acquired its main name from the devil who, jealous of its efficacy, took a bite from its root in an attempt to render it worthless. (Presumably his attempt was ineffective.) Through early colonists an American variety, *Scabiosa succisa,* also acquired the name *Devil's bit*. It was used by unspecified Native American tribes as an external remedy in the same way as *S. columbaria*.

Looking at Scabious' total therapeutic profile, it becomes clear that it can be seen as a cross between those of Pleurisy root and Ribwort plantain. It is said to be as effective as Pleurisy root for the same kind of bronchial conditions marked by **heat, pain, coughing** and **asthmatic breathing**.

Moreover, as its many names in several languages attest, Scabious was in the past considered one of the finest **skin** remedies available, dealing like Ribwort plantain with everything from wounds to abscesses to infections. It is another plant that deserves more widespread use.

Grindelia: Class 4

GRINDELIA

Pharmaceutical name: herba Grindeliae
Botanical name: Grindelia robusta WILLD. et NUTT. (N.O. Asteraceae)
Other names: Gumweed, Wild sunflower, Gumplant, Tarweed (Am)
Goldkörbchen (Ge)
Part used: the herb

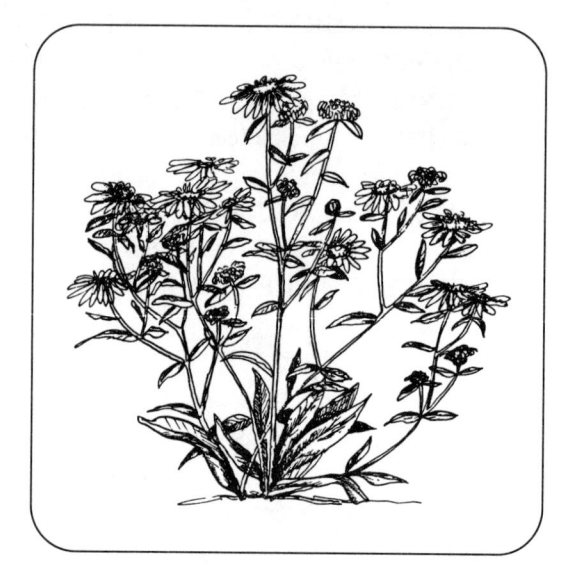

Nature

CATEGORY: mild herb with minimal chronic toxicity
CONSTITUENTS: saponins 2% (incl. grindelin), bitter alkaloid grindeline, ess. oil, resin 20% (incl. diterpenes), phytosterin, matricianol, matricarianol-acetate, tannins, laevoglucose
EFFECTIVE QUALITIES
Primary: bitter, a bit pungent, neutral with some cooling potential, moist
Secondary: stimulating, relaxing, decongesting
TROPISM: lungs, heart, arterial circulation, skin
        Air, Fluid organism
        Lung, Heart meridians
GROUND: all krases, biotypes and constitutions for symptomatic use

Functions and Uses

1. RELAXES THE HEART AND BRONCHI; OPENS THE CHEST, LEVELS ASTHMA AND RELIEVES COUGHING; LIQUIFIES AND EXPELS VISCOUS PHLEGM
   heart Qi constraint with nervous rapid heartbeat
   lung Qi constraint with asthmatic breathing, tight chest
   lung dryness with harsh dry cough
   lung phlegm dryness with coughing up scanty viscous phlegm
   BRONCHITIS, ASTHMA, dyspnea

2. STIMULATES THE HEART AND CIRCULATION, DREDGES THE KIDNEYS, PROMOTES URINATION AND RELIEVES FLUID CONGESTION
   heart/lung fluid congestion with acute pulmonary edema
   kidney Qi stagnation with cystitis, skin rashes

3. PROMOTES TISSUE REPAIR, REDUCES INFLAMMATION AND BENEFITS THE SKIN
   CHRONIC SKIN CONDITIONS (DERMATOSES) in deficient conditions
   MALIGNANT, indolent skin ulcers, running sores
   ECZEMA, dermatitis

Class 4: White Horehound

BURNS, blisters, poison ivy/oak
INSECT BITES & stings

Preparation

USE: The short DECOCTION and TINCTURE are the best preparations. The following doses should not be exceeded to avoid kidney irritation.
DOSAGE: TINCTURE: 1/2-3 ml, or 12-75 drops
DECOCTION: 6-15 g per 1/2 l (or 1 pint) of water

Notes

Grindelia is an effective lung remedy with a narrow, specific range of uses. It is basically a *circulatory stimulant* and a *respiratory relaxant* in one, similar to Inmortal, Celandine, Hyssop and Angelica in this respect. **Lung Qi Constraint** type asthma with harsh, dry, spasmodic couging with or without thick, sticky phlegm calls for Grindelia, especially where **skin rashes** are present, and secretions are at a standstill. Saponins and essential oils together go to ensure these *stimulant, secretolytic* and *relaxant* effects on the bronchials. Here as with deficiency type coughs, Grindelia could effectively replace *Chuan bei mu, bulbus Fritillariae cirrhosae,* commonly used in Chinese formulas. In acupuncture terms, Lu 7 & 5, Ki 7, CV 17 and Bl 13 would be a comparable point selection.

Grindelia's very high resin content assures a certain **moistening** effect on the lungs. In addition it is a *heart relaxant*. The comparison with *Bai he, bulbus Lilii,* is an obvious one in this connection.

WHITE HOREHOUND

Pharmaceutical name: herba Marrubii
Botanical name: Marrubium vulgare L. (N.O. Labiatae)
Ancient names: Prasion (Gr)
Marrubium albium/candidum (Lat)
Other names: Horone, Houndbene, Marvel, Marrube (Eng)
Marrube blanc/commun, Herbe vierge, Mont blanc (Fr)
Weisser Andorn, Lungenkraut, Weisser Dorant (Ge)
Part used: the herb

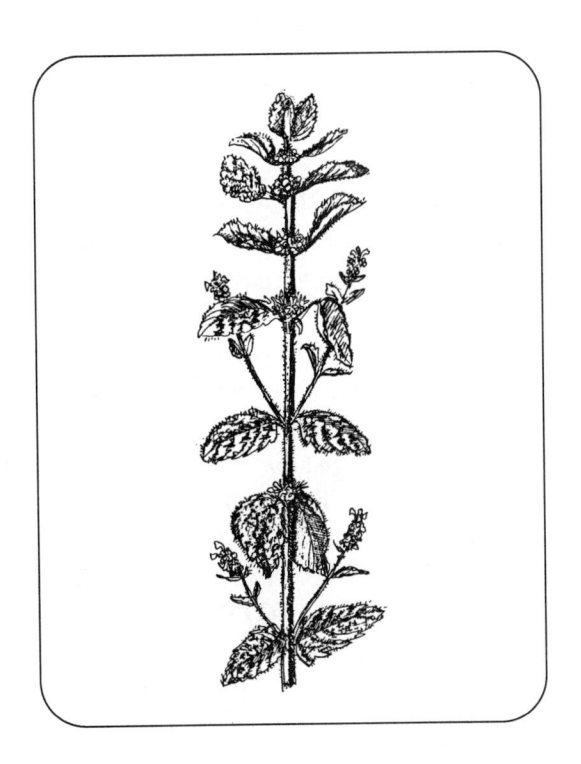

Nature

CATEGORY: mild herb with minimal chronic toxicity
CONSTITUENTS: sesquiterpene bitters (incl. marrubine), cholin, saponins, stachydrin, betonicin, flavonoids, tannins, mucilage, potassium nitrate, gallic & ursolic acid, iron, pectin, resin, ess. oil
EFFECTIVE QUALITIES
Primary: bitter, a bit pungent & salty, cool, dry

White Horehound: Class 4

Secondary: restoring, stimulating, deobstructing, relaxing
TROPISM: lungs, heart, kidneys, liver, stomach, uterus
  Air, Warmth organism
  Lung, Liver, Spleen meridians
GROUND: Phlegmatic temperament
  Dependant/Tai Yin Earth biotype
  Mixed/Phosphoric/Grey-Green Iris & Lymphatic/Carbonic/Blue Iris constitution

Funtions and Uses

1. STIMULATES THE LUNGS, EXPELS PHLEGM AND RELIEVES COUGHING; CLEARS HEAT, RESTRAINS INFECTION AND RESOLVES FEVER; BENEFITS THE THROAT

    lung wind heat: swollen sore throat, full cough with fetid sputum, thick nasal discharge, some fever
    CATARRHAL head colds
    lung phlegm heat/damp: asthmatic breathing, copious white or yellow phlegm, full cough, possible sore throat
    CHRONIC & ACUTE BRONCHITIS, laryngitis, etc.
    LUNG TB
    TYPHOID FEVER
    CHRONIC COUGH, HOARSENESS

2. RELAXES THE HEART

    heart Qi constraint: nervousness, unrest, palpitations

3. PROMOTES CLEANSING, CLEARS TOXINS AND DRAINS PLETHORA; DREDGES THE KIDNEYS, PROMOTES AND HARMONIZES URINATION AND MENSTRUATION

    kidney Qi stagnation with general toxemia: skin rashes, malaise, poor appetite, scanty urination
    GENERAL PLETHORA: obesity, cellulite, spleen & liver hardening
    DIFFICULT, painful, urgent urination
    URINARY IRRITATION
    uterus Qi stagnation: delayed, scanty clotted menstruation, PMS
    RETAINED PLACENTA

4. RESTORES THE LIVER AND STOMACH/*SPLEEN*, AWAKENS THE APETITE AND CREATES STRENGTH

    liver & stomach Qi deficiency: slow, painful digestion, constipation, jaundice
    Spleen Qi deficiency: no appetite, fatigue
    ANEMIA

5. PROMOTES TISSUE REPAIR

    WOUNDS, running sores, bites, ulcers, scabs

Preparation

USE: The INFUSION or TINCTURE will do equally well; taken warm or hot they will promote sweating and expel phlegm; taken cool they will promote urination, stop sweating and discharge.

Class 4: White horehound

In days past the European apothecary was well stocked with sundry Horehound preparations: SYRUPS, SALVES, LOZENGES, WINES, CONSERVES, SNUFFS and many others lined its shelves. Horehound was often combined with other *bronchial stimulants* such as Hyssop, Rue, Aniseed, Squills and Figs in these medicines. We could do worse than take our cue from these examples.

DOSAGE: **Smaller** than average doses stimulate Spleen and liver Qi in deficient conditions; **standard** doses work especially on the lungs; **large** doses tend to cause vomiting.

CAUTION: Horehound is contraindicated in cold and deficiency kidney conditions, especially Kidney Yang deficiency.

Notes

White horehound was a significant remedy in Egyptian and Greek medicine right up to the eighteenth century, when it fell into oblivion for two centuries or so. Today it enjoys a new scientifically accepted reputation under scientific condonement as a moderately strong *cool stimulating expectorant* and is applied to **congestive bronchial** conditions of both an **acute** and **chronic** kind. This makes Horehound very useful in hot lung patterns, i.e. acute or chronic infections, especially with unproductive coughing. In this context, it could functionally replace herbs from the Chinese pharmacy such as *Chuan bei mu, bulbus Fritillariae cirrhosae,* and *Qian hu, radix Peucedani*. Besides, White horehound's *cardiac relaxant* property is very appropriate in **lung wind heat** conditions presenting with irritability or palpitations due to stress affecting the heart; its effect is roughly like that of Bl 12 & 13, Lu 10, TH 5 and Ht 5, in this particular case. Like many a lung remedy, Horehound is also a good **throat** herb.

When used for liver/stomach/Spleen deficiency on the basis of its *bitter* taste, it has the advantage of regulating bowel movement whether constipation or diarrhea is present. Its *cleansing* effect, carried by its effective *salty* taste quality, is the result of both renal and hepatic stimulation. IBN AL-BAITAR in his monumental *Treatise on Simples* (1225) specified that "It has the properties of eliminating fluids from all the internal organs, of cleansing the lungs and chest of the fluids offending them…" Horehound specifically addresses **plethoric** conditions with languid menstruation, toxemia, acidosis, overweight and so on. This, as far as Alexandrian and Roman physicians, including GALEN were concerned, was its main function.

Coltsfoot: Class 4

COLTSFOOT

Pharmaceutical name: folium seu flos Tussilaginis
Botanical name: Tussilago farfara L. (N.O. Compositae)
Ancient names: Bechion (Gr)
    Farfara, Ungulla caballina (Lat)
Other names: Foal foot, Horsehoof, Coughwort (Eng)
    Ginger root, Bullsfoot (Am)
    Pas d'âne, Pas de cheval, Procheton, Tatonnet, Herbe de St. Quirain (Fr)
    Huflattich, Rosshub, Brandlattich, Hustenkraut (Fr)
    Kuan dong hua (Ch)
Part used: the leaf or flower

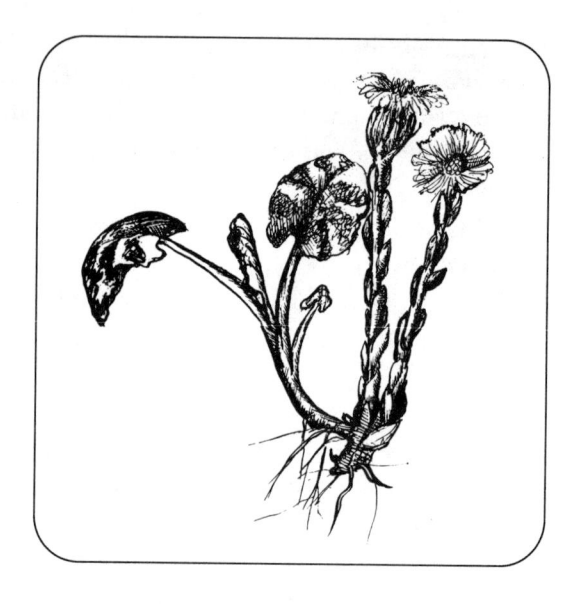

Nature

CATEGORY: mild herb with minimal chronic toxicity
CONSTITUENTS: mucilage, tannins (up to 17%), bitter glycoside, inulin, hormonal substances, gallic acid, triterpenes, pyrrolizidine alkaloids, sitosterol, ess. oil, calcium, magnesium, sodium, zinc, trace minerals
EFFECTIVE QUALITIES
Primary: a bit astringent & bitter & sweet, cool, dry & moist
Secondary: restoring, stimulating, decongesting, relaxing
TROPISM: lungs, throat
    Air, Warmth organism
    Lung meridian
GROUND: Melancholic krasis
    Sensitive/Tai Yin Metal biotype
    Lymphatic/Carbonic/Blue Iris constitution

Functions and Uses

1   STIMULATES THE LUNGS, RESOLVES MUCUS AND EXPELS PHLEGM; RELAXES THE BRONCHI, RELIEVES COUGHING AND WHEEZING
    CATARRHAL lung conditions with white or fetid yellow phlegm, with *lung phlegm damp* or *lung phlegm heat*
    ASTHMATIC and BRONCHITIC conditions of all types
    COUGHING or WHEEZING in any condition

2   CLEARS HEAT AND RESTRAINS INFECTION; RESTORES AND MOISTENS THE LUNGS, BENEFITS THE THROAT
    lung Qi deficiency with weakness, shortness of breath
    lung Yin deficiency with low fever, night sweats, coughing
    EMPHYSEMA, whooping cough, pleurisy, silicosis, TB
    lung phlegm heat with thick yellow phlegm

Class 4: Coltsfoot

ACUTE & CHRONIC lung infections
THROAT conditions in general

3   PROMOTES TISSUE REPAIR, REDUCES INFLAMMATION AND BENEFITS THE SKIN

CHRONIC WOUNDS, ulcers, scrofulous sores
skin damp heat with boils, furuncles, abscesses
INFLAMMATORY lesions & swellings, burns

Preparation

USE: Long INFUSIONS, TINCTURES, etc., are suitable for internal use. Externally, the **fresh leaf** can be applied directly, or a POULTICE made. SMOKING the dried leaves is useful in asthma (e.g. with Thyme, Lavender and Eyebright).

Former preparations included the SYRUP, CONSERVE (of the **flowers**) and the ELECTUARY (e.g. with Pine kernels and Squills).

DOSAGE: standard doses throughout

Notes

Although Coltsfoot is very versatile in its use in the whole respiratory area, it should not be dismissed as merely a symptomatic remedy by any means. It is precisely its versatility which makes it so useful in all conditions and syndromes with **coughing**, **throat inflammation**, and **wheezing** as main symptoms. A glance at the range of its analyzable ingredients testifies to the variety of bioenergetic processes at work in this plant. Coltsfoot **is** a symptomatic remedy, the ideal *antitussive,* in fact, and it is very amazing how natural living processes organize themselves in order to achieve this. We should be thankful that such herbs exist. If we are looking for a remedy for clear-cut, definable syndromes, then this is not the one. There are other, brilliant lung agents that do particular jobs better than Coltsfoot, which does virtually all. For this reason, Coltsfoot excels as a symptom focused and a supportive remedy, as also a good domestic, first aid herb.

Nevertheless, Coltsfoot is anything but a parachute standby in moments of uncertainty. Clearly, its somewhat *bitter astringent cool* energetic qualities make it suitable for dealing with **heat** of all kinds, especially **chronic** or **subacute inflammatory** conditions of the **lungs** and **throat,** and low or tidal fevers as found in empty heat/Shao Yin syndromes. In these type of conditions, its mild *Qi restoring* effects are an assest in supporting vital forces and strength.

Coltsfoot flower, *Kuan dong hua,* are used in Chinese medicine in precisely the same way.

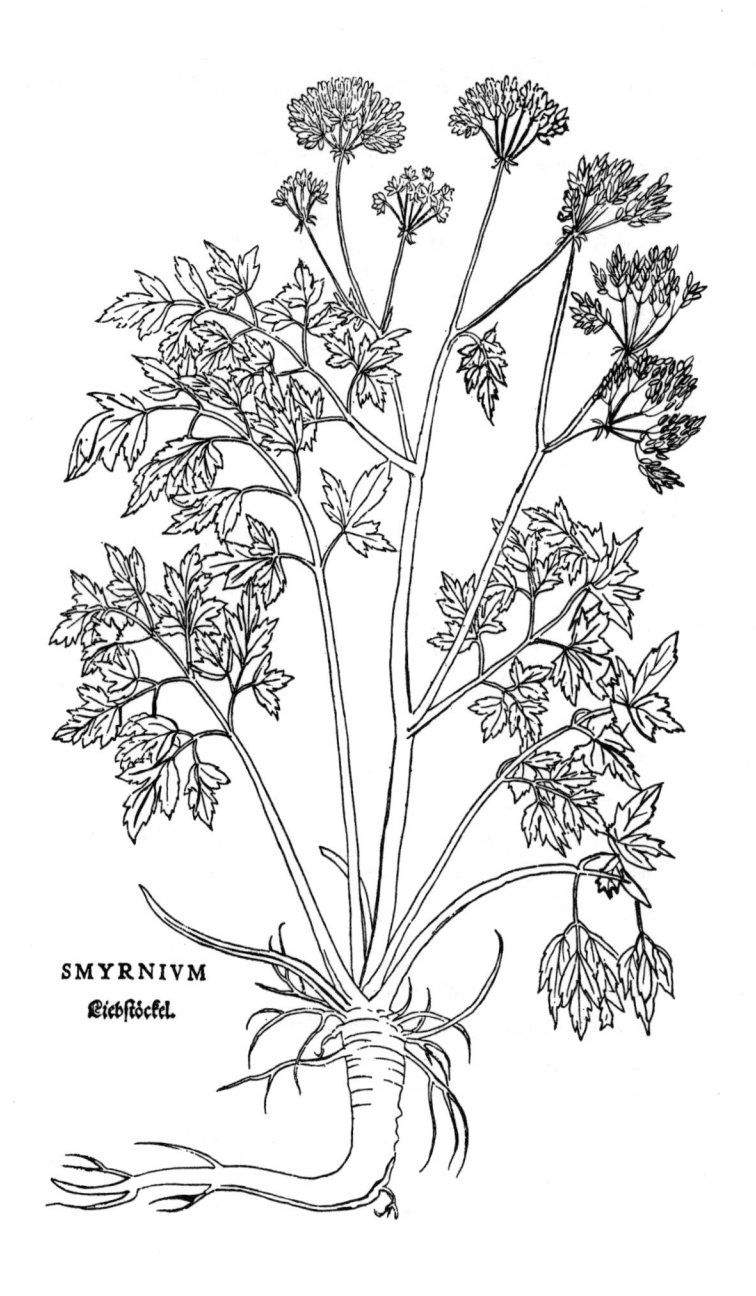

Lovage

CLASS 5

Herbs to Promote the Menses and Clear Stagnation

Herbs of this class promote the onset of menstruation by stimulating an elimination of retained menstrual blood. They are used primarily in cases of stagnation where the menses have become delayed or have ceased entirely (functional amenorrhea) because of a retention of congested uterine blood. By effectively breaking up this substantial obstruction these remedies clear stagnation and provoke an active discharge. By assisting a natural process of elimination they are able to eventually bring about regular monthly menstruation, which is the ultimate purpose of their use.

There is a basic link between woman and the blood, and the Hippokratic texts *De natura mulierum* and *De morbis mulierum* discuss her more moist quality in comparison to man's. which is more dry. All traditional medical theories state that she has more blood than man and hence menstruates the excess. When her monthly cycle becomes longer or ceases entirely outside of pregnancy, they advise eliminating this redundant accumulated blood to prevent it from causing imbalance and illness. As part of feminine hygiene they also recommend certain comportment during menstruation.[1]

In the Western tradition menstruation has always been held to have a general **draining** effect energetically. Both HIPPOKRATES and GALEN explain how menstruation is actually a *katharsis*, i.e. a radical renewal on every level. Certainly, women who suffer minor symptoms of excess, such as malaise, irritability, and water retention before or during menstruation, find that these disappear afterwards, leaving them refreshed and more grounded. Many past Galenic practitioners, such as RIVIERE *(Praxis Medica)*, POTERIUS *(Centuriae)*, CORBEIUS *(Gynaeceium)*, VARANDÉE *(Traité des Maladies des Femmes)*, FREIND *(Emmenologiae)*, KÄMPF *(Enchiridium Medicum)* and HUFELAND, affirmed that if this monthly excess is not discharged, conditions of stagnation with a variety of symptoms are liable to set in. These beliefs were held right up to the nineteenth century, when energetics based medicine was discarded.

However, since the rise of the German Nature Cure school of healing and the Protestant influenced toxemia theories in the early nineteenth century, the energetic concept of **draining** has been exchanged for the more physical tissue based idea of **cleansing**. Menstruation was now interpreted as an **eliminant cleansing act**, like sweating, urination, and bowel movement, rather than a *draining cleansing* one. Practitioners of this school and later ones, including BERNHARD ASCHNER, were convinced that menstrual retention caused systemic toxemia with symptoms such as weight gain, chronic arthritis and rheumatism, neuralgias, migraines, skin eruptions and mental/psychic imbalances (the neuroses and psychoses). As a result, they too stressed the importance of reinstating a regular monthly flow if it was lacking—but for very different reasons.

Clearly, while we can agree with Greek medicine that, energetically speaking, menstruation has a draining effect which can relieve Qi stagnation, the position of more recent practitioners that its primary action is a cleansing one is untenable. Although menstruation is a discharge of waste, it does not eliminate body wastes as do sweat, urine and stool, and the above-mentioned symptoms and signs can be attributed to hormonal imbalance equally as well as to toxemia.

The equation menstruation = elimination = cleansing is only understandable if we consider the patriarchal, male dominated character of official Galenic medicine that was ubiquitous in the past.

The Energetics of Western Herbs

From this perspective, menstrual blood is the substantial emblem of woman's basic uncleanliness, while menstruation itself represents the most feared and denigrated of all of woman's functions.[2] In consequence there arose the general tendency to believe that menstruation could only form part of a cleansing process and the obsession with promoting cleansing that unfortunately characterized much of the gynecological practice of past male physicians. These biased predispositions, then, generated more specific medical reasons to associate menstrual retention or amenorrhea with systemic toxemia. Since amenorrhea is often found together with conditions of stagnation, plethora, and toxemia, past practitioners were often unable to distinguish its consequences from its contextual energetic imbalance. After all, menstrual retention is not just a local disharmony, but also a systemic one, and the conditions in which it is found are its predisposing factors more often than its consequences.

Now that feminine and masculine values are once more seeking a balance, a more levelheaded, unbiased assessment of menstrual conditions is possible. An essential part of this is to determine the systemic conditions accompanying this imbalance.

Chinese and Greek medicine here describe syndromes such as uterus cold, liver Qi stagnation, phlegm retention in the Lower Warmer, cold in the meridians (also known as arterial blood & Qi deficiency) and general plethora. In terms of the uterus organ itself these conditions invariably entail a weakness of uterus tone, or Qi, not of uterus blood. Rather than the blood being involved, as in blood deficiency or blood congestion, implicated here in causing menstrual disharmony is the Qi. "Qi is the leader of the blood," runs an old quote from the *Huang di nei jing (The Yellow Emperor's Classic of Internal Medicine)*, which finds a new relevance here.

The more **specific triggers** of the amenorrhea should also be examined. These include emotional shock, a great weight loss or gain, going off the pill and travel, all of which affect the pituitary; ovarian tumors or cysts and early menopause; hormonal imbalance, especially estrogen insufficiency; general causes such as childbirth, poor nutrition, cirrhosis, TB, adrenal disease and thyroid insufficiency; and, more rarely, structural impairment of the reproductive organs or adrenals. These factors should be corrected at the same time as the menstruation set in motion.

The treatment of **amenorrhea** with **menstrual retention** due to **blood obstruction** has several aspects which may need consecutive or concurrent attention. First, the immediate obstruction needs breaking up and the retained menstruum eliminating. Secondly, the overall pattern of disharmony forming the context of this condition requires rebalancing. Thirdly, the *sequelae,* or consequences, of both these factors should be treated in whatever way appropriate. This differentiation of treatment is essential if menstrual retention is to be treated more than symptomatically.

There are two main types of conditions involving retained menstruation, Qi stagnation and cold stagnation. In both cases, the treatment principle underlying promoting menstruation entails a stimulation of the Qi and the Yang to mobilize the blood. In this way uterine tone is restored, the monthly elimination of excess blood occurs without delay, and a spontaneous flow of menstruation is encouraged on a more long-term basis.

Since the herbs in this class specifically stimulate an elimination of congested endometrium, they are called *stimulant emmenagogues* or *uterine stimulants.* There are two types, addressing the two basic kinds of menstrual retention.

1 HERBS TO STIMULATE THE UTERUS, CLEAR STAGNATION AND PROMOTE THE MENSES

These remedies treat all types of **uterus Qi stagnation** which result in a gradual lengthening of the cycle with possible complete menstrual cessation. Typically, this is accompanied by painful

Herbs to Promote the Menses and Clear Stagnation

menstrual onset with dark colored clots, irritability, depression, constipation, weight gain and a tight, full pulse. Other conditions, such as liver Qi stagnation and general plethora often complete the energetic picture of disharmony. Uterus Qi stagnation, as well as the above syndromes, may be produced by events such as shock and depression of feelings.

Botanicals used to clear uterus Qi stagnation are *stimulant emmenagogues* comprising herbs such as Celandine, Lovage, Blue cohosh, Blue flag, Rosemary, Rue, Arnica, Sabine, Aloes and Senna leaf. The latter two should be used only with chronic constipation present, which is frequently the case. These herbs cause uterine hyperemia that produces menstrual elimination. They should be used continuously until a period arrives, in the case of functional amenorrhea; one week before the due onset, in the case of delayed menstruation; and four days before onset and during the flow, in the case of scanty menstruation. They may be used singly, combined or, as is more usual, with other remedies to balance the overall condition.

2 HERBS TO STIMULATE THE UTERUS, GENERATE WARMTH AND PROMOTE THE MENSES

Botanicals in this category are used to provoke menstrual onset in all conditions marked by **cold stagnation**. The energy of cold always causes a slowing down of processes, a condensing and a stasis of the Qi, resulting in syndromes such as **uterus cold** (also known in Chinese medicine as cold blood). There are two types: one is characterized by deficiency (deficiency cold) and associated with a Yang deficiency (e.g. liver Yang deficiency), with fatigue, palpitations, a weak, sunken pulse, etc.; the other is typified by excess (excess cold) and linked with Yin excess or liver cold stagnation with heaviness, nausea, a tight, knotted pulse, etc. Both types may entail a delay or stoppage of the menses and cramping pains of a constant, persistent nature before menstrual onset. They may be caused by exposure to cold or dampness or by the generation of cold internally.

Uterus cold is treated with *hot stimulant emmenagogues,* with the addition of Class 7 *warm Qi tonics* in the case of deficiency cold and Class 8 *hot stimulant Yang* tonics in the case of excess cold. These *emmenagogues* are general *circulatory stimulants* as well as local *uterine stimulants*. They all have a *pungent* taste and an *active* nature, due to either a high volatile oil content, as with Pennyroyal, Juniper, Angelica, Cinnamon, Rosemary, Wild ginger and Hazelwort; due to a high resin content, as in Balm of Gilead, Myrrh, Galbanum, Guaiacum, Olibanum, Mastix, Asafoetida and Sagapenum; or due to a high terpene content, as in Turpentine and its botanical sources Pine, Thuja and other coniferous trees. They should be used in the same way as herbs from the previous category.

Since estrogen insufficiency might be implicated in causing delayed or stopped menses, *uterine Qi* and *blood tonics* from Class 7 should be added to these herbs class where appropriate. In addition to herbal medication, traditional techniques for causing menstrual flow include several important external methods.[3]

Caution: Herbs in this class are not suited to treating those types of delayed or stopped menses caused by blood deficiency of any kind, for which Class 7 and 9 *restoring* and *nourishing* herbs should be adopted. The importance of careful differential diagnosis is once more highlighted.

A summary listing of all herbs in this class is found on page 694.

Notes

1 During menstruation Galenic medicine recommends avoiding excessive work or exercise, contact with excessive cold or heat, and all strong medication and operations.

2 See *The Wise Wound* by Penelope Shuttle and Peter Redgrove, (London, 1978). It would have

The Energetics of Western Herbs

been interesting to hear the traditional view of a wise woman practitioner on this matter.

3   The main external treatments used throughout the entire history of Greek/Galenic medicine for menstrual retention caused by Qi stagnation or cold—many of which we consider worth rediscovering today—were:

- **physical therapy** such as stimulating footbaths and hipbaths (see p. 91);
- **squatting inhalations** and **vaginal fumigations** (see p. 84);
- **pessaries** made with *emmenagogue* herbs;
- **cupping**, with or without bleeding, on the sacrum, the medial proximal thigh region, the lower abdomen or the inguinal region;
- **leeching**, i.e. the setting of live leeches, a type of phlebotomy, on the *labiae majorae* or the medial upper thigh region (which is acupuncture point Li 10);
- **bloodletting** in the lower extremities, especially at the malleolus.

The last two methods were found to be invariably effective, even with the most intractable amenorrhea.

To this list Chinese medicine adds **acupuncture** and **moxibustion**.

4   Classical Greek medicine also used effectively small doses of stronger *purgative emmenagogues* such as Colocynth, Hellebore, Scammony, Water hemlock, Squirting cucumber, Stavesacre and Saffron, as well as animal remedies such as Cantharides, Millipede, Cockroach and Cockchafer.

A note is in order here on the use of animal products in medicine. Remedies prepared from animal parts have been as much part of every healing system as remedies of botanical and mineral origin. It is only more recently, during the late nineteenth century, in fact, that the concept and practice of a purely herbal medicine came about, and then solely as a reaction to the rise of synthetic medication. Most texts on remedies before 1800 list animal and mineral remedies alongside herbal ones or in a separate section. Cantharides, for example, was (and still is, in Chinese medicine) indispensable for numerous external and internal preparations (see also p. 667), and the total number of animal remedies used in Greek/Tibb Unani medicine was well over 400—more than that used in Chinese medicine.

During the sixteenth and seventeenth centuries animal products became so widely and frequently used that this practice acquired the name **filth pharmacy**. That age's insatiable exploration of natural substances, together with its obsessive preoccupation with things bizzare, exotic and obscure spilt over into medicine, and the more remote, exotic, and disgusting a remedy, the more certain it was held to cure illness. The best bezoar stone, therefore, came from the stomach of a wild Persian mountain goat, as the strongest herbal remedy was "far-fetch't and dear bought" (WILLIAM COLE, 1652). And the more horrific the remedy, such as animal feces (e.g. from the Egyptian hippopotamus or crocodile) or shavings from a dead man's skull, the more it was thought that disease could be terrified into finally leaving.

Interestingly, though, despite the naive terrors of the European late Galenic filth pharmacy, the fact remains that certain animal remedies have always proven effective. Biochemists have also been able to isolate powerful compounds from many animal remedies used in both Greek and Chinese medicine. These include Deer antler, Antelope horn, Toad secretion, Cantharides, Centipede and Scorpion.

JUNIPER

Pharmaceutical name: fructus Juniperi
Botanical name: Juniperus communis L. (N.O.
      Cupressaceae)
Ancient names: Arkeuthos (Gr)
Other names: Aiten, Gorst, Melmot berries, Horse
      savin (Eng)
   Evergreen tree (Am)
   Genevrier (Fr)
   Wacholder, Kramerstaud, Machandel,
      Reckholder, Kranewitt, Feuerbaum (Ge)
Part used: the berry

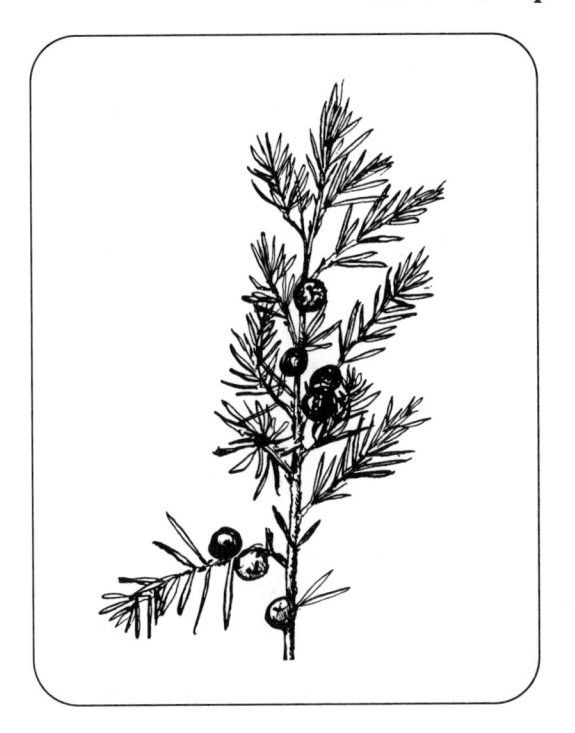

Nature

CATEGORY: mild herb with some chronic toxicity
CONSTITUENTS: ess. oil up to 2% (incl. camphene, terpineol, cendinene, alphapinene), flavonoids, resin, tannins, antitumor agent, bitter (juniperin), formic and acetic acids, pentosane, calcium, manganese
EFFECTIVE QUALITIES
Primary: *Taste:* a bit pungent & bitter & sweet
      Warmth: warm
      Moisture: dry
Secondary: stimulating, decongesting, softening, dissolving, astringing
      sinking movement
TROPISM
Organs or parts: stomach, intestines, bladder, kidneys, uterus, skin
Organisms: Warmth, Fluid
Meridians: Spleen, Kidney, Chong & Ren
Tri Dosas: increases Pita & Vayu, decreases Kapha
GROUND
Krases/temperaments: Phlegmatic & Melancholic
Biotypes: Dependant/Tai Yin Earth & Burdened/Shao Yin
Constitutions: Lymphatic/Carbonic/Blue Iris & Mixed/Phosphoric/Grey-Green Iris

Functions and Uses

1 SUPPORTS THE YANG, STIMULATES THE CIRCULATION AND CREATES WARMTH; DISPELS COLD, PROMOTES THE MENSES AND RELIEVES PAIN; ENHANCES LABOR AND DELIVERY

   arterial blood & Qi deficiency: fear of cold, weakness, chest oppression, wheezing, cold extremities or limbs

Juniper: Class 5

wind/damp obstruction: acute rheumatism or neuralgia
uterus cold: cramping pain before onset, delayed or no menstruation, scanty pink flow
SPASMODIC DYSMENORRHEA, amenorrhea
PAINFUL, DIFFICULT LABOR
TOOTHACHE

2 STIMULATES AND STRENGTHENS THE UROGENITAL ORGANS, DRIES MUCOUS DAMP AND ARREST DISCHARGE

genitourinary cold (Kidney Yang deficiency): frequent scanty or copious clear urination with irritation, lumbar pain, mental and emotional dullness
genitourinary damp cold: white leucorrhea, mucousy urine
CHRONIC MUCOUS CYSTITIS, cervical erosion
kidney fluid congestion: edema from the ankles upwards

3 WARMS AND INVIGORATES THE STOMACH AND INTESTINES/*SPLEEN*, AWAKENS THE APPETITE AND FLENZES MUCUS

Spleen Yang deficiency with intestines damp cold: abdominal swelling, diarrhea, chilliness, no appetite
CHRONIC GASTROENTERITIS
GASTRIC ULCERS due to hypoacidity
intestines mucous damp (Spleen damp): heaviness of body and head, headache, gurgling distended abdomen
INTESTINAL FERMENTATION
DIABETES (supportive)

4 PROMOTES CLEANSING, CLEARS TOXINS AND RESOLVES TOXEMIA; DREDGES THE KIDNEYS AND PROMOTES URINATION; SOFTENS DEPOSITS AND BENEFITS THE SKIN

kidney Qi stagnation with *general toxemia:* malaise, skin rashes, poor appetite
ALBUMINARIA
general fluids dyskrasia: chronic gout, rehumatism, arthritis
URIC ACID DIATHESIS
HARD DEPOSITS: urinary stones, arteriosclerosis
ACNE, PSORIASIS, ECZEMA, DERMATOSIS

5 ACTIVATES IMMUNITY, RESTRAINS INFECTION AND ANTIDOTES POISON; PROMOTES TISSUE REPAIR

PREVENTIVE IN EPIDEMICS
CHRONIC BACTERIAL & VIRAL INFECTIONS of kidneys, bladder, lungs, intestines (incl. cystitis, gonorrhea)
POISONING from food, herbs, insects
ATONIC WOUNDS, ulcers, sores
WEEPING ECZEMA, acne
SKIN PARASITES

Preparation

USE: The SYRUP or PUREE made from the sweetened inspissated JUICE is as effective a form of taking Juniper as it is pleasant. More *disinfectant* and *cleansing* is the pure ESSENTIAL OIL taken internally, inhaled or massaged with a carrier oil; while the INFUSION or TINCTURE are serviceable all-purpose preparations.

DOUCHES or HIP BATHS are used for cold and damp **gynecological** conditions. (PESSARIES cause burning of the mucous membrane, however.) *Warming, pain-relieving* LINIMENTS are used **externally**, and SALVES, CREAMS and the like in **skin** problems.

DOSAGE: ESSENTIAL OIL: 2-4 drops in a little warm water three times a day.
PUREE: 2 tsp twice or thrice daily (1 tsp for children).
OTHERS: standard doses

CAUTION: Juniper should be used cautiously during pregnancy since it may stimulate uterine contractions. (This is disputed, however.) The INFUSION drunk a few weeks prior to parturition will enhance labor.

Juniper may also irritate the kidneys and should therefore be used with a little care: the early warning sign of irritation is albuminuria. In any case, about six weeks of continuous use is the limit. In any **organic** kidney disease it is also to be avoided (nephritis, nephrosis), and certainly never used with **acute renal inflammations** of any kind. Another way of saying the above is that Juniper should be used in cold conditions only and never with full or empty heat.

Notes

The Juniper tree in its natural habitat is filled with the qualities of *warmth* and *dryness,* both Yang qualities, and produces a *spicy, warming* essential oil which forms its main chemical constituent. As a result, the most important therapeutic applications of Juniper as a remedy are conditions of **cold** and **damp**. It is a Kidney and Spleen Yang Deficiency remedy *par excellence,* dealing with every symptom depending on this pattern of disharmony in the same way as the acupuncture point selection Ki 7, Bl 23, GV 4, St 25, and Sp 3 & 5. Being a *circulatory stimulant* in addition, it improves cold limbs, fatigue and blood deficiency. It also warms and clears cold damp pervading the reproductive and urinary sphere.

Like *Wu yao, radix Linderae strychnifoliae* from the Chinese pharmacy, Juniper treats cold blood in the uterus. Both herbs treat functional amenorrhea and spasmodic dysmenorrhea due to cold, being roughly equivalent in this respect to Ki 5, Sp 10, LI 4, and CV 4, St 29 & Bl 32 with moxa. And the parallel does not end there: both share virtually all of the above functions except for Juniper's *cleansing* effect and its use as a remedy for preparing labor.

In this light it becomes clear that Juniper as a *urinary disinfectant* has severe limitations: it cannot cool and efficiently disinfect at the same time. Nor is its tannin count high enough to disinfect. For thits use must be kept to **chronic, cold infections** with low vitality or reserve, and never acute ones. In more ways than one, Juniper is also very similar to Buchu. Unlike the latter, however, Juniper in addition is a kidney oriented *resolvent cleanser,* addressing **high uric acid, depository** and **skin** condtitions with cold—conditions appropriately known in chinese nedicine as *cold obstruction.*

As a general *anti-infective* herb, however, Juniper has none of the above limitations; as might be expected from a remedy with a prime tropism for urogenital functions, it deals especially well with infections of the external genitalia.

Wild Ginger: Class 5

WILD GINGER

Pharmaceutical name: rhizoma Asari canadensis
Botanical name: Asarum canadense L. (N.O. Aristolochiae)
Other names: Canada snakeroot, Vermont snakeroot, Southern snakeroot, Black snakeweed, False coltsfoot (Am)
Part used: the rhizome

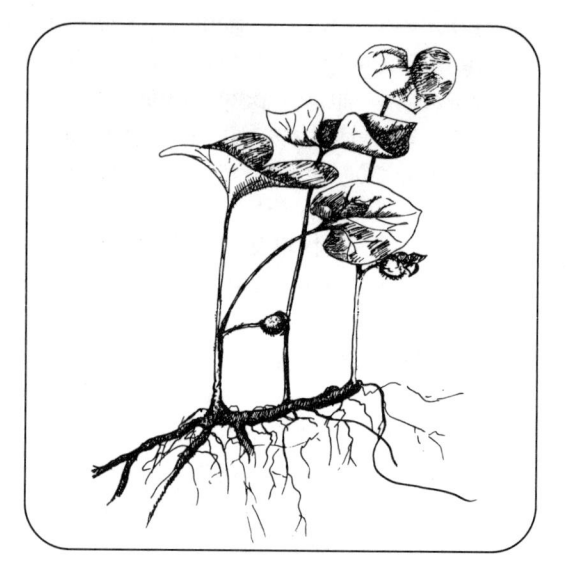

Nature

CATEGORY: mild herb with minimal chronic toxicity
CONSTITUENTS: ess. oil 4%. bitter (asarin), resin, alkaloid, mucilage, sugar, camphoraceaous substance, ß-sitosterin
EFFECTIVE QUALITIES
Primary: pungent, a bit bitter, warm, dry
Secondary: stimulating, relaxing, restoring, decongesting
dispersing movement
TROPISM: uterus, head, arterial circulation, lungs, stomach, intestines, liver
Warmth, Air, Fluid organisms
Lung, Colon, Chong & Ren meridians
GROUND: Phlegmatic krasis
Dependant/Tai Yin Earth & Self-Reliant/Yang Ming Metal biotypes
Mixed/Phosphoric/Grey-Green Tris constitution

Functions and Uses

1   STIMULATES THE UTERUS, PROMOTES AND HARMONIZES MENSTRUATION AND LABOR, EXPELS THE AFTERBIRTH
    uterus cold with delayed, cramping menstruation, stopped menses
    AMENORRHEA, SPASMODIC DYSMENORRHEA
    DIFFICULT, PAINFUL LABOR with nervous tension or depression
    STALLED LABOR
    RETAINED PLACENTA

2   CAUSES SWEATING, RELEASES THE EXTERIOR, SCATTERS WIND COLD AND PUSHES OUT ERUPTIONS; CLEARS THE HEAD AND RELIEVES PAIN
    external wind cold onset of infections with chills, head & body aches
    head damp cold with congestion, suppressed discharge
    wind/damp obstruction: acute neuralgia, rheumatism, myalgia
    ERUPTIVE FEVERS

3   STIMULATES THE HEART, CIRCULATION AND LUNGS; CREATES WARMTH, DISPELS COLD AND EXPELS PHLEGM

arterial blood & Qi deficiency with cold limbs, fatigue
lung phlegm cold with coughing, white phlegm production
CHRONIC BRONCHITIS, bronchial asthma

4   RELAXES THE NERVE, FREES SPASMS AND RELIEVES COUGHING

lung Qi constraint with spasmodic coughing
WHOOPING COUGH
intestines Qi constraint with colic

5   WARMS AND INVIGORATES THE LIVER, STOMACH AND INTESTINES/*SPLEEN*, AWAKENS THE APPETITE; SEEPS WATER AND PROMOTES URINATION

stomach & intestines cold (Spleen Yang deficiency) with no appetite, diarrhea
liver cold stagnation with jaundice, nausea, constipation, edema
fluid congestion of any type with swelling, bloating, etc.

Preparation

USE: The overnight cold water MACERATION with brief warming up before use is excellent; so are the TINCTURE or FLUID EXTRACT. Up to 1/2 teaspoon of the TINCTURE may also be taken at regular intervals **during labor** to promote general and specific relaxation and to encourage contractions with atonic action. **External uses** include SQUATTING INHALATIONS and PESSARIES.

DOSAGE: Standard dose throughout. In larger doses it makes a good *emetic* for strong constitutions.

CAUTION: If Wild ginger is used at all during pregnancy, then only as a *labor preparer* just before or as labor begins.

Wild ginger should not be used on its own in deficiency conditions.

Notes

For all practical purposes, Wild ginger and Hazelwort are identical in effect and produce the same medicine, *rhizoma Asari*. In addition, the Chinese variety, *Xi xin,* is also used in an identical, though more limited, way.

All types of *Asarum* are primarily *pungent warm stimulants, spasmolytics* and *diaphoretics*. Although not quite as strong as the Snakeroots of the *Aristolochia* family in this respect, they are still adequate for most cases. Deficiency cold conditions with **spasms, cramps, pain**, and **chilliness**, affecting menstruation, breathing or digestion, call for their use. They make superlative *hot stimulant emmenagogues* when the menses cease due to exposure to cold or damp and will treat delayed, scanty menstruation with cramps, chills and "violent pain in the small of the back on the approach of the menstrual epoch, which seems to interfere with the breathing" (ELLINGWOOD, 1898).

Wild ginger is also useful for easing labor and enhancing contractions, being both a *stimulant* and *relaxant parturient*. Of course it cannot supersede the likes of Blue cohosh, Lobelia and others during labor, yet it makes a good substitute or all-round ground support when required.

In days past, when treatment often simplistically boiled down to how strong a discharge could be provoked in a patient, the *Asarum* species Hazelwort was seen as one of the best *eliminants* in general, "carrying off the morbific matter of many inveterate disease by all ways, as vomit, stool,

Hazelwort: Class 5

urine and sweat" (WILLIAM SALMON, 1710). Contributing his small attempt at a more specific symptom conformation, JOHN QUINCY adds that "Its operation is very brisk and is therefore recommended in constitutions that are *moist and cold*."

HAZELWORT

Pharmaceutical name: rhizoma Asari europaei
Botanical name: Asarum europaeum L. (N.O. Aristolochiae)
Ancient names: Asaron, Nardos igia (Gr)
    Nardus sylvestris, Perpensa, Vulgago (Lat)
Other names: European snakeroot, Wild nard,
    Fole's root, Asarabacca (Eng)
    Asaret, Herbe de cabaret, Oreillettes, Nard commun, Rondelle, Cabaret, Panacée des fièvres quatres, Oreille d'homme (Fr)
    Haselwurz, Wilder Nard, Hasenöhrlein, Scheibelkraut, Brechwurzel, Weihrauchkraut (Ge)
Part used: the rhizome

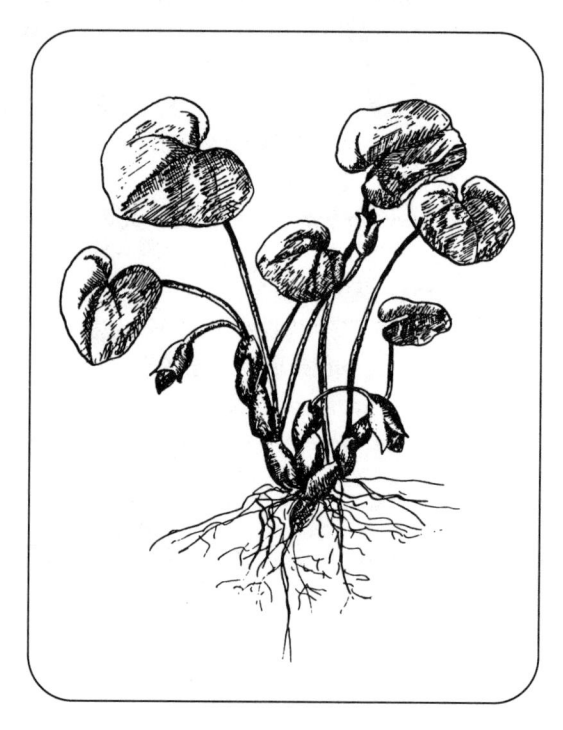

Nature

CATEGORY: mild herb with minimal chronic toxicity
CONSTITUENTS: ess. oil up to 4% (incl. asarone 30-30%), acids, glycosides, resins, tannins, mucilage, starch

This remedy is virtually identical in its nature, functions and uses to WILD GINGER, Asarum canadense (p. 216).

PENNYROYAL

Pharmaceutical name: herba Menthae pulegii
Botanical name: a) Mentha pulegium L., b) *vel Hedeoma pulegioides seu oblongifolium* Pers., *vel Monardella odorantissima* Gray (N.O. Labiatae)
Ancient names: Glechon, Blechon (Gr)
  Pulegium, Gliconus (Lat)
Other names: a) Pudding grass, Hillwort,
    Brotherwort (Eng)
  European pennyroyal, Brotherwort,
    Churchwort, Fleamint (Am)
  Menthe pouliot (Fr)
  Polei, Kleiner Balsam, Flohkraut,
    Herzminze, Hirschminze (Ge)
  b) American pennyroyal, Squaw mint,
    Tickweed, Stinking balm, Wild bergamot,
    Coyote mint, Dwarf pennyroyal/thyme,
    Poleo chino (Am)
Part used: the herb

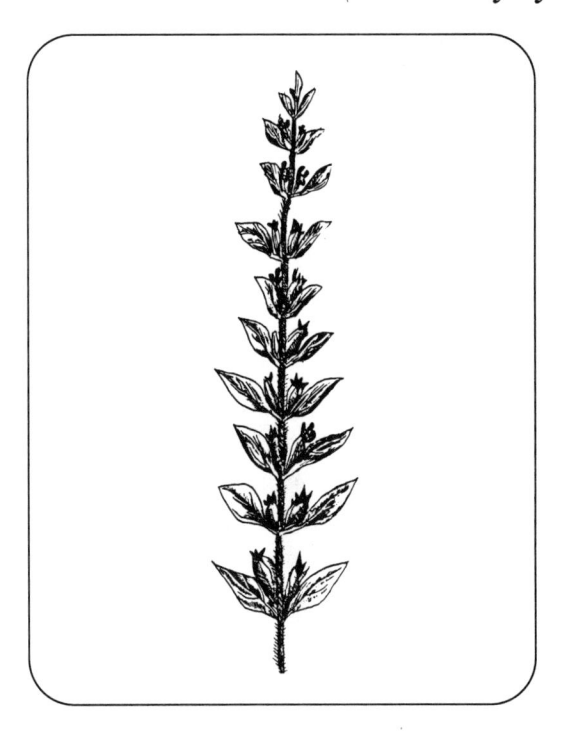

Nature

CATEGORY: medium-strength herb with some chronic toxicity
CONSTITUENTS: a) ess. oil (incl. pulegone 80-94%, isopulegone, piperitone, menthol, pinenes, limonenes, dipentenes), tannins 4%, flavonoid glycosides (diosmin & hesperidin)
EFFECTIVE QUALITIES
Primary: pungent & bitter, neutral with both cooling and warming potential, dry
Secondary: stimulating, relaxing, restoring, astringing
    sinking movement

This herb is similar in its nature, constituents, functions and uses to PEPPERMINT, herba Menthae piperitae, with the following differences:

1   Whereas Peppermint has but limited use as a *uterine stimulant,* Pennyroyal exerts several distinct effects on this organ. First, it is one of the strongest herbs to promote menstruation in conditions of **uterus Qi stagnation** with poor womb tone, whatever its origin or contextual imbalance. Secondly, it treats **uterus Qi constraint** where **spasms** and **PMS** symptoms appear, often as a result of Qi or blood stagnation. Both properties combined contribute to Pennyroyal's use as an excellent *puerperal remedy* for creating local and general *relaxation* during labor with hypertonic action, as well as or *expelling the placenta* and *promoting healing.*
2   Pennyroyal has a more marked *relaxant* effect in Qi Constraint patterns, unlike Peppermint being also effective in lung Qi constraint.
3   Pennyroyal has more actively *downward moving* and *heat clearing* effects than Peppermint and is therefore used for conditions of rising fire such as **sunstroke** (both mild and severe), **cerebral congestion, apoplexy,** etc. Also being a *diaphoretic* with both *stimulant* and *relaxant*

Pennyroyal: Class 5

properties, it is may be used for both **wind heat** and **wind cold** feverish conditions with restlessness.

4   Pennyroyal also *restrains infection, resolves ecchymosis, promotes tissue repair, antidotes poison* and *repels insects*. This indicates its use for **wounds,** ulcers, injuries, contusions, skin blemishes and itching, and insect and animal bites. The ESSENTIAL OIL is ideal for this external use in 1% dilution (no more) for SWABS, WASHES, LINIMENTS, COMPRESSES, etc., and may be used here in preference to the TINCTURE.

Preparation

USE: The TINCTURE is preferred over the INFUSION for full medicinal effects. The latter is good drunk hot in wind heat conditions, however.
DOSAGE: TINCTURE & INFUSION: standard doses
CAUTION: Being a *uterine stimulant*, Pennyroyal is contraindicated during pregnancy. Pennyroyal should not be used internally in ESSENTIAL OIL form, since it contains a high proportion of the toxic ketone pugelone. Moreover American pennyroyal (Squaw mint) has twice the pugelone content of the European variety and hence twice the toxicity.

Notes

Pennyroyal is an outstanding example of a remedy which, even more than Peppermint, vacillates between being *hot* and *cold*. A case could be made out for either, since its *pungent* taste is definitely *warming,* while its *bitter* taste has a *cooling* effect. Added to his, its *stimulant-relaxant pungency* tends to create a *cooling* effect by causing sweat. In short, although Pennyroyal has a definite overall bias for the cooling side, one might say that it has both heating and cooling potentials.

The *stimulant emmenagogue* effects of Pennyroyal, at any rate, are straightforward and to be relied upon—no matter whether the European or any of the American Southwestern *(Hedeoma),* Northeastern *(Hedeoma)* or Californian *(Monardella)* varieties are used. This remedy was not gratuitously called *Squaw mint* by early pioneers: it is a woman's remedy, one of the Squaw herbs, no less. It excels in both menstrual and childbirth situations where events are **delayed, painful, constrained** and **spasmodic**. It causes *uterine relaxation* and *relieves pain,* safely promoting the onset of tardy menstruation due to Qi stasis. Likewise, it will resume labor interrupted from tension, apprehension or just sheer exhaustion, and help prevent postpartum complications.

OREGANO

Pharmaceutical name: herba Origani
Botanical name: Origanum vulgare L (N.O. Labiatea)
Ancient names: Oreiganon (Gr)
    Golena, Cunila, Glitonum (Lat)
Other names: Pot marjoram, Argan, Organy (Eng)
    Origan, Marjolaine sauvage/batarde, Thym de berger (Fr)
    Dosten, Wilder Majoran, Kostenz, Dorant (Ge)
Part used: the herb

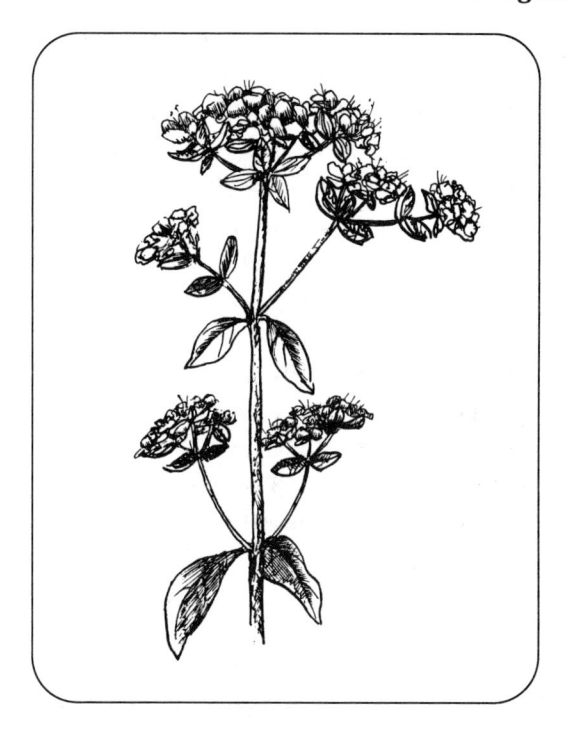

Nature

CATEGORY: mild herb with minimal chronic toxicity
CONSTITUENTS: ess. oil (incl. 16-50% phenol carvacrol), bitters, tannins, coffeeic/ursolic/rosmarinic acids, resins, gum
EFFECTIVE QUALITIES
Primary: a bit pungent & bitter, neutral with both warming and cooling potential, dry
Secondary: stimulating, relaxing, restoring
    dispersing movement

This herb is virtually identical in its nature, functions and uses to MARJORAM, folium Origani majoranae (p. 630), with the following differences:

1   Oregano's uterine *stimulant* effect for promoting the menses and expelling the afterbirth is a stronger one than Marjoram's.
2   In addition to its *relaxant* effects on the lungs, Oregano is used in syndromes such as lung phlegm dryness, lung phlegm damp and lung Yin deficiency, where it exerts a *strengthening* and *secretolytic stimulating* effect, helping to liquefy and expectorate viscous phlegm in chronic conditions especially.
3   Unlike Marjoram, Oregano has a good effect in *restraining infection, antidoting poison, relieving pain* and *ridding skin parasites,* being used for:
• mouth, gum & throat infections, tonsilitis;
• upper and lower respiratory infections (bronchitis, etc.);
• sores, ulcers;
• poisoning from herbs or insect stings/bites;
• parasitic skin diseases, itchy skin eruptions;
• acute or chronic rheumatism of muscles, joints;
• cellulite.

Oregano: Class 5

4   Drunk hot, Oregano *promotes sweating, releases the exterior and pushes out eruptions*, its main use here being for eruptive fevers and wind heat onset of infections.

Preparation

USE: The ESSENTIAL OIL and the TINCTURE of Oregano are the best preparations; the INFUSION is less effective. However, due to its hot, irritating quality the ESSENTIAL OIL should only be used externally in LINIMENTS and SALVES for conditions such as **myalgia**, **joint pain**, etc., as well as for parasitic and other skin infections, and for cellulite.

DOSAGE: ESSENTIAL OIL: 3-5 drops taken in a gelatin capsule with olive oil
                 Others: standard doses

CAUTION: Being a *uterine stimulant* Oregano is contraindicated during pregnancy. Standard doses should not be exceeded.

NOTE: Spanish Oregano has proved to yield the best *antimicrobial* essential oil, and is one of the top five essential oils used in infectious conditions in general.

Notes

Oregano was once an important medicine in Greece, where it was praised for its *stimulating, warming* and *relaxing* effects on the respiratory and reproductive organs especially. With obstructed menstruation due to **cold stasis**, it often worked wonders, effectively preventing the physician from resorting to stronger *stimulant emmenagogues* like Aloes from the island Sokotra, Water and Poison hemlock which grew wild everywhere, and Spurge laurel berries from the island Knidos (Knidos, interestingly, was the stronghold of the disease and local pathology oriented school of early Greek medicine, rather than the prevention and systemic diathesis-oriented one.

Many centuries later, the Italian natural physician PIERANDREA MATTIOLI (1610) recommended combining Oregano with Mugwort, Camomile and Fieldmint for delayed, difficult menstruation with cramps brought on by the energy of cold. Can we improve upon this formula today for a *stimulant, antispasmodic* and *relaxant* effect acting both locally on the uterus and generally on the whole system? We hardly think so, using just European botanicals. If one of the irreplaceable North American women's herbs, the squaw remedies, were substituted, however, that would be another story entirely.

RUE

Pharmaceutical name: herba Rutae
Botanical name: Ruta graveolens L. (N.O.Rutaceae)
Ancient names: Pyganon (Gr)
   Ruta domestica/sylvestris (Lat)
Other names: Herb grace, Ave grace,
   Countryman's treacle (Eng)
   Rue, Rue domestique, Herbe de grâce,
   Péganion (Fr)
   Gartenraute, Weinraute, Hexenkraut,
   Braunminze (Ge)
Part used: the herb

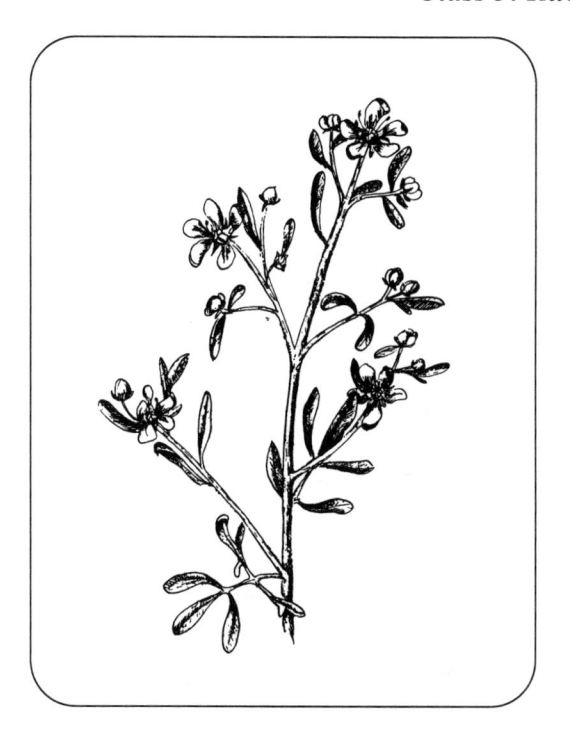

Nature

CATEGORY: medium-strngth herb with some chronic toxicity
CONSTITUENTS: ess. oil (incl. sesquiterpenes, ketones, alcohols), flavonoid glycoside (rutin), coumarin derivatives, alkaloids
EFFECTIVE QUALITIES
Primary: pungent & bitter, a bit warm, dry
Secondary: stimulating, relaxing, decongesting
TROPISM: uterus, liver, kidneys, lungs, inestines, stomach
   Air, Warmth organisms
   Lung, Small Intestine, Liver, Chong & Ren meridians
GROUND: Phlegmatic krasis
   Self-Reliant/Yang Ming Metal biotype constitution

Functions and Uses

1. STIMULATES AND WARMS THE UTERUS, PROMOTES THE MENSES AND CLEARS STASIS

   uterus Qi/cold stagnation with delayed or obstructed, painful menstruation
   AMENORRHEA, SPASMODIC DYSMENORRHEA

2. DREDGES THE KIDNEYS AND LIVER; PROMOTES URINATION AND BOWEL MOVEMENT; BENEFITS VISION

   kidney Qi stagnation with skin rashes, malaise
   liver Qi stagnation with depression, constipation
   POOR EYESIGHT

3. STIMULATES, WARMS AND INVIGORATES THE LUNGS, STOMACH AND INTESTINES; EXPELS VISCOUS PHLEGM; RIDS PARASITES

Rue: Class 5

    lung phlegm damp with productive coughing
    stomach Qi stagnation with nausea, sour regurgitation, indigestion
    intestines mucous damp (Spleen damp) with alternating loose & hard stool
    INTESTINAL PARASITES

4   CIRCULATES THE QI AND LOOSENS CONSTRAINT; RELAXES THE NERVE AND FREES SPASMS; CALMS WIND AND RELIEVES PAIN
    intestines Qi constraint with colicky pains, irritability
    lung Qi constraint with asthmatic breathing
    uterus Qi constraint with irregular painful menstruation
    kidney wind (internal wind) with spasms, tremors, convulsions
    EPILEPSY
    PAIN due to neuralgia, gout, arthritis, rheumatism, etc.

5   ACTIVATES IMMUNITY, RESTRAINS INFECTION AND ANTIDOTES POISON; BENEFITS THE SKIN
    PROPHYLACTIC in epidemics
    BOILS, carbuncles, abscesses,
    ULCERS
    VARICOSE VEINS
    SWOLLEN GLANDS, SCALY ERUPTIONS
    INSECT BITES and stings

Preparation

USE: The long INFUSION and TINCTURE are good preparations. LINIMENTS for **painful** conditions should include Rue, and WASHES, COMPRESSES and similar preparations are always appropriate.

DOSAGE: standard doses throughout

CAUTION: Being a *uterine stimulant,* Rue is forbidden during pregnancy. If used as a simple, a few days' break should be taken after two weeks or so, since its alkaloids and ketones elevate it to the rank of a medium-strength category remedy.

Notes

Greek medicine made extensive use of this plant for a variety of conditions, foremost of which was its m*enstruation promoting* effect. Today, when we look at the whole configuration that its functions and uses present, it becomes clear that uterus Qi stagnation and uterus cold are its syndromes of predilection. Menses that have ceased due to conditions of Qi stagnation and plethora demand its use, not those amenorrheas due to deficiency.

Rue contains plenty of alkaloids and volatile oils that make it an **energetic** remedy, in all senses of the word. It breaks up stasis, moves down food, and dredges phlegm and waste in the entire digestive tract, promoting bowel movement in so doing. GALEN's way of putting it was that "it discusses and digests all thick viscous fluids…it strongly resolves and dries." In language strongly reminiscent of Chinese texts he adds that "it extinguishes wind, being of subtle parts". The *relaxant* effect he is referring to is mild, on the other hand, but is usually a welcome addition. Today we would say that Rue is primarily an herb dealing with **systemic**, **chronic stagnation** of the internal organs with tendency to **cold** and **spasms** and with **mucous** and **damp** obstruction. It will shine if these conditions are met.

CLASS 6

Herbs to Cause Vomiting

Botanicals in this class are used to cause emesis, i.e. vomiting, either as part of an Eliminating treatment strategy or for use in acute poisoning. Although primarily used as part of the treatment of illness, emesis has traditionally been considered a significant prophylactic measure, assisting as it does the natural reflex of the organism's vital force; as such it is also a constitutional treatment for the ground, along with other treatment methods.

Vomiting as an eliminant therapy is traditional and universal to all systems of healing. Chinese medicine counted it among their treatment methods long before ZHANG ZI HE established his *dispelling* and *purging* school of healing. The canons of Ayurvedic medicine, the *Susruta* and the *Charak Samhita,* for example, contain the most developed presentation of emetic therapy, complete with indications, contraindications, techniques and botanicals used. For Persian physicians such as IBN SINA emesis was employed mainly in pediatrics. Greek medicine up to the nineteenth century made extensive use of it; it was considered an important treatment by physicians such as HIPPOKRATES, GALEN, RIVIERE, SYDENHAM, HUFELAND and ASCHNER.

Inducing vomiting provides perhaps the clearest example of a treatment method which can be **supportive** of the healing process while yet carrying out an *eliminant* technique. Greek doctors recognized that nature often indicates to us its tendencies and that the physician should strive to emulate her in this.[1] In the case of nausea and queasiness the natural consequence is vomiting; hence, by causing vomiting spontaneous processes are assisted. Here there is no question of forcing things against nature: rather the *virtus expulsiva naturae,* nature's eliminative power, is merely supported. Unsurprisingly, **nausea** was held to be an absolute indication for this method of treatment. The importance of only treating in the right context is thereby highlighted once again.

In this light, speaking about emetic herbs, the attitude of the Eclectic physician HERBERT WEBSTER becomes more meaningful when we read in his text of 1898: "The follower of Thomsonian methods might attempt too much with this class of remedies, and do harm by indiscriminately subjecting his patients to emesis; this, however, ought not to be employed as an argument against their proper use to fulfill important indications when so demanded." We would add that this consideration actually extends to all methods of treatment now unfashionable, such as bloodletting and external *derivative* techniques using *rubefacient, pustulant* and *vesicant* herbs (see p. 666).

The beneficial effects of emesis may be better understood when its deep influence on the nervous, circulatory, lymphatic and glandular systems are considered. Its energetic effects are *stimulant, decongestant, resorbant, softening, anti-inflammatory, antispasmodic* and *relaxant.* More importantly, however, these are a matter of direct experience. In the words of the Susruta: "When an emetic is effective it provokes a painless evacuation of phlegm and bile. Head, neck and chest feel liberated, and body and soul relieved."

Specifically, vomiting creates the following effects: it causes a local evacuation of contents from the stomach, duodenum, bile-ducts, gall bladder, liver and probably spleen and pancreas—hence its use in **stagnant, congestive** conditions of these organs, especially when **damp heat** is

The Energetics of Western Herbs

generated; it stimulates all secretions and excretions and is useful in **excess internal heat** conditions in general; it stimulates the solar plexus nerves and thus restores tone to the stomach, also adjusting faulty secretions; it stimulates the autonomic nerves in general, hence is useful in **life threatening situations** such as all types of asphyxia, lung edema, pulmonary emboly, bronchial asthma and angina pectoris, as well as in stroke and paralysis; it has a *derivative* effect that is useful for relieving inflammations, congestions and spasms in all organs above the diaphragm; finally it has a *resorbant* effect helpful with tumors, myomas, hard and fatty deposits, etc., as well as lymphatic congestion and edema above the waist.

Inducing vomiting may be summed up as a form of **shock therapy** (especially for the solar plexus) in which the trade-off is the obviation of chronic debility or hospitalization and of dangerous operations.

The Hippokratic aphorism that "pains above the diaphragm require evacuation upwards, while those below demand evacuation downwards" is a basic rule of thumb for the use of emetic therapy.

More specifically, we can say that all excess conditions of the lungs, throat and head are an indication for it, whether in the form of **stagnation, congestion, constraint** or **heat,** and whether **inflammation, catarrh** or **spasm** are involved. Disharmonies that respond best include migraine, mumps, erysipelas, anosmia, throat & mouth inflammation, bronchial asthma, bronchitis, lung TB, pneumonia, angina pectoris, gastric insufficiency, liver, gall bladder or Spleen damp heat, Spleen damp cold, Spleen fire (i.e. fever due to mucus), all skin conditions, lumbago, arthritis, mania, epilepsy and mental or psychic conditions.

Clearly, in light of the wide range of conditions addressed, it is important to use emesis as a whole method of treatment, like all other Eliminating methods. It is unfortunate to see it used purely for symptomatic effect or, worse still, reduced to a more exotic kind of cleansing method.

Remedies that provoke an emetic response when ingested operate mainly by stimulating a mechanical reflex by irritation. *Emetics* include roots such as Horseradish, Vervain root, Ipecac, Wild yam, Wild ginger and Pleurisy root; and herbs such as Melilot, Boneset, Horehound, Arnica, Lobelia and Holy thistle. They need to be taken in larger than normal doses for an emetic effect. They are found throughout the Materia Medica. Due care is taken to select the right botanical for each person according to his or her type or condition. Warm infusions of Peppermint, Yarrow and Camomile should be given to relax and settle the stomach afterwards. No food should be eaten for two or three hours following emetic treatment.

Caution: Inducing vomiting is contraindicated in deficient conditions with debility, in heart disease, high blood pressure, lung hemorrhage, during grieving and during pregnancy and menstruation.

A summary listing of all herbs in this class is found on page 695.

Notes
1   The Hippokratist THOMAS SYDENHAM especially was meticulous in distinguishing signs and symptoms which are part of the striving for balance of a person's *physis* from those which belong to the pathogenic process itself. Fever, sweating, skin eruptions, bleeding and nausea may all belong to this first type of symptom.

RESTORING

Restoring is the first of three treatment principles that address conditions of disharmony more systematically than either the Eliminating or Symptom Treatment principles. While the *eliminant* botanicals are geared primarily towards relieving stagnant and obstructive conditions of excretory organs by causing a discharge, and while the symptom remedies mainly relieve acute symptoms, Restoring, Draining, and Altering and Regulating are **constitution altering** principles and methods of treatment. Their main use is to treat the roots of disease involving long-term imbalance, both remedially, when there are existing problems, and preventively, in correcting constitutional tendencies to disharmony.

Restoring, Draining, and Altering and Regulating address every level of the human being—the Air, the Warmth, the Fluid and the Physical organisms. These treatment principles are able to rebalance disharmonies at the deepest level, whether involving nerve mediated physical, mental and emotional strength (the Air organism), warmth distribution and responses such as chill, fever and inflammation (the Warmth organism), or fluid and blood circulation and distribution (the Fluid organism). They regulate a variety of conditions not amenable to the more linear, directional Eliminating treatment methods. The Restoring principle deals with every type of **deficient** condition, while the complementary Draining method treats functional or qualitative conditions of **excess**, and the neutral Altering method affects the balance of whole systems. The combination of the excess, deficient and systematic conditions with the four organisms produces the herb classes of this section.

Herbs found under the Restoring, Draining and Altering and Regulating principles of treatment clearly represent the core materia medica for treatments directed at more than a symptomatic level: they effect the *cura generalis,* when this is possible. Their correct use represents the finest and most evolved use of botanical remedies.

Remedies that restore are classified as follows:

Class 7: Herbs to increase the Qi, restore and replenish deficiency
Class 8: Herbs to support the Yang, generate warmth and dispel cold
Class 9: Herbs to restore the blood, nourish and replenish deficiency
Class 10: Herbs to foster the Yin, provide moisture and lenify dryness
Class 11: Herbs to cause astriction, dry mucous damp, arrest discharge and stop bleeding

All remedies in the Restoring classes in one way or another cause restoration or tonification in both a structural and functional way. Because of this, they are also known as *tonics.*[1] They are used in a variety of conditions typified by global or local weakness, laxness and deficiency, which may be concisely termed **deficiency** or **empty** conditions. They are called *kenos* in Greek medicine and *xu* in Chinese. Since the deficiency consists of absence of some positive functional or structural element, it must be "replenished", as happily conveyed by the Greek term *plerosis,* and "supported" (*bu* in Chinese). The botanicals used for deficient conditions include *restorers* that generate warmth (*stimulants*), those that provide moisture (*demulcents*) and those that create astriction (*astringents*), since various types of deficiency conditions present cold, dryness or, conversely, damp, as part of their symptom configuration.

Chinese medicine in its clinical subtlety differentiates between five kinds of deficiency conditions requiring Restoring treatment: deficiency of the **Qi**, the **blood**, the **Yin**, the **Yang**, the **fluids** and the **Essence**. There are five distinct types of Restoring methods corresponding to these different types of deficiencies. Herbs that increase the Qi are discussed in Class 7; those that support the Yang are found in Class 8; those that restore the blood in Class 9; those that foster the Yin and the fluids in Class 10; while those that nourish essence belong for the most part to the *nourishing* kind (again Class 9). Other remedies that tonify the Yin and the Yang are discussed among the *systemic Yin/Yang regulators* in Class 16.

Various cultures, periods and styles of medicine have often favored one type of restoring treatment over another, a bias that arose as often from speculative considerations as from actual need. The eighteenth century, for example, saw the heyday of herbs that generate warmth using *stimulants* (Class 8); classical Greek medicine placed emphasis on remedies that restore the blood, nourish and supplement with *nutritives* (Class 9); while Chinese medicine has always favored increasing the Qi and restoring with *Qi tonics* (Class 7). On the whole, however, it is necessary to simply use the botanicals that best meet the need of the given situation. Today, given the psychic (emotional) stress and environmental pollution that many people are subject to, and the resultant weakening of the immune system, it is the herbs that increase the Qi and restore (Class 7), those that loosen constraint and circulate the Qi (Class 12) and those that promote cleansing and resolve toxemia (Class 15) that are finding a renewed currency.

Restoring or tonifying treatment methods address not only local situations of deficiency such as organ or system insufficiencies, insufficient secretions, chronic discharges and prolapse, but also more global, systemic deficiencies. Because the organism is an interplay of energies and processes, even if only one body part manifests weakness, the entire organism is usually involved in these syndromes of deficiency. This becomes even more evident when we look at the properties of *restorative* herbs that address deficiency conditions: in addition to their local action on tissues they invariably also exert a systemic effect on the whole organism, energetically affecting the individual on all levels. *Moistening* herbs relax and soothe at a distance by reflex action in addition to their purely topical tissue coating and cooling effects; *astricting* herbs restore overall tone and strength besides causing local tissue tightening; *blood restoring* remedies nourish tissues as a whole in addition to the fluid blood tissue itself; *liver/stomach/Spleen tonics* strengthen and improve global functioning by reflex action on secretory glands as well as by aiding digestion specifically.

When chosing a treatment principle, note that Restoring is used when the intention is to support the organism's vital force and to generate physical strength. Restoring supports the righteous Qi (*zheng zhi*) as opposed to correcting the disharmony or pathogenic factor itself, called the injurious Qi (*fan zhi* or *tou xie*). Supporting may often be necessary even when some excess manifests together with a deficiency, as explained in the introduction to the Eliminating section. As a result, *restoring* herbs are commonly used in conjunction with remedies from all classes that drain, alter and eliminate. Restoring is therefore the antithesis of both the Draining and Eliminating modalities in which a pathogenic factor is dealt with directly.

Ultimately, restoration or tonification has only two types of uses, preventive and curative. Although this section of the Materia Medica deals uniquely with curative application, it should be remembered that in its widest sense restoration denotes the prophylactic or preventive treatment of the person's ground with mild herbs, i.e. botanicals from the mild, nontoxic category. Many of these types of herbs will treat a person's entire psychosomatic make-up, so helping to bring the individual back to a condition of his or her own natural, innate balance, known in Greek medicine as *physis*. It is through a person's constitution, biotype and diathesis that his/her natural condition can be treated. Hawthorn, for example, can be said to be a *ground* tonic to the Charming/Yang Ming Earth type,[2] and hence will rebalance the energetic and physical functions that constitute the authentic, normal condition of that biotype.

Hippokratic medicine was possibly the biggest proponent of the Restoring method as a kind of general constitutional treatment. The physicians on the island Kos all emphasized prevention rather than cure, and health maintenance rather than the treatment of disease. *Restorative* herbs were known as **similars** to both HIPPOKRATES and GALEN, since only remedies similar to the human organism are in a position to have a restoring effect.[3] In Chinese medicine, LI DONG YUAN promoted Restoration through his emphasis on restoring the stomach and Spleen, these being the central organ functions vital for the upkeep of all others.

Notes

1   Throughout this text, the word *tonic,* used as an alternative to the term *restorative,* refers specifically to a restoring type botanical used in **deficiency** conditions. It is not used in the more usual imprecise sense.

2   The beauty of herbs of the mild category, which form the bulk of this Materia Medica, is their bivalency. While Bayberry bark is a good *ground tonic* for the Dependent/Tai Yin Earth person, it is at the same time a *stimulant astringent* for those with deficient Yang or Spleen Yang deficiency patterns of disharmony. Mild botanicals play a dual role as both preventive tonics and remedies.

3   Restoring in the past was essentially seen in the larger context of maintenance and is described in Hippokratic texts as being achieved by dietary measures, using the principle "*similia similibus*" (GALEN). In other words, nature (i.e. the righteous vital force) should be supported in deficient conditions by providing a type of nourishment similar to the body. In contrast, the treatment of actual illness was always carried out by **contraries,** according to *contraria contrariis*. The medical historian GEORG HARIG (1974) correctly points out that "the Homeopathy of modern times as a method of treating disease processes themselves is not to be found in Galen, nor anywhere in the entire history of ancient medicine." This simple historical evidence effectively undermines the claims which homeopaths since HAHNEMANN have made, namely that their healing art is based on Hippokratic therapeutic principles. This does not invalidate Homeopathy as a valid and effective procedure, of course. Homeopathy merely shifts the Greek application of treating *similia similibus* (by tonifying the vital force) over to HAHNEMANN's application of treating the entire pattern of disharmony with remedies causing symptoms similar to the illness.

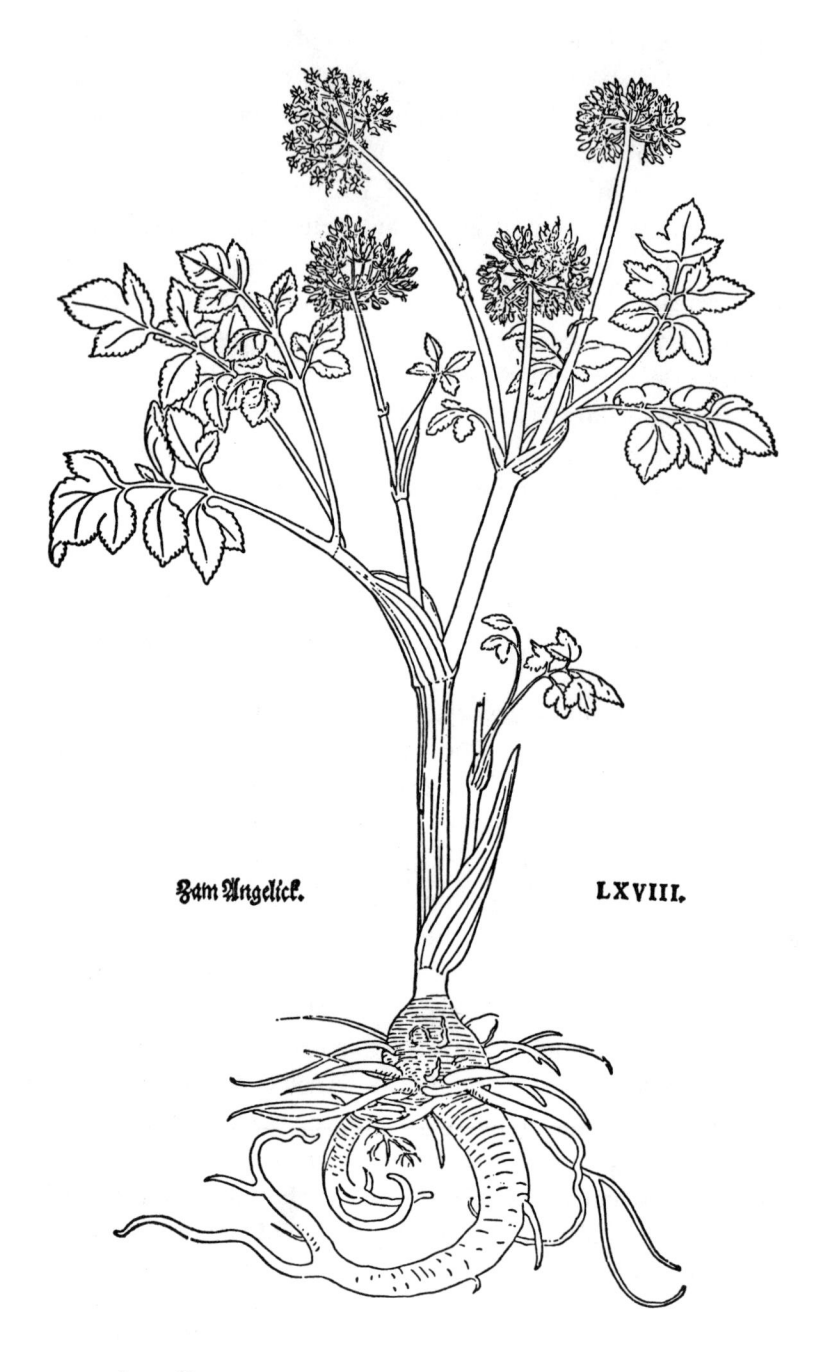

Angelica

CLASS 7

Herbs to Increase the Qi, Restore and Replenish Deficiency

The function of botanicals in this class is to treat conditions known in Chinese medicine as Qi deficiency. In Qi deficiency conditions the active, configurating forces of the Qi, or vital breaths, become weakened, causing typical signs of deficiency such as weakness, fatigue and hypofunctioning. Qi deficiency conditions are usually endogenous and chronic, may be either systemic or local, and generally represent a lack of tone (hypotonia) or stimulation (hyposthenia). When the Qi's organizing activities in the human organism diminish, a passive, weak condition of the organ(s) or part(s) concerned results. Herbs in this class have the ability to increase the Qi (*yi Qi*) and restore (*bu*) in a large variety of Qi deficiency conditions, and hence replenish (*ying*) or make good this deficiency. In so doing they not only generate physical strength, but also enhance immune potential as part of their overall action.

In general terms, a Qi deficiency represents a weakness in an individual's vital spirit (*spiritus vitalis* in Greek medicine), and specifically the *zhen qi* or *authentic Qi* in Chinese medicine. Qi deficiency may include a weakened nervous system with insufficient neuromuscular activity and poor immunity and may entail reduced innervation and poor tissue tone. Hence Qi deficiency conditions are generally characterized by **weakness, looseness** and **collapse.** While they might be sparked off by events such as sudden physical exertion, emotional jolts such as grief and worry, and sudden mental stress, they are more significantly engendered by predisposing factors such as poor constitution, chronic physical or mental overwork, childbearing, excessive sexual activity or long-term emotional disharmony.

Qi deficiency may be found systemically or locally. When systemic, it entails global hypofunctioning and atonicity, causing symptoms such as fatigue, worry, listlessness, nervous behavior, weakness, excessive sweating and urination, a pale complexion, shallow breathing, poor appetite, shallow sleep, a weak, empty or thin pulse and a puffy, scalloped, often furless tongue. Found locally, Qi deficiency entails local atonicity and asthenia of one or more organs or systems with corresponding symptoms. Chinese medicine describes a variety of syndromes such as lung Qi deficiency, Spleen Qi deficiency and Kidney Qi deficiency to account for these local emphases. The first two of these are the most important, since lung and Spleen activity are responsible for generating and maintaining the Qi.

Qi deficiency is clearly a preclinical state from the biomedical perspective, since usually no actual lesions are present, and it may not entail any Western disease entity. However, this is not to diminish its energetic physiological presence as an imbalance, especially since Qi deficiency can easily progress to other, more serious conditions. Qi constraint and toxemia are the most common follow-ons. These are both forms of stagnation, one on the level of the soul, the other on the physical level; they are described in Classes 12 and 15 respectively. On a simpler level, Qi deficiency often entails a blood deficiency in which nutrition becomes impaired (Class 9), and sometimes Yang or Yin deficiency that points to systemic autonomic nervous imbalance (Class 16).

Individual biotypes in which Qi deficiency conditions are inherent are the Sensitive/Tai Yin Metal, dominated by the Lung meridian, and the Dependant/Yai Yin Earth, dominated by the

The Energetics of Western Herbs

Spleen meridian. More than other types, they are candidates for treatment with herbs from this class, with the treatment objective of increasing the Qi and restoring.

Increasing the Qi and restoring is, of all treatment methods, the one best suited to a **preventive** application more than to a remedial one. Preventive treatment will maintain health by enhancing the body's defenses against illness and will specifically bolster deficient constitutional potentials (*yuan qi*)—especially in the above-mentioned biotypes—and optimize maximum functioning of the healthy vital forces (*zhen qi*), including immunity, in the face of pathogens and general stress. Traditional Greek medicine was/is especially concerned with maintaining these righteous life forces (*zheng qi*) which it called *pneuma,* and many texts specifically deal wih the treatment of deficiency conditions through appropriate diet supplemented by *restorative* herbs, as well as through suitable exercise. *Plerosis* is the Greek medical term for the treatment objective in deficiency conditions, which is one of **filling** or **replenishing**. The relevance today of building up our innate resources, irrespective of what name we actually give them, cannot be overemphasized; immune integrity itself is only a part, if a major part, of the normal expression of our individual life force (*zong qi*). At this time, when immune-deficiency diseases such as MS, Aids and Epstein-Barr are on the increase, and viruses are increasingly capable of mutation (in turn due to pollutants such as radiation and chemicals), restoring and strengthening with *Qi tonics* is indicated on a virtually continuous basis.

However, when used to restore and tonify organs, systems or tissues, increasing the Qi and replenishing deficiency becomes part of **remedial** or **curative** treatment. As well as treating general debility caused by excessive physical, emotional or mental activity, it especially addresses chronic deficiency conditions, including those found with immune deficiency diseases, with low-grade fevers, during convalescence, after an acute illness, and following childbirth or an operation.

Clearly, treatment will be more effective if a specific and comprehensive assessment of the individual condition is made. Consequently, treatment should first address immediate symptoms (e.g. debility, copious sweating, depression, anxiety, prolapse of an internal organ due to Central Qi sinking); secondly should adjust or remove immediate or predisposing factors such as mental or physical overwork, stress or emotions; and thirdly should rebalance the Qi deficiency (and any other condition involved) as well as take into account constitutional factors. In this connection, it is important to create lifestyle modifications that will encourage changes in this direction.

Herbs that increase the Qi, called *Qi tonics, restoratives* or simply *tonics,* represent the purest type of *mild* herbs, i.e. herbs with virtually no toxicity, even when ingested over long periods of time (see p. 52). The *Shennong ben cao jing,* the oldest extant Chinese herbal, classifies *restorative* botanicals as the most superior type of herb known. They cause an increase of physical strength, a greater sense of well-being and other unspecific and unquantifiable positive effects. This is especially true of remedies in the first two subclasses below. By impressing the higher nerve centers in the brain, they are able to influence all processes on all levels in long-range terms. They achieve this mainly through their neuroimmunological influence which tones or enhances nonspecific immunity, i.e. builds up immune potential.

The influence of the the mind (as well as feelings) on physical health in general, and immunity in particular, has always been recognized; however, this influence has only begun to be actually charted in recent years. This information helps us to understand and account for the overall immune boosting effects of *Qi tonics* such as Elecampane, American ginseng, Sage and

Herbs to Increase the Qi, Restore and Replenish Deficiency

Thyme. It places these botanicals squarely alongside other big *immunity potentizers* such as Siberian ginseng (*Eleutherococcus senticosus*), Korean and Chinese ginseng (*Panax ginseng*), *Astragalus* and *Schizandra*. *Immunity potentizers*, then, should not be reduced to or defined by the *adaptogenic* properties of these last mentioned herbs; for they do more than specifically reduce the body's energy wasteful reaction to stress.

Botanicals that increase the Qi, restore, and replenish deficiency are dominated by the *bitter* taste. There are notable exceptions to this pattern, e.g. Licorice, which is intensely *sweet,* while some herbs have a *sweet, pungent* or *astringent* taste in addition to a *bitter* taste. Bitterness is known to stimulate glandular secretions throughout the entire system, beginning with saliva in the mouth when this taste is first perceived. Bitterness thus activates not only digestive functioning, but, in ways not understood, cardiac and respiratory functions (which Greek, Chinese and Ayurvedic pharmacology described millenniums ago), and moreover strengthens and invigorates the whole organism, though again through unclear mechanisms.

The restoring action of *Qi tonics,* although immediately initiated, does not produce immediate results. Ideally *Qi tonics* should be used over a period of time to allow their fullest potential to unfold. A ten day course should be viewed as a minimum period for this restoring treatment to take effect, and a period of three months or over, with small breaks, is common. Hence, *restoratives* are best used for chronic rather than recent or acute deficiencies. Newly developed deficiencies on the other hand are better treated by Class 8 *stimulants*.

Remedies in this class are commonly combined with a variety of other herbs when Qi deficiency is found together with other conditions. When Qi deficiency leads to catarrhal damp cold in the head, intestines or urogenital organs, *Qi tonics* in this class are combined with *astringent* from Class 11. When Qi deficiency causes Qi constraint, these *tonics* are combined with relaxants from Class 12. When Qi deficiency engenders general toxemia causing obstruction of a channel of excretion, *eliminants* from Classes 1 through 6, and especially *diaphoretics, diuretics* and *laxatives,* are used additionally. If toxemia is a chronic condition manifesting as a general fluids dyskrasia, *antidyskratic* remedies from Class 15 are used in conjunction.

Since various organ systems may be involved in any Qi deficiency condition, this class is defined by five kinds of *Qi tonic* herbs, each with its own nature, functions and uses.

1 HERBS TO INCREASE THE QI AND RESTORE THE LUNGS, RESTORE THE NERVE, ENHANCE IMMUNE POTENTIAL AND CREATE STRENGTH

Botanicals in this category address **Qi deficiency** patterns with signs such as shallow breathing, a low gruff voice, pale complexion, spontaneous daytime perspiration, fatigue, despondency or depression, mental dullness, poor appetite, low resistance to infections, a weak, empty pulse, and a pale, puffy tongue with scalloped edges. Since Qi deficiency consists of **lung Qi deficiency** and **Spleen Qi deficiency**, these herbs can in fact also treat either syndrome separately. In Western terms they also address neuromuscular weakness, i.e. nerve deficiency, and low blood pressure, as well as specific lung conditions such as chronic bronchitis and emphysema, and gastrointestinal disorders.

These remedies provide the deepest, most encompassing and long-term tonification possible. Many belong to the Labiates, the Mint family, which includes Sage, Thyme, Rosemary and Basil; those from other families include American ginseng and Prickly ash. These herbs have a moderately *sweet, bitter* or *pungent* taste, or a combination of these, and the majority are known as *nerve tonics* in the West. They tend to work through the autonomic nervous system, primarily

The Energetics of Western Herbs

restoring nervous and respiratory functions and secondarily aiding digestive ones, which include the functions of the Spleen in Chinese medicine. Most of them effectively increase immune potential as a result of their systemic actions and produce a noticeble increase in physical strength. Many are known to also increase blood pressure, and those are known as *hypertensives*.

Moreover, since Qi deficiency is closely linked to blood deficiency, herbs that restore the Qi also tend to assist in restoring the blood. If chronic depression is found in this context, *nerve trophorestoratives* from Class 21 should additionally be used.

2 HERBS TO RESTORE, STRENGTHEN AND SUPPORT THE HEART, HARMONIZE THE CIRCULATION, LIFT THE SPIRIT AND RID DEPRESSION

Although botanicals in this category are used in a variety of heart syndromes and heart conditions, their primary function is to address **heart Qi** and **heart Yang deficiency**. They are therefore used when symptoms present such as palpitations, chest oppression, shortness of breath aggravated by exercise, cold extremities and cyanosed lips, mental depression and dullness, a thin, weak or knotted pulse and a pale, sometimes purplish (cyanosed), moist tongue. These two syndromes usually involve cardiac insufficiency and arrhythmia, and may be found in the context of a large variety of Western diseases.

The treatment of these deficiencies involves restoring and strengthening the heart; heart Yang deficiency also needs a stimulation of the heart. *Cardiac tonics* and *cardiac stimulants* are the remedies of choice. They have a moderately *sweet* taste which is a qualitative aspect of their restoring functions. Hawthorn, Cowslip flower, Lily of the valley, Cereus, Valerian and Arnica are the most important remedies in this category, and most of them are flowers. They are joined by the Chinese herb Rehmannia which, although not a flower, is typically also *sweet* in taste.

One of the primary actions of these herbs is to lift the spirit and dispel mental gloom or depression. Because of this, they are sometimes used together with botanicals in Class 21 that lift the spirit.

Most important of all perhaps, botanicals of this type are able to **support** and **stabilize** the heart in its function of keeping a balance between the nerve-sensory pole above the heart and the metabolic pole below it. This in itself commends their use in all ailments where the heart is affected, especially in excess conditions involving liver fire and Qi constraint.[1]

3 HERBS TO RESTORE THE LIVER, STOMACH AND *SPLEEN/ INTESTINES*, AWAKEN THE APPETITE, PROMOTE DIGESTION AND CREATE STRENGTH

Herbs of this type are used, first, in **liver and stomach Qi deficiency** syndromes with upper gastric and hepatic insufficiency. Typical symptoms are slow, painful digestion, poor appetite, constipation, and a weak, tight pulse. Secondly, they are used in **Spleen Qi deficiency** patterns with fatigue, no appetite, abdominal distention and rumbling, loose stool, weak or thin pulse and a pale tongue with thin white moss. In Western terms this may be gastroenteritis, chronic dysentery and other functional gastrointestinal problems.

In the first case of liver and stomach Qi deficiency, the treatment method is to stimulate the liver and stomach by restoring liver and stomach Qi. In the second case, the objective is to stimulate and harmonize the gastrointestinal tract by restoring stomach/Spleen Qi. In both cases, *hepatic* and *gastro-intestinal stimulants* with a *bitter pungent* taste are used. Many of these botanicals, such as Tansy, Holy thistle, Yarrow, Wormwood and Feverfew, belong to the

Composite family. In character, they belong to the Chinese element Earth, thus influencing all organs and the body as a whole, both in the short and long term. Specifically, they stimulate glandular secretions by reflex action, enhancing overall metabolism and strengthening the physical body as a result.

If liver and stomach Qi deficiency is accompanied by severe constipation, Class 3 *choleretic laxatives* should reinforce herbs from this category. If Spleen Qi deficiency is accompanied by severe diarrhea, suitable Class 11 *astringents* should be added. In addition, Class 19 contains three types of *digestive remedies* often used in combination with the herbs in this category. *Carminatives* are useful when gas and distention are prominent, *digestive stimulants* when abdominal pain and nausea are uppermost, and enzymatic remedies when *enzyme secretions* specifically are lacking.

All herbs with a *bitter* taste are known to have a *restoring* effect on liver & stomach Qi. It should be noted, however, that intensely bitter botanicals such as Gentian, Wormwood, Bogbean, Chicory and Centaury, when used as *restoratives*, are best taken in small dosages. In normal or large doses they have a *draining, heat clearing* and *detoxifying* effect, which explains their placement in this Materia Medica in Class 13.

4 HERBS TO RESTORE AND STRENGTHEN THE UROGENITAL ORGANS

Herbs of this type treat weakness in the urinary or reproductive system, and in Chinese medicine are said to "restore Kidney Qi." Symptoms of **urogenital Qi deficiency**, or **Kidney Qi deficiency**, include clear, frequent, scanty (or copious) urination, urination at night, bedwetting, prostate irritation, leucorrhea, premature ejaculation, lumbar soreness, heavy knees, a deep, thin pulse and a pale, white coated tongue. Some of these botanicals will also rectify Kidney Yang deficiency, which in addition to the above symptoms may present low vitality, fatigue, cold limbs, water retention in the legs, infertility, impotence, lack of sexual desire, mental dullness or stupor, and emotional insensitivity. In Western terms there might be insufficient functioning of the adrenal cortex and sympathetic nervous system, in addition to conditions such as chronic nephritis.

Treatment aims at restoring urogenital functioning through a tonification of Kidney Qi or Kidney Yang, using *urinary* and *urogenital tonics*. These remedies tend to have a *gentle, bitter* or *sweet* taste, as well as a specific tropism for the reproductive and urinary system which they strengthen structurally and functionally. They include Fennel, Sea holly, Poplar, Buchu, Saw palmetto, Jasmin and Damiana. Being true *tonics,* like their equivalent *Ze xie* in the Chinese pharmacopoeia, they also impart strength and may be used preventively.

If dryness is associated with these genitourinary or Kidney deficiency conditions, as in Liver and Kidney depletion, then appropriate Class 10 *demulcents* are added. If general urinary irritation presents, then herbs from Class 2 or 10 should also be selected. If discharges are severe, Class 11 *astringents* should also be adopted.

5 HERBS TO RESTORE THE UTERUS AND RETURN THE MENSES

There are two types of deficiency conditions requiring the use of *uterine restorative* remedies. One is uterus Qi deficiency, the other is uterus blood deficiency. Each is treated by specific botanicals. Both conditions may be triggered by events such as childbirth, breastfeeding, emotional upsets and approaching menopause, as well as being generated by the same predisposing factors that cause Qi deficiency and blood deficiency in general.

Herbs used in conditions of **uterus Qi deficiency** have a specific restoring action on weakened uterine tone, resulting in scanty, delayed or irregular menstruation. This is often

The Energetics of Western Herbs

found in the context of other, more global deficiency conditions such as Qi deficiency and Liver & Kidney depletion, where weakness, fatigue and other typical symptoms present. By restoring the tone of the womb, these herbs naturally promote a return to regular menstruation. Their final effect is actually *emmenagogue,* although they are not termed as such, in order to distinguish them from the *uterine stimulants* in Class 5. They include Helonias, Blue cohosh, White deadnettle, Squaw vine, Raspberry, Black haw and Life root—most of them outstanding botanicals from the Native American tradition. They do not belong to any single family, their only common factor being their tropism for woman's reproductive organs.

If uterus Qi deficiency causes passive bleeding, resulting in copious, long periods (menorrhagia), or even intermenstrual bleeding (metrorraghia), then *hemostatics* from Class 11 and 14 should be used to treat this symptom. At the same time *uterine tonics* from this class should be used to restore uterine tone.

These botanicals may also be used in conditions of uterus Qi constraint and uterus cold with painful, copious or delayed menses. They will restore the uterus Qi deficiency condition often found at the root of these syndromes.

Equally, and for the same reason, they should be used to back up more specific herbs in syndromes of liver Qi stagnation and general plethora exhibiting menstrual disharmonies.

Botanicals used for **uterus blood deficiency** treat uterine blood where the menses become delayed or more scanty and gradually cease altogether. Since this is often the case in context of patterns such as genitourinary Qi deficiency, blood deficiency and liver blood deficiency, uterus blood deficiency often presents signs of fatigue, inordinately scanty or copious urination, aching lumbars, dizziness, a deep, thin pulse and a pale tongue. By restoring womb blood, therefore, these remedies naturally encourage regular menstruation to resume as an expression of a flourishing blood condition. Helonias, Mugwort, Parsley root, Artichoke and the Chinese Dang gui (*Angelica sinensis*) belong to this select set.

Both types of *uterine restorers* should be used with more general *nutritives* from Class 9 if this condition is found in the context of blood or fluids deficiency syndromes. They should be supplemented by other *estrogenic* herbs if, as is usually the case, an estriol insufficiency is implicated.

Infertility is often found together with delayed or absent periods and also represents a uterus Qi or blood deficiency. It too is essentially treated with herbs in this category.

Caution: In both deficient uterus blood and deficent uterus Qi types of amenorrhea, where there are no signs of obstructed or retained menses, Class 5 *stimulant emmenagogues* that promote menstruation are contraindicated. The periods should be encouraged to return by restoring the deficiency, not by forcing an elimination that may cause further deficiency.

A summary listing of all herbs in this class is found on page 695.

Note

1   The concept of the heart maintaining a balance between nervous functions centered in the head and metabolic activities in the abdomen (or Lower Warmer in Chinese medicine) is not a well understood one, although it has clinical as well as theoretical relevance. All traditional medical theories see the heart as being the most central organ of all, but this particular idea of balance goes back to RUDOLF STEINER in this century, if not to earlier writers. From this perspective, the heart represents an effective transformer or equalizer which softens the blow of the disharmonies of the one system over the other (the nervous over the metabolic or vice versa). As a result, the heart becomes stressed whenever disharmonies arise where one system is

encroached upon by the other: Qi constraint, general plethora, Yang excess, liver fire, Yin excess are examples of some possible syndromes. In all cases, the heart is eventually weakened, resulting in additional heart blood deficiency or heart Qi constraint and calling for botanicals that will support it in its harmonizing, balancing functions.

For an in-depth study of this subject, see the works of WERNER CHRISTIAN SIMONIS.

Licorice: Class 7

Herbs to Increase the Qi, Restore the Lungs and Nerve, Enhance Immune Potential and Create Strength

LICORICE

Pharmaceutical name: radix Glycyrrhizae
Botanical name: Glycyrrhiza glabra L. (N.O. Papilionaceae)
Ancient names: Glykyrizza (Gr)
    Liquirita (Lat)
Other names: Réglisse, Herbe-aux-tanneurs, Bois doux (Fr)
    Süssholz, Likrize (Ge) Gan cao (Ch)
Part used: the root

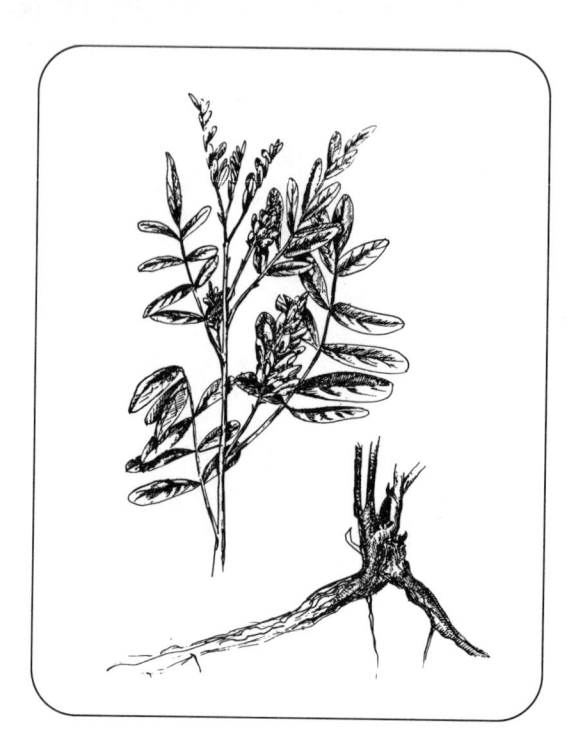

Nature

CATEGORY: mild herb with minimal chronic toxicity
CONSTITUENTS: glycoside glycirrizin 5%, glycirrhizic acid as calcium & magnesium salts 2-15%, flavonoids, steroid hormones (oestrogens), triterpenoid saponins, flavonoids (incl. liquiritoside, isoliquritoside), resinous oil 15%, starch 20%, saccharose 3%, glucose 3%, asparagin 2-6%, mannitol, atropin, coumarins, cholin, betain, progesterone-related substances, steroids analagous to ACTH, triterpenoids, bitters
EFFECTIVE QUALITIES
Primary: very sweet, slightly bitter, cool, moist
Secondary: restoring, calming, relaxing
    stabilizing movement
TROPISM: lungs, stomach, intestines, bladder, adrenal cortex, pituitary
    Warmth, Air organisms
    twelve main meridians
GROUND: Phlegmatic & Melancholic krases
    Dependant/Tai Yin Earth & Sensitive/Tai Yin Metal biotypes
    all three constitutions

Funtions and Uses

1 INCREASES THE QI, SUPPORTS THE YANG AND REPLENISHES DEFICIENCY; RESTORES THE PITUITARY AND ADRENALS, ENHANCES IMMUNE POTENTIAL AND GENERATES STRENGTH; INCREASES ESTROGEN AND PROMOTES MENSTRUATION; FREES SPASMS AND RELIEVES PAIN

Class 7: LIcorice

Spleen Qi deficiency: weakness, poor appetite, epigastric pain
Spleen & Kidney Yang deficiency: no appetite, exhaustion, loose stool, lumbar pain, lack of sexual desire, impotence, stopped menstruation
DEBILITY, fatigue due to overwork, stress or illness
ADRENOCORTICAL INSUFFICIENCY with vagotonia or gonadal insufficiency; Addison's disease
ESTROGEN INSUFFICIENCY with delayed menses or amenorrhea
LOW BLOOD SUGAR
HIGH BLOOD CHOLESTEROL
AUTOIMMUNE DISEASE in general
intestines Qi constraint: indigestion, cramping intestinal pains & spasms

2 ACTIVATES IMMUNITY, RESTRAINS INFECTION AND PROTECTS THE LIVER; CLEARS HEAT, RESOLVES FEVER, REDUCES INFLAMMATION, CLEARS TOXINS AND ANTIDOTES POISON; BENEFITS THE SKIN

PREVENTIVE in epidemics
BACTERIAL & VIRAL INFECTIONS of lungs (incl. TB, pneumonia), intestines, liver (INFECTIOUS HEPATITIS), urogenital system
fire toxin: boils, furuncles, abscesses with fever
stomach fire: great appetite, thirst with desire for cold water, swollen painful gums
MOUTH, TONGUE & EYE INFLAMMATIONS, incl. apthous sores, stomatitis
CHRONIC JOINT INFLAMMATIONS
POISONING of food, herb, mineral or animal origin
SKIN ERUPTIONS incl. dermatitis, eczema, pruritus; cysts

3 PROVIDES MOISTURE AND LENIFIES DRYNESS; LIQUIFIES AND EXPELS PHLEGM, RELIEVES COUGHING AND WHEEZING

lung dryness: dry cough with some viscous phlegm, dry mouth, nose and throat with tickle in throat
lung heat dryness: head & body aches, fever, dry cough,
thirst FEBRILE LUNG INFECTIONS, whooping cough
lung phlegm dryness: difficult breathing and coughing, coughing up plugs of phlegm, wheezing
ALLERGIC ASTHMA, flu
IRRITABLE & CATARRHAL lung conditions
COUGHING due to dryness, irritation or nervousness
HOARSENESS, sore throat
GASTRIC & DUODENAL ULCER due to hyperacidity
URINARY IRRITATION or PAIN due to sand, stone or uric acid

Preparation

USE: The DECOCTION and TINCTURE are both suited to put Licorice's potentials into practice, although the first is preferable in hot or **hyperacidic stomach** conditions, with or without ulcer, and taken **after** meals. The sliced root should be **toasted** first before decocting for greater *Spleen restoring* effects.

The SYRUP was and still is a favorite for **lung** conditions of all kinds; Schroeder's Dispensatory gives a SYRUP recepy which both stimulates and restores the lungs, consisting of Licorice,

Licorice: Class 7

Coltsfoot, Elecampane, Hyssop, Yarrow, Scabious, Speedwell, Lungwort, Meadow saffron petals, Dates and Jujubes. Excellent WASHES can be made where there is **inflammation** in external parts.
DOSAGE: standard doses throughout
CAUTION: Licorice should be avoided in excess adrenal conditions such as hypertension, water retention (esp. around the heart); in hyperglycemic states; in osteoporosis; and with excess secretions generally, such as is found in stomach Qi stagnation, for example.

Some individuals are naturally sensitive to Licorice extracts and preparations such as true Licorice candy (as found mainly in Europe), laxatives containing a large proportion of Licorice extract, and anti-ulcer medicines made from its concentrated derivatives. (For these DGL—deglycyrrhizinated Licorice—should be used instead in ulcer treatment.) At any rate, the untreated root itself prepared in DECOCTION or ingested directly has **never** produced any symptoms of toxicity in anyone, even when used on a daily basis.

Notes

Licorice is one of the botanicals where Western and Chinese uses intersect, resulting in an interesting assortment of uses. Looking over some of the pharmacological and clinical research, it becomes clear that *Glycyrrhiza uralensis* is interchangeable with *G. glabra,* so any claims about different uses arising out of different botanical specimens are unjustified. Here the traditional Chinese medical emphasis on describing herb functions in terms of physiopathology in a purely phenomenological way comes to the fore, forming a sharp contrast to the more analytical, experimental approach of current Western pharmacy. Nevertheless, when digging back through Western botanical literature, it becomes apparent that the similarity of uses outweighs the differences: once again, the key lies in Galenic medicine. In addition, Western research (which has been enormous) fully consolidates Licorice's position in the traditional Chinese pharmacopoeia as a *Qi tonic.*

The differences can be quickly appreciated: whereas Chinese practice emphasizes Spleen Qi deficiency as calling for its use, a Western practitioner, seeing its *adrenal cortex* and *medulla* and *gonadic stimulant* properties, would rather put it under Spleen Yang, as well as Kidney Yang. Certainly the symptomatology of the deficiencies of both syndromes justifies this. Its *estrogenic* effect is another reason for making Spleen & Kidney Yang deficiency in women a firm indication for its use. Moreover, as a result of Western research, Licorice has emerged as an *immune enhancer* (as well as *immune activator*) through the pituitary/adrenal axis, which merely reinforces its place among the full-fledged *Qi tonics.* Like these, it is a **maintenance** botanical in the completest sense. To document its very complex, interrelated and comprehensive pharmacological effects in a way that would do it justice would require a separate study; suffice it to mention that exciting evidence has appeared indicating its use in autoimmune disease. However, the net result of these *restoring* and *regulating* effects also makes Licorice a global *enhancer* of the effective functions of other remedies: it stands alone in this capacity of intensifying any other herb it may be combined with.

Both Galenic and Chinese herbal traditions see Licorice as having *moderating, tempering* and *smoothening* energetic qualities—largely derived from its intense *sweet* taste. This applies on one hand to conditions of **irritability, hypersensitivity** of the **lungs** and **throat, stomach** and **urinary organs,** where its *lenitive demulcent* effects prevail over dry and inflammatory symptoms.
JOHANN SCHROEDER (1610), in fact, devotes quite some space to explaining how and why Licorice "linders the sharpness of urine" (refering to excess uricosuria), "tempers the sharpness of the fluids causing urinary stones" and "heals bladder ulcers." Both traditions have made use of Licorice's *anti-infective, anti-inflammatory* and *antiseptic* effects for a long time; only today do we also know of its *protecting* and *detoxifying* effect on liver cells which highlights its use for

infectious hepatitis, for example.

On the other hand, Licorice's smooth quality rubs off on the very remedies it is combined with: it uniformly softens any harshness in their effects, of whatever nature (warmth, taste, moisture, toxicity); in this context it is an important *antidote* and *temperer* to a variety of toxic plants or their extracts, including strychnine, caffeine, cocaine, pilocarpine, nicotine, Aconite. Moreover, it is a very common ingredient in many formulations not only for this reason, but also because "it makes them more acceptable to the stomach" (DIERS RAU, 1968). The Chinese theme of protecting and strengthening the Spleen/stomach once again raises its head.

If it was felt neccessary to assign a planet to this remedy, it would assuredly be Venus.

AMERICAN GINSENG

Pharmaceutical name: radix Panacis quinquefolii
Botanical name: Panax quinquefolium L. (N.O. Araliaceae)
Other names: Five fingers, Tartar root, Cherokee root, Red berry, Sang, Jinshard, Garantogen, Ninsin, Manroot (Am)
  Xi yang shen (Ch)
Part used: the root

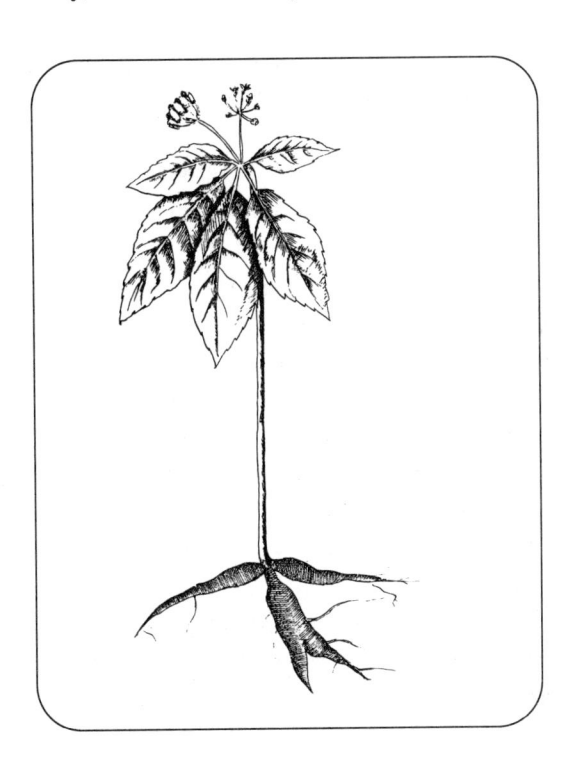

Nature

CATEGORY: mild herb with minimal chronic toxicity
CONSTITUENTS: saponin glycosides ginenodide & panaxoside, ess. oil 3%, camphoraceaous substance, resin, arabinose, mucilage, starch, glucose, panaxin, panacic acid, panaquilin, panacen, ginsenin, sapogenin, trace minerals
EFFECTIVE QUALITIES
Primary: a bit bitter & sweet, neutral, dry
Secondary: restoring, relaxing
TROPISM: lungs, stomach, intestines, adrenals, nerves
       Air organism
       Lung, Spleen meridians
GROUND: Melancholic krasis
       Sensitive/Tai Yin Metal biotype

American Ginseng: Class 7

Functions and Uses

1. INCREASES THE QI AND REPLENISHES DEFICIENCY; ENHANCES IMMUNE POTENTIAL AND GENERATES STRENGTH, RESTORES THE LUNGS, STOMACH/*SPLEEN*, LIVER AND ADRENALS, AND AWAKENS THE APPETITE

    Qi deficiency with fatigue, weakness
    lung Qi deficiency with shallow or difficult breathing, dry cough
    ADRENAL INSUFFICIENCY
    liver & stomach Qi deficiency with slow painful digestion, no appetite
    DEBILITY due to chronic illness, childbirth, constitution

2. RESTORES AND RELAXES THE NERVE, BENEFITS THE BRAIN AND INDUCES REST

    nerve deficiency with weakness, dull thinking, unrest
    CEREBRAL ANEMIA
    heart blood & Spleen Qi deficiency with palpitations, insomnia, poor appetite
    INSOMNIA, unrest, nervous exhaustion
    RHEUMATISM, gout

3. FOSTERS THE YIN AND CLEARS DEFICIENCY HEAT

    lung Yin deficiency with low afternoon fever, voice loss
    LUNG TB in initial stages
    LUNG IRRITATION due to cold

Preparation

USE: American ginseng is best DECOCTED or TINCTURED. With occasional breaks of several days, it may be used continuously for maintenance in Qi deficiency and Yin deficiency prone individuals.

DOSAGE: standard doses throughout

Notes

With American ginseng as with other botanicals used in both Western and Chinese herbal medicine (such as Licorice, Ginger, and Cinnamon), an interesting interface between the two uses is created—and a dialogue is set up between the strictly **therapeutic** orientation of the Oriental system and the pharmacologically based Western one whether traditional or modern. This dialogue is now possible since biochemical research has at long last established a medicinal value for this root, which has been known and used therapeutically in China for three hundred years or more.

American ginseng has for many centuries been a sought after botanical. At the turn of this century, for example, Chinese sea ports received over 400,000 pounds of dried roots from the North American continent.

Outstanding in this Tartar root from the Chinese perpspective is its ability to enhance the Yin, and especially lung Yin, where deficiency heat, irritation, dry coughing, insomnia, etc. present. For this reason, American ginseng is classed among the *Yin tonics* in Chinese pharmacopoeias, unlike Chinese and Korean ginseng which are put under the *Yang tonics*. Modern investigation has in fact revealed a far higher proportion of both glycosides and adaptogens in the Oriental varieties (the Japanese ginseng excepted, which is closer to the American one) in support of this differentiation.

Although the American use of this remedy goes back to the eighteenth century, it never got beyond the status of a good domestic medicine then: in the days of the dramatics of eliminating and stimulating therapies using brisk mineral and vegetable remedies, the unobtrusively *restoring, relaxing* and *strengthening* Ginseng never had a chance. Nor did Native Americans make much use of it; Cherokees in Georgia were one of the few peoples acquainted with it (although they are said to have recognised its *tonic* qualities). Even Eclectic practitioners underestimated its importance: despite knowing about its being a "mild sedative and tonic to the nerve centers" and mainly "prescribed in the failure of digestion incident to nervous prostration and general nerve irritation," a practitioner as prominent as (ELLINGWOOD, 1898) still felt the need to add, "If combined with other tonics [it] is capable of doing some good." However, and more importantly, Eclectic physicians missed perhaps the central point of *restoring remedies* in general, namely, the treatment of the personal ground and biotype in order to correct constitutional tendencies and so to **maintain** an individual's unique *physis*. From this perspective, American ginseng is probably the best sweet-jar *tonic* to the Sensitive and the Burdened biotypes.

With its *adaptogenic* qualities, which enhance long-term immunity and reduce stress-induced damage by influencing higher nerve centers, and with its *restoring* and *adjusting* influence over gastric, hepatic and renal metabolic events (among many other things), there is not an inkling of doubt that American ginseng is one of the best *Qi tonics* in existence. From the energetic approach, its *sweet bitter* taste qualities fully substantiate this. The reluctance of Chinese medicine to recognize it as such has perhaps more than a little to do with cultural and philosophical considerations. This, however, should not deter us from using it as a *Qi tonic* above all, as we would use acupuncture points CV 6 & 12, St 36 and Bl 24 & 38.

ELECAMPANE

Pharmaceutical name: rhizoma Inulae
Botanical name: Inula helenium L. (N.O.
         Compositae)
Ancient names: Elenion (Gr)
         Enula, Helenium (Lat)
Other names: Elfwort, Elfdock, Horseheal,
         Scabwort, Horse elder (Eng)
         Grande aunée, Inule aunée, Herbe d'Hélène,
         Hélèniaire, Lionne, Oeil de cheval,
         Aillaume (Fr)
         Echter Alant, Lungenwurz, Stickwurz,
         Beinerwell, Odenkopf (Ge)
Part used: the rhizome

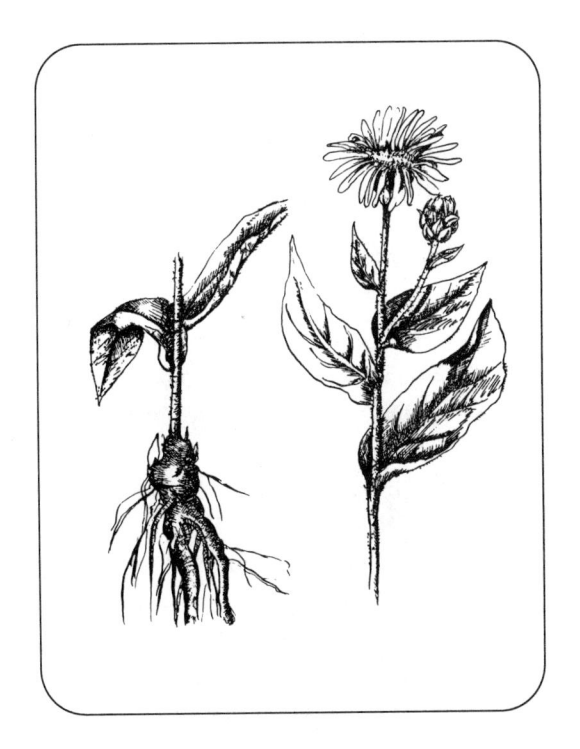

Nature

CATEGORY: mild herb with minimal chronic toxicity
CONSTITUENTS: inulin (40%), bitters, triterpenes, ess. oil helenin (incl. camphor), alkaloid, helinin, synanthrose, inulic acid, bitter resin, sodium, calcium, magnesium

Elecampane: Class 7

EFFECTIVE QUALITIES
Primary: *Taste:* a bit bitter & pungent
  Warmth: warm
  Moisture: dry
Secondary: Restoring, astringing, stimulating, decongesting
TROPISM
Organs or parts: lungs, stomach, spleen and pancreas, liver, bladder, kidneys, uterus, nerve
Organisms: Air, Water
Meridians: Lung, Spleen, Liver, Triple Heater
Tri Dosas: increases Vayu, decreases Pitta
GROUND
Krases/temperaments: Phlegmatic & Melancholic
Biotypes: Dependant/Tai Yin Earth, Self-Reliant/Yang Ming Metal & Burdened/Shao Yin
Constitutions: all three

Functions and Uses

1. INCREASES THE QI AND REPLENISHES DEFICIENCY; BENEFITS THE HYPOTHALAMUS, ENHANCES IMMUNE POTENTIAL, RESTORES THE LUNGS AND GENERATES STRENGTH

    Qi deficiency: tiredness, debility, daytime sweating; proneness to exogenous & endogenous llnesses, poor immunity
    lung Qi deficiency: shortness of breath, feeble low cough, weakness, low resistence to colds, melancholy
    heart & lung Qi deficiency: as above with palpitations worse on exertion, chronic coughing
    LOW BLOOD PRESSURE, syncope
    AUTOIMMUNE DISEASES of all kinds
    DEBILITY, EXHAUSTION physical or mental

2. STRENGTHENS AND STIMULATES THE LUNGS, OPENS THE CHEST, RELIEVES COUGHING AND EXPELS PHLEGM; EXPELS PARASITES

    lung Yin deficiency: night sweats, dry unproductive cough, emaciated appearance
    LUNG TB lung phlegm cold: full cough with coughing up white sputum
    CHRONIC BRONCHITIS, bronchial asthma

3. RESTORES THE THE *SPLEEN*/STOMACH AND PANCREAS, CREATES ASTRICTION AND DRIES MUCOUS DAMP

    Spleen Qi deficiency: loss of appetite, distended painful abdomen, diarrhea
    ANEMIA
    genitourinary damp cold: white leucorrhea, mucous cystitis
    DIABETES (supportive)
    INTESTINAL WORMS

4. STIMULATES THE LIVER AND UTERUS, DREDGES THE KIDNEYS AND CLEARS STASIS; PROMOTES URINATION AND MENSTRUATION AND EXPELS THE AFTERBIRTH

    liver Qi stagnation: tender swollen right flank, slow digestion, constipation, jaundice
    kidney Qi stagnation: unease, irritability, painful scanty urine, headache, edema

Class 7: Elecampane

uterus Qi stagnation: delayed scanty menses with clots, cramps with onset, skin rashes
ESTROGEN & PROGESTERONE INSUFFICIENCY with deficiency menstrual conditions
RETAINED LOCHIA

5 RESTRAINS INFECTION AND CLEARS TOXINS, BENEFITS THE SKIN AND RELIEVES PAIN

INFECTIONS of the LUNG, TRACHEA, KIDNEY & BLADDER, esp. chronic
NERVE INJURY, wounds, damp sores, chronic ulcers
SKIN CONDITIONS: dermatosis, eczema, rashes, cankers, atonic skin ulcers, scabies, scurf, pruritis
wind damp obstruction: acute pain from sciatica, gout, arthritis, paralysis, urination

Preparation

USE: Elecampane can be used continuously for **general maintenance** with only positive results. For this the DECOCTION is ideal. For remedial purposes, the TINCTURE is more stimulating, and will in addition bring out Elecampane's *antiseptic* quality better.
Either may be used for preparing SALVES, WASHES etc., for skin conditions including ulcers and wounds: it is also known as Scabwort. The SYRUP comes into its own with this *Lungwort* (Germany), and Elecampane WINE has for centuries been a household cordial which "cheers the heart and revives the spirits" (SALMON). An old-fashioned CANDY—Roman Empress Julia Augustas' favorite, according to PLINIUS—using Cane sugar, Cinnamon, Cloves and Nutmeg was made with this root, as later with the roots of Angelica, Eryngo, Ginger and Calamus.
DOSAGE: standard doses throughout
CAUTION: Elecampane is contraindicated in pregnancy, being a *uterine stimulant*.

Notes

When comparing the *tonics* presented in this class, it is striking that more than any other remedy, Elecampane corresponds to the Oriental ideal of a *Qi tonic*. First, it fulfills all the symptomatological requirements of such a remedy, restoring both lung and Spleen Qi, and even heart Qi besides. Secondly, this remedy is a **root** like all Chinese *Qi tonics*—an consideration from the Chinese point of view—therapeutically resembling *Dang shen, radix Codonopsis pilosulae*.

In another sense also Elecampane stands out among other herbs that increase the Qi and restore: it has been shown to beneficially affect the hypothalamus, thus creating a long-term *enhancement* of **immune potential**. Besides this, and connected with it, there is the bitter substance which stimulates the liver/stomach/Spleen as well as increasing overall strength. But Elecampane is also a *dry warm stimulant expectorant* and *emmenagogue*, useful where **cold** and **damp** have set in, causing stasis and catarrhal discharge. Being a **lung remedy** above all, and *antiseptic*, it has always been used in formulas for chronic cold lung infections, as well as lung Yin deficiency patterns, where its mucilage also helps. In the urinary area its *diuretic* effect is very certain, and the *antiseptic* property is still active.

Elecampane is clearly a remedy for **chronic deficient** conditions resulting in **Qi stagnation** of one or more internal organs, especially with symptoms of fatigue and weakness due to lung, heart and Spleen Qi deficiency. In this sense, its general *restorative* and *destagnating* action on the Qi corresponds to an acupuncture point selection such as Bl 13, 18, 20, 22 & 38, Li 13, and CV 6 & 12. Elecampane is an excellent main herb when combined with others for various deficiencies. Named after the Greek heroine Helen of Troy, *Helenium* in modern times yet awaits the true clinical usage for which it was designed.

Sage: Class 7

SAGE

Pharmaceutical name: folium Salviae
Botanical name: Salvia officinalis L.
 (N.O.Labiatae)
Ancient names: Elelisphagon (Gr)
  Lilifagus, Elbium, Lingua humana, Salvia
   salvatrix (Lat)
Other names: Red sage, Garden sage, Save (Eng)
  Sauge, Thé de France/de Grèce, Herbe
   sacrée (Fr)
  Salbei, Edel-Salbei, Garten-Salbei, Scharlei,
   Sachsedenkraut (Ge)
Part used: the leaf

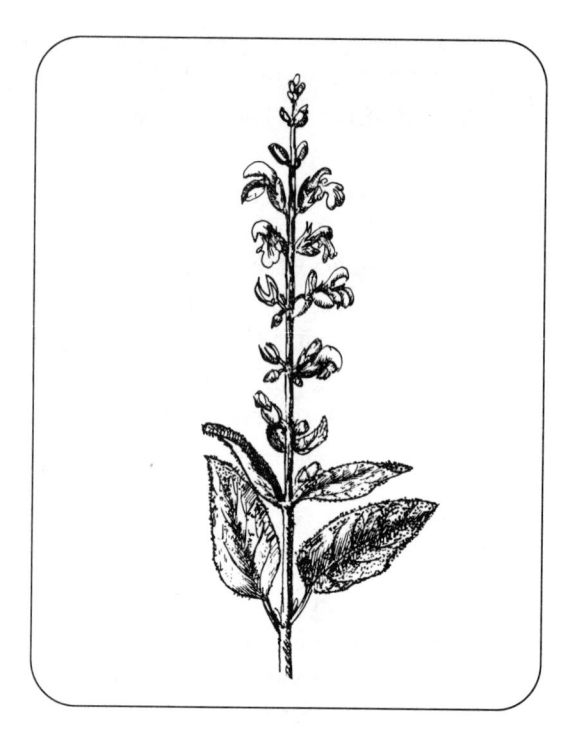

Nature

CATEGORY: medium-strength herb with some chronic toxicity
CONSTITUENTS: ess. oil (incl. thujone, borneol, salviol, cineol, salvene), saponins, tannins, flavonoids, bitter, resin, estrogenic substances, glycoside, calcium oxalate, phosphoric acid salts
EFFECTIVE QUALITIES
Primary: *Taste:* a bit pungent & bitter & astringent
   Warmth: cool
   Moisture: dry
Secondary: astringing, solidifying, restoring, relaxing
   stabilizing movement
TROPISM
Organs or parts: stomach, intestines, lungs, uterus, brain, nerve, pituitary, fluids
Organisms: Air, Fluid
Meridians: Spleen, Lung, Chong & Ren
Tri Dosas: decreases Kapha, regulates Vayu
GROUND
Krases/temperaments: Phlegmatic & Melancholic
Biotypes: Dependant/Tai Yin Earth & Self-Reliant/Yang Ming Metal
  Sensitive/Tai Yin Metal
Constitutions: Lymphatic/Carbonic/Blue Iris & Mixed/Phosphoric/Grey-Green Iris

Functions and Uses

1. INCREASES THE QI AND REPLENISHES DEFICIENCY: ENHANCES IMMUNE POTENTIAL, RESTORES THE PITUITARY, NERVE, LUNGS, INTESTINES AND STOMACH, AND GENERATES STRENGTH

   Qi deficiency: exhaustion, excessive daytime sweating, shortness of breath
   Spleen Qi deficiency: no appetite, indigestion, diarrhea

Class 7: Sage

    nerve & brain deficiency: vertigo, nervous exhaustion, poor memory, coma, paralysis
GENERAL IMMUNE DEFICIENCY, autoimmune disease
PITUITARY INSUFFICIENCY or imbalance
LOW BLOOD PRESSURE
CHRONIC DEBILITY due to constitution or overwork, during convalescence, etc.
LUNG TB with night sweats, debility, tidal fever
RICKETS

2. **CREATES ASTRICTION, RESOLVES MUCUS AND DRIES DAMP; ARRESTS DISCHARGE AND RESTRAINS SECRETIONS**

    Spleen Yang deficiency with *intestines damp cold:* chilliness, loose mucousy stools, fatigue
    CHRONIC ENTERITIS, mucous colitis
    intestines mucous damp (Spleen damp): loose mucousy stool alternating with hard distended gurgling abdomen
    genitourinary damp cold: white leucorrhea, urethrtis, scanty urination
    head damp cold: nasal and sinus cogestion, watery discharge
    EXCESSIVE PERSPIRATION in any condition, esp. from hands and armpits
    BREAST MILK: for weaning

3. **STIMULATES THE LUNGS, EXPELS VISCOUS PHLEGM AND RELIEVES WHEEZING**

    lung phlegm damp: asthmatic breathing, full cough with thin white phlegm
    CHRONIC BRONCHITIS, bronchial asthma

4. **CIRCULATES THE QI AND LOOSENS CONSTRAINT: RELAXES THE NERVE, STOPS SPASMS AND CALMS WIND**

    Qi constraint with deficiency:
    intestines Qi constraint: abdominal cramps and flatulence worse with eating or emotional tension
    kidney Qi constraint: nervous restlessness, agitated depression, abdominal cramps, lumbar pain
    uterus Qi constraint: irregular, painful menses
    kidney wind (internal wind): tremors, shaking or cramping up of limbs, stroke

5. **RESTORES THE UTERUS AND RETURNS THE MENSES; PROMOTES ESTROGEN AND HARMONIZES THE MENOPAUSE; PROMOTES CONTRACTIONS AND LABOR**

    uterus blood deficiency: delayed, scanty or no menstruation with cramps, dry skin or dry vagina
    ESTROGEN INSUFFICIENCY and resultant scanty menses
    AMENORRHEA, INFERTILITY, sterility
    MENOPAUSAL SYNDROME
    PROPHYLACTIC & REMEDIAL for labor

6. **ACTIVATES IMMUNITY AND RESTRAINS INFECTION; PROMOTES TISSUE REPAIR AND BENEFITS THE SKIN**

    PREVENTIVE in epidemics
    CHRONIC WOUNDS, ulcers, sores, abscesses

Sage: Class 7

    INFECTIONS of mouth, throat, gums, incl. stomatitis, tonsilitis, thrush
    MOUTH ULCERS, loose teeth
    INSECT BITES & STINGS
    SKIN CONDITIONS: eczema, scrofula, hairloss
    SORE MUSCLES, toothache

Preparation

USE: The daily strong INFUSION of Sage leaves (keeping the tea covered with a lid in Chinese fashion) is the simplest preparation for health maintenance, Sage being an outstanding *Qi tonic* and *immune enhancer.*

However, if, as RICHARD BREUSS recommends, the tea is simmered or infused a few minutes without a lid, Sage's *disinfectant* and some other qualities diminish as its essential oil content evaporates in steam. The trade-off, however, is that a ferment essential to the glands, intervertebral discs and bone marrow is supposedly released. Certainly, Sage's *astringent* properties are also thereby enhanced. (The longer preparation time pushes out the tannins.)

Still, the essential oil is very much part of Sage's active properties, especially its *nerve relaxing, disinfectant* and *mucolytic* ones, and it is retained in its entirety if the lid is kept on while the INFUSION is sitting. The ESSENTIAL OIL itself comes into its own with external WASHES, LINIMENTS, SQUATTING INHALATIONS, DOUCHES, PESSARIES, and for GARGLING (combine with a more tannic herb such as Tormentil, Selfheal or Lady's Mantle). The less effective TINCTURE is nevertheless still very viable in all respects.

DOSAGE: INFUSION: 20 g or 2/3 oz to 1/2 l or 1 pint of water, drunk in three doses over a day
                 TINCTURE: 1-3 ml or 25-75 drops
                 ESSENTIAL OIL: 2-4 drops twice daily

CAUTION: Since being a *uterine stimulant* and *dry astringent,* Sage is contraindicated during pregnancy and nursing. If the ESSENTIAL OIL is used, as it safely can be on a daily basis with intermittent small breaks of a few days (SCHNAUBELT, 1985), the dosage must not be exceeded, because the essential oil contains the ketone thujone.

Sage's thujone content also makes it forbidden to those prone to epileptic fits.

Notes

The very name of this plant, derived from the Latin word *salvus,* meaning well-being, indicates the unsurpassed esteem which Sage enjoyed at the time of ecclesiastical European medicine. It figures in the opening verses of Abbot WALAFRIED STRABO's twelfth century work on botanical remedies, for example, and there are many reports that Sage was a main ingredient in longevity prescriptions and elixirs of life that were routinely concoted throughout the Middle Ages —exactly as was wild Ginseng from the Korean mountains in the days of the Chinese Empire. The medical verses of the eleventh century Salerno medical college cryptically state that the *supertonic* effects of Sage are only limited by death itself. Much later(1532), humanist herbalist HIERONYMUS BOCK praises it even higher than his beloved Nettle; and in 1688 a 414 page book comprehensively covering all known aspects of Sage appeared under the pen of the Danish physician CHRISTIAN PAULLINI.

Today we know that Sage, through the powerful action of the essential oils found mainly in its leaf, directly *tonifies* the pituitary, the gonads and non-specific immunity (DURRAFOURD et al, 1982). But what more evidence do we need, apart from that of our own experience, that this plant does indeed possess long-lasting *restorative* effects that reach deeply into the penetralia of the human being, the higher endocrine and nerve centers ?

The energetics of Sage are mainly *dry* and *astringent,* with strong *Kapha reducing* and some *Vayu stimulating* effects, to use the Ayurvedic idiom. In addition to treating deficiencies of the Qi and the nervous system as *nerve* and *Qi tonic* rolled into one, it *mucolytically* resolves and expels unwanted phlegm through all possible channels. But Sage is a *restorer* to the mucous membrane as well—in this sense a *Spleen tonic* in Chinese medicine, like its similars *Bai shu, rhizoma Atractylodis albae,* and *Cang shu, rhizoma Atractylodis*—going for deep, systemic tonification here as elsewhere. Body and tissue strength is increased by its *astringent* effects, which in practice overlap with fairly strong *antiseptic* and *vulnerary* properties where infections, especially respiratory ones, and injuries are concerned.

Sage's effect of *restraining excessive sweating,* which should be used clinically in deficient Qi and deficient Yin patterns, is well documented. However, more accurately we can say it has a regulating effect on the sweat glands, since Sage also *induces sweat* where the skin has stopped breathing—and is *diaphoretic* if drunk hot. All glands, in fact, are affected by Sage.

Nor should Sage be forgotten as a **gynecological** remedy, not only being an *antispasmodic* for irregular, painful menstruation and a uterine *oxytocic* remedy facilitating labor contractions when hypertonic, but also, paradoxically, an *estrogenic uterine blood tonic* and, like Savory, a possible cure for infertility and sterility due to pituitary/gonadic disharmony.

THYME

Pharmaceutical name: herba Thymi
Botanical name: Thymus vulgaris L. (N.O. Labiatae)
Ancient names: Thymon (Gr)
　　　Serpillium hortense (Lat)
Other names: Garden thyme (Eng)
　　　Thym (Fr)
　　　Thymian, Römischer/Welscher Quendel,
　　　　Immenkraut, Demut, Kuddelkraut, Zimis,
　　　　Jungfernzucht (Ge)
Part used: the herb

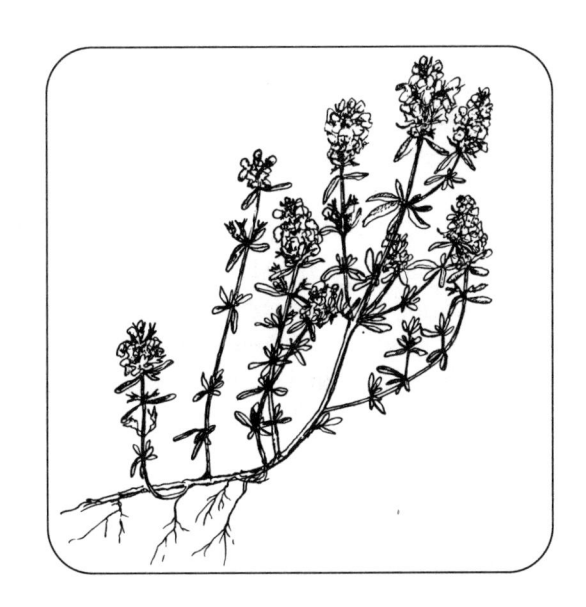

Nature

CATEGORY: mild herb with minimal chronic toxicity
CONSTITUENTS: ess. oil min.1% (incl. terpenoid phenol thymol & isomer carvacrol up to 60%, cymol, linalool, borneol, pinene), bitter, tannin 10%, flavonoids, triterpenoids, saponins, resins
EFFECTIVE QUALITIES
Primary: a bit pungent & bitter & astringent, warm, dry
Secondary: restoring, astringing, stimulating
TROPISM: lungs, stomach, intestines, uterus, nerves, adrenals
　　　Air, Warmth organisms
　　　Lung, Spleen meridians
GROUND: Melancholic & Phlegmatic krases
　　　Sensitive/Tai Yin Metal & Dependant/Tai Yin Earth biotypes
　　　Lymphatic/Carbonic/Blue Iris constitution

Thyme: Class 7

Functions and Uses

1. **INCREASES THE QI AND REPLENISHES DEFICIENCY: ENHANCES IMMUNE POTENTIAL, RESTORES THE LUNGS, NERVE AND ADRENALS AND GENERATES STRENGTH**

   Qi deficiency: fatigue, shallow breathing, pale complexion
   lung Qi deficiency: shortness of breath, low resistance to infections
   Spleen Qi deficiency: no appetite, loose stool, abdominal distension
   ANEMIA, low blood pressure
   nerve deficiency: weakness, nervous exhaustion, depression
   ADRENAL INSUFFICIENCY

2. **STIMULATES AND WARMS THE LUNGS, LIQUIFIES AND EXPELS VISCOUS PHLEGM AND RELIEVES COUGHING; RELAXES THE BRONCHI AND RELIEVES WHEEZING**

   lung phlegm cold: full productive cough with thin white phlegm, wheezing
   lung & Kidney Yang deficiency: chilliness, exhaustion, wheezing
   CHRONIC BRONCHITIS, emphysema, lung TB
   lung dry phlegm: dry, difficult cough, difficult breathing, coughing up plugs of phlegm
   lung Qi constraint: irritating, spasmodic dry cough, severe wheezing, obsessive thinking
   SPASMODIC & ALLERGIC ASTHMA
   WHOOPING COUGH

3. **CAUSES SWEATING, RELEASES THE EXTERIOR AND SCATTERS WIND COLD; CLEARS THE HEAD AND RELIEVES PAIN**

   external wind cold: onset of infections with stiff muscles, aches and pains, chills, fatigue
   head damp cold & lung wind cold: watery nasal discharge, congested sinuses, sore throat
   wind/damp obstruction: with acute neuralgia, rheumatism

4. **WARMS AND INVIGORATES THE STOMACH AND INTESTINES/*SPLEEN* AND REMOVES STAGNANCY; STIMULATES THE UTERUS AND PROMOTES THE MENSES**

   Spleen Yang deficiency with intestines damp cold: chilliness, watery stool with undigested food, colic, flatulence
   intestines mucous damp (Spleen damp): nausea, slow digestion, gurgling abdomen
   INTESTINAL FERMENTATION, enteritis, mucous colitis
   uterus damp cold: no or delayed menstruation, cramps, white leucorrhea
   LACK OF SEXUAL DESIRE

5. **ACTIVATES IMMUNITY, RESTRAINS INFECTION, ANTIDOTES POISON AND CLEARS PARASITES; PROMOTES TISSUE REPAIR AND RESOLVES CLOTTING**

   PREVENTIVE IN EPIDEMICS (low white blood cell count)
   VIRAL, FUNGAL & BACTERIAL INFECTIONS of all kinds, esp. of sinuses, mouth, throat, lung, urinary, intestines & skin, incl. candidiasis, tonsilitis, pyelitis, typhus, mycosis, etc.
   SKIN INFECTION & IRRITATION, incl. psoriasis, scrofula, dermatosis
   INFECTED, PUSSY WOUNDS, contusions
   INTESTINAL PARASITES of all types, esp. tapeworm

Class 7: Thyme

POISONOUS ANIMAL BITES
ANESTHETIC
HAIR LOSS

Preparation

USE: As a first class *Qi tonic* Thyme may be taken extensively for maintenance and prevention, the best way being a daily INFUSION of the herb, on its own or with other herbs such as Camomile and Orange flowers. On the other hand, when it comes to remedial uses, the ESSENTIAL OIL wins out by far since it makes up at least three quarters of Thyme's properties (but see caution below). The TINCTURE is less *antiseptic, warming* and *immune-stimulant,* and more *astringent* than the ESSENTIAL OIL.

Whatever preparation is chosen, it is certain that a variety of uses are open to us: MOUTHWASHES, GARGLES, DOUCHES, INHALATIONS for both **upper** and **lower mucous membrane infections,** with or without discharge. SALMON (1710) recommends a SNUFF which "purges the head of pituitous humours". The MOUTHWASH is a stronger mouth, gum and tooth *anesthetic* than Clove. BODY BATHS may be taken in **debile** or **arthritic**, gouty conditions (also with the addition of Lavender and Rosemary essential oil). **Skin** conditions can be treated with OINTMENTS, LOTIONS and the like; **lung infections** with a warm COMPRESS or with the SALVE. Acute **neuralgias** and **pain** will benefit from a LINIMENT (e.g. with Eucalyptus, Marjoram or Black pepper). Finally, since Thyme is one of the main remedies for all lung complaints, Thyme SYRUP can play an important part in therapy.

DOSAGE: ESSENTIAL OIL: 2-5 drops in a gelatin capsule with some olive oil
              Others: standard doses

CAUTION: Thyme is forbidden during pregnancy, being a *uterine stimulant,* and with hyperthyroid conditions.

Due to its skin and mucous membrane irritating nature, the ESSENTIAL OIL should be taken in a gelatin capsule and only used on the skin for the conditions specified above.

Notes

Like Rosemary, Sage, Marjoram and several others, Thyme is yet another remedy from the Mint family kitchen herb department whose seemingly dowdy and mundane potential only blossoms when the essential oil itself is used: when extracted by distillation or by alcoholic tincture, the nice common garden Thyme becomes transformed into a superior *Qi tonic* with *adrenal stimulant* and *immune potential enhancing* properties.

Thyme's *warm, dry, bitter* and *pungent* energetic qualities make it ideally suited to most cases of Qi and Yang deficiencies of both lung and Spleen. **Cold** and **damp** are removed from the entire **digestive** and **respiratory** organs, while the underlying **deficiency** is replenished. Thyme's deeply *restoring* and *stimulating* action is enhanced on one hand by *astriction* as damp symptoms go, with *tonic anticatarrhal* effects along the mucosa, and on the other hand by *spasmolytic* effects on cramping or spasmodic symptoms. In the bronchial area a *relaxant* affect is especially evident in addition to a *secretolytic stimulant expectorant* action, elevating the humble garden Thyme to the ranks of the finest herbs for the lungs. By combining it with more specifically and narrowly-acting plants to reinforce one or other of its actions, a greater therapeutic effect may be achieved in severe cases—not that Thyme actually needs reinforcing in most simple conditions.

Clearly, in terms of its overall *expectorant* and *lung tonic* properties, Thyme resembles *Jie geng, radix Platycodi,* from the Oriental pharmacopoeia, while its *mucolytic* and *diaphoretic* effects addressing wind cold afflicting the head and lungs, as well as damp cold in the intestines, call to

Cardamom: Class 7

mind *Zi su ye, folium Perillae acutae,* also known as Chiso leaf. Thyme is thus able to treat the whole range of external wind/cold conditions, from the most superficial and uppermost beginning in the sinuses, to the most internal and lowest ending up in the bronchioles—again, quite a broad spectrum for such a modest plant. In the acupuncture idiom, it runs the gamut of points from Lu 5 through Lu 9, depending on how it is used, and definitely has a Bl 13, Bl 20 and Bl 38 kind of push about it.

As *anti-infective* and *antiseptic* botanical for treating bacterial, viral and fungal infections of a large variety, when used in essential oil form, Thyme has consistently proved itself as one of the strongest essential oils known, with Spanish thyme in the lead above the French.

CARDAMOM

Pharmaceutical name: fructus Elettariae
Botanical name: Elettaria cardamomum L. (N.O. Zingiberaceae)
Ancient names: Kardamomon (Gr)
    Grana paradisi (Lat)
Other names: Grains of paradise (Eng)
    Kardamomlein, Pariskörner (Ge)
Part used: the fruit

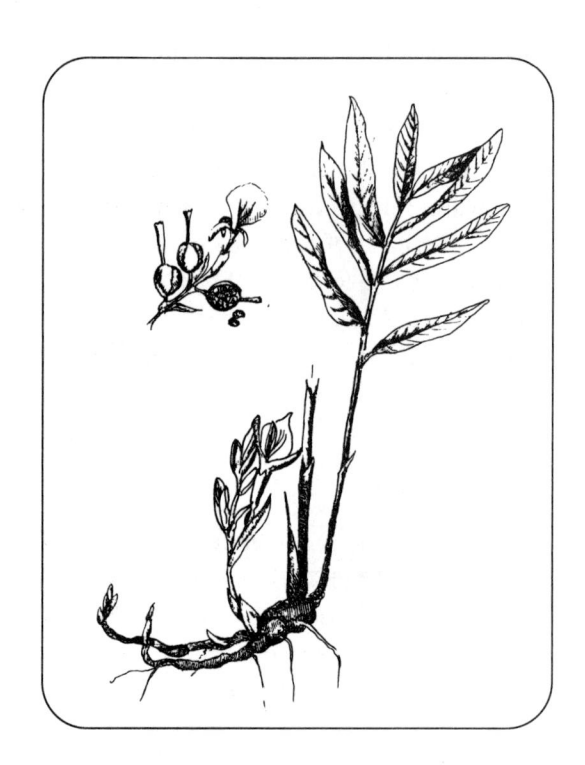

Nature

CATEGORY: mild herb with minimal chronic toxicity
CONSTITUENTS: ess. oil 3-8% (incl. terpenes & terpineol, cineol, limonenes, borneols, sabines), manganese, iron
EFFECTIVE QUALITIES
Primary: pungent, a bit bitter & sweet, warm, dry
Secondary: restoring, stimulating, relaxing
TROPISM: lungs, stomach, intestines, nervous system, brain
    Warmth, Air organisms
    Lung, Spleen meridians
GROUND: Melancholic & Phlegmatic krases
    Sensitive/Tai Yin Metal & Dependant/Tai Yin Earth biotypes
    Lymphatic/Carbonic/Blue Iris constitution

Functions and Uses

1   INCREASES THE QI AND REPLENISHES DEFICIENCY; RESTORES THE LUNGS, *SPLEEN* AND NERVE AND GENERATES STRENGTH; LIFTS THE SPIRIT AND RIDS DEPRESSION

Class 7: Cardamom

Qi deficiency with fatigue, mental depression or stupor
Spleen Qi deficiency with loose stool, no appetite
lung Qi Deficiency with shallow breathing, fatigue
nerve deficiency with dizziness, poor memory, listlessness
NERVOUS EXHAUSTION or DEPRESSION in deficiency conditions

2 WARMS AND INVIGORATES THE STOMACH AND INTESTINES; FREES SPASMS AND DRIES MUCOUS DAMP; AWAKENS THE APPETITE, SETTLES THE STOMACH AND QUELLS VOMITING

intestines mucous damp (Spleen damp) with gurgling abdomen, epigastric pain & distention
NAUSEA & VOMITING due to *stomach Qi reflux* or *stomach cold*

3 STIMULATES THE LUNGS, EXPELS PHLEGM AND CLEARS THE HEAD

lung phlegm damp with coughing up copious white phlegm
CHRONIC BRONCHITIS
head damp cold with nasal & sinus congestion

4 ANTIDOTES POISON AND RESOLVES CONTUSION
POISONOUS STINGS
CONTUSIONS, bruises, sprains, paralysis

Preparation

USE: The most effective way to use Cardamom for the above range of effects is in ESSENTIAL OIL form. It may be combined with a carrier oil and massaged into the skin externally, or taken internally. An INFUSION of the **crushed fruits**, or a TINCTURE are only fair alternatives.
DOSAGE: ESSENTIAL OIL: 2-5 drops in a little warm water
               Others: standard doses

Notes

Cardamom is one of the most esteemed essential oil bearing spices used in Ayurvedic medicine and is also known in Chinese medicine as *Bai dou kou*. Greek physicians were not slow in picking up on its use, as fourth century B.C. records of importation of this fruit from India show. Its status as the "chief of all seeds" (WILLIAM COLE) is underlined by Renaissance herbalists, who insisted on getting to authentic, original sources of information.

Cardamom has *warm, pungent bitter sweet* energetics which qualify *restoring* and *stimulating* properties. In light of its restoring effect on the Qi, lungs and Spleen, and the nerve in the Western sense, Cardamom definitely secures itself a place among the Qi tonics—all the more so when its essential oil is used. In this context Cardamom has an effect on the spirit or mind similar to Basil, removing the listless gloom often found in chronic Qi deficiency syndromes, similarly to acupuncture points Bl 15, P 4 and GV 20.

All this distinguishes Cardamom from other spicy fruits such as Coriander and Fennel. However, in the absence of these effects, it would still be a fine *digestive stimulant* and *mucolytic* remedy for damp catarrhal conditions of the respiratory and digestive tract, for Spleen damp in other words. As the Oxford dean WILLIAM COLE put it in typical seventeenth century Galenic language: "it draweth forth flegmatick humours both from head and stomach."

Arnica: Class 7
Herbs to Restore, Strengthen and Support the Heart, Harmonize the Circulation, Lift the Spirit and Rid Depression

ARNICA

Pharmaceutical name: flos Arnicae
Botanicals name: Arnica montana L., vel A. cordifolia L. (N.O. Compositae)
Ancient names: Alisma/Caltha alpina (Lat)
   Engel Trank (Old Ge)
Other names: Leopard's bane, Wolfsbane, Mountain tobacco (Eng)
   Arnica, Tabac des Vosges, Herbe aux chutes, Souci des alpes, Bétoine des montagnes (Fr)
   Arnika, Bergwohlverleih, Waldblume, Donnerblume, Wolfsblume, Wolfstöterin (Ge)
Part used: the flower; also the whole plant, *planta tota Arnicae*

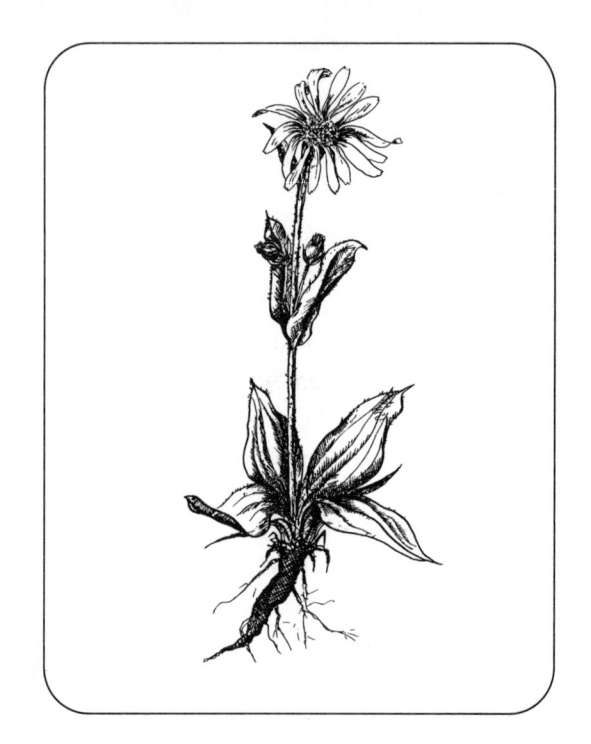

Nature

CATEGORY: medium-strength herb with some chronic toxicity
CONSTITUENTS: ess. oil (incl. two triterpenoid alcohols arnidiol & faradiol, thymol esters, sesquiterpene arnicolide), flavonoid heterosides kempferol & quercetol, malic & tannic acid, arnicin, bitter, sesquiterpene lactones (incl. autumnolide, helenanin), astragalin, isoquercitrin, adrenal-like substance, cardioactive substance, volatile alkaloid, silicic acid, luteolin, phulin, tannin, cholin, inulin, resins, potassium, calcium
EFFECTIVE QUALITIES
Primary: *Taste:* a bit sweet & bitter & pungent
   Warmth: neutral with a secondary cooling effect
   Moisture: neutral
Secondary: restoring, relaxing, simulating
TROPISM
Organs or parts: medulla and spinal cord, nerves, heart, lungs
Organisms: Warmth, Air
Meridians: Heart, Pericardium
Tri Dosas: increases Vayu, decreases Pitta & Kapha
GROUND
Krases/temperaments: all
Biotypes: all
Constitutions: all

Class 7: Arnica

Functions and Uses

1. **STIMULATES THE HEART, CIRCULATION AND LUNGS; RELIEVES BLOOD CONGESTION AND FREES SPASMS, OPENS THE CHEST AND RELIEVES WHEEZING**

    heart Yang deficiency: chilliness, cold limbs, purple lips, scanty urine, weak breathing, depression, anemia

    heart blood deficiency: stabbing ccardiac pain, chest discomfort, palpitations, fatigue

    heart Qi constraint: anxiety, worry, nervousness, unrest, palpitations

    HIGH BLOOD PRESSURE, angina pectoris

    CORONARY HEART DISEASE, arterial spasms, arteriosclerosis

    SUPPORTIVE in *heart Qi deficiency* in typhoid & other infections, and in old age

    WHEEZING

2. **RESTORES THE NERVE AND BRAIN, LIFTS THE SPIRIT AND RIDS DEPRESSION**

    nerve deficiency: slow response, mental dullness, fatigue, local numbness or paralysis

    PARAPLEGIA, hemiplegia after acute stage, poliomyelitis, medullary degeneration

    COMA & COLLAPSE of the Yin type, incl. hyperglycemic coma

    GENERAL DEBILITY and NERVOUS DEPRESSION, esp. due to chronic illness

3. **RESOLVES FEVER, CLEARS DEFICIENCY HEAT AND CALMS THE SPIRIT**

    LOW TIDAL FEVERS in Shao Yin stage

    Yin deficiency: low afternoon fever, night sweats, insomnia, irritability, restlessness

    AGITATION in any condition

4. **PROMOTES TISSUE REPAIR AND ACTIVATES IMMUNITY; REDUCES INFLAMMATION, SWELLING AND CONTUSION, RELIEVES PAIN**

    TRAUMATIC INJURIES with unbroken skin: contusions, bruises, atomic messy wounds, sprains, pulled sinews, chilblains

    SURFACE INFLAMMATIONS incl. skin, vein and joint inflammation, neuritis

    fire toxin with flat boils, abscesses, furuncles, low fever

    CHRONIC THROAT & larynx infections with pain, hoarseness or catarrh, in deficiency conditions

    MUSHROOM POISONING

    SORE MUSCLES due to strain, labou, surgery, rheumatism

    BACKACHE, headache, any aches or pains

    HAIR LOSS

Preparation

USE: Externally, both the INFUSION and TINCTURE give equally good results, being used mainly in SWABS and WASHES. It is important to use Arnica only on an unbroken skin surface and not to cover or bandage up the injured or inflamed surface after application, since for best results evaporation should occur. Repeated applications are also usually neccessary. Arnica OINTMENT is often sufficient, however.

Arnica may be used internally if dosages are followed to the letter. With traumatic injury or shock, the person should sip the tea until the complexion and pulse return to normal and then stop (until later use, if required).

Arnica: Class 7

Excellent GARGLES and DOUCHES can be made for chronic and catarrhal conditions (one of the best sore throat and hoarseness herbs). Arnica is also available homeopathically prepared.

DOSAGE: INFUSION of the **dried, chopped flowers**:
- **internal use**: 1/2-1 tsp
- **external use**: 2 tsp

DECOCTION of the **whole plant**:
- **internal use**: 2-5 g to 2 cups of water for three doses
- **external use**: the same or slightly more

TINCTURE of the **flowerheads**:
- **internal use**: start with 10 drops three times a day; all being well graduate to a maximum of 40 drops four days later
- **external use**: 30-60 drops (or 1/4-1/2 tsp) in 1/2 cu of water (i.e. 1 part tincture to 6 parts water)

CAUTION: Having some toxicity, Arnica should be used with care if taken internally, and the dosage never exceeded. In addition, some people are naturally sensitive to this plant, while others are not: therefore reactions (even with external use) should be watched for. Negative reactions may include dizziness, nervous twitches or trembling, gastric irritation, edema and skin rashes or other allergic reactions.

Notes

Life in the European Alps is intimately connected with Arnica, where it has represented the main (and sometimes only) wound and injury remedy for thousands of years. In this setting it has served not only to heal wounds, but also to check bleeding, to allay neuralgic and muscular pains (especially due to damp), to abort the onset of colds and flus (as does Echinacea) and to relieve venous congestion including varicosis. It was additionally used for cerebral or spinal concussion, colic, blood poisoning and, last but not least, for threatened miscarriage and for postpartum conditions when the local wise woman, witch or wildcrafter was not within reach to dispense her stronger, more certain remedies. The unofficial Arnica symptomatology! Here we have an example of the many uses that an herb may be put to if needed.

Native American medicine has in all probability used Arnica for an equally long time. And today we can say that both European and American species are virtually identical in their makeup and uses. Passing on, however, from the universal use of this superlative *vulnerary,* we will see that Arnica has much more to offer, both as a simple and in combination with other botanicals.

Clearing heat in the sense of both **deficiency heat** and **fire toxin** is one of its strengths. In Yin deficiency syndromes with either low fever or hot flushes, it matches up well with the likes of Hawthorn, Rehmannia, Mistletoe and Valerian (all *cardiac tonics,* too). Then Arnica is both nerve and cardiac tonic, like Cereus and Lily of the valley, as also a depression ridder (*antidepressant*). Here silicic acid as light bearing bioenergy plays into the minerals, producing a remedy that restores the light vehicle, the nervous system. As *nerve restorative*, Arnica should again be supported with similar herbs for a balanced effect on the overall condition. Elderly people and the chronically ill usually stand to benefit the most here.

Finally, it is as a **heart remedy** that Arnica's deep secrets are revealed. Here it displays astonishing *stimulating, decongesting* and *relaxing* properties which have been qualified as positively "Napoleonic". The heart is both stimulated in deficient conditions and relieved in excess ones, depending on the case presented. In short, the vital spirits housed in the heart are regulated and given a new lease of life. The essential oils and cardioactive substances thought responsible for these effects are merely the artifacts of the bioenergies involved: the latter translate the original blueprint of Arnica as a **spiritual idea** into its final design as a **material actuality**; they embody the forces that go into its creation. Arnica's bioenergies have always been likened to the forces of the sun itself, in the same way that the vital spirits are the sun forces of the whole organism.

Small wonder that GOETHE, as depicted by WILHELM PELIKAN, waxes lyrical, nay spiritually enkindled, after a stiff draught of Arnica tea, and consecrates this plant to the sun god Helios.

HAWTHORN

Pharmaceutical name: fructus seu flos Crataegi
Botanical name: Crataegus oxyacantha L. (N.O. Rosaceae)
Ancient names: Arbustus, Spina alba, Ornus, Sorbus aculeata (Lat)
Other names: Hedgethorn, Maybush, Whitethorn, Red Haw, Hogberry Wickens, Quickset, Bread and cheese, Aggles (Eng)
Aubépine, Epine blanche, Pain d'oiseau, Hague de cochon (Fr)
Weissdorn, Hagendorn, Dornstrauch, Hühnerbeere, Mehlbeerstaude, Vogelbeer (Ge)
Part used: the berry or the blossom

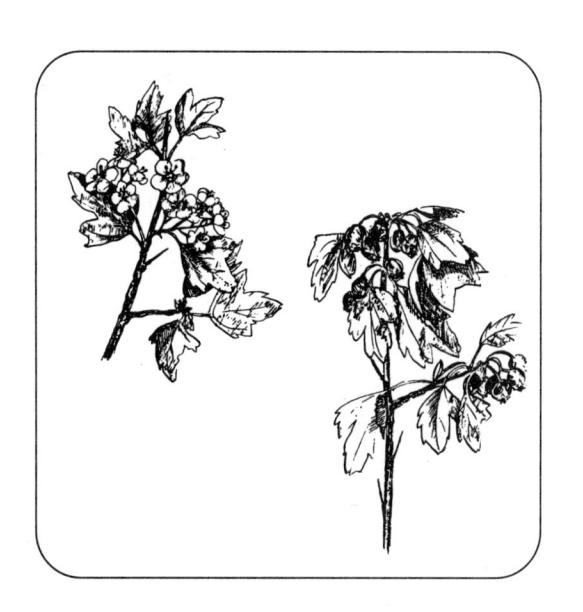

Nature

CATEGORY: mild herb with minimal chronic toxicity
CONSTITUENTS: flavonoid glycosides (hyperoside & vitexin-rhamnoside), oxyacanthin, saponins, procyanidins, trimethylamin, ursolic and oleanolic acids (crataegus lactones), condensed tannins, flavones (quercitrin, quercetin), ß-sitosterin, pectin, aluminium, calcium, phosphoric acid
EFFECTIVE QUALITIES
Primary: *Taste:* a bit sweet & bitter & astringent
Warmth: a bit cool
Moisture: dry
Secondary: nourishing, restoring, calming, astringing, softening, dissolving
TROPISM
Organs or parts: heart, arteries, intestines, blood, nerve
Organisms: Warmth, Fluid
Meridians: Pericardium, Heart, Small Intestine, Kidney
Tri Dosas: increases Vayu, decreases Pita & Kapha
GROUND
Krases/temperaments: Sanguine & Choleric
Biotypes: Charming/Yang Ming Earth & Industrious/Tai Yang
Constitutions: all three

Hawthorn: Class 7

Functions and Uses

1. **STRENGTHENS AND RESTORES THE HEART, BALANCES AND HARMONIZES THE CIRCULATION**

    heart Qi deficiency: fatigue, difficult breathing, palpitations, chest oppression, spontaneous sweating
    ORGANIC DEGENERATIVE HEART DISEASE of all kinds
    CIRCULATORY, esp. arterial conditions in general
    HIGH or LOW BLOOD PRESSURE
    MYOCARDIAL WEAKNESS following infections, e.g. pneumonia, influenza, scarlet fever, diptheria
    MYO/ENDO/PERICARDITIS, valvular insufficiency
    AFTERTREATMENT of myocardial infarct

2. **TONIFIES THE YIN AND CLEARS DEFICIENCY HEAT; SUPPORTS AND STABILIZES THE HEART AND CALMS THE SPIRIT**

    Yin deficiency: flushed feeling in palms, soles and sternum, night sweats, physical and mental restlessness
    Kidney & heart Yin deficiency: palpitations, insomnia, anxiety, paranoia, feverishness
    GLOBAL PARASYMPATHETIC INHIBITION with passive vasodilation
    HIGH BLOOD PRESSURE, DIABETES in children, menopausal syndrome

3. **STIMULATES THE HEART, PROMOTES URINATION AND RELIEVES CONGESTION; SOFTENS DEPOSITS AND CAUSES WEIGHT LOSS**

    heart blood congestion: stabbing cardiac pain radiating down left inner arm, shortness of breath, cyanosed lips, face & nails
    ANGINA PECTORIS, CORONARY SCLEROSIS or thrombosis
    heart fluid congestion: fatigue, nausea or vomiting, general muscular weakness, peripheral or central edema
    TACHYCARDIA, ARRHYTHMIA
    HARD DEPOSITS: arteriosclerosis, gallstones, urinary sand & stones
    ADIPOSITY, general plethora

4. **REMOVES STAGNANCY AND RELIEVES DISTENSION; CREATES ASTRICTION AND ARRESTS DISCHARGE**

    INTESTINAL STAGNATION due to *intestines mucous damp or intestines Qi stagnation,* with painful distension
    heart blood & Spleen Qi deficiency: loose stools, no appetite, insomnia, restlessness
    DIARRHEA, LEUCORRHEA

Preparation

USE: The optimum medication, here as with the majority of mild remedies whose herb, leaves or berries we use, is the fresh JUICE made from ripe Hawthorn berries. The FREEZE-DRIED EXTRACT comes a close second, and the short DECOCTION (10 minutes) or TINCTURE of the **berry**, or the INFUSION or TINCTURE of the **blossom** are not poor substitutes. All apply to the spectrum of uses outlined above.

Functional heart disorders register a more rapid influence of this herb than do organic ones: for these, as for systemic parasympathetic nerve inhibition, a course of upwards of 2 months is recommended. Of course, even simple cases of empty heat will not be cured in a week! In any event, the wholly positive effect of **continuous** taking of Crataegus is grounded in the complete absence of any accumulative toxic activity or dependence.

DOSAGE: Standard doses are used throughout. It is possible that **smaller** doses are more effective than larger ones in cardiac syndromes. However, **larger** doses are needed for causing astriction and for food stagnation (function 4).

Notes

Hawthorn berry is an outstanding example of a remedy that has very different uses in the West and in the Orient. This demonstrates clearly how the basic assumptions about the nature of herbal medicines and their preparation forms go to shape the very uses that an herb is put to. In the West the plant parts **above ground** are valued as much as those **below;** while in China the bulk of remedies consists of **roots**. The medicinal parts of the lovely Hawthorn tree being its flowers and fruits, in China this remedy automatically is disqualified from the class of serious remedies, let alone the *tonics*. Hence Hawthorn finds a niche among botanicals that relieve food stagnation (a use that Western herbalism has yet to appreciate). In the West on the other hand, all parts of plants have been found to exhibit *restorative* effects: it is precisely as a *tonic* that Hawthorn is valued, to the confutation of deep running Chinese beliefs.

The origins of using Hawthorn as a heart remedy are lost in European folk medicine of the Middle Ages. That it was then used in a variety of ways is very probable, given the insights of women healers in those days—insights that were acquired through their activities in natural magic and witchcraft as much as through direct experience. The first written record of Hawthorn seems to be by PETRUS DE CRESCENTIS around 1305, who used it for gout; in 1695 an anonymous healer is recorded to have used it for symptoms of hypertension (HENRI LECLERC, 1935), and in the nineteenth century in Lorraine, France the infusion of the flowers were used for insomnia and palpitations. In short, countless centuries elapsed before male professional doctors took any notice of it.

Hawthorn is not a neglected folk remedy by mere accident since as prime emblem of the beauty and harmony loving Rose family, it is a feminine type of plant. Besides, physiologically it **tonifies the Yin!** Medicine, herbalism included, since Renaissance days has seen the rise of more masculine, active remedies like the array of imported toxic *eliminants* from the Americas, as well as the narrow focused alkaloidal herbs such as Digitalis and Bryony. A subtle, gentle yet highly effective remedy such as Hawthorn simply found no part in this trend.

The first article on Hawthorn, quoted by FINLEY ELLINGWOOD in 1907, was written in 1896 by a doctor JENNINGS of Chicago. ELLINGWOOD is the first to give it the attention it deserves (writing more on Hawthorn than on Digitalis, but less than on Cereus!). From here its use spread back to Europe where it has been extensively researched in the biochemical method. This research has hardly thrown more light on its use than was discovered by the Eclectic physicians of the early twentieth century: it has merely confirmed and embellished it.

Since it restores heart tissue, Hawthorn may be called a *cardiac trophorestorative*, and as such should be used in all organic heart conditions. It also has a functional *restoring, stimulating* effect on the heart and circulation, of which the net result is a **balancing** effect: balancing because it is the heart's basic energetic role as central organ to balance the metabolic area with the neurosensorial area both functionally and structurally. Hawthorn has been found to improve **deficiency, congestive** and **depository** conditions affecting it either chronically or acutely.

Moreover, given both its symptom sign complex and its physiological action, Hawthorn

Cereus: Class 7

emerges as a *Yin tonic*; its special emphasis is the type of Yin deficiency where the Kidneys are said to loose contact with the heart, resulting in feelings of anxiety, anguish or paranoia (compare with Pasque flower), and for which acupuncture would select points Bl 15, 24 & 39, Ht 7, P 7 and Kd 3. Its mild *sedative* effects are merely an aspect of its overall restoring of the Yin. Significantly, from the Western viewpoint Hawthorn is a leading remedy for essential hypertension. At the very least, Hawthorn should be used in all conditions where Yin deficiency is attended by cardiac symptoms of whatever kind.

Oriental herbalists have always considered Hawthorn an integral part of formulas for relieving food stagnation and have also appreciated its mild *astringency*. This use, far from being unworthy of this great heart tonic, has been vindicated by modern pharmacology: Austrian researchers found that it decreases free fatty acids and lactic acid, a fact rightly interpreted by MOWREY (1987) as indicating a stimulation of digestive enzymes with decreased oxygen and energy demands; the resultant picture of Hawthorn is as an *anabolic,* upbuilding remedy as far as metabolism is concerned.

As with the several other *Qi tonics* of this class which are not roots, Hawthorn is both a *tonic* remedy for the heart and the Yin, and a *stimulating, dispersing* one in terms for the digestion. It can comfortably live with both images, if we let it.

CEREUS

Pharmaceutical name: caulis et flos Cerei
Botanical name: Cereus grandiflorus Mill. (syn.
    Seleniceras grandiflorus Britt. *et* Rose
    (N.O. Cactaceae)
Other names: Night-blooming cactus, Vanilla
    cactus, sweet-scented cactus (Am)
    Cièrge à grandes fleurs (Fr)
    Königin der Nacht (Ge)
Part used: the stem and flower

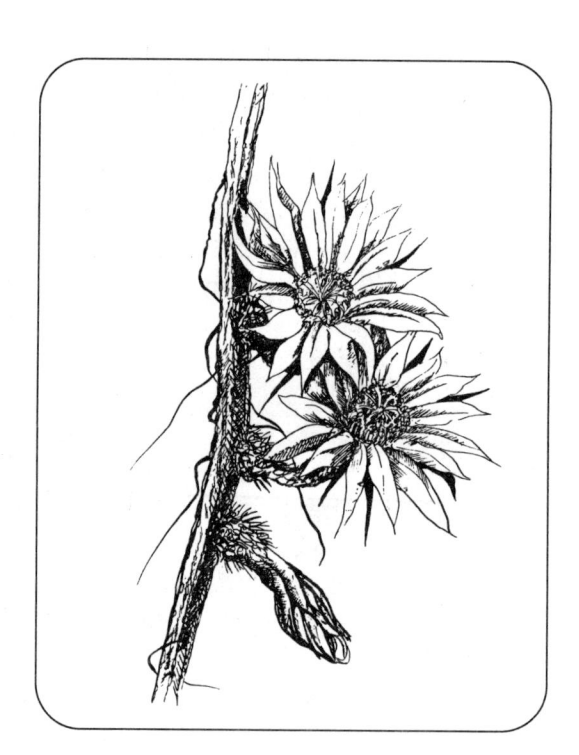

Nature

CATEGORY: medium-strength herb with some chronic toxicity
CONSTITUENTS: alkaloid cactine, cardioactive flavonoid glycosides (incl. narcissin, rutin, resinoid, cacticin, kaempferitrin, grandiflorin), resinoid glucoside, digitalis-like substances, resin
EFFECTIVE QUALITIES
Primary: a bit sweet & bitter, cool, dry
Secondary: restoring, relaxing, stimulating, decongesting
TROPISM: heart, pericardium, vascular system, kidneys, uterus
    Air, Fluid organisms

Class 7: Cereus

Heart, Pericardium, Chong & Ren meridians
GROUND: all krases, biotypes and constitutions for symptomatic use

Functions and Uses

1 STRENGTHENS AND RESTORES THE HEART AND CIRCULATION; RESTORES THE HEART, BRAIN AND ADRENALS; LIFTS THE SPIRIT AND RIDS DEPRESSION

   heart Qi deficiency with severe chest oppression, palpitations, despondency, mental depression
   FUNCTIONAL CARDIAC & VALVULAR INSUFFICIENCIES of all types
   LOW BLOOD PRESSURE
   THREATENED HEART FAILURE
   nerve deficiency with depression, fatigue, neuralgia
   ADRENAL INSUFFICIENCY
   heart & Kidney Yang deficiency with difficult breathing, chest oppression or constriction, no sexual desire
   CARDIAC DYSPNEA and arrhythmias
   ENDO/PERICARDITIS due to chronic disease

2 STABILIZES AND SUPPORTS THE HEART, HARMONIZES MENSTRUATION AND MENOPAUSE AND BANISHES FEAR

   heart Qi constraint with deficiency with nervous tension, worry, anguish, anginal chest pains
   STENOCARDIAC FIT, angiona pectoris
   Liver Yang rising with deficiency with hot flushes, visual disturbances, vertex headache, tinnitus
   MENOPAUSAL SYNDROME
   uterus Qi constraint with painful, irregular menstruation, PMS
   GASTROCARDIAC SYNDROME with heartburn, palpitations
   CHOKING & FEAR (e.g. of suffocation, of death) before sleep

3 SEEPS WATER, PROMOTES URINATION AND RELIEVES CONGESTION; STIMULATES AND DREDGES THE KIDNEYS AND BENEFITS THE SKIN

   kidney fluid congestion with ankle or leg edema, malaise
   kidney Qi stagnation with skin rashes, malaise, bladder or prostate irritation, poor vision
   MENORRHAGIA: early, copious periods due to uterus blood congestion
   SKIN ERUPTIONS

Preparation

USE: Cereus should be used in TINCTURE or FREEZE-DRIED extract form for good results. Less effective is the short DECOCTION.
DOSAGE: TINCTURE: 10-50 drops, or 0.66-2 ml
             DECOCTION: 2-8 g per cup of water
CAUTION: Cereus is contraindicated in all Qi constraint conditions with excess such as high blood pressure and excessive cardiac force.

Notes

This remedy is furnished by a cactus growing in places such as the American Southwest, northern Mexico, Hawaii, the West Indies and the Bay of Naples. It is called a night-blooming cactus, since flowering only at night. Its large, satiny cream flowers exude a heavy perfume that the fine nose of WILHELM PELIKAN (1962) found reminiscent of jasmine, vanilla, violets and benzoin. With the dawning sun, the short-lived gifts of this *Queen of the night* fade.

It is difficult to imagine a more perfect remedy for deficiency conditions of the heart, being without doubt "the heart tonic *par excellence*" (ELLINGWOOD, 1898). Cereus is by no means the equivalent of Hawthorn, being entirely different in application. However, in one essential point these two botanicals touch: both are *cardiac trophorestoratives.* Cereus as much as Crataegus produces "improved nutrition of the entire nervous and muscular structure of the heart" (ELLINGWOOD), hence qualifying as the formost agent in the treatment of **deficiency heart** conditions in all their variations and sequelae. Cardiac insufficiencies found with advancing age, in wasting disease, in all heart conditions with fatigue and exhaustion demand its use, as they would acupuncture points Ht 7 & 9, P 6 and Bl 15.

But Cereus has a trump card which not only enhances its *cardiotonic* effects, but also puts it among the herbs that lift the spirit, the *antidepressants.* It is a first class *nerve restorative,* toning and regulating the entire sympathetic branch. Clearly, this means nothing less than a balancing effect on the body's Yang, like the Yang qiao extra meridian in acupuncture. It is not difficult to see that this is a superb enhancement of its action on the heart: as a result, deficiency states of both the heart and nerve with depression and debility are best served by Cereus. While Eclectic writers recommended support with other *tonics* such as Oats and Pasque flower in the presence of Qi constraint, herbs such as Rosemary, Melissa and Lily of the valley would be better for simple deficiency. Moreover, specific to the Cereus pattern of disharmony is also a "sensation of a band or cord around the body or chest or head" (ELLINGWOOD) or of the heart bounding as if trapped in a cage, sometimes found with nervous exhaustion. Excess Liver Yang conditions (as found during the menopause, for example) with oppressive headache at the vertex and hot flushes will also benefit from its use; as will a varieties of menstrual disharmonies.

Also like Hawthorn, Cereus is a great *regulator* and *balancer,* assisting that central organ the heart in its striving to maintain a balance between the nervous sytem above it and the metabolic system below it, between gravity and levity. In light of this, the conclusion of our much cited Eclectic writer comes as no surprise: "Those who have used all the heart remedies unite in the belief that for breadth of action, for specific directness, for reliability and smoothness and general trustworthyness, Cereus takes preference over all the rest."

LILY OF THE VALLEY

Pharmaceutical name: folium seu flos Convallariae
Botanical name: Convallaria maialis L. (N.O. Liliaceae)
Ancient names: Lilium convallium, Ephemerum non lethale, Callionym, Chamaecytinus (Lat)
Other names: May lily, Wood lily, Liriconfancy, Our Lady's tears, Jacob's ladder (Eng)
Muguet des bois, Lis de mai/des vallées, Passerolle (Fr)
Maiglöckchen, Mai Blümlein, Mayenriss, Zaucken, Zweiblatt (Ge)
Part used: the leaf or flower

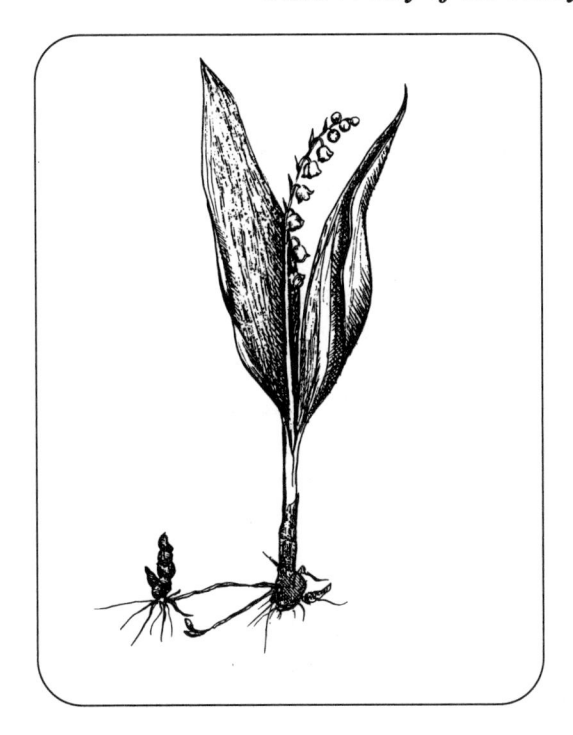

Nature

CATEGORY: medium-strength herb with some chronic toxicity
CONSTITUENTS: cardioactive glycosides (convallatoxin, convallamarin etc.) saponins, ess. oil, asparagin, convallarinic & chelidonic acid, malic & citric acid, carotene, 8 flavonoids
EFFECTIVE QUALITIES
Primary: a bit sweet & bitter, neutral, moist
Secondary: restoring, stimulating, decongesting, softening, dissolving
TROPISM: heart, pericardium, circulation, nerves, brain,
Air, Fluid organisms
Heart, Pericardium meridians
GROUND: Melancholic krasis
Sensitive/Tai Yin Metal biotype
Lymphatic/Carbonic/Blue Iris constitution

Functions and Uses

1 STRENGTHENS AND SUPPORTS THE HEART; RESTORES THE NERVE AND BRAIN AND BENEFITS THE MEMORY; LIFTS THE SPIRIT AND RIDS DEPRESSION

   heart Qi deficiency: tiredness, palpitations, chest oppression, shortness of breath, frequent sweating
   SENILE HEART, arrhythmia, mitral insufficiency or stenosis, low blood pressure, bradycardia
   heart blood deficiency: lethargy, exhaustion, insomnia, palpitations, poor memory, depression
   nerve deficiency: chronic depression, mental dullness, confusion
   VALVULAR DISEASE, endo/pericarditis
   SPEECH LOSS, PARALYSIS

Lily of the valley: Class 7

2 STIMULATES THE HEART, PROMOTES URINATION AND RELIEVES CONGESTION; DREDGES THE KIDNEYS AND SOFTENS DEPOSITS

heart Yang deficiency: mental depression, dizziness, chilliness, weak respiration
heart & Kidney Yang deficiency: wheezing, chest constricton palpitations
CARDIAC ASTHMA
heart blood congestion: cardiac pain, chest oppression, cyanosed face, lips & nails
ANGINA PECTORIS, coronary thrombosis
COMA, SHOCK, STROKE
heart fluid congestion: irregular heart beat, dyspnea, hepatic fullness, edema, dizziness
ACUTE or CHRONIC NEPHRITIS
HARD DEPOSITS: ARTERIOSCLEROSIS, RHEUMATISM (acute or chronic), gout

3 DISSIPATES TUMORS, RESTRAINS INFECTION AND ANTIDOTES POISON, REDUCES INFLAMMATION AND CLEARS TOXINS

TUMORS, cancer; eye cataract
INFECTED WOUNDS, ulcers, gangrene
INSECT & animal bites, esp. wasps & bees

Preparation

USE: In addition to ready-made preparations, INFUSIONS and TINCTURES may be made and used for all the above purposes. For **chronic heart deficiency** conditions, long-term use is needed for a good accumulative effect that, moreover, will carry on long after stopping use of the remedy. External WASHES and COMPRESSES may also be made.

A traditional SNUFF to provoke sneezing was, and still is, being used for stubborn **headaches**, **earaches** and **epileptic fits** (Switzerland). In Renaissance times Lily of the valley was a much used, popular remedy; apothecaries prepared an array of distilled waters based on it, such as *Aqua aurea*.

DOSAGE: INFUSION: 2-7 g twice a day
TINCTURE: 0.3-2 ml or 10-50 drops twice a day

CAUTION: Although a safe medium-strength remedy in therapeutic doses, if these are exceeded poisoning may occur. For the same reason, if taken on its own, a break of ten days is advisable after ten days of continuous use.
Avoid using in deficient Yin conditions and with fatty heart degeneration.

Notes

If Renaissance medical manuscripts are any guide, Lily of the valley must be a *cephalic* panacea for all ills. Pages fairly teem with receipts for "waters for the head" to be used in any number of ailments afflicting the **head** and **brain**, from dizziness to stroke. WILLIAM COLE (1657), for example, affirms that it "recrutes a weak Memory." Unfortunately, although some of these formulas are interesting—those of the Italian herbalist PIERANDREA MATTIOLI (1611), for example, which combine *stimulants* and *antispasmodics*—they betray a lack of rigor where differential diagnosis is concerned. Rather than treat certain organ symptoms by rebalancing underlying dishamonies, they usually attempt to treat all symptoms of an organ in one fell swoop. However, their reliance on the swift scimitar stroke of an Arabian style prescription is clearly a misguided one. Then already, sadly enough, the approach was symptom relief as often as it was syndrome treatment.

Still, Convallaria can be seen as a *nerve restorative* as much as a *cardiac* one even today. In this respect it is the nearest thing in temperate zones to Cereus from the tropical ones. Both botanicals will deal effectively with both **nerve** and **heart Qi deficiency** causing mental confusion and depression, palpitations, etc., and for which acupuncture would select points such as P 4 & 6, Ht 7 and Bl 15. The very scent of the small white "bells", delicate and evocative of cool, shady summer woods, is naturally *antidepressant*—although "spirit lifting" is a more positive way of putting it.

Lily of the valley's second function, however, is like Hawthorn's: a *cardiac stimulant* with *decongestant* and *diuretic* effects. Through a stimulation of heart Yang both **cardiac fluid** and **blood congestion** are relieved and anginal attacks effectively prevented. Like Hawthorn too, it is one of the best remedies where the heart is "invaded" by metabolic processes from below (rather than by nervous ones from above): in this sense it also supports the heart in its general function of maintaining a balance beween the two. In short, Lily of the valley is called for where the heart is affected due to a tendency to either a deficient Yang or an excess Yin condition.

Again like Hawthorn, Lily of the valley will tend to soften **deposits**, whether in the arteries, joints, muscles, or in the blood itself, hence is a good ingredient in combinations for general fluids dyskrasia with cardiac symptoms, for example, as well as an effective preventer of thrombosis (EDWARD SHOOK, 1932). Its beneficial effect in tumors and even forms of cancer are again an advantage where excess conditions of the metabolic organs present.

VALERIAN

Pharmaceutical name: rhizoma Valerianae
Botanical name: Valeriana officinalis L. (N.O. Valerianaceae)
Ancient names: Phu (Gr)
 Amantilla, Dacia, Genicularis, Marcinella (Lat)
Other names: All-heal, Capon's tail, Setwell, Cut-heal, Treacle (Eng)
 Fragrant valerian, Dysentery root, Tobacco root (Am)
 Valériane, Herbe aux chats (Fr)
 Baldrian, Speerkraut, Denmark, Augenwurz, Balderbracken (Ge)
Part used: the rhizome

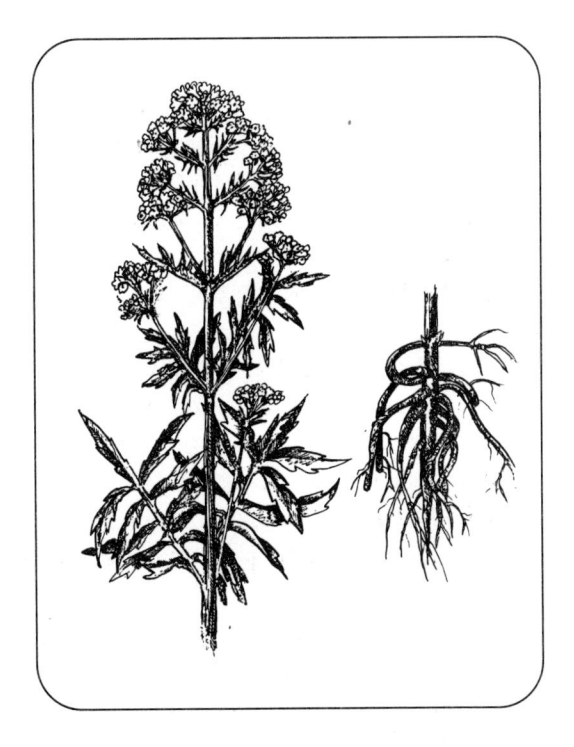

Nature

CATEGORY: medium-strength herb with some chronic toxicity
CONSTITUENTS: ess. oil (incl. valerianic acid, borneol, camphene, pinene, sesquiterpenes), volatile alkaloids, valepotriates, terpenoid alcohols/acids/aldehydes/esters/ketones up to 1.4%, cholin, glycosides, ferments, tannic acid, glucose & fructose, resin
EFFECTIVE QUALITIES
Primary: a bit sweet & bitter & pungent, warm with some cooling potential, dry
Secondary: restoring, stimulating, relaxing, decongesting
TROPISM: heart, arterial circulation, nerves, brain, spine, lungs,

Valerian: Class 7

>>uterus, kidney, bladder, stomach, pancreas
>>Air, Fluid organisms
>>Heart, Pericardium, Lung, Spleen meridians
>**GROUND:** Sanguine krasis
>>Charming/Yang Ming Earth & Expressive/Jue Yin biotypes
>>Lymphatic/Carbonic/Blue Iris constitution

Functions and Uses

1. STIMULATES THE HEART, CIRCULATION AND LUNGS; RESTORES THE NERVE, BRAIN AND SPINE; LIFTS THE SPIRIT AND RIDS DEPRESSION
   heart Yang deficiency: palpitations, shortness of breath, cold limbs, mental depression
   heart blood congestion: chest pain, cyanosed face, lips, nails
   heart & Kidney Yang deficiency: wheezing, exhaustion, chilliness
   lung & Kidney Yang deficiency: wheezing, grief, depression
   nerve & brain deficiency: mental stupor, headache, dizziness
   NERVOUS DEPRESSION and despondency in chronic deficiency conditions
   SPINAL WEAKNESS

2. CIRCULATES THE QI AND LOOSENS CONSTRAINT; RELAXES THE NERVE, ALLAYS IRRITABILITY AND INDUCES REST
   heart Qi constraint: anxiety, worry, chest pain
   lung Qi constraint: wheezing, dry nervous cough
   kidney Qi constraint: agitated depression, kidney or sacral pain
   uterus Qi constaint: irregular, painful menstruation
   bladder Qi constraint: difficult, painful scanty urination
   MIGRAINE, HYSTERIA, EPILEPSY, MENOPAUSAL SYNDROME

3. FOSTERS THE YIN, RESOLVES FEVER AND CLEARS DEFICIENCY HEAT; SUPPORTS THE HEART AND CALMS THE SPIRIT
   heart Yin & Kidney deficiency: fear, mental & nervous unrest, night sweats, low afternoon fever
   heart blood & Spleen Qi deficiency: insomnia, fatigue, poor memory
   LOW TIDAL FEVERS with empty heat in Shao Yin stage

4. RESTORES THE LIVER, STOMACH AND PANCREAS; DREDGES THE KIDNEY AND PROMOTES URINATION, STRENGTHENS THE EYES AND BENEFITS VISION
   liver & stomach Qi deficiency: poor appetite, epigastric pain, constipation
   DIABETES (supportive)
   kidney Qi stagnation: nervousness, fatigue
   POOR EYESIGHT

5. ACTIVATES IMMUNITY AND RESTRAINS INFECTION; ANTIDOTES POISON, CLEARS PARASITES AND PROMOTES TISSUE REPAIR
   PROPHYLACTIC in EPIDEMICS
   WOUNDS, injuries, fractures, chronic ulcers (all internal or external)
   FOOD or HERB POISONING
   INTESTINAL WORMS

BITES & STINGS
SPLINTERS (drawing)

Preparation

USE: The simplest preparation is an overnight (or overday) cold water MACERATION (stirring occasionally). The TINCTURE is somewhat stronger. Valerian WINE is definitely more *stimulating* than the rest (for function 1). All should be made from the **fresh root** if possible—a sound Swiss folk custom.

ENEMAS have proved useful in the type of menstrual and kidney conditions outlined above. Externally Valerian is an effective *vulnerary* in WASHES, FOMENTATIONS and the like for injuries, fractures and for drawing splinters.

Homeopathic preparations are also used for the same indications as above, with an emphasis on the empty heat and Qi constraint symptomatology.

DOSAGE: Valerian being the fussy, selective remedy it is, the dosage varies with the effect required as well as with the individual taking it: some people respond more quickly or intensely to it than others. As a general rule, three dosage levels may be defined: a **low dosage** for *restoring* (functions 1 & 4); a **medium dosage** for *stimulating* and *relaxing* and promoting rest (functions 1,2 & 3); a **high dosage** for *greater calming* effects. The problem with the high dosage is that there is a 50/50 chance that Valerian may produce the opposite effects, namely excess symptoms such as excitation, headache, vision disturbances, etc. Valerian can be unpredictable as well as variable!

Low dose:
> TINCTURE: 5-25 drops, or up to 1/5 tsp or 1 ml
> MACERATION: 2 tsp. of finely chopped root steeped in two cups of cold water at least 8 hrs. for a one-day supply; this may be gently warmed before drinking

Medium dose:
> TINCTURE: 25-50 drops, i.e. 1/5-1/2 tsp or 2 ml
> MACERATION: 4 tsp prepared as above for a one-day supply

High dose:
> TINCTURE: 50-130 drops, i.e. 1/2-1 tsp or 2-5 ml

CAUTION: Being a medium-strength herb with low-level toxicity, Valerian should be discontinued for a week after 2 to 3 weeks of continuous usage if taken as a simple, and the dosage should not exceeded. It can produce a mild dependence and eventually create the same symptoms that it initially treated (an example of spontaneous homeopathic proving). Extreme excessive use can cause paralysis and cardiac problems.

In tincture form, the use of Valerian should be restricted to conditions of Qi constraint and Yin deficiency or empty heat and never applied with any excess, full heat, sthenic fever or inflammation. The exception is acute situatons such as migraine epileptic or hysteric fits.

Valerian should not be taken with any sleep inducing drugs, since it has a potentizing effect on these.

Notes

It is significant that in German speaking countries Valerian has been given well over 500 distinct names, and that the Romans already graced it with a string of feminine names. This reflects perhaps on the amount that it has always been talked about, and also confirms an impression that one gets from the plant when catching sight of it in sunny clearings in woods: tall and upright, crowned with tiny pale pink blossoms, and exuding its delicate scent, it seems a somewhat vain, conceited plant.

Valerian: Class 7

Valerian is a good example not only of versatility and fickleness as regards its names, but also as regards its therapeutic use: here too it has undergone several fashions—a term appropriate enough to this plant! Before the germ theory was conceived in the last century, Valerian was regarded essentially as a *tonic remedy* to the heart, the eyes, the mind, to drooping spirits—in brief, to well-being in general. It was a main ingredient of the thick, dark all-purpose Theriack paste which bequeathed it with yet another name, Treacle. The image of Valerian today, chameleon being that it is, has changed to its exact opposite: it is popularly seen as a heavy *sedative* in the pharmaceutical sense of the word.

Clearly, it is time to seriously come to grips with this elusive, paradoxical herb, to cut through the images that it has generated. For a start, the myth of its *nerve sedative* action has been dispelled (MILLS, 1980), so that terms such as *tranquillizer* and *calmative* are now more appropriate. Valerian does not interfere with activity and coordination in the manner of true *nerve sedative* such as Wild lettuce and Gelsemium. Furthermore, a more secure basis for understanding this plant is gained when seen in the light of Chinese and Galenic pharmacology: these provide a therapeutic basis that is anything but ephemeral or speculative.

Valerian's gentle *sweet bitter* taste clearly indicates a *restoring* ability, a general strengthening and harmonising power. As a result, Valerian is not only a *restoring digestive tonic* applicable in liver and stomach Qi deficiency and low tidal fevers with prostration, but also, and more fundamentally, a *nerve and brain tonic*. WILHELM HUFELAND in the early 1800's, for example, used this remedy for "chronic weakness of the nerves". It has been suggested (SIMONIS, PELIKAN) that Valerian's real identity is the result of **phosphorus** bioenergies. This element (meaning in Greek *light-bearer*) is intimately connected with the substance of the nervous system which brings us the light of sensation and consciousness. Clearly, there is something to be said for the traditional belief that Valerian restores the **brain** and benefits **thinking** and **memory**, strengthens the **spine** and improves **vision**. For two thousand years, Valerian was in fact considered the main herb for failing eyesight.

Since phosphorus has *cool, dry, contracting* qualities, Valerian by analogy enhances these when used to foster the Yin and clear empty heat. By impressing the cool, calm, deep and hidden sphere of the nerve and brain, it effectively proves useful in syndromes such as **Kidney and heart Yin deficiency**, like Arnica and Hawthorn in this class of *cardiac tonics*. It has proven a specific for emotional insecurity, mental restlessness and paranoia in this context, as well as for the attendant empty heat symptoms.

Closely connected with its *nerve and Yin restoring* function is Valerian's *relaxant* effect, which is a systemic one. Energetically speaking, this is evident in its pungent taste, and structurally in its content of essential oil, valepotriates and (iso)valerianic acids. *Antispasmodic* effects are also evident, not only on smooth but on visceral muscles as well. **Qi Constraint** syndromes with deficiency causing tension and restlessness are addressed in addition to Yin deficiency ones, inviting a comparison with botanicals such as Marjoram, Skullcap and Mistletoe—with all of which it makes congenial combinations.

But the *pungent* taste also has *stimulating* dynamics, and here Valerian shows its true colors in its use in the rhythmic region of the chest. Like Rosemary and Prickly ash bark, the unlikely Valerian stimulates **heart** and **lung Yang** into action, turning around mental apathy, depression and gloom in so doing. This function is significant to the point where congested heart blood is effectively cleared (Qi moves blood), and asthmatic conditions due to lung & Kidney Yang Deficiency are improved. Far from throwing a monkey wrench in its pharmacological works, therefore, Valerian's mild *pungency* creates a link between its tropism for the nervous system and the heart and between the heart/lungs and the kidneys (through hormonal linkage). Small wonder that WEISENBERG in 1853 summed up Valerian as a *"stimulating nervine"*. As such, a comparison with Pasque flower is inevitable: both combine *restoring, stimulating* and *relaxing* effcts on virtually the same organs.

Nevertheless, Valerian creates a stronger impression on the heart and lungs than Pasque flower. This not only merits it a firm place among the *restoring* remedies, but, more significantly, serious considerations in its use as a *relaxant*. Since it is a *circulatory stimulant* and *stimulant/relaxant expectorant,* Valerian cannot successfully be used for excess conditions of any kind. The reports of it causing a groggy kind of alertness with insomnia due to excess conditions (e.g. in children) are legion. Only deficiency heat and deficiency Qi constraint are amenable to its influence. Anything else is liable to fail. The only exception to this is purely symptomatic use with migraine, epilepsy and hysteric fits.

On balance, Valerian is a perfect remedy for chronic stress or illness affecting the heart and nerves, with fatigue, tension and any of the other symptoms already singled out. It promotes rest and sleep when there is exhaustion—when a person simply needs to recuperate.

COWSLIP FLOWER

Pharmaceutical name: flos Primulae
Botanical name: Primula veris L. (syn. *Primula off.* Hill.), *vel Primula elatior* L. (N.O. Primulaceae)
Ancient names: Paralysio, Palladium, Sanamunda, Verbascum odoratum, Herba arthritica, Tradella, Clavis S. Petri (Lat)
Other names: White betony, Palsywort, Bear's ears, Fairy cups, Horse buckles, Galligaskins, Mayflower, Herb Peter, Our Lady's keys, Culverkeys (Eng)
Primevère, Coucou, Oreille d'ours, Herbe à la paralysie (Fr)
Schlüsselblume, Himmelsschlüssel, Weisse Betonie, Frühlingsprimel, Lerchenblume (Ge)
Part used: the flower

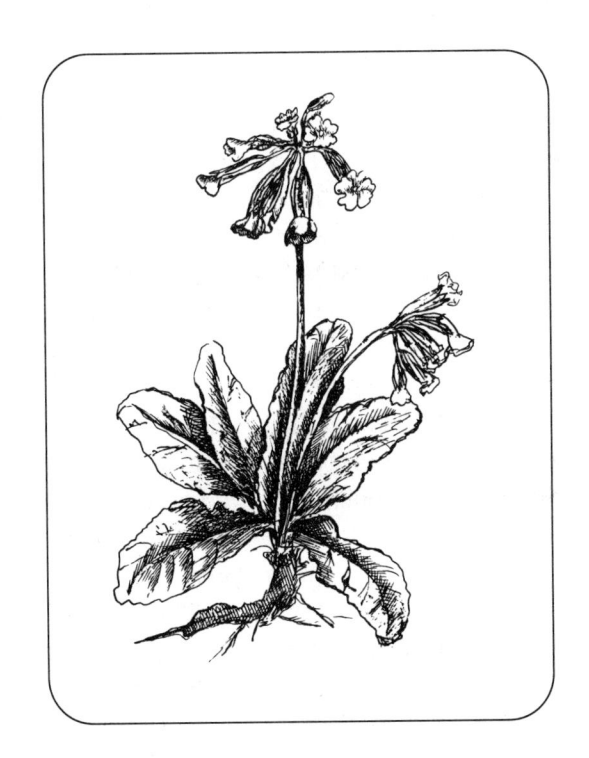

Nature

CATEGORY: mild herb with minimal chronic toxicity
CONSTITUENTS: ess. oil, primulic camphor, glycoside, zyclamine, yellow pigment, bitter extractive substances
EFFECTIVE QUALITIES
Primary: a bit sweet & bland, neutral, dry
Secondary: restoring, relaxing
TROPISM: heart, pericardium, vascular systm, nerves, lungs
Air organism
Heart, Pericardium, Lung meridians
GROUND: Melancholic krasis

Cowslip flower: Class 7

Sensitive/Tai Yin Metal biotype
Lymphatic/Carbonic/Blue Iris constitution

Functions and Uses

1. RESTORES THE HEART AND NERVE; CIRCULATES THE QI, FREES SPASMS AND CALMS WIND; RELIEVES PAIN AND INDUCES REST

   heart Qi deficiency with chest oppression, palpitations
   nerve deficiency with weakness, fatigue, local paralysis, numbness
   NEURALGIA, NEURITIS, HEADACHE, MIGRAINE VERTIGO, dizziness, tendency to fainting
   heart Qi constraint with anxiety, chest oppression, cardiac pains
   PERICARDITIS, cardiac edema
   lung Qi constraint with wheezing, dry cough
   WHOOPING COUGH, lung infections
   internal wind with convulsions in children
   INSOMNIA, unrest

2. CAUSES SWEATING, RELEASES THE EXTERIOR AND SCATTERS WIND HEAT; REDUCES INFLAMMATION AND CLEARS THE HEAD

   external wind heat onset of infections with fever, headache, aches and pains, delirium
   head damp heat with nasal discharge & head congestion
   UPPER RESPIRATORY INFECTIONS

Preparation

USE: The INFUSION or TINCTURE of the entire **flowerheads** (including the calyx, which is high in vitamin C) is best. These should be immediately dried to ensure that they don't loose their color, and with the same care as Marigold flowers (WILLFORT, 1972). For incipient **colds** or **flus** the INFUSION should be sipped hot to cause sweating. Being one of Cowslip's main ingredients, the ESSENTIAL OIL can be extracted through either steam distillation or enfleurage. Cowslip flower was a standard item in the European pharmacy until the eighteenth century and was used **externally** in LINIMENTS, COMPRESSES etc. for neuralgic conditions, paresthesia, paralysis, etc., i.e. for wind/damp obstruction.
DOSAGE: standard doses throughout.
NOTE: *Primula vulgaris* L., or Primrose, is not used in herbal medicine.

Notes

Cowslip flower could be placed equally well with the Class 1 herbs that scatter wind heat and the *restorers* of this class. The choice was made in favor of the latter since in Western terms Cowslip flower has traditionally been one of the main nerve *restorative* botanicals. As such it deals superbly with local neuralgic and paralytic conditions due to nerve deficiency, especially in the head. It was called White betony in the past since it was considered second only to Wood betony in treating maladies of the head. These include severe vertigo and fainting spells, of the kind found in Liver Yang rising syndromes due to deficiency.

Cowslip flower also has a reputation for *restoring, relaxing* and *stabilizing* the **heart** in both **deficiency** and **Qi Constraint** conditions and reminds one of Pasque flower in this respect. For heart Qi constraint conditions due to chronic cardiac weakness—a diathesis common with Lymphatic constitutions—Cowslip flower is clearly the equivalent of an acupuncture point selecion such as Ht 5 & 9, P 4 & 7 and Bl 15. Its *relaxant* effect extends to the bronchial region and to the peripheral circulation, implying usage in wind heat onsets of upper respiratory infections in addition to dry, spasmodic lung conditions. The essential oil and glycoside are probably "responsable" for these effects. Key symptoms calling for its use here are **pain, congestion, inflammation** and general **irritability**.

The overall profile of Cowslip flower as medicinal plant clearly matches *Man jing zi, fructus Viticis,* used in Chinese medicine. Both are used for damp paralysis, wind heat conditions with headache, and "dull mentality". Only the cardiac component is missing from the overall gestalt.

Calamus: Class 7

Herbs to Restore the Liver, Stomach, *Spleen* and Intestines, Awaken the Appetite, Promote Digestion and Create Strength

CALAMUS

Pharmaceutical name: rhizoma Acori
Botanical name: Acorus calamus L. (N.O. Araceae)
Ancient names: Akoron (Gr)
    Acorus verus, Calamus aromaticus, Canna persidis (Lat)
    Beewort, Sweet flag/myrtle/rush, Myrtle sedge/grass, Wild iris (Eng)
    Acore vrai, Roseau aromatique, Jonc odorant (Fr)
    Kalmus, Ackerwurz, Magenwurz (Ge)
Part used: the rhizome

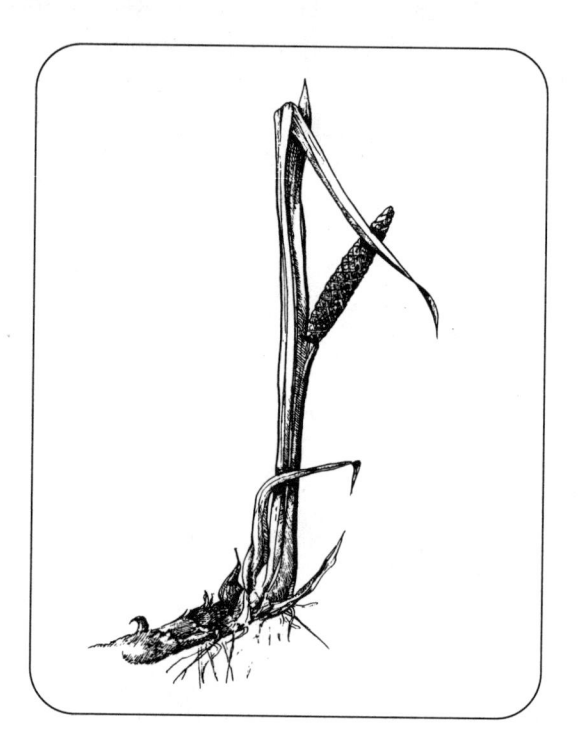

Nature

NATURE: mild herb with minimal chronic toxicity
CONSTITUENTS: mucilage, bitter, ess. oil up to 3.5% (incl. asarone, eugenol, asamyl alcohol), tannin, glycoside acorin
EFFECTIVE QUALITIES
Primary: *Taste:* a bit pungent & bitter & sweet
        Warmh: warm
        Moisture: dry
Secondary: restoring, stimulating, astringing, decongesting, relaxing, dissolving
TROPISM
Organs or parts: stomach, intestines, uterus, liver, urinary organs
Organisms: Warmth, Air
Meridians: Spleen, Stomach, Lung, Liver
Tri Dosas: decreases Kapha, increases Pitta
GROUND
Krases/temperaments: Phlegmatic & Melancholic
Biotypes: Dependant/Tai Yin Earth, Self-Reliant/Yang Ming Metal & Burdened/Shao Yin
Constitutions: Lymphatic/Carbonic/Blue Iris

Functions and Uses

1   WARMS, INVIGORATES AND RELAXES THE STOMACH AND INTESTINES; AWAKENS THE APPETITE, SETTLES THE STOMACH AND LEVELS VOMITING
   Spleen Yang deficiency (intestines cold): fatigue, no appetite, diarrhea

ANOREXIA NERVOSA, chronic gastritis
intestines Qi constraint: flatulence, abdominal colic worse with emotions or stress
ACUTE GASTRITIS, mucous colitis
stomach dryness: oppressive feeling of lumps in stomach, dry mouth & tongue, anxiety
GASTRIC HYPO or HYPER-ACIDITY, PEPTIC ULCER, heartburn
NAUSEA & VOMITING due to *stomach Qi reflux*

2 CREATES ASTRICTION, RESOLVES MUCUS AND DRIES DAMP; EXPELS AND DRAINS PHLEGM AND CLEARS THE HEAD; PROMOTES THE MENSES AND ARRESTS DISCHARGE

head damp cold: head colds with stuffed nose and sinuses, watery discharge, headache
lung phlegm damp: coughing up thin white phlegm, wheezing
BRONCHITIS
intestines mucous damp (Spleen damp) gurgling distended abdomen, epigastric pain, heavy body and head
genitourinary damp cold: white leucorrhea, mucous cystitis
uterus damp cold: delayed or scanty menstruation with cramps before onset, white vaginal discharge

3 STIMULATES THE LIVER, DREDGES THE KIDNEYS AND CLEARS STASIS; PROMOTES URINATION AND SOFTENS STONES

liver Qi stagnation: right flank distention & pain, slow painful digestion, constipation
kidney Qi stagnation: headache, skin rashes, fatigue
URINARY SAND or STONES

4 RESOLVES FEVER

LOW TIDAL FEVERS in Shao Yin stage

5 ACTIVATES IMMUNITY, RESTRAINS INFECTON AND ANTIDOTES POISON; RESOLVES CONTUSION, SOFTENS SWELLING AND RELIEVES PAIN

PREVENTIVE IN EPIDEMICS
BONE DISEASE, e.g. osteonecrosis
CHRONIC ABSCESSES, hard cold boils, cysts
ANIMAL BITES, INTESTINAL PARASITES
BRUISING, contusions, superficial wounds, internal ruptures
SCROFULA, tumors
SKIN eruptions and blemishes
RHAUMATIC & GOUT PAINS, teething pains
HAIRLOSS

Preparations

USE: Calamus may be prepared and used in a variety of ways in order to enhance one or other of its many properties. The overnight cold water MACERATION preserves its mucilage content while loosening out the bitter substances, hence is suited to **hyperacidic, spasmodic** and **chronic inflammatory gastric** conditions above all. The warm long INFUSION and the TINCTURE bring out its essential oil in addition to the bitters, result in a loss of mucilage, and open up its application to the full. The DECOCTION leaves us with the tough tannins and bitters for *astricting tissue* as

Calamus: Class 7

well as for *restoring*.

Calamus CANDY, made from the tender rhizomes boiled first in water and then in sugar, was popular in the eighteenth century on both sides of the Atlantic.

Calamus is traditionally one of the top remedies for external use, as function 5 evinces. It may substitute for Arnica and can be used in BATHS *(restorative)*, SWABS, LOTIONS, SALVES, LINIMENTS (neuralgias) and the like. **Chewing** the fresh or dried root helps infants while teething and helps adults to stop smoking.

DOSAGE: standard doses throughout

CAUTION: ESSENTIAL OIL of Calamus should be avoided unless the North American variety is used, since all four chemotypes of Calamus except for the North American one contain toxic amounts of the compound asarone.

Notes

The Arabian physician IBN AL-BAITAR, in his masterly work *Collection of Simple Remedies* (ca. 1225), comments on Calamus in the folloing way: "It warms the stomach and dissolves phlegm of that organ. It warms up phlegmatic blood and is useful for cold temperaments." With this he touches on the essential use of this remedy as a *warm mucous* and *phlegm expeller*. Chinese medicine would use the terms Spleen damp and phlegm fluids (tan yin) to point to the same phenomenon of phlegm—as it does with the main botanical used for these in its own pharmacy, *Ban xia, rhizoma Pinelliae*.

Calamus is virtually an all-purpose digestive remedy, acting at once in a *lenitive, demulcent, stimulant* and *relaxant* way on the whole intestinal tract. Respectively, mucilage, bitters, glycosides and tannins may be noted in support of these effects. For this reason Calamus can be used in **dry, deficient, cold** or **excess** conditions involving **digestion**, combining well with more directional remedies such as Marsh mallow on one hand and Wild yam on the other. Ulcers of all types, for example, will benefit from its use, as will colic and gas due to its *carminative, antispasmodic* effect. In short, with its mild *pungent bitter sweet* tastes, Calamus represents as ideal a *Spleen tonic* as may be found in the Western mataria medica. Besides, the similarity in the core egestalt of its uses with *Ban xia* is so close that interchangeability is fairly justified. In this sense, Calamus is the equivalent of needling acupuncture points St 40, Sp 3 & 5, St 41, CV 12 & Bl 20.

Metabolic slow-down with accumulation of physical and toxic excess is another way of characterizing the conditions most meet for its use. In this sense Calamus is a gentle *cleansing eliminant*. This and its *tonic* properties, which increase all glandular scretions, conjoin to deal effectively with low, endless fevers with depleted vital response. Here also, Calamus has always enjoyed a stellar reputation.

Today we have the advantage (or disadvantage, depending on our attitude) of knowing some of the mechanisms involved in this remedy's effects. We may talk about the *mucolytic* effect of its essential oil and of its *tonic astringent* or *anticatarrhal* effect on the mucosa, both of which will remove and resolve toxic mucous. But we have to tread carefully, lest we simply reduce this botanical to its biochemical make-up. The **bioenergies** must be kept in mind, forces which, although hidden to our direct experience, produce a physical substance such as essential oil as a result of their activities. Since constituting a plant as a living organism (not a chemical one), these bioenergies equally need to be understood. And begin to understand them we can through an inspection of its chemical ingredients, for one thing.

ANGELICA

Pharmaceutical name: radix Angelicae archangelicae
Botanical name: Angelica archangelica L. (N.O. Umbelliferae)
Ancient names: Radix Sancti Spiritus, Angelica imperatoria (Lat)
Other names: Garden angelica (Eng)
Angélique, Racine du Saint-Esprit (Fr)
Engelwurz, Heiligenbitter, Brustwurzel, Angelick (Ge)
Part used: the root; also the fruit, *fructus Angelicae,* and the leaf, *folium Angelicae*

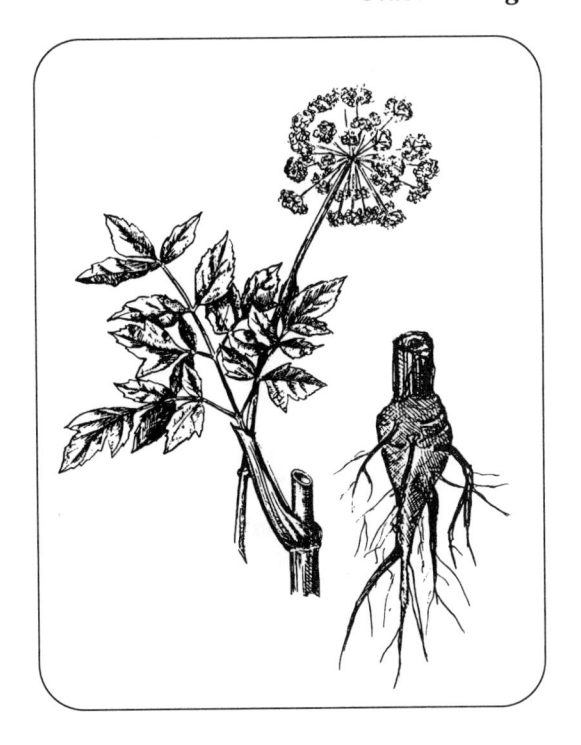

Nature

CATEGORY: medium-strength herb with some chronic toxicity
CONSTITUENTS: ess. oil 0.35 to 1.3% (incl. α & ß-phellandrenes, α-pinenes), furocoumarins (bergapten, isoimperatorin, xanthotoxin, angelicin, archangelicin), coumarins (incl. umbelliferon), phenol-carbonic acids, flavanoid (archangeleron), bitter, sitosterol, tannins, angelic/bernstein/malic/acetic/valerianic/
oxalic acids, pectin
EFFECTIVE QUALITIES
Primary: *Taste:* pungent & bitter & sweet
Warmth: warm
Moisture: dry
Secondary: stimulating, relaxing, decongesting, restoring
TROPISM
Organs or parts: lungs, intestines, stomach, urinary organs, uterus, head
Organisms: Air, Warmth, Fluid
Meridians: Colon, Lung, Spleen, Chong & Ren
Tri Dosas: increases Pitta & Vayu, decreases Kapha
GROUND
Krases/temperaments: Phlegmatic
Biotypes: Dependant/Tai Yin Earth
Constitutions: Lymphatic/Carbonic/Blue Iris

Functions and Uses

1 DRAINS THE YIN, GENERATES WARMTH AND RESTORES STRENGTH: WARMS AND INVIGORATES THE STOMACH/*SPLEEN* AND INTESTINES; AWAKENS THE APPETITE, ABATES DISTENTION AND FLENZES MUCOUS DAMP

Yin excess: chilliness, cold limbs, lethargy, timidity

Angelica: Class 7

stomach cold: persistant dull epigastric pain better with eating or massage
CHRONIC GASTRITIS, chronic ulcer
intestines cold (Spleen Yang Deficiency): lack of appetite, weakness, swollen painful abdomen
CHRONIC ENTERITIS, chronic colitis, anorexia, weightloss
intestines mucous damp (Spleen damp): heavy body & head, mucousy stool, gurgling distended abdomen
DEBILITY or exhaustion due to physical or mental strain or stress, in convalescence

2 STIMULATES AND WARMS THE LUNGS AND EXPELS PHLEGM; RELIEVES WHEEZING AND CLEARS THE HEAD

lung phlegm cold: full cough with thin white phlegm, wheezing
CHRONIC BRONCHIAL ASTHMA, bronchitis
head damp cold: stuffed nose and sinuses, headache, running nasal discharge, toothache

3 CAUSES SWEATING, RELEASES THE EXTERIOR, SCATTERS WIND COLD AND MOVES THE LYMPH

external wind cold: onset of infections with stiff neck, aches and pains, headache, restlessness, dislike of cold
wind/damp obstruction: acute flitting or stationary pains
SWOLLEN GLANDS in head and neck

4 STIMULATES AND WARMS THE UTERUS, HARMONIZES AND PROMOTES MENSTRUATION AND URINATION, PROMOTES LABOR AND EXPELS THE AFTERBIRTH

uterus damp cold: delayed, scanty menses with persistent cramps before onset, leucorrhea
uterus Qi deficiency: delayed, short menses with pain during flow, weakness, restlessness
ESTROGEN INSUFFICIENCY
DIFFICULT LABOR, RETAINED PLACENTA (preventive and remedial)
GENERAL BLADDER IRRITATION with difficult, dribbling urination or anuria

5 LOOSENS CONSTRAINT AND RELAXES THE NERVE; FREES SPASMS, OPENS THE CHEST AND LEVELS ASTHMA

Qi constraint: tension & unrest, vertigo, fainting, migraine
lung Qi constraint: dry coughing with scanty sticky or no sputum, asthmatic breathing
SPASMODIC ASTHMA

6 ACTIVATES IMMUNITY AND RESTRAINS INFECTION; ANTIDOTES POISON; RESOLVES CONTUSION

PREVENTIVE in epidemics
CUTS, wounds, ulcers, abscesses
POISONING from food, toxic herbs or alcohol
INTERNAL or EXTERNAL INJURIES, contusions with congealed blood

Preparation

USE: The cold-water MACERATION of the root is as effective as the TINCTURE for all treatment purposes. It should be soaked overnight, or for about 10 hours anyway, and then heated up and strained for immediate drinking. The DECOCTION is still valid, however, especially in all conditions with deficiency with discharge, and combines well with other *restoring* herbs. The ESSENTIAL OIL (from **seed**, root or leaf) may also be used for greater *diaphoretic, relaxant* and *diuretic* effects, applied externally in a base oil or used internally.

External uses include DOUCHES for menstrual complaints, INHALATIONS, WASHES, SALVES, etc. Traditionally WINES, LIQUEURS, CONSERVES and CANDIES were very popular, and not only with the religious fraternity. The CANDY was a more *tonic* kind of sweet than those of today; the whole washed root was embedded in raw sugar to candy for at least three months.

DOSAGE: MACERATION and DECOCTION: use up to 14 g (1/2 oz) of the dried root.
TINCTURE: 1-3 ml
ESSENTIAL OIL: 2-4 drops in a little warm water.

CAUTION: Angelica is contraindicated in pregnancy, as it is uterine stimulant; with diabetes; and in hot conditions of any kind. Breaks of four days are advised every two weeks or so if full doses are taken continuously. If the ESSENTIAL OIL is used externally, exposure to ultrqviolet light should be avoided (e.g. sunbathing), since its *bergapten* content increases photosensitivity,

Notes

When the medical popularizer WILHELM RYFF in 1573 writes of Angelica "that through such a remedy all poison is effectively expelled from the Heart, and eliminated through sweating," he touches not only on the essence of the significance of Angelica for physicians and lay people of those days, but also on the core of the treatment of externally triggered disease. His statement reveals that *anti-infective* effects through immune stimulation were considered to proceed through a stimulation of the vital spirit housed in the heart and to be activated primarily through sweating. Now this Angel root had long since been revealed to mankind as a specific in the prevention and treatment of epidemics, along with Juniper berries, Gentian and Tormentil. It becomes clearer, as a result, why along with Theriac it had become the single most important medicinal agent of the times.

But, perhaps by coincidence, there are other "reasons" for its name. Angelica belongs to the element Air in first place, like all umbel bearing plants of its family. Its morpholgy and its liking for dry, spacious and mountainous places attest to this. In harmony with this, its sphere and method of action when used medicinally have likewise to do with Air, for Angelica works on the nervous system, on the Qi, and on energy transformation generally. Angelica's *spicy bitter* taste further defines a *Qi circulating* botanical: by inhibiting the vagus nerve it is useful for freeing nervous tension and spasms caused by Qi Constraint with excess, for example. It is definitely more airy than its Chinese relative *Dang gui* which, being *spicy* and *sweet*, is more earthy, and deals with the blood, metabolism and menstrual problems. The two roots are as different, therefore, as the polarity of Qi and blood itself; they are distinct in almost every therapeutic application.

Angelica is both a *sympathetic* and a *parasympathetic nerve inhibitor* and in practice this is borne out by its use in Yin excess conditions of all kinds with **cold, damp, phlegm congestion** and **plethora**—in the **lungs, intestines** and **uterus** mainly. Its *restoring, stimulant* and *relaxant* effects obtain it a place among the *restoratives,* while its very application for digestive conditions earn it a place among the *Spleen tonics*. Here, Angelica root excels at turning around **chronic cold** conditions with underlying **Spleen Qi deficiency**, regardless of whether any of the above-mentioned excess injuries are involved, and regardless of what the actual symptoms are and of what the Western diagnosis may be. As long as these energetic conditions are fulfilled, Angelica will shine.

The overall resemblance is to the Chinese herbs *Du huo, radix Angelicae tuhuo,* and *Bai zhi,*

Holy thistle: Class 7

radix *Angelicae dahuricae*—even though both these actually belong to other therapeutic categories.

Only as a warm *estrogenic menstrual tonic/stimulant* is Angelica similar to *Dang gui,* relieving cramps with delayed, short or stopped menses, like acupuncture points Sp 6, Kd 8, CV 4, St 29 and Bl 32.

HOLY THISTLE

Pharmaceutical name: herba Cardui benedicti
Botanical name: Carduus benedictus Bruns (syn. *Cnicus benedictus* L.) (N.O. Compositae)
Ancient names: Benedicta, Senation, Carduncellus, Cnicus sylvestris, Atractylis hirsurtior (Lat)
Other names: Blessed thistle, Lady's thistle (Eng)
 Chardon béni (Fr)
 Benediktendistel, Kardobenedikte, Bitterdistel (Ge)
Part used: the entire herb; also the fruit or root, fructus seu radix Cardui benedicti

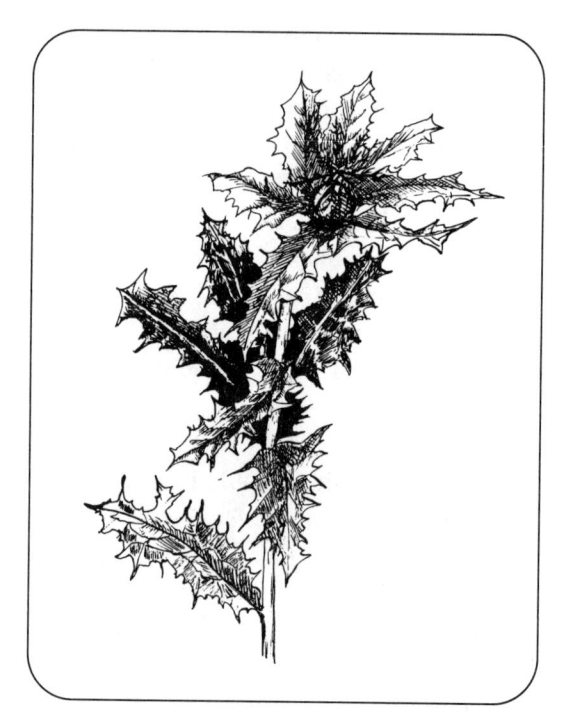

Nature

CATEGORY: mild herb with minimal chronic toxicity
CONSTITUENTS: bitter glycosides (incl. cnicin), alkaloids, flavonoids, ess. oil, tannins, sesqiterpenoid lactone, resin, nicotinic acid, mucilage, iodine, potassium, calcium, magnesium
EFFECTIVE QUALITIES
Primary: bitter, a bit pungent & astringent, neutral with secondary cooling effects, dry
Secondary: restoring, stimulating, decongesting
TROPISM: stomach, liver, intestines, kidneys, lungs brain, nerves
 Air, Fluid organisms
 Spleen, Liver, Lung meridians
GROUND: Phlegmatic & Melancholic krases
 Dependant/Tai Yin Earth, Self-Reliant/Yang Ming Metal & Sensitive/Tai Yin Earth biotypes
 all three constitutions

Functions and Uses

1 RESTORES THE STOMACH/*SPLEEN*, INTESTINES, LIVER AND NERVE; AWAKENS THE APPETITE AND RESTORES STRENGTH; DRIES MUCOUS DAMP, ENHANCES THE MEMORY, LIFTS THE SPIRIT AND RIDS DEPRESSION

liver & stomach Qi deficiency: fatigue, lack of appetite, painful digestion
intestines mucous damp (Spleen damp): gurgling distended abdomen, alternating, constipation and diarrhea

nerve deficiency: dull thinking, memory loss, dizziness, poor hearing, tinnitus, nervous depression
EXHAUSTION or DEBILITY due to overwork, illness, e.g. anemia

2 CLEARS STASIS, SEEPS WATER AND PROMOTES URINATION; STIMULATES THE LIVER AND DREDGES THE KIDNEYS; PROMOTES CLEANSING AND PROMOTES LACTATION
liver fluid congestion: edema from waist down, nausea
liver Qi stagnation: depression, constipation, headache
JAUNDICE
kidney Qi stagnation: headaches, dry skin, poor appetite, intermittent pains
general toxemia with rheumatism, arthritis, gout
POOR EYESIGHT
DEFICIENT or poor quality BREASTMILK

3 CAUSES SWEATING, RELEASES THE EXTERIOR AND SCATTERS WIND COLD; RESOLVES FEVER AND PUSHES OUT ERUPTIONS
external wind cold: onset of infections with fatigue, feverishness
ERUPTIVE FEVERS: measles, chickenpox, etc.
REMITTENT FEVERS in Shao Yang stage, incl. malaria

4 DRAINS AND EXPELS VISCOUS PHLEGM, OPENS THE CHEST AND RELIEVES COUGHING
head phlegm congestion: difficult breathing or hearing, sinus congestion, dizziness, heavy head
lung phlegm damp: full cough, wheezing, coughing up thick viscous phlegm
CHRONIC BRONCHITIS, bronchial asthma

5 RESTRAINS INFECTION, ANTIDOTES POISON AND DISSIPATES TUMORS
SLOW HEALING WOUNDS, sores, internal ulcers
INTESTINAL INFECTIONS
TUMORS, CANCER
STINGS, bites
CHILBLAINS

Preparation

USES: The whole herb, including the seeds, drunk in hot INFUSION, will cause sweating to chase wind cold conditions and will bring out eruptions in measles, etc. For all other uses the TINCTURE or FLUID EXTRACT is the optimum preparation.
WASHES and COMPRESSES come into their own in the external treatment of chronic wounds, stings, chilblains and, by traditional use, local inflammations.
DOSAGE: Standard doses are recommended. **Large** doses may cause vomiting and nosebleeds.
CAUTION: Avoid using in acute kidney inflammations or with high gastric acidity.

Notes

Holy thistle, or Blessed thistle, as it is also known, is very much the European equivalent of the American remedy Boneset. Both possess a pronounced *bitter* taste and *stimulate sweating*, among

Yarrow: Class 7

other things. Both these energetic factors have traditionally been used—in all medical systems—to *clear heat* and *resolve fever*. Holy thistle is therefore an important fever herb, and all the more called for where there is **weakness, poor digestion**, and **phlegm** or **damp accumulation.** Like Boneset it is both a Tai Yang and a Shao Yang type **fever** herb when the temperature runs high and the pathogen is severe; it was classically always used for **remittent fevers**, as well as for goading timid surface eruptions into full expression during the course of eruptive fevers.

Equally important, however, and connected with these functions, is Blessed thistle as an important **liver** and **gastrointestinal** remedy, regulating **Spleen** functions in Chinese medicine. It belongs to the Composite family after all, and is a thistle at that. It is adequately equipped with tannins, mucilage, essential oil and various minerals to cope with most types of **deficiency** and **stasis** conditions of these organs. Liver Qi stagnation and liver fluid congestion are vigorously taken command of, the kidneys are dredged and the whole fluid organism, as a result, is regulated. Mucus and phlegm, wherever it is found, are also loosened, thinned and eliminated under its active influence: in the head, lungs, intestines, the urogenital and possibly the lymphatic system. Where mucous damp affects the head, causing dizziness and other neurological symptoms, Holy thistle is the remedy. It was termed *cephalick* and *nervine* by past physicians for this reason, being used additionally to lift depressions and treat severe headaches caused by hepatic congestion.

Being called blessed is a pale reminder of the esteem which this remedy at one time enjoyed.

YARROW

Pharmaceutical name: herba Achilleae
Botanical name: Achillea millefolium L. (N.).
    Compositae)
Ancient names: Chiliophyllon (Gr)
    Ambrosia, Ballusticum, Centifolia,
      Supercilium veneris, Sideritis (Lat)
Other names: Milfoil, Thousandleaf, Nosebleed,
    Devil's nettle, Cammock (Eng)
    Millefeuille, Achillée, Herbe aux
      charpentiers (Fr)
    Schafgarbe, Garbenkraut, Tausendblatt,
      Jungfernaugen, Blutstillkraut (Ge)
Part used: the herb

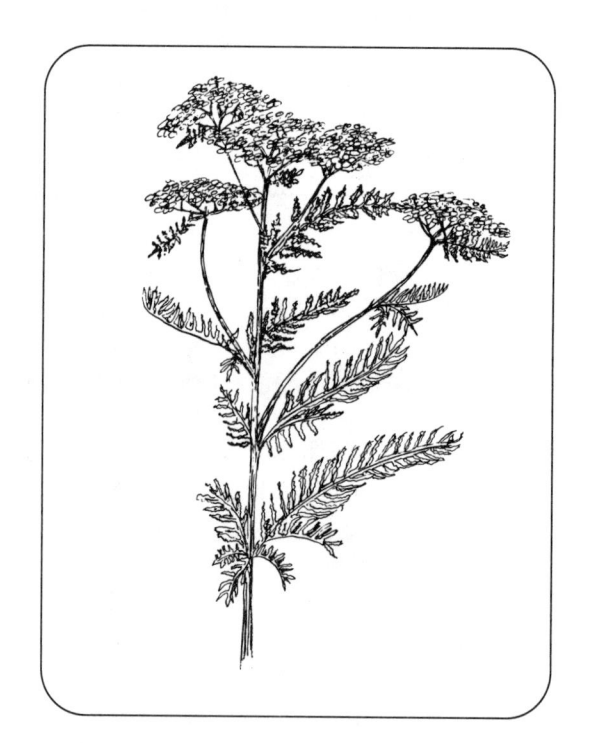

Nature

CATEGORY: mild herb with minimal chronic toxicity
CONSTITUENTS: essential oil (incl. pinenes, borneolic esters, thujones, chamazulene), alkaloidal achillein, anthocyane, apigenin & glucoside, tannins, aconitic/salicilic/acetic/isovalerianic acids, asparagin, inulin, ferment, resin, glycoside, hormonal substance, vit. C, chlorophyll, potassium 48%, calcium, magnesium, iron, phosphoros, silicon
EFFECTIVE QUALITIES
Primary: *Taste:* a bit bitter & astringent & sweet

Class 7: Yarrow

> *Warmth:* neutral with some cooling potential
> *Moisture:* dry

Secondary: restoring, stimulating, relaxing, astringing, decongesting

TROPISM

Organs or parts: circulation, liver, spleen, intestines, kidney, bladder, uterus, blood, endocrine system
Organisms: Air, Fluid
Meridians: Spleen, Liver, Bladder, Kidney, Chong & Ren
Tri Dosas: increases Vayu, decreases Pitta & Kapha

GROUND

Krases/temperaments: Sanguine & Choleric
Biotypes: Expressive/Jue Yin & Tough/Shao Yang
Constitutions: Hematic/Sulphuric/Brown Iris & Mixed/Phosphoric/Grey-Green Iris

Functions and Uses

1 RESTORES THE LIVER, STOMACH/*SPLEEN*, KIDNEYS, BLADDER AND BONE MARROW; REDUCES INFLAMMATION AND LENIFIES IRRITATION

  liver & stomach Qi deficiency: painful slow digestion, no appetite, abdominal distension
  GASTROENTERITIS, COLITIS, CYSTITIS
  genitourinary Qi deficiency (Kidney Qi infirmity): frequent scanty urination, lumbar pain
  NEPHROSIS
  BLADDER IRRITATION in general
  URINARY STONE or SAND
  BONE MARROW DISEASE

2 CLEARS STASIS AND PROMOTES CLEANSING: STIMULATES THE LIVER, DREDGES THE KIDNEYS AND PROMOTES URINATION; PROMOTES THE MENSES, HARMONIZES PREGNANCY AND MENOPAUSE

  liver Qi stagnation: moodiness, sore right side, constipation
  kidney Qi stagnation: headache, fetid stool and urine
  general toxemia: chronic skin rashes, rheumatism of back & shoulders
  uterus Qi stagnation: irregular, delayed or scanty menstruation, breast swelling & tenderness
  ESTROGEN or PROGESTERONE INSUFFICIENCY
  MENOPAUSAL SYNDROME

3 CAUSES SWEATING, RELEASES THE EXTERIOR AND SCATTERS WIND COLD/HEAT; RESOLVES FEVER AND PUSHES OUT ERUPTIONS

  external wind cold/heat: onset of flu or cold with chills, feverishness (either predominant); unrest
  ERUPTIVE FEVER, e.g. measles, chickenpox

4 CIRCULATES THE QI AND LOOSENS CONSTRAINT: RELAXES THE NERVE AND FREES SPASMS

  heart Qi constraint: stabbing cardiac pains, fatigue, palpitations, shortness of breath
  ANGINA PECTORIS
  intestines Qi constraint: abdominal colic and distention, flatulence, kidney or sacral pain
  Liver Yang rising (liver/endocrine disharmony): migraine or headache, vertigo, palpitations, painful eyes
  bladder Qi constraint: scanty, dribbling and frequent urination, anxiety, bedwetting

Yarrow: Class 7

uterus Qi constraint: tension & irritability before onset of menses, dysmenorrhea, PMS

5   CREATES ASTRICTION, ENLIVENS THE BLOOD AND REMOVES CONGESTION; MODERATES THE MENSES AND STAUNCHES BLEEDING; RESOLVES MUCUS, DRIES DAMP AND ARRESTES DISCHARGE

venous blood stagnation: varicose veins, hemorrhoids, phlebitis, thrombosis
uterus blood congestion: pelvic weight and dull pain, copious menstruation
PASSIVE HEMORRHAGING internally or externally, incl. from mouth and nose, in urine or stool; intermenstrual bleeding (metrorrhagia)
LEUCORRHEA, esp. in young women, cervical erosion, spermatorrhea

6   PROMOTES TISSUE REPAIR AND BENEFITS THE SKIN

PUSSY WOUNDS
ULCERS of mouth, throat, leg; peptic ulcers, fistulas, cracked nipples
EYE SORENESS or inflammation
SKIN CONDITIONS in general, dandruff

Preparations

USE: As with so many other herbs, the fresh plant JUICE is the optimal preparation form for Yarrow, with the fresh FREEZE-DRIED a close second. The hot INFUSION is especially good to cause sweating at the early stage of **respiratory infections**, while the TINCTURE serves best for general purposes.

The INFUSION is also much used externally for **women's problems** (HIP BATH, DOUCHE, etc.), for **wounds and ulcers** (SWABS, COMPRESSES, WASHES...). In all cases the best results are obtained with combined internal and external application and with repeated small doses. This is especially true of acute situations like hemorrhage, of course.

DOSAGE: standard doses throughout

CAUTION: Sensitive people in rare cases may present an allergy to Yarrow in the form of rashes. Also, prolonged use on its own over several months may lead to increased skin photosensitivity.

Notes

This ubiquitous wayside plant far exceeds its present position among the herbs that restore the liver/stomach/*Spleen*. Nevertheless, as one of many Composites in this class it excels here simply for its net *regulating* effect on the entire digestive tract. With its *bitter* and *sweet* taste induced *restoring* effects and its tannin caused *calming* action, Yarrow is useful in virtually all possible **digestive** problems, whether used on its own or as support to other botanicals with more specific, one-sided properties. Its *tonic astringent* action which stops both **intestinal** and **genital mucous damp discharges** is merely another aspect of its identity as an all-round *restoring* remedy.

Still, using this Ambrosia is no excuse for bailing out under the wide parachute canopy of its effects. Yarrow is above all a botanical for the **liver**, addressing liver & stomach Qi deficiency, as well as tension caused intestines Qi constraint. As such it fits the Chinese concept of **Liver/Spleen disharmony** to absolute perfection, untangling as it does every possible type of stagnation the liver may be subject to—digestive, menstrual, emotional and urinary. Where Liver Yang rises to the head causing visual and brain disturbnmces, Yarrow will effectively lower it.

It has to be admitted that Yarrow is one of those very versatile, multidirectional agents that would have been forgotten as an "old wives' tale" a long time ago had it not consistently proved effective through use. Moreover, whereas past herbalists such as JOHANN SCHROEDER (1611) valued it as "among the *wound remedies* one of the most egregious," its full scope has only been fully appreciated in modern times. It is gentle, true enough, but reliable. As a *diaphoretic* in fevers it is often combined with other stronger *circulatory stimulants* in wind cold, or *vasorelaxants* in wind heat. Moreover it also *promotes cleansing* and *elimination* through the kidneys (with a gamut of trace minerals to account for it), hence is traditionally used in both acute and chronic **rheumatic** and **neuralgic** complaints, especially of the upper trunk. As *nerve relaxant* Yarrow is used in Qi constraint patterns of many organs, especially of the heart. Here vascular spasms are relieved and cardiac neurosis eased (due to its achillein content).

Reliable is also the key word for Yarrow as a **gynecological** remedy. As much as White deadnettle or Life root it qualifies as a universal *regulator* of female reproductive functions from pre-puberty to postmenopause. It is an outstanding woman's ally, constant like the plant itself, which endures into the autumn months. Besides the direct hormonal influence of estrogen, Yarrow achieves this regulating effect through a comprehensive action on the uterus, the blood and circulation. As a *uterine stimulant* it relieves delayed, painful menses with swollen breasts. As an *astringent venous tonic* and *uterine decongestant* Yarrow not only enlivens and thins the venous return, but also relieves uterine and pelvic blood congestion, restraining flooding periods and metrorrhagia in so doing. As a local *relaxant* in Qi constraint type syndromes, it assists spasmodic dysmenorrhea with painful periods. The end result is a rebalancing of menstrual functions in almost every way possible, bringing relief in all types of premenstrual syndromes with their long retinue of symptoms.

TANSY

Pharmaceutical name: herba seu flos Tanaceti
Botanical name: Tanacetum vulgare L. (N.O. Compositae)
Ancient name: Artemisia, Lepophyllo, Athanasia, Tanesia (Gr)
   Athanasia vulgaris, Ambrosia, Sanacum (Lat)
Other names: Bitter buttons, Bachelor's buttons, English cost, Parsley/Scented fern, Ginger plant, Hindheal (Eng)
   Tanaisie, Herbe amère, Barbotine, Herbe d'effort (Fr)
   Rainfarn, Wurmkraut, Mutterkraut, Kraftkraut Donnerblume (Ge)
Part used: the herb or flower

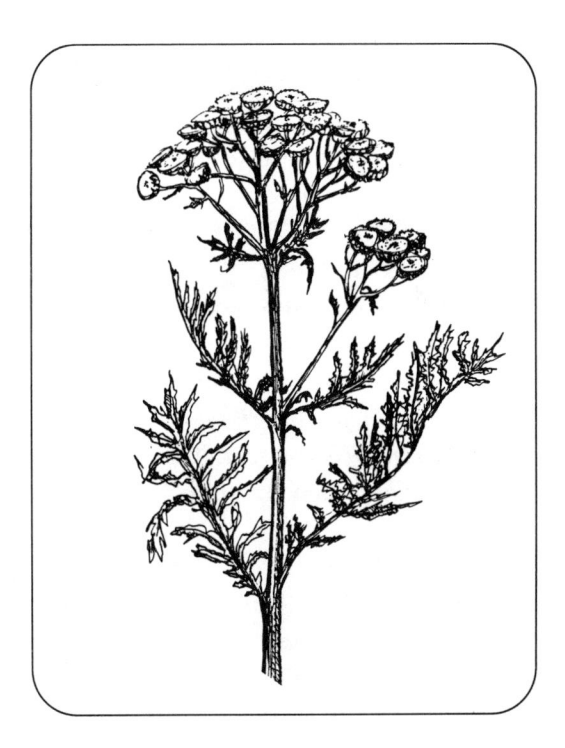

Nature

CATEGORY: medium-strength herb with some chronic toxicity
CONSTITUENTS: ess. oil (incl. thujone 70%), bitter resin (tanacetin), bitter extractive gum, chlorophyll, borneol, stearine, wax, tannin, lead oxydes, tanacetic/gallic/citric/malic/oxalic/arabinic acid
EFFECTIVE QUALITIES
Primary: bitter, a bit pungent, cool, dry
Secondary: restoring, stimulating, relaxing

Tansy: Class 7

TROPISM: stomach, intestines, liver, kidneys, bladder, nerves, skin
Air, Fluid organisms
Spleen, Liver, Kidney, Bladder, Chong & Ren meridians
GROUND: Choleric & Sanguine krases
Tough/Generous & Expressive/Jue Yin biotypes
Hematic/Sulphuric/Brown Iris constitution

Functions and Uses

1. **RESTORES THE STOMACH/*SPLEEN*, AWAKENS THE APPETITE AND RESTORES STRENGTH; RESOLVES MUCUS AND DRIES DAMP; KILLS AND EXPELS PARASITES**

    Spleen Qi deficiency: fatigue, no appetite, loose stool
    genitourinary damp cold: white leucorrhea, backache
    WEAKNESS, debility, due to overwork, convalescence, etc.
    PINWORMS, tapeworms, especially in children

2. **STIMULATES THE LIVER AND DREDGES THE KIDNEYS; STIMULATES THE UTERUS, PROMOTES AND HARMONIZES MENSTRUATION**

    liver Qi stagnation: painful swollen abdomen and side, nausea, fatigue, jaundice
    liver fluid congestion: water retention from waist downward, or generalised, nausea
    uterus Qi stagnation: scanty or delayed menses with purple clots, dull pain before onset; breast swelling
    DYSMENORRHEA, amenorrhea
    kidney Qi stagnation: malaise, skin rashes, smelly urine
    BLADDER SAND or stones

3. **CIRCULATES THE QI AND LOOSENS CONSTRAINT: RELAXES THE NERVE AND FREES SPASMS**

    Qi constraint with excess conditions: emotional or mental tension, nervousness, irritability
    kidney & intestines Qi constraint (Liver/Spleen disharmony): abdominal cramps or spasms, indigestion with flatulence, worsening with emotion
    uterus Qi constraint: pelvic cramps before and during menstruation, tension, agitation, PMS
    bladder Qi constraint: difficult, obstructed, or frequent scanty urination
    nerve excess conditions (sthenia) in general, incl. sciatica, epilepsy, convulsions

4. **CAUSES SWEATING, RELEASES THE EXTERIOR, SCATTERS WIND HEAT AND RESOLVES FEVER**

    external wind heat: onset of cold or flu with fever, restlessness, irritability
    REMITTENT FEVERS in the Shao Yang stage

5. **REDUCES INFLAMMATION AND SWELLING, PROMOTES TISSUE REPAIR, CLEARS CONTUSION AND BENEFITS THE SKIN**

    INFLAMMATON of eyes, skin; sunburn
    TUMORS, lumps (e.g. breasts)
    WOUNDS, ulcers, abscesses, varicose veins
    BRUISES, contusions, sprains
    ERUPTIVE SKIN conditions incl. acne
    SKIN deformities and blemishes incl. freckles

Class 7: Tansy

Preparation

USE: Tansy is a valuable remedy both internally and externally. Either the **herb** or **flowerhead** may be used; the latter contains up to 1.5% of the essential oil, more than four times the amount found in the herb without flowers. The whole flowers, if these are used, should therefore be TINCTURED or INFUSED fresh or the ESSENTIAL OIL itself extracted through distillation or maceration. The latter would place Tansy squarely among the botanicals that circulate the Qi and loosen constraint (function 3 here), and could be used like Wormwood essential oil, and with the same caution. The TINCTURE (of herb or flower) is overall more effective than the INFUSION; even so, the latter makes an invaluable *bitter tonic* in all **digestive deficient** conditions. Either may be used to make LOTIONS, WASHES, DOUCHES, SQUATTING INHALATIONS, etc., as required. Tansy **seeds** are more effective against **worms** than the herb: both may be used for hot abdominal COMPRESSES and SUPPOSITORIES in addition to oral taking in this condition. Alternately, the POWDER may be taken on an empty stomach. In all these cases it is better combined with a *laxative,* and with another *vermifuge* such as Wormwood.

Tansy was traditionally used to SMUDGE or FUMIGATE places for protection. Tansy and Elder leaves together can distance flies, as well as afford topical pain relief in general.

DOSAGE: TINCTURE of **herb**: 2-4 ml or 50-100 drops
            INFUSION of **herb**: 20-30 g/ (2/3-1 oz) for a day's supply
            INFUSION of **seed** for worms: 1 tsp per cup, taken before breakfast
            POWDER of seeds for worms: 1/2 to 1 tsp before breakfast

While standard doses are safe for the **herb**, 1/2 or 1/4 doses are advised for the **flower**—esp. at the beginning.

CAUTION: If taken continuously in full doses on its own, several days' break are advised every ten days, as Tansy is a medium-strength herb. Its thujone content also commends it for strict dosage: overdoses have caused vomiting, coma, convulsions and even death.

Being *uterine stimulant,* Tansy is contraindicated during pregnancy.

Notes

Tansy with its striking yellow "buttons" is therapeutically multifaceted and has similar uses to other members of its family. Nothing quite replaces it, however, when a certain combination of disharmonies coalesces. These are of a more **chronic** nature, involving **deficiency**, **stagnation** and **constraint** at the same time.

A typical case where Tansy would be appropriate involves elements of chronic Spleen Qi deficiency with exhaustion, Qi constraint with emotional tension and internal spasms, and poor liver and kidney functioning. Tansy is a *digestive bitter tonic* more than anything else, perhaps, with an *astringent tonic* influence on the mucosa with chronic damp cold catarrhal discharges; where these involve chronic infections, it is also useful, like Blessed thistle. At the same time its *nervine relaxant* properties allow it to treat painful spasms and cramps, especially digestive and menstrual. In most cases of emotional holding with nervous unrest, Tansy's *diaphoretic relaxant* effects should be activated by drinking it hot to cause free perspiration, also excellent for fevers with the same conditions (essential oil + bitters + acids). It is not as strong as Black cohosh in similar conditions, but adequate for average cases.

Nor should Tansy be forgotten as a woman's friend, as one of the *Motherworts,* no less. Not only menstrual disharmonies with **Qi constraint** and **stagnation** come under its beneficial influence, but also, as with Yarrow, breast lumps and masses, and possibly tumors. Like Yarrow, Tansy is ideal for those poor quality estrogen conditions, so prevalent in Brown Iris Jue Yin or

Feverfew: Class 7

Shao Yang types, presenting mental and emotional unrest and anxiety in addition to physical PMS symptoms, for which acupuncture would select points such as Li 2, Kd 5, Sp 8, Gb 41, CV 3 and Bl 32. In tincture form, both Tansy and Yarrow are no mean stand-ins for the Chinese *Xiang fu, rhizoma Cyperi,* where spasmodic dysmenorrhea is concerned.

FEVERFEW

Pharmaceutical name: herba Chrysanthemi parthenii
Botanical name: Chrysanthemum parthenium L.
    (N.O. Compositae)
Ancient names: Parthenion (Gr)
    Matricaria, Febrifuga (Lat)
Other names: Featherfew, Featherfowl,
    Midsummer daisy, Bertram, Nosebleed,
    Mayweed, Whitewort (Eng)
    Espargoutte (Fr)
    Bertram, Mutterkraut, Metram (Ge)
Part used: the herb; also the root

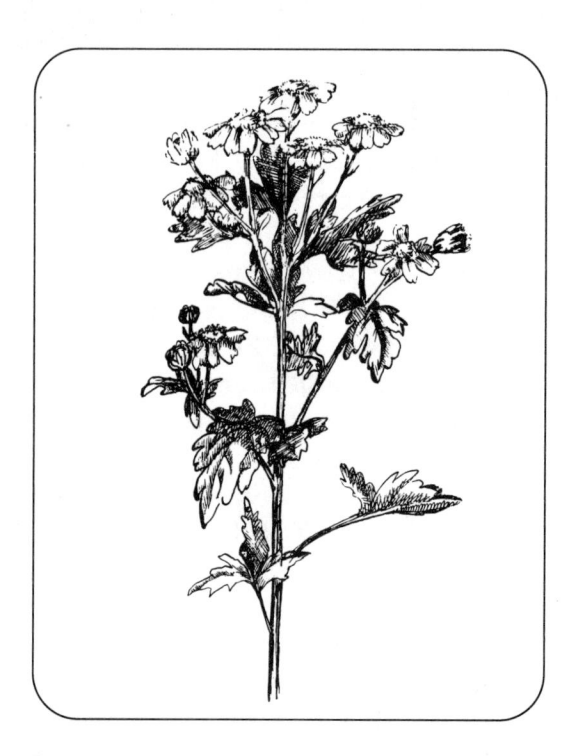

Nature

CATEGORY: mild herb with minimal chronic toxicity
CONSTITUENTS: essential oil, bitter resin, inulin (in root), pyrethrin

This remedy is virtually identical with TANSY, herba Tanaceti, (p. 282) in its nature, functions, uses and preparations, with the following differences:

1   Feverfew has in recent years been shown to have specific *antimigraine* activity, unlike Tansy. While both plants are used for treating **liver Qi stagnation**, Feverfew has this extra bonus to offer in the context of treating the liver.

2   Feverfew herb and root are used in **neuralgic** and **myalgic** or **damp/cold** obstruction conditions such as trigeminal neuralgia, sciatic neuralgia, as well as other nerve related disorders such as paralysis, epilepsy and convulsions.

3   Feverfew's *anticatarrhal* property is most noticeable when applied to treating **head damp cold** and **genitourinary cold** patterns.

Notes

Featherfew, as this plant was originally and most widely known in England from the delicacy of its corolla, is one of the many Composites used in herbal medicine since Greek days. Like Yarrow, Camomile and Tansy (among others), it was also called *Motherwort* in Europe since it treats disharmonies of the mother, meaning *womb*. The herbalist JOHN PARKINSON in his major herbal of 1629 makes this clear: "It is chiefly used for the diseases of the mother, whether it be the stranglings or the risings of the mother, or the hardness or inflammations of the same." We must remember that he is speaking not only as a medical practitioner, but also as an extraordinary researcher in ancient texts who devotes up to half a folio page or more, if neccessary, to discussing the identification and taxonomy of plant remedies.

Featherfew should be seen primarily as a **woman's friend**. Like Tansy it is able to treat uterus Qi constraint ("stranglings or risings") with painful, cramping periods and other possible PMS symptoms, and uterus Qi stagnation ("hardness"), mainly with irregular or delayed clotted flow. PARKINSON also advises a SQUATTING INHALATION at this time, using a hot infusion. Clearly the same *stimulant, relaxant,* and *antispasmodic* properties that are found in Yarrow are also here in evidence.

Nevertheless we are dealing also with a *febrifuge* plant, witness its name as also its pronounced bitter taste. Containing as it probably does essential oil in addition to bitter compounds, it is best used in wind heat acute fevers and Shao Yang remittent ones. Like Tansy it is a *relaxant cooling diaphoretic.*

Energetically speaking, however, the *bitter* taste is two-edged. It not only clears heat but also restores the entire system via the Spleen, or digestive activity, all the more so since it is somewhat *pungent* as well as *bitter,* and therefore a more versatile *Spleen tonic*. It is here that its liver opening activity also unfolds, with the much publicized *antimigraine* effect. Clearly, its *nerve relaxant* effect, so useful in Qi constraint and wind damp/cold type conditions, here also comes into play.

BARBERRY

Pharmaceutical name: cortex radicis Berberis
Botanical name: Berberis vulgaris L. (N.O. Berberidaceae)
Ancient names: Crespinus, Spina acida, Oxycantha (Lat)
Other names: Barbaryn, Guild tree, Jaundice berry, Pipperidge bush, Woodsour, Maiden barberry (Eng)
   Epine-vinette, Vinettier commun (Fr)
   Sauerdorn, Berberize, Reisselbeeren, Versich (Ge)
Part used: the root bark, also the berry, *fructus Berberis,* and the leaf, *folium Berberis*

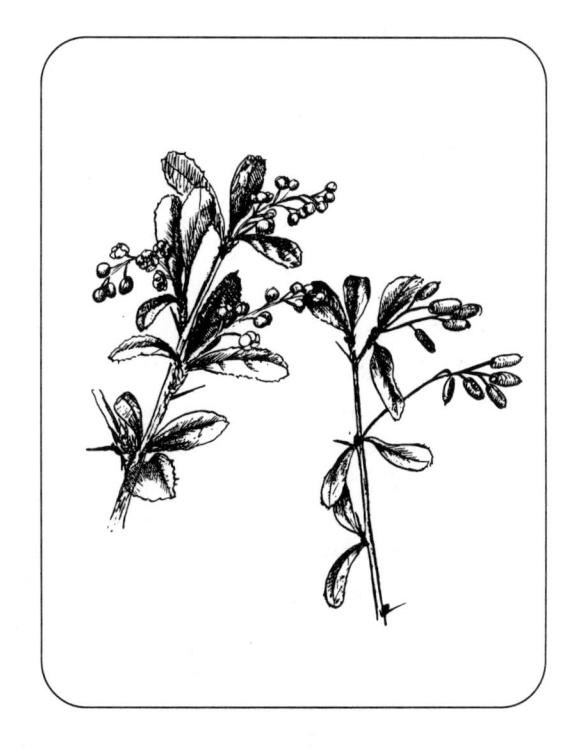

Nature

CATEGORY: mild herb with minimal chronic toxicity
CONSTITUENTS: alkaloids (incl. berberin, oxycanthin, berberrubin, palmatin, isotetrandin), chelidonic acid, tannins, gum, resin, wax
EFFECTIVE QUALITIES
Primary: *Taste:* bitter & astringent
   Warmth: cold
   Moisture: dry

Barberry: Class 7

Secondary: astringing, decongesting, relaxing, restoring
sinking movement

TROPISM

Organs or parts: liver, gall bladder, spleen, intestines, blood
Organisms: Warmth
Meridians: Spleen, Stomch, Liver, Gall Bladder
Tri Dosas: decreases Pitta & Kapha, increases Vayu

GROUND

Krases/temperaments: Choleric & Sanguine
Biotypes: Industrious/Tai Yang, Expressive/Jue Yin & Charming/Yang Ming Earth
Constitutions: all three

Functions and Uses

1 RESTORES THE LIVER, STOMACH AND INTESTINES/*SPLEEN*, AWAKENS THE APPETITE AND RESTORES STRENGTH

Spleen Qi deficiency: weakness, poor appetite, stuffy chest and abdomen, diarrhea
liver & stomach Qi deficiency: slow painful digestion, constipation, lethargy
FATIGUE due to anemia, convalescence, malnutrition, etc.

2 BREAKS UP OBSTRUCTION, PROMOTES BOWEL MOVEMENT AND REMOVES STAGNANCY: STIMULATES THE LIVER AND GALL BLADDER, PROMOTES BILE FLOW; DREDGES THE KIDNEYS, PROMOTES URINATION AND CLEANSING

liver Qi stagnation: moodiness, swollen sore right flank, midback pain, jaundice, constipation
kidney Qi stagnation: skin rashes, scanty urination, static or migratory pains
general toxemia with arthritis, rheumatism, gout
BILLARY & KIDNEY STONES

3 CREATES ASTRICTION, DRIES MUCOUS DAMP AND ARRESTS DISCHARGE; REDUCES INFLAMMATION, RESTRAINS INFECTION AND CLEARS TOXINS; ENLIVENS THE BLOOD, REMOVES CONGESTION AND MODERATES THE MENSES

intestines damp heat: urgent defecation with burning, blood in stools
ENTERITIS, dysentery
genitourinary damp heat: veneral infections with purulent yellow discharge
MOUTH, THROAT & GUM INFECTIONS, loose teeth, spongy sore gums, mouth ucers and sores, sore throat
venous blood stagnation: varicose veins, hemorrhoids, constipation
uterus blood congestion: early or copious menses with dull pelvic pain and weight

4 CLEARS HEAT, CALMS THE LIVER, GALL BLADDER AND STOMACH

liver fire: bursting headache, thirst, irritability
INFECTIOUS HEPATITIS, jaundice, cholecystitis, biliary colic
stomach fire: ravenous hunger, thirst for cold water, mouth ulcers, bleeding gums

Preparation

USE: The DECOCTION is suitable for WASHES, GARGLING and for *cooling* and *astringing* purposes generally; the TINCTURE and FLUID EXTRACT have the widest range of effects.
The **berry** and **leaf** are *astringent sour cool* in quality and would probably be useful with genital

Class 7: Barberry

discharges to "consolidate sperm" and other discharges in deficient Qi and deficient Yin conditions. They are also used in lung phlegm heat patterns with purulent yellow expectoration, etc.

DOSAGE: standard doses throughout

Smaller doses taken unsweetened are sufficient for the *bitter tonic* effect of function 1.

CAUTION: Use of this herb on its own should be avoided during pregnancy, as its energy is strongly downward moving. Discontinue if—as in rare cases possible—the TINCTURE causes nosebleeding or dizziness.

Notes

Having accepted the considerations detailed under *Oregon grape,* both Barberry and Oregon grape root may in general be considered therapeutically identical.

Berberis primarily is a good *bitter* liver stomach *digestive restorative,* a *Spleen tonic* in short. Here its action is not a cooling one, but rather a *stimulating* one on the **digestive** and **glandular system**, promoting nutrient assimilation and generating strength, both basic functions of the Chinese Spleen.

However, Barberry is more than a sweet and simple *tonic:* it will treat the results of Spleen Qi deficiency as much as its root causes. By stimulating all secretions it helps break up and move out toxic intestinal obstructions of whatever kind, addressing **stagnant** and **congestive** syndromes of the **liver, gall bladder**, **stomach** and **intestines**. In short, it is suited for chronic conditions that through **deficiency** have turned into **stagnation**. Even when stagnation and its concommitant irritation turns into **heat**, as in stomach or liver fire, Barberry is still in the league.

In second place, Barberry represents an excellent *(sour) cold astringent* and *blood decongestant* à la Class 14, dealing not only with **infections** with **inflammation** and **discharge** of the **damp heat** variety, but also with **blood stagnation** in general. Here it enlivens the blood, relieves venous or pelvic blood congestion, and even lends tone to the veins themselves. The alkaloid *berberin* in particular is thought responsible for these effects, with a little help from the tannins. The similarity of some of these uses with the Chinese root *Huang lien, rhizoma Coptidis,* which also contains the alkaloid berberin, should not be overlooked. Inferences can be made about both when their remaining indications are considered—inferences, however, that await the actual evidence of use before any definite conclusions can be reached.

Barberry and Oregon grape combine well with other herbs that either restore the Spleen, promote bowel movement or clear heat. With Spleen Qi deficiency with damp cold in the intestines and with loose stool and fatigue, for example, Barberry may be combined with Angelica root or Lovage root; with liver stasis with constipation it would go well with a *cold laxative* such as Cascara sagrada; in full heat conditions with intestinal stasis stronger *laxatives* such as Senna or Rhubarb may be combined with it.

Oregon grape root: Class 7

OREGON GRAPE ROOT

Pharmaceutical name: cortex radicis Mahoniae
Botanical name: Mahonia repens Webber (syn. *Berberis aquifolium* Pursh. (N.O. Berberidaceae)
Other names: Mountain grape, Holly grape, Creeping/Trailing mahonia, California barberry (Am)
Part used: the root bark

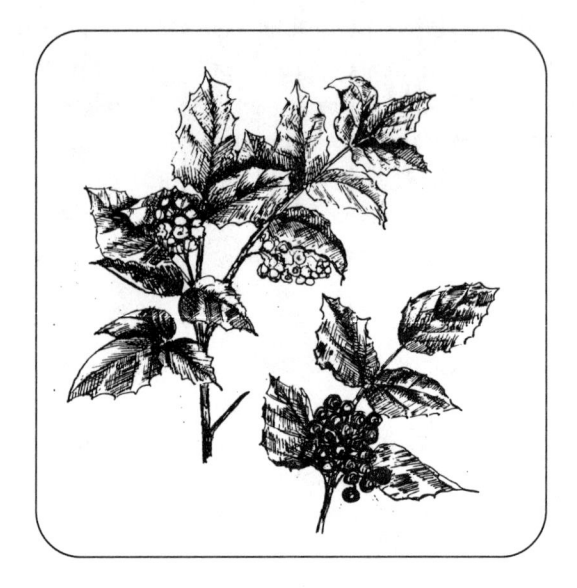

Nature

CATEGORY: mild herb with minimal chronic toxicity
CONSTITUENTS: alkaloids (incl. berberine, oxyberberine, oxyacanthin, berbamine), tannins, resins
EFFECTIVE QUALITIES
Primary: bitter & astringent, cold, dry
Secondary: restoring, astringing, decongesting

This remedy is identical to BARBERRY, *cortex radicis Berberis* (p. 285) in all its nature, functions, uses and preparations, with the following significant differences:

1   Oregon grape is somewhat more strongly *restorative* on the entire sytem than Barberry. This on one hand is due to its gentle *thyroid stimulant* effect which will increase metabolic rate (MOORE, 1986). On the other hand, it has a greater *liver restorative* effect which increases anabolic functions as much as catabolic ones. Hence Mountain grape in small doses should be used especially in liver, stomach & Spleen Qi deficiency conditions with **chronic fatigue.**

2   Oregon grape is more **liver centered** than Barberry, being used in both deficient and excess type liver conditions. As a result it also excels in **dry skin eruptions** due to liver congestion, especially with excess alkalinity present. It is also said to be specific to **chronic hepatitis B,** where it may be combined with others such as Dandelion, Milk thistle or Celandine according to sign and symptom conformation.

3   Oregon grape root is less effective in clearing infectious conditions, such as intestinal damp heat, and venous blood stagnation than Barberry due to a lesser quantity of the alkaloid berberine. In other words its *antiseptic, anti-inflammatory* and *blood decongestive* actions are weaker; this again confirms Oregon grape as a primarily *restorative* botanical.

CAUTION: Avoid in hyperthyroid conditions, e.g. with rising Liver Yang syndromes, and on its own during pregnancy.

Class 7: Fennel

Herbs to Restore and Strengthen the Urogenital Organs

FENNEL

Pharmaceutical name: fructus Foeniculi
Botanical name: Foeniculum vulgare Miller (N.O. Umbelliferae)
Ancient Names: Marathoron (Gr)
    Foeniculum, Maratrum (Lat)
Other names: Sweet fennel, Wild fennel, Large fennel (Eng)
    Fenouil (Fr)
    Fenchel, Brotanis (Ge)
Part used: the fruit; also the root, *radix Foeniculi*

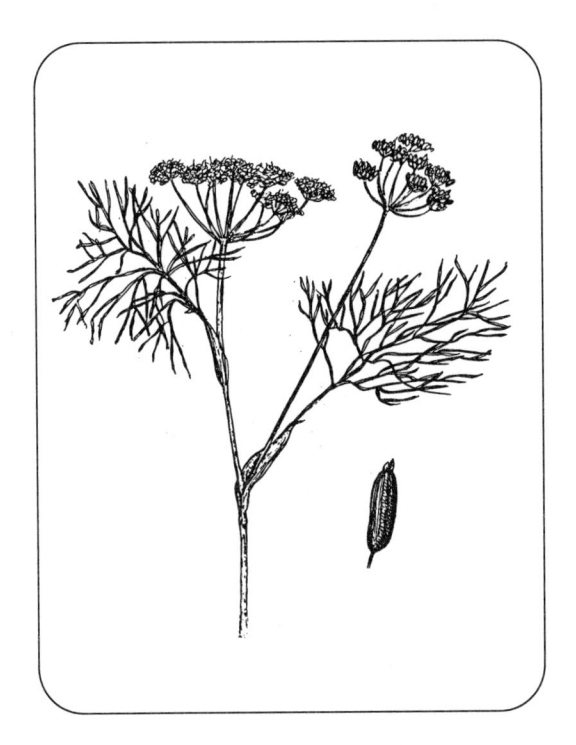

Nature

CATEGORY: mild herb with minimal chronic toxicity
CONSTITUENTS: ess. oil 2-6% (incl. anethone, fenchone, estragol, terpenes, fenone, anesic aldehyde), fixed oil 12-28%, sugar, silica
EFFECTIVE QUALITIES
Primary: a bit pungent & sweet, warm, dry
Secondary: stimulating, relaxing, restoring, astringing
TROPISM: bladder, kidney, stomach, intestines, lungs, uterus
    Air, Fluid organisms
    Kidney, Bladder, Spleen, Chong & Ren meridians
GROUND: Melancholic krasis
    Sensitive/Tai Yin Metal biotype
    Lymphatic/Carbonic/Blue Iris constitution

Functions and Uses

1 RESTORES AND DREDGES THE URINARY ORGANS, LENIFIES IRRITATION, PROMOTES URINATION AND EXPELS STONES; BENEFITS VISION AND CLEARS THE EYES

bladder Qi deficiency (Kidney Qi infirmity): frequent scanty urination, bedwetting, urination at night, lumbar backache
kidney Qi stagnation: headaches, poor appetite, malaise, fetid orange urine
GOUT, OBESITY
GENERAL BLADDER IRRITATION due to high uric acid or stone
HIGH URIC ACID in urine
URINARY SAND or STONE

Fennel: Class 7

        POOR EYESIGHT, spots in vision
        EYE INFLAMMATIONS, e.g. conjunctivitis

2   STIMULATES THE UTERUS, PROMOTES MENSTRUATION AND LACTATION, BENEFITS THE BREASTS

uterus Qi stagnation: irregular or delayed menstruation with clots
uterus cold: absent or delayed scanty menses, cramps
ESTROGEN INSUFFICIENCY with deficiency menstrual problems
AMENORRHEA
INSUFFICIENT BREAST MILK
BREAST CONDITIONS: engorged breasts, breast lumps, curdled breast milk

3   WARMS AND INVIGORATES THE STOMACH/*SPLEEN* AND INTESTINES; DRIES MUCOUS DAMP, REMOVES STAGNANCY AND FREES SPASMS, CLEARS FLATUS AND SETTLES THE STOMACH

stomach cold: constant dull abdominal pain better with food, regurgitation of sour clear liquid
intestines mucous damp (Spleen damp): no appetite, gurgling abdomen, colic
intestines Qi stagnation: swollen painful abdomen, hiccups, nausea, slow digestion
NAUSEA & VOMITING in all conditions
GASTROCARDIAC SYNDROME

4   STIMULATES THE LUNGS AND EXPELS PHLEGM, RELAXES THE BRONCHI, OPENS THE CHEST AND RELIEVES WHEEZING

lung phlegm damp: productive full cough with thin white phlegm, wheezing
BRONCHIAL ASTHMA, WHEEZING, asthmatic breathing in any condition
HOARSENESS, VOICE LOSS

5   ACTIVATES IMMUNITY, ANTIDOTES POISONS AND CLEARS PARASITES; RESOLVES CONTUSION AND BENEFITS THE SKIN

PREVENTIVE in influenza
POISONING from mushrooms or herbs
INTESTINAL PARASITES
CONTUSIONS, bruises, sprains
SKIN DEFORMITIES or blemishes
LOOSE, spongy gums
DEAFNESS

Preparation

USE: Fennel **root** in DECOCTION or TINCTURE should be used for best effects on the urinary system. If the **fruits** (i.e. seed) are used, these should be crushed in a mortar and pestle or ground in a coffee-grinder to make an INFUSION (always covered to retain the volatile oils). They make an excellent EYEBATH for inflamed conditions.

If available, the pure ESSENTIAL OIL (itself made from the fruit) is no mean alternative, since it is Fennel's main active constituent. It excels at functions 5 above, which include *immune stimulation* when flu spreads around.

SALVES, LOTIONS, MOUTHWASHES, etc., can also be prepared.

DOSAGE: DECOCTION or TINCTURE of the **root**: standard doses

ESSENTIAL OIL: 1-5 drops in some warm water
INFUSION: one tsp of ground seeds per cup, after or between meals.
CAUTION: Fennel is forbidden during prgnancy as it stimulates the uterus.

Notes

In Mediterranean countries every part of this lovely plant has played as large a role in healing as it still does in cooking. It is not surprising, then, that a popular Italian physician such as PIERANDREA MATTIOLI devotes so much space in his herbal of 1611 to his native plant Fennel. He fills several large folio pages with excellent formulas based on this remedy for **urinary, bronchial** and **digestive** complaints.

Due to its successful use in a variety of conditions, Fennel is a difficult botanical to pin down to one category. In the last 200 years Fennel seed has usually found a place among the *carminatives* that relieve flatus and distention, as one of the Galenic four greater warming seeds. However, we feel this does this important remedy injustice. Here an earlier emphasis is preferred: GALEN, after all, established Fennel **root** as one of the four opening roots, with Asparagus, Parsley and Celery. Since its fruit has much in common both biochemically and therapeutically with the root, it is equally an important remedy for obstructed urination (anuria). With its *sweet* taste, Fennel is a *urogenital restorer, stimulant, lenifier* and *cleanser,* used especially in bladder Qi deficiency with difficult urination, irritation and stones, and with *lao lin* type urinary disharmony, acting along the lines of acupuncture points Bl 22 & 28, CV 3, St 28 and Lu 7. In this area, sluggish or deficient menstrual syndromes also benefit all the more due to its estrogenic effect.

And there is further reason to regard Fennel in first place as a kidney and bladder tonic: its property of improving eyesight, clearing floaters in vision, and so on. Historical texts fully document this, giving vision strengthening formulas besides. Eye inflammations are also resolved with its external use.

Like Aniseed, Fennel is also a **lung** and **throat** herb, a *lenitive* and *stimulant expectorant,* and may be used symptomatically for hoarseness or wheezing or in cold phlegm conditions. Likewise, its *pungent warm dry* qualities also come to effect in the intestinal tract, where **stagnation** and **cold** predominate. Key symptoms here are a feeling of fullness with griping or dull abdominal pains. WILLIAM SALMON's comments at the turn of the eighteenth century are flowery but accurate when he says, "It is a singular stomachick and cordial; it refreshes, comforts and strengthens the Stomach after an admirable manner, taking away Vomiting, Nauseating, want of Appetite and Indigestion…"

Saw palmetto: Class 7

SAW PALMETTO

Pharmaceutical name: fructus Serenoae
Botanicals name: Serenoa serrulata L. (syn.
      Sabal serrulata L.) (N.O. Palmaceae)
Other names: Dwarf palm, Sabal berries (Am)
Part used: the fruit

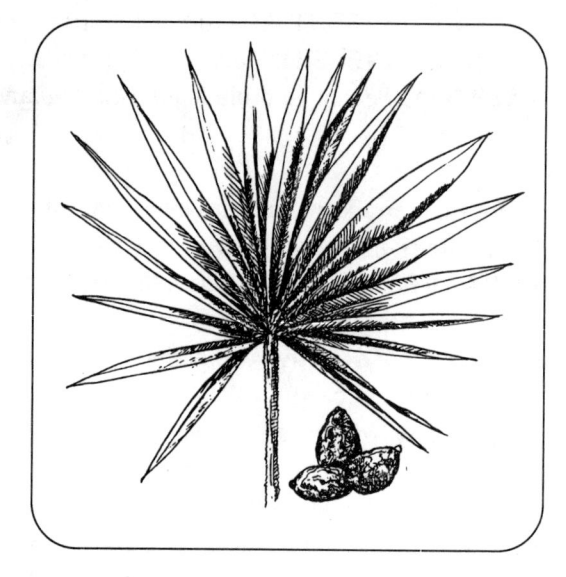

Nature

CATEGORY: mild herbs with minimal chronic topxicity
CONSTITUENTS: ess. oil 1%, steroids (incl. ß-sitosterol), alkaloid, resins, tannins, fixed oil
EFFECTIVE QUALITIES
Primary: a bit sweet & oily & astringent & pungent, warm, dry
Secondary: restoring, stimulating
TROPISM: reproductive & urinary organs, nerves, thyroid
      Air organism
      Kidney, Spleen, Chong & Ren meridians
GROUND: Melancholic krasis
      Sensitive/Tai Yin Metal & Burdened/Shao Yin biotypes
      Lymphatic/Carbonic/Blue Iris constitution

Functions and Uses

1 RESTORES AND STRENGTHENS THE GENITAL ORGANS; ENHANCES SEXUAL DESIRE AND PROMOTES CONCEPTION; CLEARS INFLAMMATION AND RELIEVES PAIN; PROMOTES LACTATION
   Kidney Yang deficiency with no sexual desire, fatigue
   uterus Qi deficiency with scanty, delayed menstruation
   Liver & Kidney Qi depletion with backache, fatigue, irregular, variable, scanty menses
   IMPOTENCE, FRIGIDITY, INFERTILITY, STERILITY
   PROSTATE & OVARIAN ENLARGEMENT with throbbing pain
   SALPINGITIS, ovaritis, orchitis, etc.
   SCANTY BREAST MILK, small breasts

2 RESTORES THE *SPLEEN*, NERVE AND THYROID; AWAKENS THE APPETITE, PROMOTES WEIGHT GAIN AND GENERATES STRENGTH
   Spleen Qi deficiency with no appetite, fatigue, loose stool
   WEIGHT LOSS
   nerve deficiency with fatigue, nervousness, weakness
   THYROID INSUFFICIENCY

3   RESTORES THE LUNGS AND OPENS THE VOICE; EXPELS PHLEGM AND RELIEVES WHEEZING

CATARRHAL LUNG CONDITIONS with or without infection and wheezing
VOICE LOSS

Preparation

USE: Sabal berry may be DECOCTED or, better still, TINCTURED for best results.
DOSAGE: standard doses throughout

Notes

The dark red berries of the small Saw palmetto tree of the Southeastern American States have long been valued for their *tonic* properties. Exactly what kind of *restorative* they are now needs some redefining.

The observation that animals grow heavier and stronger when feeding on these berries goes back to Southern Black experience with livestock. Having made the same experience themselves when taking these berries, the Blacks were soon copied by the Whites in this lucky find. By the 1870's JOHN LLOYD, GOSS, HALE and other practitioners were busy documenting the therapeutic effects of this plant. They reported on its ability to increase **nutrient assimilation**, promote **weight gain**, *restore* and *relax the* **nerves** (as *nerve trophorestorative*), restore the **reproductive** system and the **respiratory mucosa**. Moreover, at the present time **thyroid** *toning* properties seem evident, at least as regards sexual development and behaviour (MOWREY, 1987).

Given all this, Saw palmetto emerges very much as a general *tonic* in a variety of deficiency conditions. Energetically speaking, however, and using the language of Chinese syndromes, the two conditions that most require its *sweet astringent warm* qualities are Spleen Qi deficiency and Liver & Kidney depletion. In both syndromes the whole gamut of symptoms are relievd, with a special emphasis on relieving fatigue and gently arousing the digestive and sexual appetite. With the latter syndrome Saw palmetto acts in the same way as acupuncture points Kd 5, Li 5, CV 3, Kd 13 and Bl 23 would in treating irregular or scanty periods.

Whatever deficiency conditions it is used for, Saw palmetto combines easily and well with other botanicals of this class. With inflammatory conditions of the reproductive organs it may be backed up with others such as Marigold, Pipsissewa and Echinacea.

Buchu: Class 7

BUCHU

Pharmaceutical name: folium Barosmae
Botanical name: Barosma betulina L. (N.O. Rutaceae)
Other names: Buchu (Fr)
　　Buchublätter, Duftstrauch, Starkduft (Ge)
Part used: the leaf

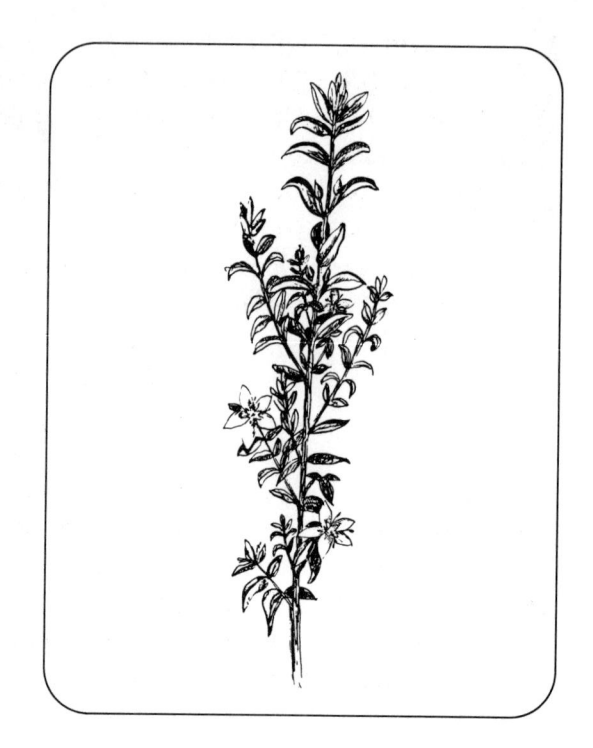

Nature

CATEGORY: mild herb with minimal chronic toxicity
CONSTITUENTS: ess. oil up to 2.5% (incl. diosphenol 25-40%, limonene, menthone, barosma camphor), mucilage, gum, flavonoid (hesperidin), resin, glycoside (diosmin or barosmin), vit. B1, phosphorus, magnesium
EFFECTIVE QUALITIES
Primary: pungent & bitter, a bit astringent, hot, dry
Secondary: stimulating, restoring, astringing
　　stabilizing movement
TROPISM: urinary & reproductive organs, intestines
　　Warmth, Air organisms
　　Kidney, Spleen, Bladder meridians
GROUND: Melancholic krasis
　　Burdened/Shao Yin biotype
　　Lymphatic/Carbonic/Blue Iris constitution

Functions and Uses

1 RESTORES, STRENGTHENS AND RELAXES THE UROGENITAL ORGANS, LENIFIES IRRITATION AND HARMONISES URINATION

　genitourinary Qi deficiency (Kidney Qi infirmity) with frequent, scanty, dribbling or incontinent urination, bedwetting
　bladder Qi constraint with frequent painful urination
　BLADDER IRRITATION due to any cause incl. gravel & stone
　PROSTATE IRRITATION and congestion, aching penis

2 WARMS AND INVIGORATES THE UROGENITAL ORGANS AND INTESTINES
　genitourinary cold (Kidney Yang deficiency) with lumbar pain, copious pale urination,

Class 7: Buchu

leucorrhea, chilliness
intestines cold (Spleen Yang deficiency) with poor digestion, flatus and colic
Spleen & Kidney Yang deficiency with digestive & urogenital symptoms above

3   RESTRAINS INFECTION AND CLEARS TOXINS, DRIES MUCOUS DAMP AND ARRESTS DISCHARGE

bladder & kidney damp heat in the chronic phase
CHRONIC URINARY INFECTIONS: urethritis, nephritis, prostatitis, pyelitis
CHRONIC VENEREAL INFECTIONS of all kinds
UROGENITAL DISCHARGES with damp heat or damp cold, incl. spermatorrhea

Preparation

USE: Buchu leaf, like Bearberry leaf, contains an essential oil that must be preserved in the preparation; for this reason the overnight cold water MACERATION, TINCTURE or long INFUSION are best.
DOSAGE: standard doses throughout
CAUTION: Breaks of several days are advisable every two weeks, as continuous use may produce slight kidney inflammation.
Being *hot* and *irritant*, Buchu is contraindicated in all excess heat or acute inflammatory conditions.

Notes

Derived from a heavily scent laden and essential oil saturated South African shrub (*buchu* means "odiferous"), Buchu leaf has proved an invaluable remedy for genital and urinary functions. Like Damiana, Asparagus and Jasmin, this remedy is a *warm* natured *restorative* in this area, and where overall *stimulation* is required in addition to local restoration of functions. **Deficient Yang** conditions with fatigue, cold limbs, spasms and discharges therefore best meet its use—as found in Shao Yin biotypes, for example. The comparison with the Chinese botanical *Bu gi zhi, fructus Psoraleae,* is a manifest one, seeing the close therapeutic resemblance between these two, both in terms of their qualities and their functions. Using Buchu leaf is thus similar to using acupuncture points Bl 20, 23 & 26, CV 4 & 6 and GV 3 in treating Spleen & Kidney Yang deficiency with corresponding symptoms in the digestive, urogenital and lumbar regions.

Buchu's essential oil content is also highly *bacteriocidal,* and so this herb is appropriate in all **chronic urinary** and **genital infections** where the basic condition is a **deficiency cold** one. Here it will combine well with Juniper or Elecampane, for example, as well as with gentler, moister *antiseptic* and *anti-inflammatory* herbs from Class 10 such as Cornsilk.

Jasmine: Class 7

JASMINE

Pharmaceutical name: flos Jasmini
Botanical name: Jasminum officinalis L., *seu grandiflorum* L. (N.O. Oleaceae)
Other names: Jasmin (Fr)
Jasmin (Ge)
Part used: the flower

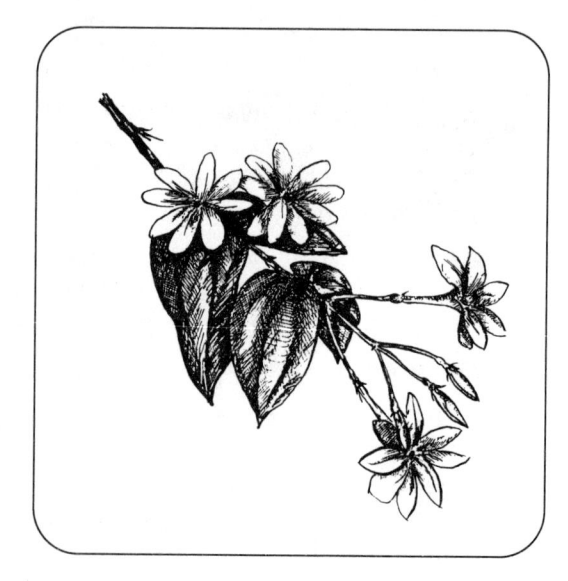

Nature

CATEGORY: mild herb with minimal chronic toxicity
CONSTITUENTS: ess. oil (incl. linalol, benzyle acetate & other sterols & esters), salicilic acid, alkaloids (jasminine), astringent substance
EFFECTIVE QUALITIES
Primary: pungent, a bit sweet, warm, moist
Secondary: restoring, stimulating, relaxing, calming, astringing
TROPISM: reproductive organs, kidneys, bladder, nervous system, lungs, intestines
Warmth, Air organisms
Liver, Kidney, Spleen, Chong & Ren meridians
GROUND: Melancholic & Phlegmatic krasis
Burdened/Shao Yin, Sensitive/Tai Yin Metal, Self-Reliant/Yang Ming Metal & Dependant/Tai Yin Earth biotypes

Functions and Uses

1 RESTORES, WARMS AND RELAXES THE UROGENITAL ORGANS, DRIES MUCOUS DAMP AND ARRESTS DISCHARGE; HARMONIZES THE MENSES AND ENHANCES CHILDBIRTH; ENHANCES SEXUAL DESIRE AND PROMOTES LACTATION

genitourinary cold (Kidney Yang deficiency) with scanty frequent urination, lower backache, lack of sexual desire
IMPOTENCE, FRIGIDITY
Liver meridian cold with painful swollen genitals
uterus cold with stopped, or delayed painful difficult menstruation
PROPHYLACTIC & REMEDIAL for difficult, painful delivery
LEUCORRHEA and all genital discharges with damp cold
INSUFFICIENCT BREASTMILK

2 SUPPORTS THE YANG, GENERATES WARMTH AND DISPELS COLD; RESTORES THE NERVE, LIFTS THE SPIRIT AND RIDS DEPRESSION

Yang deficiency with apathy, chilliness, depression
nerve deficiency with fatigue, weakness, restlessness

Class 7: Jasmine

NERVOUS DEPRESSION or ANXIETY in all conditions

3   WARMS AND LENIFIES THE LUNGS, BENEFITS THE VOICE, RELIEVES COUGHING AND WHEEZING; WARMS THE INTESTINES AND ARRESTS DISCHARGE

lung phlegm cold/dryness with full catarrhal or dry cough, wheezing, dry itchy throat
COUGHING, hoarseness, voice loss in any condition
intestines cold (Spleen Yang deficiency) with diarrhea, abdominal pain, listlessness
MUCOID DIARRHEA, mucous colitis due to damp cold

4   PROMOTES TISSUE REPAIR, RELIEVES PAIN AND BENEFITS AND MOISTENS THE SKIN

WOUNDS, ulcers, sores
INJURIES and pain in general
DRY, irritable skin, eczema, dermatitis, pruritus

Preparation

USE: The widely available ESSENTIAL OIL extracted from the flowers is used both internally and externally. In the latter case it should be massaged into the skin either locally or globally with the help of a carrier oil.

A TINCTURE from the **fresh** flowers is possibly more *anodyne* and *astringent*. However, both make excellent LINIMENTS and OINTMENTS.

DOSAGE: ESSENTIAL OIL: 2-5 drops in some warm water

Notes

Like many herbal remedies used in essential oil form, Jasmine has a double therapeutic advantage: its suave, elegant scent and its physiological effects. This combination is clearly a benefit in the various types of **cold deficiency** syndromes that Jasmine addresses, where mental lethargy, depression and insensitivity are as much part of the picture as physical symptoms such as backache, white discharges, urinary problems and cold extremities. Scent is known to influence the hypophysis and hence trigger a variety of reactions which cause rebalancing on the mental, affective, vital and physical bodies. The essential oil from this Mediterranean flower therefore acts as a totality on an individual's being. Jasmine has been aptly called a *depression fighter* and is equal to Melissa, Basil and Ylang-ylang in this respect. However, we would also want to know what **type** of depression it will dispel. When the totality of its therapeutic imprint is considered, the answer is that Jasmine acts best on depression of the **Yang deficiency** kind. When treating delayed or painful periods and leucorrhea in context of this condition, it will mimic acupuncture points Bl 23 & 32, Kd 2, Gb 26 and CV 4 & 6 with moxa.

The scent of Jasmine, on the other hand, has no likeness.

Damiana: Class 7

DAMIANA

Pharmaceutical name: herba Turnerae
Botanical name: Turnera diffusa **Willd.** (N.O. Turneraceae)
Other names: Mexican damiana (Am)
Part used: the herb

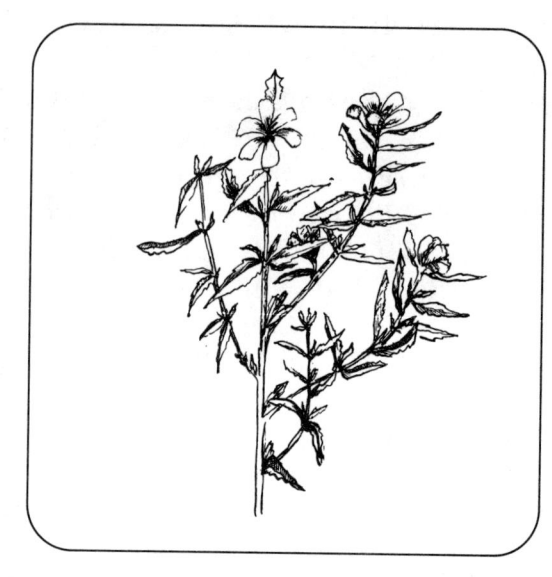

Nature

CATEGORY: mild herb with minimal chronic toxicity
CONSTITUENTS: ess. oil 0.5-2% (incl. α & ß-pinene, cineol, cymol, arbutin, cymene, ß-cadinene, α-copaene), alkaloids, bitter (damianin), flavonoid (gonzalitosin), cyanogenic glycoside, tannins, resins, albuminoid, chlorophyll
EFFECTIVE QUALITIES
Primary: bitter, a bit pungent, neutral, dry
Secondary: stimulating, restoring, astringing
TROPISM: reproductive organs, stomach, liver, nerves, pituitary
    Air organism
    Kidney, Liver, Chong & Ren meridians
GROUND: Melancholic krasis
    Sensitive/Tai Yin Metal & Burdened/Shao Yin biotypes
    Lymphatic/Carbonic/Blue Iris constitution

Functions and Uses

1. **TONIFIES THE YANG, STRENGTHENS AND RESTORES THE NERVE AND BRAIN, LIFTS THE SPIRIT AND GENERATES STRENGTH**
   Yang deficiency: fatigue, weakness, chilliness, depression
   nerve deficiency: debility, nervous exhaustion, numbness, paralysis
   CHRONIC DEBILITY due to physical or mental overwork, illness, childbirth, etc.
   ANXIETY, neurosis

2. **RESTORES AND SOOTHES THE UROGENITAL ORGANS, HARMONIZES URINATION AND ENHANCES SEXUAL DESIRE**
   Kidney Yang deficiency (genitourinary cold): mental dullness or stupor, lumbar aching, premature ejaculation, frigidity, infertility, frequent scanty or incontinent urination
   LACK OF SEXUAL DESIRE in both sexes, impotence & frigidity in all conditions
   LEUCORRHEA
   URINARY IRRITATION and irregularity
   CHRONIC URINARY INFECTIONS in deficiency cold conditions

3 RESTORES THE LIVER AND STOMACH, PROMOTES MENSTRUATION AND BOWEL MOVEMENT

liver & stomach Qi deficiency: slow painful digestion, constipation, no appetite
uterus Qi stagnation: painful, delayed menstruation with purple clots, moodiness, skin rashes

4 REGULATES THE PITUITARY, HARMONIZES THE MENSES AND MENOPAUSE

general hormone disharmony (Chong/Ren disharmony) due to pituitary dysfunction with chronic variable and irregular menstruation in all respects
MENOPAUSAL SYNDROME

Preparation

USE: Damiana is a good, safe maintenance tonic in the right dosage. The INFUSION and TINCTURE are equally good, the latter being more suited to **stagnant digestive** and **menstrual** conditions. As a hormonal regulator it may be taken every morning before breakfast for several weeks, or until menstruation normalizes.

DOSAGE: Standard doses throughout. Severe depletion requires up to twice the amount.

CAUTION: Do not overdose, as this overstimulates in every sense.

Notes

It is difficult not to lavish praise on the gentleness yet efficacy of this medicinal plant from the American tropics and sub-tropics. In the intense heat of these regions Damiana develops caffeine-like alkaloids and an essential oil which are responsible for much of its physiological effect. As a result of these, Damiana is one of the few remedies that deserves the status of *Yang tonic* from both the Chinese and Western point of view—whether one accepts that a truly systemic tonification of the Yang amounts to global sympathetic nervous stimulation or not. The **Kidney Yang** is boosted, and every imaginable symptom found under its syndrome relieved, including leucorrhea, premture ejaculation and prostate discharge (tannins, glycoside). A Chinese herbalist would not even think about placing Damiana in any other category than the *Yang tonics*—even were it not *sympathomimetic* in action! An acupuncturist, moreover, would definitely see this botanical as the nearest thing to Ki 2 & 7, GV 4 and Bl 23, 28, 31 & 53. Damiana's *genitourinary tonic* effects include the relief of urinary irritation and incontinence, as well as the treatment of bladder infections with **empty cold** conditions (arbutin, tannins).

From the Western perspective there is more to the Damiana story, however. For the central nervous system it also has a tonic influence, and specifically a *trophic nerve restorative* one. This simply means that Damiana nourishes and regenerates nerve cells with more **long-term** *tonic* effects—not undesirable in stress related and chronic conditions with depressive tendencies. Moreover, to this is added the strengthening effect of its *bitter* substance/taste which ensures a more immediate and experienceable global *tonifying* effect via glandular secretions.

Another, and related side to Damiana is its *hormonal regulation* effect through the pituitary. This ensures a wide ranging *rebalancing* of secretions responsible for menstrual and menopausal changes. Damiana is perhaps not as strong as Chasteberry or Watercress in this respect; but in the context of its overall enhancement of sexuality on all levels, and of its thorough nervous restoration, its rebalancing effect is highly significant, adding icing to a remedy already full of tonic potential.

POPLAR

Pharmaceutical name: cortex Populi tremuloides
Botanical name: Populus tremuloides Michx., *seu candicans* L. (N.O. Salicaceae)
Other names: Quaking aspen, American aspen/poplar, Aspen poplar, Trembling poplar, White poplar, Alamo, Cottonwood (Am)
Peuplier tremble, Trémole (Fr)
Zitterpappel, Espe, Lybischer Pappelbaum (Ge)
Part used: the bark

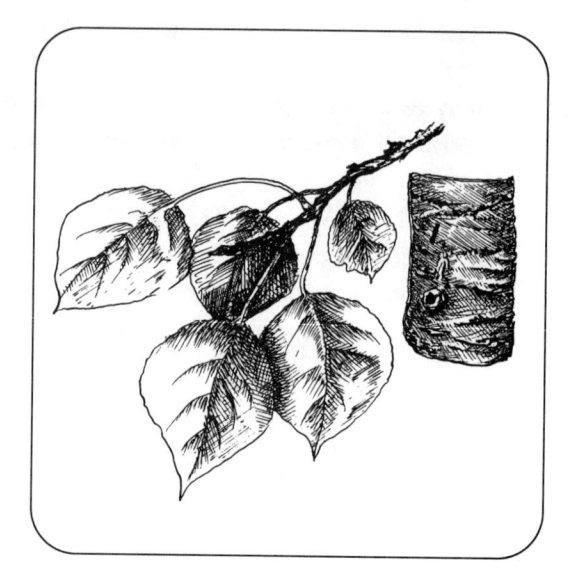

Nature

CATEGORY: mild herb with minimal chronic toxicity
CONSTITUENTS: populin, ess. oil, glycosides (incl. salicocortin, salicin, tremulacin, tremuloidin, grandidentotin, riciresinol-ß-glucoside), acids, coloring matter, mannitol, fixed oil
EFFECTIVE QUALITIES
Primary: a bit bitter & astringent, cool, dry
Secondary: restoring, astringing
TROPISM: urinary & reproductive organs, stomach, intestines
Air organism
Kidney, Bladder, Spleen meridians
GROUND: all krases, biotypes and constitutions for symptomatic use

Functions and Uses

1 RESTORES THE UROGENITAL ORGANS, ARRESTS DISCHARGE AND CREATES STRENGTH
genitourinary Qi deficiency (Kidney Qi infirmity): lumbar pain, weak knees, scanty or copious frequent urination, chronic white leucorrhea
MUCOUS CYSTITIS, PROSTATE ENLARGEMENT

2 RESTORES THE *SPLEEN*/INTESTINES; CLEARS HEAT, RESOLVES FEVER AND REDUCES INFLAMMATION
Spleen Qi deficiency with fatigue, poor appetite, diarrhea
DEBILITY in chronic disease or convalescence, after childbirth
REMITTENT & TIDAL FEVERS in Shao Yang & Shao Yin stage, incl. malaria
MILD URINARY INFLAMMATIONS

Preparation

USE: The standard DECOCTION and TINCTURE are good preparation forms, and should be used over a long time—unless given specifically for intermittent fever.
DOSAGE: standard doses throughout

Notes

The bark of both the Quaking aspen and the Cottonwood was used by Native Americans and early settlers alike for its *pain relieving, anti-inflammatory* and *febrifuge* effects, long before anything about salicic glycosides was known. Its *bitter* taste effectively restores strength to the whole organism, allowing low, lingering Shao Yin type hectic fevers with deficiency heat to be thrown off, and a more rapid convalescence to ensue. With its use appetite and assimilation are restored as an integral part of the process. Poplar bark thus links up, through similar uses, with other barks, such as those from the Willow, Alder, Wild cherry, Wafer ash, Wahoo and other trees.

Nevertheless, it is Poplar's focus on the urogenital organs that makes it distinctive. Here its *restoring* effect both functionally and structurally works on Kidney Qi, which makes it a suitable remedy for mild cases of Liver and Kidney depletion in Chinese medicine (in severe ones it should be combined with stronger botanicals such as Helonias and Oats).

In combining digestive and urogenital *restorative* effects, Poplar bark is similar to Gravel root. The two herbs make a natural, mutually reinforcing pair.

GRAVEL ROOT

Pharmaceutical name: radix Eupatorii purpurei
Botanical name: Eupatorium purpureum L. (N.O.
    Compositae)
Other names: Motherwort, Queen of the meadow,
    Joe pye weed, Feverweed, Kidney root,
    Purple boneset, Trumpetweed (Am)
Part used: the root

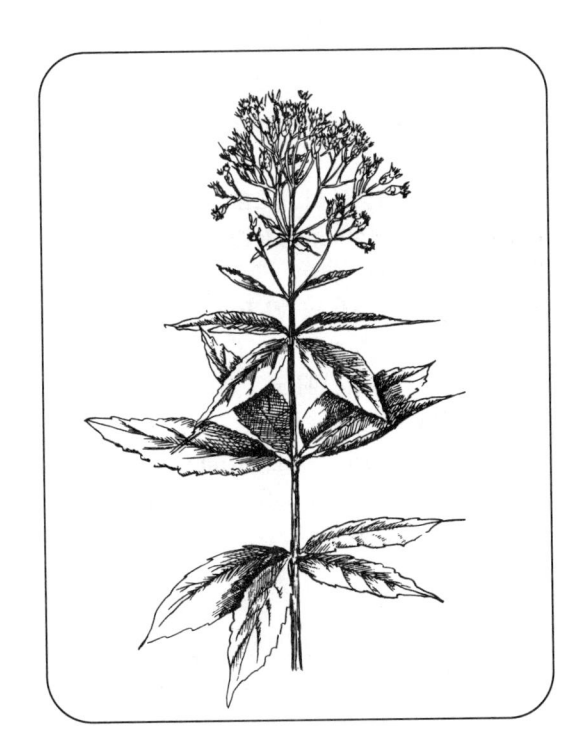

Nature

CATEGORY: mild herb with minimal chronic toxicity
CONSTITUENTS: resins (incl. eupatorin, euparin), oleoresin 'eupurpurin', saponins, tannins
EFFECTIVE QUALITIES
Primary: bland, a bit bitter, neutral with cooling potential, dry
Secondary: astringing, restoring, cleansing, relaxing
TROPISM: reproductive & urinary organs
    Fluid, Air organisms
    Kidney, Liver, Bladder, Chong & Ren meridians
GROUND: Melancholic & Phlegmatic krasis

Gravel root: Class 7

Sensitive/Tai Yin Metal, Burdened/Shao Yin,
Self-Reliant/Yang Ming Metal & Dependant/Tai Yin Earth biotypes
Lymphatic/Carbonic/Blue Iris & Mixed/Phosphoric/Gray-Green Iris constitutions

Functions and Uses

1 RESTORES THE UROGENITAL ORGANS, LENIFIES IRRITATION AND PAIN, HARMONIZES URINATION AND ARRESTS DISCHARGE

genitourinary weakness (Kidney Qi infirmity) with frequent scanty urination, incontinence, prostate problems, delayed or absent menses
genitourinary depletion (Liver & Kidney depletion) with lumbar pain, variable, irregular or painful menstruation
BLADDER IRRITATION due to any cause, with urgent, difficult urination
UROGENITAL DISCHARGES, incl. those due to acute & chronic infections

2 RESTORES THE UTERUS, HARMONIZES THE MENSES, PREVENTS MISCARRIAGE AND ENHANCES LABOR

uterus Qi deficiency with delayed, scanty menses
PROPHYLACTIC & REMEDIAL for HABITUAL MISCARRIAGE
PROPHYLACTIC for DIFFICULT LABOR

3 CLEARS HEAT, REDUCES INFLAMMATION AND RESOLVES FEVER

bladder damp heat with cutting urinary pain, thirst
CYSTITIS
LOW TIDAL FEVER in Shao Yin stage with night sweats

4 DREDGES THE KIDNEYS, CLEARS STASIS, PROMOTES URINATION AND CLEANSING

kidney Qi stagnation with chronic mucous cystitis
general toxemia with gout, chronic rheumatism
URIC ACID DIATHESIS

Preparation

USE: The DECOCTION is suited for more *restoring* and *cleansing* effects, whereas the TINCTURE is a good all-round preparation. To ensure problem free labor and childbirth in women prone to genitourinary weakness or miscarriage, Gravel root may be taken in small doses both early in pregnancy and a few weeks before labor is due, as well as intermittently in between.

DOSAGE: TINCTURE: 1-3 ml (25-75 drops)
DECOCTION: up to 3/4 oz per pint of water for a day's supply

Notes

This *Purple boneset,* which is botanically closely related to both Boneset in the US and *Pei lan* in China, is therapeutically used in a way very different from both. Its field of action is almost entirely the urinary and reproductive system, where it *restores, strengthens* and *disinfects*. In this it has much in common with Bearberry, Cornsilk and Pipsissewa on one hand, and with *Ze xie, rhizoma Alismatis,* and *Di fu Zi, fructus Kochiae,* on the other. It is used in **deficient** and **depleted** conditions in this area with **discharge**, as well as for **acute** (or **chronic**) **damp heat** infections such as Stone Lin. In severe infections, however, it should be combined with more *cold astrigent* herbs from Class 13 and *urinary demulcents* from Class 10, as required. With general urogenital weakness with scanty, urgent, dribbling urination, a syndrome known as *Kidney Qi infirmity* in Chinese medicine, Gravel root is the nearest thing for an herbalist to what points Bl 23, 28 & 53, Kd 11, CV 3 and Li 4 would represent for an acupuncturist.

On the womb itself Gravel root exerts a *toning* and *normalizing* influence, somewhat like Helonias. Its applications are both menstrual and puerperal ones in this respect, and could be used simply for this alone since it is a gentle acting, safe remedy whose benefits only increase when taken continuously, hence its use as *childbirth preparator*. It was suitably called *Motherwort* somewhere along the line. In this context, Gravel root was also a love medicine to one Native American tribe.

Eclectic physicians were emphatic about Gravel root in altering high uric acid conditions and its *sequelae*—not an unlikely proposition in view of its saponin and resin content. Here a comprehensive regulating effect in treating general toxemia is obtained.

SEA HOLLY

Pharmaceutical name: radix Eryngii
Botanical name: Eryngium maritimum, seu
    campestre L. (N.O.Umbelliferae)
Ancient names: Cardus onarinus, Centum capita
    (Lat)
Other names: Eryngo, Field eryngo (Eng)
    Panicaut, Chardon Roland, Cents têtes (Fr)
    Mannstreu, Brackendistel, Seichdistel (Ge)
Part used: the root

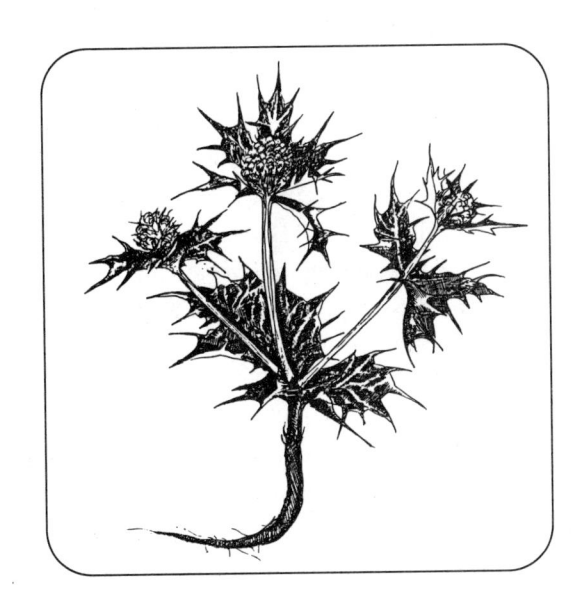

Nature

CATEGORY: mild herb with minimal chronic toxicity
CONSTITUENTS: saponins, ess. oil, minerals & trace minerals (incl. potassium, sodium), mucilage, resin
EFFECTIVE QUALITIES
Primary: bland, a bit salty & pungent, neutral, dry
Secondary: restoring, astringing, stimulating, decongesting
TROPISM: urogenital organs, uterus, lungs, liver, nerves
    Air, Fluid organisms
    Kidney, Bladder, Chong & Ren meridians
GROUND: Melancholic krasis
    Sensitive/Tai Yin Metal biotype
    Lymphatic/Carbonic constitution

Sea holly: Class 7

Functions and Uses

1 STRENGTHENS AND RESTORES THE UROGENITAL ORGANS, LENIFIES IRRITATION, HARMONIZES URINATION AND ARRESTS DISCHARGE

   genitourinary Qi deficiency (Kidney Qi infirmity) with irregular, dribbling urination, backache, diarrhea
   FRIGIDITY, impotence, lack of sexual desire in *Kidney Yang deficiency*
   genitourinary depletion (Liver & Kidney depletion) with irregular menses, weak knees & legs
   BLADDER IRRITATION, obstructed or painful urination
   URINARY INFECTIONS in deficient conditions
   genitourinary damp cold with white discharges
   CHRONIC NEPHRITIS

2 STIMULATES THE UTERUS, PROMOTES MENSTRUATION AND LABOR

   uterus Qi stagnation with delayed menstruation
   DIFFICULT, slow chidbirth
   STALLED LABOR

3 CLEARS STASIS, SEEPS WATER, PROMOTES URINATION AND CLEANSING; STIMULATES THE KIDNEYS AND LIVER

   liver & kidney fluid congestion with local or global water retention
   liver Qi stagnation with jaundice
   general toxemia with skin rashes, malaise, cystitis

4 STRENGTHENS THE LUNGS, RELIEVES COUGHING AND WHEEZING

   lung Yin deficiency with profuse expectoration
   WHEEZING, asthmatic breathing due to *lung & Kidney Yang deficiency*

5 RELAXES THE NERVE AND CALMS WIND

   internal wind with spasms, convulsions

6 PROMOTES TISSUE REPAIR AND EXTRACTS SPLINTERS

   WOUNDS, injuries, fractures
   SPLINTERS

Preparation

USE: the DECOCTION of the sliced root or its TINCTURE should be used. For enhancing labor it shoud be taken every day beginning several weeks before.
DOSAGE: standard doses throughout

Notes

Sea holly and Field eryngo, both being *Eryngium* species, are used interchangeably, and what is said here about Sea holly applies equally to the land variety.

Sea holly is yet another innocent looking, though today very relevant *tonic* remedy with special application to the urogenital organs. Yet depths lie undisclosed within it. Its German name *Mannstreu* refers to its ability to retain a husband's faithfulness, and an Arabian variety was used in a similar way to revive flagging sexual vitality. Clearly, there is no doubt about Sea holly's abilities

Class 7: Sea holly

with Kidney Qi or Yang deficiency, even if there is enormous ambiguity about whether it affects a husband or his wife; and even if it has fallen out of favor for more tropical herbs such as Damiana and Saw palmetto. Yet it is doubtful that whether with its almost *nutritive* edge it could be any less certain in effect than Gravel root or Pipsissewa in enlivening and stabilizing reproductive and urinary functions. Its slight *astringent* quality serves catarrhal **damp cold** discharges in these conditions well. All in all, Sea holly could serve as proxy for Chinese remedies such as *Tu si zi, semen Cuscutae,* and *Yi zhi, fructus Alpiniae oxyphyllae.*

Sea holly's baroquely elegant thistle-like appearance along the dunes of Western European ocean shores must have had tremendous meaning for many a wildcrafter, wise woman and herbalist. As **gynecological** remedy, it must have been used for many thousands of years by countless nameless women healers, especially those living within easy reach of the sea. Besides, its German name also suggests that it is a woman's remedy, not a man's, in every respect! Leaving more symptomatic uses aside, Sea holly was, and still can be, used as *uterine stimulant* both where **deficiency** or **stagnation** of menstrual functions prevail (e.g. with Mugwort or Pennyroyal), as well as for easing labor.

An American variety, the Button snakeroot (or Rattlesnake master, Corn snakeroot), *Eryngium aquaticum* L., is used in a very similar way. Being *stimulant, diaphoretic* and *expectorant* in the urogenital and repiratory areas it is basically more of an *eliminant* remedy than Sea holly, which is more *restoring*. At the same time it has most of Sea holly's toning properties, somewhat amplified: its effect of drying mucous damp, and of calming sexual erethism (nymphomania, satyriasis) is a strong one, whereas it is less pronounced in the European species. Its ability to remove **phlegm damp** in the lungs was said to equal that of Seneca snakeroot.

Helonias: Class 7

Herbs to Restore the Uterus and Return the Menses

HELONIAS

Pharmaceutical name: rhizoma Chamaelirii
Botanical name: Chamaelirium luteum Gray (syn.
　　Helonias dioica Pursh. (N.O.Liliaceae)
Other names: Fairy wand, Blazing star, False
　　unicorn root, Starwort, Studflower,
　　Devil's bit, Dwarf lily (Am)
Part used: the rhizome

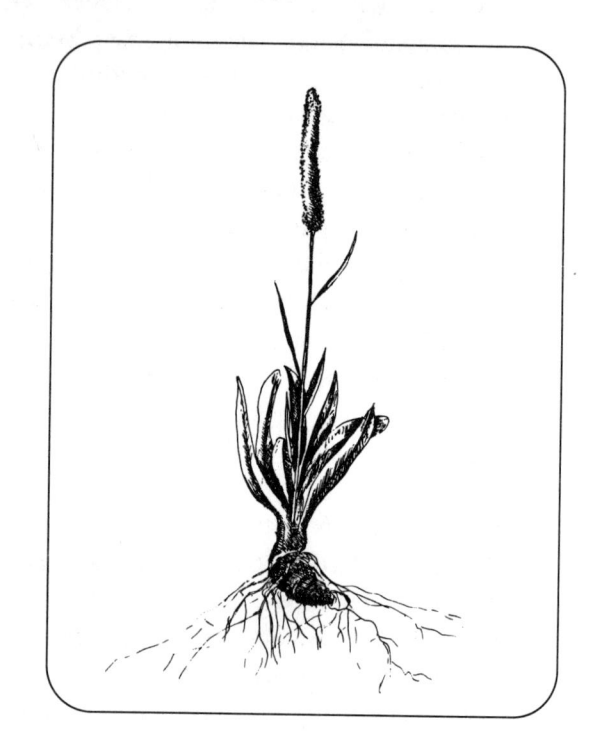

Nature

CATEGORY: mild herb wih minimal chonic toxicity
CONSTITUENS: steroidal saponins, saponaceaous diosgenin glucoside (chamaelirin 9.5%), helonin, diosgenin, oleoresin, bitter
EFFECTIVE QUALITIES
Primary: *Taste:* bitter, a bit astringent
　　　　　Warmth: cool
　　　　　Moisture: dry
Secondary: restoring, astringing, solidifying
　　　　　stabilizing movement
TROPISM
Organs or parts: uterus, kidneys, intestines, brain, mucous membrane
Organisms: Fluid, Air
Meridians: Liver, Spleen, Kidney, Chong, Ren & Dai
Tri Dosas: increases Kapha
GROUND
Krases/temperaments: Melancholic
Biotypes: Burdened/Shao Yin & Sensitive/Tai Yin Metal
Constitutions: all three constitutions

Functions and Uses

1 RESTORES THE UTERUS, UROGENITAL ORGANS AND LIVER AND HARMONIZES THE MENSES; CREATES ASTRICTION, ARRESTS DISCHARGE AND RAISES CENTRAL QI

uterus blood deficiency (e.g. with liver blood deficiency): scanty, delayed or absent menses,

dry vagina, skin or hair, fatigue
AMENORRHEA
uterus Qi deficiency: copious menstruation, intermenstrual bleeding, pelvic weight and fullness
MENORRHAGIA
PASSIVE HEMORRHAGE
ESTROGEN & PROGESTERONE INSUFFICIENCY
INFERTILITY, IMPOTENCE
genitourinary depletion (Liver & Kidney depletion): lumbar pain, weak knees and legs, irregular or scanty menses, pale flow, water retention in legs, prostate irritation, enuresis
GENITAL DISCHARGES, incl. leucorrhea, seminal or urethral discharge
ALBUMINURIA
central Qi sinking: prolapse of internal organs, esp. uterus, dragging sensation in lower abdomen
liver & stomach Qi deficiency: no appetite, fatigue, painful slow digestion

2 HARMONIZES PREGNANCY AND LABOR; PREVENTS MISCARRIAGE AND SETTLES THE STOMACH
PROPHYLACTIC & REMEDIAL during the last trimester of pregnancy
HABITUAL or THREATENED MISCARRIAGE
NAUSEA or VOMITING of pregnancy

Preparation

USE: Both the DECOCTION and the TINCTURE are very viable preparations for **gynecological** conditions. Helonias may be taken as a prophylactic in small doses during the last three months of pregnancy. To prevent **habitual miscarriage** it should be taken in medium doses starting two or three weeks before the anticipated miscarriage. For **threatened miscarriage** up to 1/2 tsp should be taken every hour (possibly in combination with e.g. Black haw, Wild yam or Vervain.
DOSAGE: standard doses throughout

Notes

One may be forgiven for wondering about the karma of this plant, since over the years Helonias has not only gathered quite a collection of unfortunate misnomers, but has also been confused with several other plants—an unfortunate situation for the practitioner who above all has to know with complete assurance the identity of the remedies at his disposal. Poor plant identification and fanciful naming together have conspired, then, to produce this taxonomic mess, which until fairly recently has led to erroneous properties being ascribed to some of the plants it was confused with.

Perhaps the only name really appropriate to this herb is *Fairy wand,* as it very much does look like a small Parma blue wand when in bloom, especially when swaying in the wind. All its other names are undescriptive of either its appearance or its use—a pity for one of the finest *reproductive tonics* available. Blazing star is its most common name in the areas where it grows, but there is nothing blazing or star-like about it; this is a confusion with *Liatris spicata* and *Liatris squarrosa,* which are only superficially similar in ppearance. It was also called *Devil's bit* or *bite* as a result of its similarity wih the latter (a name already attached to *Scabiosa succisa*). On the other hand, its similar appearance to *Aletris farinosa* (called *Star grass* or *Unicorn root*) also led to a confusion between these two, and our poor plant was also called *False unicorn root* as a result. Needless to say, both types of *Liatris,* as well as *Scabiosa* and *Aletris,* are quite different medicinally to

Helonias: Class 7

Helonias. Moreover, Helonias has also been called *Dwarf lily*, yet although belonging to the Lily family, there is really nothing very lily-like about its appearance. Further, its Latin name *luteum* is an absurdity since its flowers are white, not yellow; the only possible redemption for the name *luteum* is the fortuitous connection with the *corpus luteum*, whose activities Helonias' estrogenic properties enhances. Finally, as if these were not enough misnomers for our by now totally dizzy plant to bear, Helonias is not even a true *Helonias!* Although also growing in the Eastern American coastal plain, it is entirely different from *Helonias bullata*, also known as *Swamp pink*. As far as suitable naming goes, therefore, we are left with a plant that is almost enirely orphaned—almost, since it does have one name that concretely and sensually describes its actual appearance: Fairy wand.

Leaving behind the tangles of its popular botanical nomenclature and turning to its medicinal value, it becomes clear that Helonias is "peculiarly tonic," as one Eclectic writer puts it. The focus of Helonias is the **reproductive**, **urinary** and **digestive** system. On these it has an excellent *restoring* and somewhat *astricive* effect, which comes into its own in patterns such as Liver and Kidney depletion, liver blood deficiency and liver and stomach Qi deficiency. In the first syndrome its effect is not merely a local one, which would only qualify it for Kidney Qi weakness; it is a systemic one that influences **nervous, digestive** and **hepatic** activities in a way reminiscent of Rosemary. ELLINGWOOD (1898) rates it as being a "liver remedy of rare value," improving overall anabolism and nutrition. Helonias addresses syndromes of **chronic urogenital weakness** with **exhaustion, amenorrhea** or **menorrhagia, lumbar pains, discharges**, etc. It is, in fact, one of the best candidates for this syndrome in the materia madica. Moreover, being *estrogenic* both quantitatively and qualitatively on an endocrine level (containing steroidal saponins), Helonias will restore uterine blood where this is dry and, as a result, in Chinese terms nourishes liver blood.

Helonias' comprehensive *uterine restorative* functions are what clearly make it a cut above others in this class. In this capacity it restores the tone as well as the blood of the uterus. Uterus Qi deficiency is addressed, with its possible short cycles, its discharges, etc. Like Birthroot its *astrictive* effect not only redresses Spleen Qi deficiency menorrhagia but also uterine prolapse. Chronic miscarriage with Dai mai weakness is directly treated in this connection.

It is fair to say that all of Helonias' properties in concert go to create a superb *tonic* during later pregnancy.

A comparison of Helonias with *Dang gui, radix Angelicae sinensis,* is appropriate. There is a solid area of overlap, as well as differences, which must be recognized in spite of descriptive differences in Western and Chinese medicine. Both plants have the same *restoring* effect on the womb, liver and metabolism. Both clearly work on **uterus blood** and **Qi,** increasing uterine blood and tone; both increase estrogen and progesterone secretions; both will treat Blood deficiency (strictly in the Chinese sense) and its ensuing menstrual problems.

However, Helonias with its *bitter* and somewhat *astringent* taste is more of a *Qi tonic* than *Dang gui*, strengthening as it does the Spleen, restoring energy, raising central Qi and stopping bleeding. Unlike *Dang gui* it also restores Kidney Qi, i.e. urogenital functions.

Dang gui, on the other hand, with its *sweet* and *pungent* taste is more of a *blood tonic,* is *stagnation moving* in the metabolic area and *calming* in its central nervous effect.

Replacing one for the other is certainly fine if these considerations are respected.

Class 7: LIfe root

LIFE ROOT

Pharmaceutical name: herba Senecionis aurei
Botanical name: Senecio aureus L. (N.O. Compositae)
Other names: Squaw weed, Golden ragwort, Female regulator, Golden groundsel, Golden Senecio, Cough weed, Uncum (Am)
Sénéçon (Fr)
Goldenes Kreuzkraut (Ge)
Part used: the herb

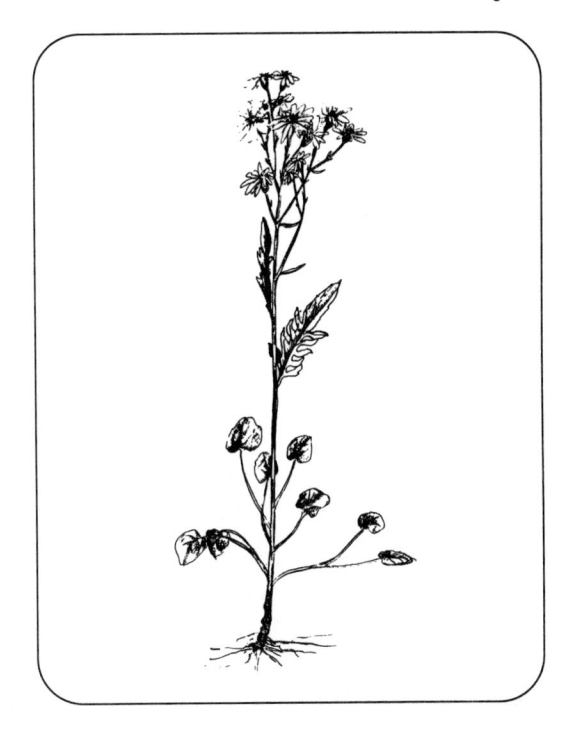

Nature

CATEGORY: mild herb with minimal chronic toxicity
CONSTITUENTS: alkaloids (incl. senecine & seneciofoline), resins, saponins, tannins, bitter, mucilage
EFFECTIVE QUALITIES
Primary: a bit bitter & astringent, cool, dry
Secondary: restoring, astringing, consolidating
stabilizing movement
TROPISM: urogenital & reproductive organs, liver, skin
Air & Fluids organisms
Kidney, Bladder, Chong, Ren & Dai meridians
GROUND: Melancholic & Phlegmatic krasis
Burdened/Shao Yin, Self-Reliant/Yang Ming Metal & Dependant/Tai Yin Earth biotypes
Lymphatic/Carbonic/Blue Iris & Mixed/Phosphoric/Grey-Green Iris

Functions and Uses

1   RESTORES AND STRENGTHENS THE UTERUS AND UROGENITAL ORGANS, PROMOTES AND HARMONIZES MENSTRUATION AND URINATION; RAISES CENTRAL QI

uterus Qi deficiency with delayed, painful menses
kidney Yang deficiency with backache, impotence, early or delayed menstruation
central Qi sinking with uterine or vaginal prolapse
bladder Qi constraint with painful, difficult frequent urination
URINARY IRRITATION, anuria

Life root: Class 7

2   STIMULATES THE UTERUS, PROMOTES CONTRACTIONS AND LABOR AND RELIEVES AFTERPAINS
    STALLED or DIFFICULT LABOR
    POSTPARTUM PAIN

3   CREATES ASTRICTION, ENLIVENS THE BLOOD AND REMOVES CONGESTION; MODERATES THE MENSES AND ARRESTS BLEEDING; DRIES MUCOUS DAMP AND ARRESTS DISCHARGE
    uterus blood congestion with pelvic weight & dragging, copious early menstruation
    genitourinary damp cold with leucorrhea, prostate enlargement & discharge
    PASSIVE HEMORRHAGE from upper & lower orifices, from internal organs, esp. uterus

4   STIMULATES AND DREDGES THE LIVER AND GALL BLADDER, PROMOTES BOWEL MOVEMENT; BENEFITS THE SKIN
    liver Qi stagnation with constipation, abdominal & flank pain
    SKIN ERUPTIONS (dermatosis)

Preparation

USE: The INFUSION and TINCTURE are the most common and effective forms in use.
DOSAGE: Standard doses throughout. If used to prepare for childbirth, only very small doses should be used—e.g. 10-20 drops of tincture once a day—starting two weeks before. It is best to save its use until labor is actually due, however.
CAUTION: Life root herb is contraindicated during pregnancy as it is a *uterine stimulant*.
NOTE: Life root belongs to the Groundsel family, of which there are hundreds of members all over the world. In Europe there are over thirty to be found, of which *Senecio vulgaris* (Birdseed, Simson, Grinning swallow) and *S. jacobaea* (Bindweed, Ragged robin, Kadle dock) especially have been used in the traditional pharmacy (mainly for skin damp heat, liver fire, wounds and vomiting). Today *Senecio fuchsii* is used for its strong hemostatic properties, especially of the pelvic organs—in exactly the same way that this American variety of Life root is used. Unfortunately there is no information about whether *S.fuchsii* is succesful in meeting the entire range of Life root's functions; the likelihood is a strong one, however.

Notes

Squaw weed, as this plant was appropriately known, was extensively used by Native Americans not only for **menstrual** problems, but also for **obstetrical** ones: it was used not only to enhance labor generally, but also specifically to restart stalled labor and to reduce afterpains.

Life root herb is one of those rare remedies that are applicable in almost any menstrual disharmony or disrhythmia. Still, it excels specifically with **relaxed, atonic, congestive** and somewhat **prolapsed** conditions of the **womb** and **pelvic organs,** involving in Chinese medicine either a deficiency of Kidney or Spleen Yang, or blood stagnation. As a result it will both adjust tardy, scanty painful periods and restrain early, flooding ones. Its ability to stop bleeding is dependant not only on tannins but also on its toning effect on the womb, like *S. fuchsii* in fact.

Being useful in the **urogenital** area, Life root will also regulate painful, difficult urination as well as stop white discharges of the damp cold variety.

WHITE DEADNETTLE

Pharmaceutical name: planta tota Lamii
Botanical name: Lamium album L. (N.O. Labiatae)
Ancient names: Galiopsis (Gr)
  Galeopsis, Urtica iners seu mortis, Apiago, Barocus (Lat)
Other names: Archangel, Bee/Dummy/Blind nettle, Suckie Sue, Suckbottle, Snakeflower (Eng)
  Lamier blanc, Ortie Blanche/morte, Lamion (Fr)
  Weisse Taubnessel, Tote Nessel, Bienenfang (Ge)
Part used: the whole plant

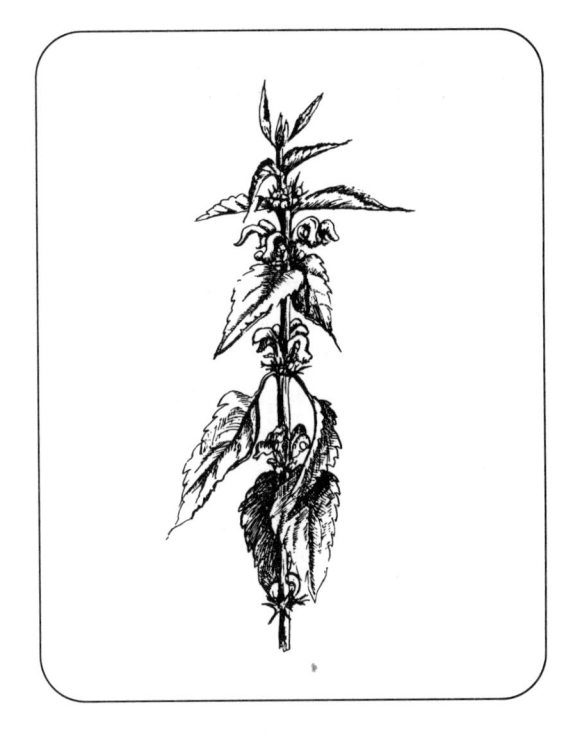

Nature

CATEGORY: mild herb with minimal chronic toxicity
CONSTITUENTS: gallic acids, potassium, tannin, sugar, saponins, ess. oil, mucilage, monoamiones, cholin, hystamine, tyramin, flavonic heterosides (isoquercitrin, kaempferol), yellow xanthophyll, glycoside
EFFECTIVE QUALITIES
Primary: a bit astringent & pungent, cool, moist with a secondary drying effect
Secondary: restoring, astringing, decongesting
TROPISM: uterus, urogenital organs, heart, intestines
  Air, Fluid organisms
  Kidney, Bladder, Lung, Chong & Ren meridians
GROUND: Melancholic & Phlegmatic krases
  Burdened/Shao Yin & Dependent/Tai Yin Earth biotypes
  Mixed/Phosphoric/Grey-Green & Lymphatic/Carbonic/Blue Iris constitutions

Functions and Uses

1   <u>RESTORES AND STRENGTHENS THE UTERUS AND UROGENITAL ORGANS, PROMOTES THE MENSES AND HARMONIZES URINATION</u>
  uterus Qi deficiency: irregular, delayed, copious or painful menstruation
  uterus blood deficiency: absent, scanty or irregular menses, dry skin & hair, cystitis, fatigue
  ESTROGEN & PROGESTERONE INSUFFICIENCY menstrual conditions
  genitourinary Qi deficiency (Kidney Qi infirmity): lumbar pain, scanty, frequent urination, prostate irritation, bedwetting
  ALBUMINURIA

White deadnettle: Class 7

2   CREATES ASTRICTION, ENLIVENS THE BLOOD AND REMOVES CONGESTION; MODERATES THE MENSES AND ARRESTS BLEEDING; DRIES MUCOUS DAMP AND ARRESTS DISCHARGE

uterus blood congestion: pelvic weight and dragging with dull pain, early or copious menses
MENORRHAGIA
LEUCORRHEA & DIARHHEA due to damp cold

3   CLEARS HEAT, RESOLVES FEVER, REDUCES INFLAMMATION AND CLEARS TOXINS; PROMOTES TISSUE REPAIR, RESOLVES SWELLING AND RELIEVES PAIN

intestines damp heat: urgent burning defecation, blood & mucous in stool
ENTERITIS, DYSENTERY
blood heat: spontaneous bleeding, fever, copious bright red menstruation
fire toxin: sores, boils, fever
BURNS, skin inflammations, rashes or blemishes
WOUNDS, chronic ulcers, bites
SWOLLEN GLANDS (incl. spleen) due to any condition
CYSTS, lipomas
GOUT, sciatica, painful joints

4   SUPPORTS THE HEART AND LUNGS, INDUCES REST

heart blood deficiency: anxiety, exhaustion, insomnia
ASTHMA, shallow breathing

Preparations

USE: Although traditionally the **flowers** alone were used, contemporary practice favors using the **entire plant** including the **root**, since the saponin content increases towards the root. White Deadnettle is mainly for internal use in **gynecological**, **urinary** and **respiratory** conditions: the INFUSION, TINCTURE and FLUID EXTRACT are best. WASHES and COMPRESSES are also useful for external conditions.

White deadnettle is also prepared homeopathically for the same complaints.

DOSAGE: standard doses throughout

Notes

Like Lady's mantle, with which it has much in common, Deadnettle is one of the plants rescued from oblivion earlier in this century by the German "herbal fathers" KNEIPP and KÜNZLE. It must have played a significant role in the tradition of the wise women too… all of it unrecorded, yet significant history, not least from the perspective of the healing arts.

Among the several types of Deadnettle (yellow, pink, spotted, Melissa-leaved…) the white variety has always been considered the most effective therapeutically. Growing up to 2,000 meters in the European Alps in cool damp environments, it is characterized by large, baroque lipped blossoms. The Abbess, botanist and physician HILDEGARD VON BINGEN, was already cultivating this plant in her physic garden during the 1100's, and in her *Physica* states that it "causes mirth since it tonifies the Spleen and therefore the heart through its warmth…" The Chinese syndrome Heart Blood deficiency where stress and anxiety affect the heart, exemplifies this application very well.

We must beg to differ with this physician on the point of White deadnettle's warmth grade, however. With its acids and tannins it is probably *neutral* if not *cool,* in spite of its slight *pungent* taste. It is *anti-inflammatory, decongestant, detoxifying* and *damp drying*, after all, especially in the region of woman's reproductive organs, and is used successfully in not too severe lower warmer **damp heat** and **fire toxin** conditions.

White deadnettle really shines as a **woman's friend**. Its hormonal influence is both *estrogenic* and *progesteronic*, hence useful in most **deficiency menstrual conditions** with late, irregular or scanty periods. For the uterine blood it is a restorer, improving late, spasmodic painful periods especially if connected with liver Qi stagnation. Moreover On the level of uterine tone it is an *astringent decongestant*, moderating flooding and intermenstrual uterine bleeding. In both these respects it closely resembles not only Life root in this class of *uterine tonics*, but also *Qian cao gen, radix Rubiae*, used in Chinese practice. In covering a large field of menstrual disharmonies, White deadnettle is one of the best menstrual remedies available where a complex disharmony above all needs *regulating*.

This central application of White deadnettle is supported by a *toning* and *soothing* of the genitourinary system, where urinary problems are resolved; and *expectorant, relaxant* effects in the respiratory area—again, as with *Qian cao gen*.

MUGWORT

Pharmaceutical name: herba Artesmisiae vulgaris
Botanical name: Artemisia vulgaris L. (N.O.
    Compositae)
Ancient names: Artemisia (Gr)
    Mater herbarum, Valentina (Lat)
Other names: Motherwort, Apple pie, Fat hen, St.
    John's plant, Fellon herb, Green ginger
    (Eng)
    Armoise, Herbe/Couronne de St. Jean (Fr)
    Beifuss, Buck, Sonnenwendgürtel,
    Himmelkehr (Ge)
Part used: the herb

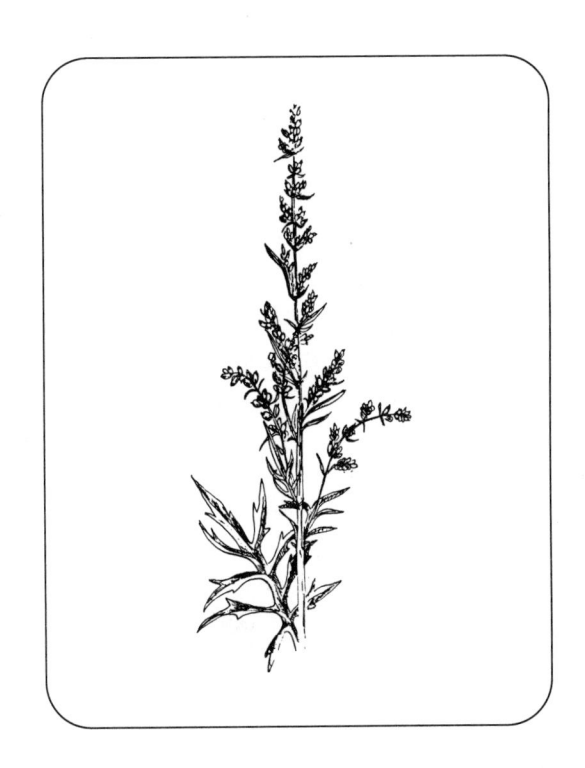

Nature

CATEGORY: medium-strength herb with some chronic toxicity
CONSTITUENTS: ess. oil (incl. thujone, cineol), bitter glycosides, quebrachite, tauremisin, sitosterin, tetracosanol, farneol, inulin 9%, flavonoids, tannins
EFFECTIVE QUALITIES
Primary: a bit pungent & bitter, cool, dry
Secondary: restoring, relaxing, stimulating, decongesting
TROPISM: uterus, liver, stomach, intestines, blood
    Warmth, Air, Fluid organism
    Chong, Ren, Liver, Bladder meridians

Mugwort: Class 7

Functions and Uses

1   RESTORES AND STIMULATES THE UTERUS; PROMOTES AND HARMONIZES MENSTRUATION AND LABOR AND EXPELS THE AFTERBIRTH
uterus blood deficiency with delayed, scanty or absent menses
uterus Qi deficiency with long menses, uterine bleeding
uterus Qi stagnation with cramps, delayed menstruation
ESTROGEN or PROGESTERONE INSUFFICIENCY menstrual conditions
INFERTILITY, sterility PREVENTIVE & REMEDIAL in difficult, slow labor
RETAINED PLACENTA

2   STIMULATES THE LIVER, RESTORES THE STOMACH AND AWAKENS THE APPETITE; SEEPS WATER AND PROMOTES URINATION
liver & stomach Qi deficiency with painful, slow digestion
liver Qi stagnation with constipation, painful digestion
liver fluid congestion with general water retention

3   CAUSES SWEATING, RELEASES THE EXTERIOR, SCATTERS WIND COLD AND RELIEVES PAIN
external wind cold with onset of flu or cold, aches & pains
wind/damp obstruction with acute pains or neuralgias

4   REDUCES INFLAMMATION AND CLEARS TOXINS; EXPELS PARASITES
bladder damp heat with painful dark urine
URINARY & INTESTINAL INFECTIONS BOILS, ulcers, sores, scrofula, tumors (?)
INTESTINAL WORMS

Preparation

USE: Standard doses are used internally in INFUSION and TINCTURE form mainly. Externally, WASHES, PESSARIES & HIP BATHS etc. are used.
DOSAGE: standard doses for all preparations.
CAUTION: Mugwort is best avoided during pregnancy and nursing as it stimulates the uterus and tends to dry up secretions.
Normal doses should not be exceeded to avoid the possibility of toxic effects from its thujone content.
NOTE: This variety of Mugwort should not be confused with a native Californian variety, *Artemisia heterophylla* Nutt. Californian mugwort was used by the Native Americans for colic, diarrhea, fevers, headache and rheumatism; external poultices arrest hemorrhage, relieve red, sore eyes and poison ivy rashes. It is also said to intensify the dreaming process when taken internally or through smelling the fresh plant.
The Chinese herb *Ai ye* is also a different species, *Artemisia argyi*. Only its gynecological uses are the same as Mugwort's, except that the emphasis is on *stopping uterine bleeding* rather than promoting the menses; it has *antiasthmatic, antitussive, expectorant* and *antiallergic* properties besides.

Notes

Most Greek and Latin authors on herbal medicine specify Mugwort as being a good *uterine restorative* and *stimulant;* Renaissance writers still see this as its main function. Today we can claim *estrogenic* properties for it as validating its former status, and hence place it among similar remedies of this class.

Mugwort is used for a deficiency of both **uterine blood** and uterine **tone**, especially where these are due to low levels of estrogen. The former may involve insufficient estrol and may be found with blood deficiency type patterns (esp. Liver Blood deficiency) where the periods over time diminish in quantity and frequency or may stop entirely, and for which acupuncture points such as Sp 6 & 10, Li 8, St 36, CV 4, Bl 17, 18 & 20 would be used. The latter, on the other hand, may entail high progesterone and may manifest as Liver Qi stagnation or general plethora with repeatedly delayed, painful clotted periods, for which points LI 4, Sp 6, 8 & 10, Li 9, St 29 and Bl 32 mighyt typically be selected. In both cases Mugwort clearly owes its action to a *uterine tonic*, not to a *stimulant emmenagogue,* effect (in the vein of Wild ginger and Pennyroyal).

The combination of Mugwort's *antiseptic, anti-inflammatory* and *bitter* properties combine to make a good remedy for intestinal as well as for kidney and bladder infections. Containing a similar essential oil as Wormwood, it is also a good *vermifuge*.

ROSMARINVS   Roßmarin.

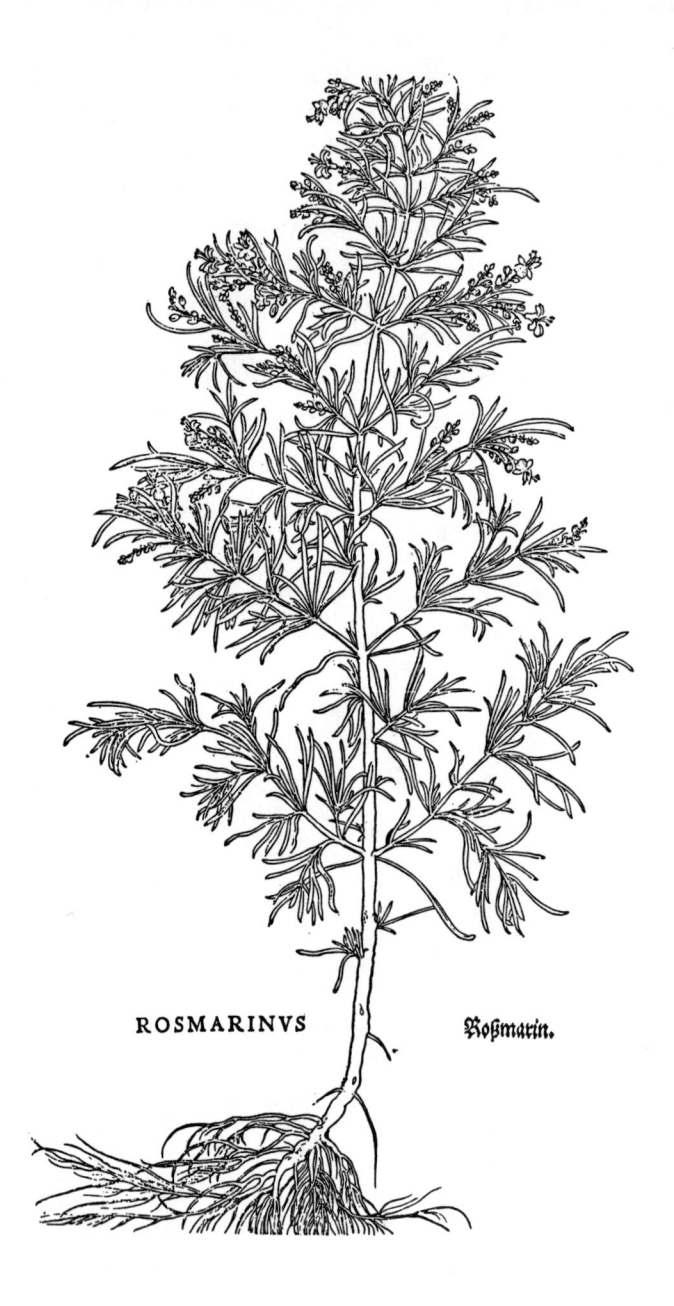

Rosemary

CLASS 8

Herbs to Support the Yang, Generate Warmth and Dispel Cold

Remedies in this class clear injurious cold through their ability to generate internal warmth. This they achieve by supporting the body's Yang forces (*fu Yang*) or energies, the *yang qi,* through stimulation of the circulation. They are used to treat cold conditions in general. Cold conditions involve the autonomic nervous system and weakened arterial circulation, and are associated with a slow metabolic rate. They usually arise endogenously, though they are sometimes triggered by exogenous pathogenic influences, such as weather that suddenly turns cold. Cold conditions belong to the **exhaustion** stage of adaptation to stressors, and in Chinese medicine to the three Yin stages of illness when the Yang is in progressive decline, namely the Tai Yin, Jue Yin and Shao Yin stages. They all represent chronic or degenerative phases of the disease process and signal nothing less than a disease crisis.

Whatever the origin or type of cold in the body, it is a condition whose severity should not be underestimated: coldness invariably signals the ebb of vitality and of life itself, since the root of human life is warmth. In Greek medicine this warmth is called **innate warmth**, and is said to reside in the heart. In Chinese medicine it is known both as the **authentic Yang** (*zhen yang*) and as **destiny gate fire** (*ming men huo*) and is seated in the lower warmer in the lower abdomen. In Ayurvedic medicine it is the **fire of life**, *agni,* also housed in the lower abdomen. Today the term **warmth organism** is often used, more specifically denoting the sum total of dynamic, adaptive, homeostatic functions to maintain the warmth responsible for the internal environment responsable warmth: these functions originate in metabolism, are based in the blood and circulation, and are controlled by the heart, circulation and a center in the hypothalamus.

No matter what aspect of its economy we look at, this warmth or Yang organism, together with the Yin and fluid organism, is the basis of all functions and activities in the human being.[1] Warmth is the only base on which the human spirit, the *shen,* which includes consciousness, the mind and the self, can develop and thrive. A fluctuation of a mere few degrees above or below the normal temperature produces a decrease and, ultimately, a loss of consciousness. The warmth organism or Yang is supported in general by maintaining an ideal body temperature through factors such as clothing and diet suited to the climate, season and environment; by appropriate activity and exercise, which keep it alive through stimulation; and by a balanced emotional and mental life. Physiologically speaking, it is maintained and balancd by all Yin functions in the organism, particularly those relating to the Fluid organism.

As was recognized in all vitalist medical systems, including Galenic medicine, supporting the Yang and generating warmth is basically a Restoring type method of treatment. It is coupled with clearing heat, its opposite Draining type treatment method. Both concern a fundamental physiological balance dealing with the two primary of the four qualities, namely heat and cold. (Similarly, Classes 10 and 11 deal with an imbalance of the secondary qualities dryness and damp, which arise from the body's Yin.)

The method of generating warmth using *stimulant* botanicals was particularly well developed in the eighteenth century by JOHN FLOYER who, independently of Chinese medicine, saw the importance of regulating the warmth organism through either stimulation with *warming* remedies

The Energetics of Western Herbs

or sedation with *cooling* ones. Hot on his tracks, the popular health practitioner SAMUEL THOMSON, the nineteenth century practitioners THURSTON and COOK and this century's JOHN CHRISTOPHER, among others, also put great store on circulatory stimulation. For example, in his simple, and simplistic, system of healing THOMSON considered all disease a failing of the warmth organism and consequently built his entire therapy around a single treatment strategy. One of his students, THURSTON, founder of the Physiomedical school of herbal medicine, which is still going strong today, developed a complete rationale based on circulatory dynamics in support of this theory of the preeminence of **stimulation** in therapy. Warming stimulation and cleansing were then the two dominant therapeutic methods in popular Western herbal treatment, and still are so today.

Chinese medicine has for milleniums utilized the terms Yin and Yang to include definitions of an insufficiency or an excess of either heat or cold in human physiology and has developed the concepts Yin/Yang to a higher degree of clinical sophistication than any other medical system. It defines two basic types of cold conditions which require warming to be used as a treatment strategy: Yang deficiency and Yin excess. Both conditions involve poor arterial circulation which may be caused by factors such as anemia, thyroid deficiency and arteriosclerosis, and which usually present symptoms such as listlessness, chilliness, cold hands and feet, pale or bluish skin, shortness of breath, lack of thirst, thin white tongue moss and a delayed, hidden, tight or knotted pulse. Both conditions may originate from insufficient activity, inadequate nutrition, excessive intake of cooling foods and of high protein and starch foods, excessive exposure to cold during childhood, and a weak constitution. Both signal a failing vital force, or *zhen qi,* with impeded defense response.

Yang deficiency entails a lack of metabolic warmth and may involve the liver, kidneys, uterus and intestines, and, if systemic, will involve the nervous system (see p. 620). It manifests cold patterns of disharmony such as Kidney Yang deficiency (also genitourinary cold), Spleen Yang deficiency (or intestines cold), liver Yang deficiency and uterus cold. Typical symptoms found in these syndromes are apathy, mental dullness, introversion, cold limbs, weakness, diarrhea, cramping or colicky pains in the abdomen or before the periods, delayed or scanty periods, occipital headache, lumbar pain, a pale wet tongue with thin white moss and a slow, thin or deep pulse. This symptom picture is often termed deficiency cold.

Conversely, symptoms of excess cold are associated with a **Yin excess** condition, which may be the result of parasympathetic nerve activity if advanced (see p. 619). In addition to cold extremities, fatigue and cramps, typical symptoms of excess cold are ones of stagnation and accumulation of physical matter and toxins, such as a tendency to overweight, water retention and catarrhal discharges of a damp cold nature; the tongue may be purplish at the edges and is moist with thick white coating, while the pulse is slow and tight.

The fundamental treatment of all **cold conditions** is to generate warmth by stimulating the arterial branches of circulation. This effectively means supporting or increasing the proportion of Yang Qi in body functions over those of the Yin. In **Yang deficiency** conditions this will make good the cold deficiency, while in **Yin excess** ones the cold stagnation will be broken through and the redundant stagnating substances transformed and eliminated.

The herbs used for this are generally known as *stimulants,* and are *circulatory stimulants* first and foremost. Their nature is *warm, stimulating* and *penetrating,* with a *pungent* taste and a *dispersing* movement. They are essentially identical with the *stimulant diaphoretics* in Class 1 and owe their effects mainly to their high content of essential oil. This is exceptionally high in the sun loving Mint family, the *Labiates,* as well as in parts of tropical plants (including many tree barks)

Herbs to Support the Yang, Generate Warmth and Dispel Cold

such as Sassafras, Prickly ash, Cassia, Cinnamon, Camphor, Ginger and Cayenne. Many of the herbs in this class, such as Bayberry bark and Hyssop, also have a *systemic* tonifying effect on the Yang by increasing sympathetic activity, and this justifies all the more their being called *Yang tonics*. However, botanicals in this class should in general be clearly distinguished from the *sympathetic stimulants* of Class 16 that systemically tonify the Yang.[2]

Stimulating the circulation is used not only to generate warmth, but also to remove stagnation of internal processes and organ functions. In this sense it complements the *eliminant* type of herbs which deobstruct eliminative functions. *Stimulants,* therefore, find much use in conjunction with the more specific *restorative* remedies in classes 8 through 11, with *cleansing* herbs in Class 15, and with *eliminants* from classes 1 through 6. Most *stimulants* will enhance the effect of these other treatment methods if carefully chosen and correctly dosed. In all toxemic conditions, for example, especially those of a chronic cold nature, including for chronic dyskrasias or systemic fluid imbalances, *stimulants* are useful in enhancing the work of the various types of Class 15 *cleansing* remedies. Similarly, when added in small quantities to the main herbs in a formula, they lend active support to all *eliminant* remedies from Classes 1 through 6 in all their functions, not only in their capacity as *cleansers*. *Circulatory stimulants* are also used for their *stimulant diaphoretic* effect at the onset of fevers in external wind cold conditions, overlaping with herbs from that class.

Similarly, these *circulatory stimulants* may be used in very small proportions (between 10 and 20 %) as adjuncts in all conditions of Qi or blood deficiency and blood congestion without signs of heat. They will amplify the effect of both Class 8 and 9 *restorers* and Class 14 *decongestants*. Cinnamon, Ginger, Prickly ash and Cayenne are particularly suited to this kind of use.

Clearly, generating warmth through stimulation is most often used in conjunction with other treatment methods or, if not used this way, is used only intermittently. Although an important method in preventing and treating illness, it cannot replace other treatments when called for. Its limits as well as its right place in therapy should be recognized.

Caution: All herbs in this class are contraindicated in conditions of Yin deficiency, fluid depletion with dryness, hemorrhage, chronic high blood pressure, and with any conditions or signs of heat. They should not be overused or taken continuously.

A summary listing of all herbs in this class is found on p. 698.

Notes

1   Recognizing this, and deriving his inspiration from Hippokratic texts discussing the ***innate warmth***, JOHN FLOYER in the early 1700's based his entire system of pathology and therapeutics on, and limited it to, an individual's clinical manifestations of hot and cold. For diagnosis he relied heavily on the pulses, and mainly their frequency, to assess hot and cold conditions. He explains this and documents the completely satisfactory results achieved in adjusting the warmth organism in his *The Physician's Pulse-Watch*. See also p. 23.

2   Nor, on the other hand, should they be too closely identified with the type of remedy termed *Yang tonic* in today's Chinese herbal classification. The unfortunate tendency to class Oriental herbs as *Yang tonics* because they address symptoms of *Kidney Yang deficiency* such as impotence, seminal incontinence and backache clearly betrays a chauvinistic cultural bias. Granted, the Kidney Yang is the basis of the the body's Yang, and many of the *Yang tonics* proposed here, such as Cinnamon, Black pepper and Rosemary, do in fact also work on the Kidney Yang; still, there is no real reason why we should exclude the heart Yang, liver Yang, and the Yang of all other organs. Today it is time to recognize that **warming the interior and generating warmth**, a separate herb class in the Chinese classification, is actually inseparably part and parcel of **supporting the Yang**.

Cayenne: Class 8

CAYENNE

Pharmaceutical name: fructus Capsici
Botanical name: Capsicum annuum L. (N.O. Solanaceae)
Ancient name: Siliquastrum (Lat)
Other names: Guinea pepper, Chillies, African pepper, Bird pepper (Eng)
Piment rouge, Poivron, Poivre de Cayenne, Capsique, Poivre d'Inde (Fr)
Paprika, Spanischer/Indischer Pfeffer, Schlotenpfeffer (Ger)
Part used: the fruit

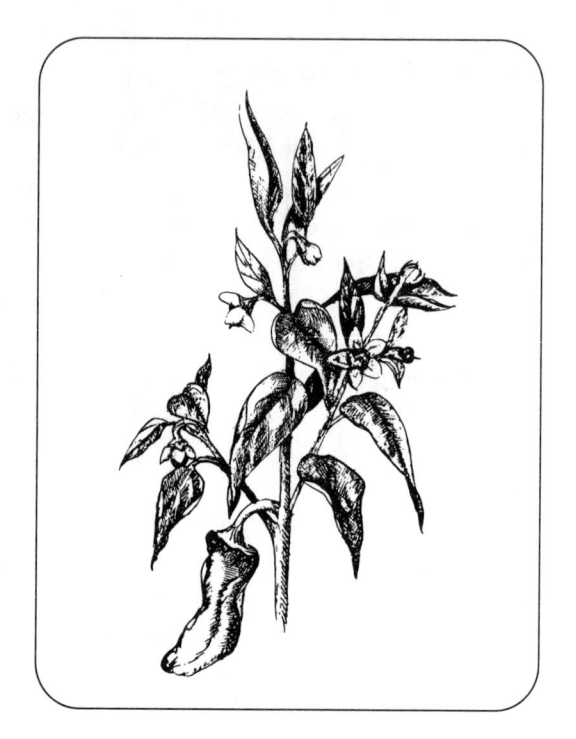

Nature

CATEGORY: mild herb with minimal chronic toxicity
CONSTITUENTS: alkaloid (capsaicin 0.1-0.22%), vanillyl amides (eg dihydrocapsai-cin), flavonoid glycosides, sapogenins, glucose, galactose, xylose, spicy oil (anuin), solanin, oleoresin, proteins, acids, carotene pigment, ess. oil, lecithin, calcium, phosphorous, iron, vitamins A, B1
EFFECTIVE QUALITIES
Prpmary: very pungent, hot, with secondary cooling effect, dry
Secondary: stimulating, restoring, relaxing
dispersing movement
TROPISM: arterial circulation, heart, stomach, intestines, lungs
Warmth organism
Lung, Spleen meridians
GROUND: Melancholic krasis
Burdened/Shao Yin biotypes
all constitutions for symptomatic uses

Functions and Uses

1 SUPPORTS THE YANG, GENERATES WARMTH AND DISPELS COLD: STIMULATES THE HEART AND CIRCULATION, BALANCES THE CIRCULATION

arterial blood & Qi deficiency: cold limbs, weakness, palpitations, slow response, melancholic depression

vanquished Yang: shock or collapse due to injury or trauma, cold limbs, clammy sweat

Yin excess conditions in general

2 CAUSES SWEATING, RELEASES THE EXTERIOR AND SCATTERS WIND COLD; RESOLVES FEVER AND BENEFITS THE THROAT

external wind cold: onset of colds and flu with chills, aches and pains, fear of cold, possible

feverishness
SUPPRESSED, LOW or REMITTENT FEVER, typhoid fever, scarlet fever, diphtheria
SORE THROAT in deficient conditions, hoarseness, quinsy, tonsillitis, laryngitis
wind damp obstruction: chronic static or wandering pains worse on cold days

3   RESTORES AND INVIGORATES THE STOMACH AND INTESTINES/*SPLEEN*; AWAKENS THE APPETITE AND ABATES DISTENTION

stomach cold: poor appetite, nausea, indigestion
intestines cold (Spleen Yang deficiency): pale white face, diarrhea, abdominal pains, chilliness
DYSENTERY

4   PROMOTES TISSUE REPAIR, RESOLVES CONTUSION AND RELIEVES PAIN
FRESH WOUNDS
MUSCULAR pains, sprains, bruises, injury, bursitis, backache, hair loss, toothache
PARESIS and paralysis (local and general) due to local nerve deficiency
BRONCHITIS, acute or chronic, with cold or heat

Preparation

USE: Cayenne is very versatile in its use. The fine POWDER, INFUSION and TINCTURE may all be used: all are good and form bases for a variety of internal and external preparations. For the onset of flu or fever in Tai Yang syndromes they should be prepared as tea and drunk hot, possibly with other herbs of that class; here as with other acute conditions such as stomach cramps or sore throat, a little may be sipped every 1/2 hour.

A LINIMENT or EMBROCATION (using diluted TINCTURE) is used externally in rheumatism, pain, numbness, sprains, congealed blood etc., or as a *rubefacient counterirritant* in bronchitis. The OINTMENT is ideal for preventing cramps, cold feet, etc., and can treat unbroken chilblains. The reason for these external uses is partly that Cayenne is an *irritant stimulatant,* activating and warming the area it comes into contact with. GARGLING with Cayenne is excellent for throat conditions in deficient conditions.

DOSAGE: In deficient stomach and Spleen conditions (function 3) **small** doses are sufficient, while deficient cold conditions need the **standard** dose.

>INFUSION: using 1 tsp per cup, 2-4 tsp of the tea
>TINCTURE: 5-10 drops
>POWDER: in acute conditions: between 4-10 grains (or 1/3 to 1 g), in chronic conditions: between 1 and 4 grains (up to 1/2 g)
>LINIMENT: 1 : 8 or 1 : 16 base oil

CAUTION: Being a *hot stimulant,* Cayenne is contraindicated in all conditions of internal *excess heat,* during pregnancy and in all acute conditions with irritation or inflammation with the exception of *external wind heat.* It should also be avoided when there is bladder involvement.

If left on the skin for a long time it may raise blisters or cause dermatitis: use carefully when in direct contact, unless using specifically as a *vesicant* in painful *obstruction* conditions.

Notes

Little did the celebrated German apothecary JOHANN SCHROEDER suspect the change of attitude towards this shiny scarlet fruit from the American tropics, a change that was to fairly sweep herbal medicine after the 1750's. Some pharmacists of his day, he noted in 1647, were quite partial to its use in replacing the conventional Pepper from the East Indies. He sounded the warning

Cayenne: Class 8

that "it has a toxic nature and quality that can cause great damage to the liver and other internal organs:" to no avail. Not only did more experimentally minded practitioners after him, such as JOHN FLOYER in England, find the opposite, but with this plant they actually initiated a trend that was to dominate herbal medicine in the U.S. for many years to come and that is still a strong force today: it was the two pronged treatment method of *stimulating* and *causing sweating*.

Propagated in the early 1800's by the popular practitioner SAMUEL THOMSON and the schools that followed, the method itself was not anything new: the Native Americans that he mimicked had been using it on this continent all along, as had Galenic medicine itself. It was THOMSON, however, who consistently put stimulation and sweating into practice, before resorting to the usual techniques of vomiting and purging. It worked for the day, and it ousted purging, vomiting and bloodletting as the dominant eliminant catch-all cure.

As a result, Cayenne has become emblematic of stimulation itself, and well it deserves to be, since it is the purest, most neutral *stimulant* known. Using the qualities of Ayurvedic pharmacology to describe its properties, we can say that it has the finest *Pitta* and *Vayu* qualities combined: mobility *(sara)*, penetration *(tikshna)*, lightness *(laghu)*, subtility *(sukshma)* and heat *(ushna)*. Above all it is a perfect addition to other herbs when a stimulating edge is required: Cayenne actually increases their effectivity, makes them more active, gives them the same added Yang that, say, the addition of LI 4 or GV 14 adds to an acupuncture point formula. The effect is similar to adding a touch of *Gui zhi* (Cassia twigs) in a Chinese prescription. For this a very small part of Cayenne is added, the same dose as is used to stimulate stomach Qi, especially after fevers, in convalescence and in older people. Cayenne, therefore, not only enhances the main herbs used for **deficiency cold** syndromes, but is also an ideal adjunct, e.g., in chronic renal congestion with chronic inflammation or chronic pelvic and uterine congestion—wherever there is blood or fluids congestion in fact. This qualifies Cayenne as one of the best sore throat herbs, as well as one of the best to resolve fevers of all kinds, from acute fevers with wind cold to chronic adynamic kinds.

The **Burdened/Shao Yin** type with his cold, deficiency and stagnation caused complaints stands to benefit most from Cayenne. His ground is basically Yang deficient, and Cayenne can be said to *support the Yang,* as the Chinese medical phrase goes. Being a *hot stimulant* to the central arteries, Cayenne circulates Yang Qi. The innate warmth of the vital spirits is kindled, using Greek terminology, and the fire of *ming men* or of the *Kidney Yang,* using Chinese. For this reason Cayenne is **the** assistant herb for all conditions due to low vitality (*zheng qi*), and used especially in ***deficient cold*** patterns with weakened circulation, including Spleen and Kidney Yang deficiency.

HORSERADISH

Pharmaceutical name: radix Cochleariae
Botanical name: Cochlearia armoracia L. (N.O. Cruciferae)
Ancient names: Rafanus albus/niger/sylvestris (Lat)
Other names: Mountain radish, Radcole, Raifort (Eng)
  Raifort, Moutarde des Allemands/des Capucins, Cransun, Ravenelle, Cranson de Bretagne (Fr)
  Meerrettich, Kren, Märek, Bauernsenf (Ge)
Part used: the root

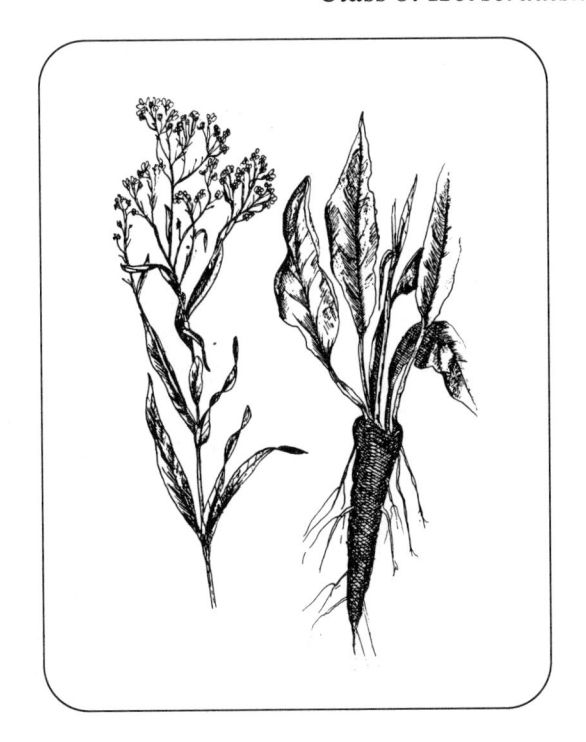

Nature

CATEGORY: medium strength herb with some chronic toxicity
CONSTITUENTS: pungent substance sinigrin, sulphur glycoside, myrosin, ess. oil, bitter resin, albumin, starch, calcium/allyle/potash acetates, asparagin, arginin, oxydase, peroxydase, sulphur, magnesium, vit. C
EFFECTIVE QUALITIES
Primary: very pungent, hot, dry
Secondary: stimulating, decongesting, dissolving
  dispersing movement
TROPISM: vascular system, heart, lungs, stomach, intestines, kidneys, lymph, pancreas, thyroid
  Warmth, Fluid organisms
  Lung, Spleen, Kidney meridians
GROUND: Phlegmatic & Melancholic krases
  Dependent/Tai Yin Earth, Self-Reliant/Yang Ming Metal &
  Burdened/Sentimental biotypes
  Lymphatic/Carbonic/Blue Iris constitutions

Functions and Uses

1 SUPPORTS THE YANG, GENERATES WARMTH AND DISPELS COLD: STIMULATES THE CIRCULATION, ENLIVENS THE LYMPH AND RELIEVES PAIN
Yang deficiency with *arterial blood & Qi deficiency* with chilliness, fatigue
ANEMIA
wind/damp obstruction with acute rheumatic/neuralgic pain
Yin excess with blue capillaries, somnolence, cold limbs
PAINFUL arthritis, gout, insect stings, etc.
LOCAL PARALYSIS
LYMPHATIC CONGESTION

Horseradish: Class 8

2. **WARMS AND INVIGORATES THE LUNGS AND INTESTINES/*SPLEEN*; DRIES MUCOUS DAMP, EXPELS VISCOUS PHLEGM AND RELIEVES WHEEZING**
   lung phlegm cold with copious white phlegm, wheezing, coughing
   intestines cold (Spleen Yang deficiency) with loose stool, no appetite, chilliness
   intestines mucous damp (Spleen damp) with nausea, epigastric swelling, fetid breath & stool
   INTESTINAL FERMENTATION

3. **SEEPS WATER, PROMOTES URINATION AND RELIEVES FLUID CONGESTION, STIMULATES THE KIDNEYS AND UTERUS, PROMOTES MENSTRUATION AND EXPELS THE AFTERBIRTH**
   kidney Qi stagnation with difficult, painful urination
   kidney fluid congestion with ankle and leg swelling
   ANURIA, urinary stones
   genitourinary damp cold with leucorrhea, mucous cystitis
   uterus cold with obstructed or cramping delayed menses
   RETAINED PLACENTA
   heart fluid congestion with central or peripheral edema
   CARDIAC EDEMA

4. **RESTRAINS INFECTION, PROMOTES TISSUE REPAIR, RESOLVES CONTUSION AND BENEFITS THE SKIN; CLEARS PARASITES AND ANTIDOTES POISON**
   CHRONIC INTESTINAL, KIDNEY, BLADDER & RESPIRATORY INFECTIONS, incl. influenza
   CHRONIC WOUNDS, ulcers, chilblains
   SKIN BLEMISHES, acne, freckles
   CONTUSIONS, bruises
   POISONING from food or herb, esp. mushrooms
   INTESTINAL PARASITES

5. **INHIBITS THE THYROID AND RESTORES THE PANCREAS**
   HYPERTHYROIDISM, goitre
   CHRONIC high or low blood sugar

Preparation

USE: Apple cider vinegar is reputedly the best solvent of Horseradish (of which the **fresh** root should always be used). It can be made into an INFUSION or an overnight MACERATION. Water preparations are still less effective than the TINCTURE, however. Freshly grated, it may also be EATEN. The best preparation is the freshly expressed JUICE, which is *colibacilluscidal*. SYRUPS are used for lung & throat conditions.

External preparations are also used for most of the above functions. They include PLASTERS to alleviate **chronic pains** and **paralysis**, WASHES and POULTICES to **promote healing.**

The **leaf juice** is *anti-inflammatory* and *cooling* when used on the skin.

DOSAGE: FRESH JUICE: 15-20 drops
          GRATED ROOT: 2-4 g
          TINCTURE: 0.5-1.5 ml, or 6-12 drops (or min)

CAUTION: Do not overdose, as Horseradish's *hot stimulant* quality may irritate the kidneys or the gastric mucosa. For the same reason, it is contraindicated in **acute inflammations** and **excess heat**

conditions, during pregnancy and with thyroid insufficiency. Its use should be discontinued if it causes diarrhea or nightsweats.

Notes

More than any other remedy, perhaps, Horseradish fills the role of a native European *circulatory stimulant* in the "pure" and systemic sense of Cayenne—although Butterbur, Oregano and Hazelwort all come close. Like all botanicals in this class, Horseradish is nothing less than a restorer of the **innate warmth**, in HIPPOKRATES' sense, with all that this implies. In today's parlance of energetic medicine, its whole action revolves around *supporting the Yang, generating warmth* and *mobilizing stagnation*.

The extremely *pungent* and *hot* taste of Horseradish is ample proof of its *Yang increasing* and *decongestant* property. It performs best in conditions of **excess** or **deficiency cold** due to sluggish circulation, of **mucous** or **phlegm damp congestion**, and of **discharges** and **chronic putrefaction**. Its complementary and reliable *anodyne, anticatarrhal* and *antiseptic* properties mean that infection and inflammation, as well as chronic pains of any type at all, will be relieved. Its action on boosting *Spleen Yang* and removing damp in conditions involving abdominal swelling, pain and gurgling, chilliness and alternating constipation and diarrhea, for example, corresponds to the action of acupuncture points Bl 20 & 25, CV 9, St 25, Sp 9 & 3 (with liberal use of moxa).

Since stimulation in second place causes elimination, as the vital force or *zheng qi* is mobilized to react against irritants, Horseradish is an excellent support with eliminating treatment methods addressing **obstructive excess** conditions, such as phlegm in the lungs or leucorrhea. Here it can replace more tropical remedies such as Sassafras, Bayberry, Camphor and Cajeput. In this context, its potent action on the urinary system must be singled out. Its efficacy in *provoking urination* with obstructed or difficult urination, for example, is shown in BERNHARD ASCHNER's anecdote of a boy with nephritis terminally threatened with anuria, whose last request was to eat some beef broth and frankfurters with horseradish: no sooner finished with these than he passed floods of urine, and his life was effectively saved.

Black Pepper: Class 8

BLACK PEPPER

Pharmaceutical name: fructus Piperis
Botanical name: Piper nigrum L.(N.O. Piperaceae)
Ancient names: Peperi, Stroggylon (Gr)
Other names: Poivre noir (Fr)
    Schwarzer Pfeffer (Ge)
Part used: the fruit

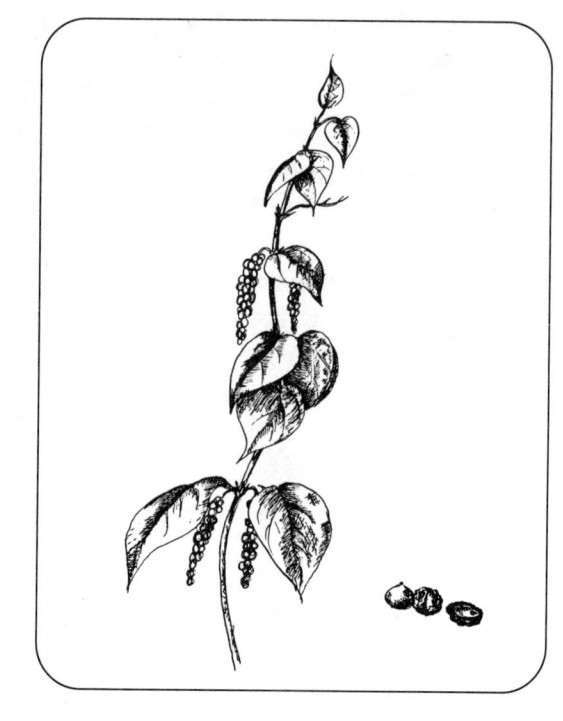

Nature

CATEGORY: mild herb with minimal chronic toxicity
CONSTITUENTS: ess. oil 1-2.5% with about 130 components (incl. pinenes, camphene, alcohols, esters, ethers, aldehydes, ketones), pungent substances piperin & piperettin, resin, starch 30-40%, ferments, minerals 5-6%
EFFECTIVE QUALITIES
Primary: very pungent, hot, dry
Secondary: stimulating, restoring, astringing
TROPISM: Stomach, heart, kidneys, nervous system
    Warmth, Air, Fluid organisms
    Spleen, Kidney, Heart meridians
GROUND: Melancholic & Melancholic krasis
    Dependant/Tai Yin Earth & Burdened/Shao Yin biotypes
    Lymphatic/Carbonic/Blue Iris constitution

Functions and Uses

1   SUPPORTS THE YANG, GENERATES WARMTH AND DISPELS COLD: WARMS AND INVIGORATES THE STOMACH, INTESTINES AND UROGENITAL ORGANS; AWAKENS THE APPETITE, CLEARS FLATUS AND FLENZES MUCUS
    intestines cold (Spleen Yang deficiency) with chilliness, no appetite, flatus & colic
    intestines mucous damp (Spleen damp) with nausea, gurgling abdomen
    genitourinary cold (Kidney Yang deficiency) with fatigue, backache, impotence
    central Qi sinking with prolapse of intestines or uterus

2   SEEPS WATER, PROMOTES URINATION, RELIEVES FLUID CONGESTION AND STIMULATES THE HEART, CIRCULATION AND KIDNEYS
    heart fluid congestion with edema, palpitations

Class 8: Black Pepper

kidney fluid congestion with leg edema, fatigue

3   CAUSES SWEATING, RELEASES THE EXTERIOR AND SCATTERS WIND COLD; CLEARS THE HEAD, RELIEVES COUGHING AND PAIN

external wind cold onset of infections with headache, chills, fatigue
head damp cold with nasal catarrh, coughing
wind/damp obstruction with acute neuralgias & rheumatism

4   RESTORES THE NERVE AND BRAIN, RESTORES EYESIGHT

nerve deficiency with weakness, vertigo
POOR VISION in all deficient conditions

5   RESTRAINS INFECTION AND ANTIDOTES POISON

INFECTIONS IN GENERAL, incl. skin infections
FOOD or HERB POISONING
ANIMAL BITES

Preparation

USE: The pure ESSENTIAL OIL itself is needed to make full use of Black pepper's therapeutic range. It is taken internally (see below) or used with a carrier oil and MASSAGED into the skin. INHALATIONS are especially good with, e.g., Cajeput or Thyme for head colds. An INFUSION of the **crushed corns** can be made for milder results. Chewed, they relieve toothache.
Used on the skin in FRICTION or LINIMENT, the ESSENTIAL OIL warms, tones and restores the muscles, and may help in skin blemishes and infections.
DOSAGE: ESSENTIAL OIL: 3 or 4 drops in a little warm water (or hot in the case of beginning colds & flus), three times a day.
       Other preparations: standard doses
CAUTION: This herb should not be used in any condition with heat or inflammation.

Notes

The fruit of this tropical spice tree, as of so many, contains a pungent volatile oil which makes for most of this remedy's medicinal properties. As such, Pepper is another deeply **warming** and **cold clearing** botanical that in the final analysis **supports the Yang** to achieve its systemic effects. The Kidney, Spleen and heart Yang are tonified and corresponding symptoms in the urogenital, digestive and cardiovascular systems improved, symptoms essentially characterized by coldness, spasms, weakness, and discharge. Like the Chinese white pepper, *Hu jiao,* Black pepper also clears damp and mucus and warms the Middle (the Middle in Chinese medicine being digestive functions), acting here in the same way as acupuncture points CV 12, Sp 5, St 41 and Bl 20 (with moxa).

In addition, as a result of its *hot stimulant* effects, Black pepper also makes a good *stimulant diaphoretic* when used in wind cold conditions at the Tai Yang stage with fatigue and chills. It relieves head congestion into the bargain, especially with coughing and headache, like *Ze su ye, folium Perillae,* in Chinese medicine. Like Cardamom, Rosemary and Basil, also, Black Pepper deals very much with the **head** area, *restoring* and *stimulating* the brain and nerves as part of its overall functions. On the other hand, like Valerian and Fennel, it is specifically for **poor vision** in the context of any deficiencies with low vitality.

Rosemary: Class 8

ROSEMARY

Pharmaceutical name: folium Rosmarini
Botanical name: Rosmarinus officinalis L. (N.O. Labiatae)
Ancient names: Libanotis, Sephanomatike, Polion, Kachrys (Gr)
Rosmarinum coronarium, Libanotis coronaria, Herba salutaris (Lat)
Other names: Romarin, Herbe aux couronnes, Encensier (Fr)
Rosmarin, Keime, Weihrauchkraut, Brautkraut (Ge)
Part used: the sprig

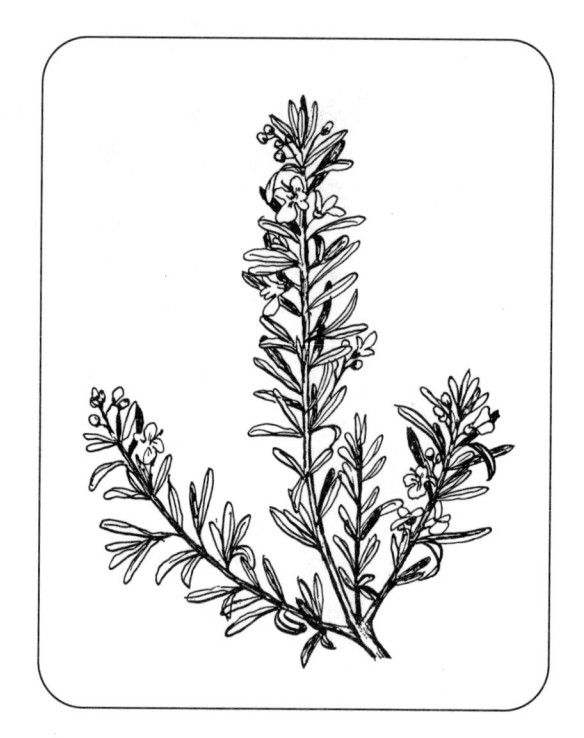

Nature

CATEGORY: mild herb with minimal chronic toxicity
CONSTITUENTS: ess. oil (incl. terpenes: cineol, camphor, borneol, esters, pinene), saponin, flavone, triterpene alcohols and acids, organic acids, tannins, resin, bitter, flavone heteroside, nicotinic acid, calcium, phosphorous, magnesium, potassium
EFFECTIVE QUALITIES
Primary: *Taste:* a bit bitter & pungent
Warmth: warm
Moisture: dry
Secondary: stimulating, restoring, astringing, dissolving
TROPISM
Organs or parts: brain & nerves, heart, lungs, intestines, uterus, urogenital organs
Organisms: Warmth, Air
Meridians: Lung, Spleen, Heart, Liver, Chong & Ren
Tri Dosas: increases Vayu & Pitta, decreases Kapha
GROUND
Krases/temperaments: Phlegmatic & Melancholic
Biotypes: Dependant/Tai Yin Earth, Self-Reliant/Yang Ming Metal
Burdened/Shao Yin & Sensitive/Tai Yin Metal
Constitutions: all three

Functions and Uses

1 SUPPORTS AND TONIFIES THE YANG, GENERATES WARMTH AND DISPELS COLD; STIMULATES THE HEART AND CIRCULATION AND DISPELS COLD

Yang deficiency: weakness, cold limbs, depression, shyness, complacency, mental stupor
arterial blood & Qi deficiency: chills, dizziness, cold limbs
ANEMIA, LOW BLOOD PRESSURE

Class 8: Rosemary

LYMPHATISM, ADENITIS

2 CAUSES SWEATING, RELEASES THE EXTERIOR AND SCATTERS WIND COLD

external wind cold: onset of infections with fatigue, aches and pains, fear of cold
wind/damp/cold obstruction: acute rheumatic or neuralgic pains

3 INCREASES THE QI AND REPLENISHES DEFICIENCY: RESTORES THE HEART AND LUNGS, RESTORES THE NERVE, BRAIN, ADRENALS AND SPLEEN; GENERATES STRENGTH AND LIFTS THE SPIRIT

heart & lung Qi deficiency: spontaneous sweating, chest oppression, shortness of breath, palpitations
nerve deficiency: fainting, headache, depression, loss of speech, vision or memory, paralysis
heart blood & Spleen Qi deficiency: poor appetite, anxiety, dream disturbed sleep
ADRENAL & SPLEENIC INSUFFICIENCY
DEBILITY or EXHAUSTION due to mental or physical overwork, chronic illness, poor constitution, etc.

4 WARMS AND INVIGORATES THE LUNGS, INTESTINES AND UROGENITAL ORGANS; EXPELS PHLEGM, CLEARS THE HEAD AND DRIES MUCOUS DAMP

head damp cold: stuffed head and sinuses, watery nasal discharge, headache
lung phlegm cold: full cough with white frothy phlegm, wheezing
lung & Kidney Yang deficiency: fatigue, depression, wheezing
CHRONIC BRONCHIAL ASTHMA, bronchitis, whooping cough
intestines damp cold: cold limbs, swollen gurgling abdomen, fatigue
CHRONIC ENTERITIS, colitis
genitourinary cold (Kidney Yang deficiency): weak knees, lumbar pain, low sexual energy, impotence or sterility, scanty or copious clear urine
uterus damp cold: delayed, painful menses, amenorrhea, leucorrhea

5 CLEARS STASIS, PROMOTES BILE FLOW, URINATION AND CLEANSING AND BENEFITS VISION

liver cold stagnation: right flank soreness, alternating constipation and diarrhea, frontal headache, chilliness
JAUNDICE, CHOLECYSTITIS, liver cirrhosis, gallstones due to damp &/or cold
kidney Qi stagnation with *general toxemia:* poor eyesight, gout, rheumatism
HIGH BLOOD CHOLESTEROL, atherosclerosis
MIGRAINE

6 ACTIVATES IMMUNITY AND RESTRAINS INFECTION; PROMOTES TISSUE REPAIR
PREVENTIVE in EPIDEMICS
INFECTIONS in general
LICE, scabies
WOUNDS, sores, burns

Preparation

USE: Rosemary is a big maintenance tonic and should be used as such. It should be taken as a long INFUSION or in TINCTURE or ESSENTIAL OIL form. If the last is used, it may be massaged

Rosemary: Class 8

into the skin with the aid of a carrier oil or taken internally.

A variety of DOUCHES and BATHS are prepared using the ESSENTIAL OIL.

DOSAGE: ESSENTIAL OIL: 3 or 4 drops in a little warm water
Others: standard doses

Notes

A look at Rosemary's two main tastes, *bitter* and *pungent,* will solve the problem of its seemingly divergent energetic qualities, dynamic properties that seem to go at once to the interior and the exterior, and to the head as well as to the genitals. On one hand, its bitter taste moves things **downward** an **inward** (as seen in its *choleretic, digestive,* and *mild laxative, diuretic* and *emmenagogue* effects); while on the other hand its *pungent* taste disperses energy **upwards** and **outwards** (as seen in its *cephalic, nervine, diaphoretic* and *antirrheumatic/neuralgic* actions).

Between these two energetic movements that, like branches of the Yin/Yang symbol, spiral in opposite directions, lies Rosemary's true center or point of departure: the **rhythmic region** of heart, lungs and circulation. Here Rosemary is a rare *heart* and *lung tonic* that should be used when both are deficient and when fatigue, palpitations, shallow breathing, mental depression, lack of self-esteem, etc., prevail—virtually a deficiency of the *zong qi,* or the thorassic **ancestral Qi**, in Chinese medicine. The Renaissance herbalist of Strasburg, WILHELM RYFF, describes the effects of a Rosemary preparation as follows: "The spirits of the Heart and entire body feel joy from this drink, which dispels all despondency and worry." The more down-to-earth medic across the Swiss border in Basel, OTTO BRUNFELS, puts it more succinctly: "It creates pluck and courage."

Rosemary's essential function is intimately connected to the warmth organism and the blood: as *circulatory stimulant* it permeates the whole organism internally and externally with warmth and movement. In other words, beginning from the rhythmic center, it dynamically and systemically supports the body's Yang, the innate warmth housed in the blood. **Yang deficient** and **deficiency cold** conditions of the internal organs therefore respond best to its use. The fact that Rosemary is also a *Yang tonic* in the sense of being an *adrenal* and *sympathetic nerve stimulant* merely reinforces its use for Spleen, Kidney and liver Yang deficiency syndromes. The full impact on the organism of a Mediterranean plant drenched in cosmic warmth and light, producing powerful, active volatile oils, is here manifested.

There is another aspect to this remedy, however, which also qualifies it as a *Qi tonic*. Rosemary is very much an archetypal *restoring* remedy as well as a *stimulating* one, due to the action of its essential oil on the glandular system, notably both adrenals and spleen. Certainly, it was seen to compete with Sage in terms of "slowing down aging, drunk on a daily basis" (BRUNFELS). Its *nerve restorative* property, allied to its *cardiotonic* effects, create an ideal remedy for that particularly Chinese syndrome known as Heart Blood and Spleen Qi deficiency, where loss of appetite and fatigue mingles with more mental symptoms such as poor memory, hazy thinking and the like. Clearly, Rosemary in the acupuncture idiom is the LI 9 of herbs for mental fatigue, and the botanical P 4 for treating amnesia. In addition, it was much used for failing eyesight, like Valerian and Eyebright (probably the result of its *renal cleansing* effect), and hence could be described as an herbal Gb 14.

PRICKLY ASH

Pharmaceutical name: cortex Xanthoxyli
Botanical name: Xanthoxylum ramiflorum
      Michx., syn. *Zanthoxylum fraxineum*
      Willd. (N.O. Rutaceae)
Other names: Toothache tree/bush, Angelica tree,
      Pellitory, Yellow wood, Suterberry (Am)
      Frêne épineux, Chevalier (Fr)
      Zahnwehholz, Gelbholz (Ge)
Part used: the bark

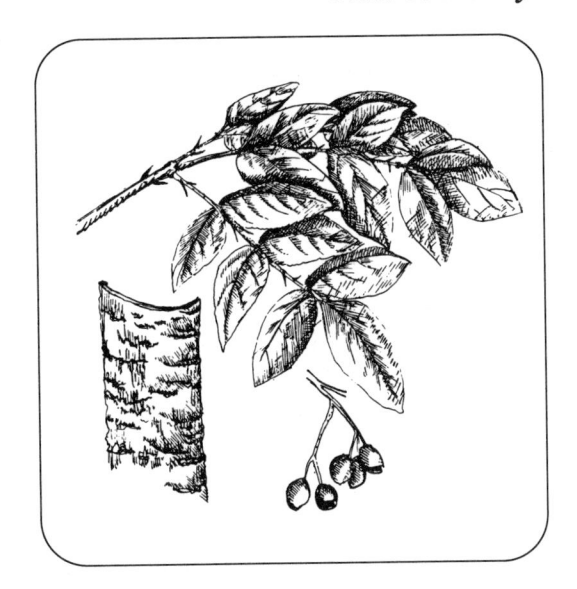

Nature

CATEGORY: mild herb with minimal chronic toxicity
CONSTITUENTS: xanthoxylin, ess. oil, bitter alkaloid, glucosides, malic acid, acrid resins, fat, fat, gum, berberin, tannin, coumarins, lignans (incl. asarinin)
EFFECTIVE QUALITIES
Primary: *Taste:* a bit pungent & bitter & sweet & astringent
        Warmth: hot
        Moisture: dry
Secondary: stimulating, restoring
TROPISM
Organs or parts: nerves, lungs, heart & circulation, intestines, uterus, skin, pituitary, hypothalamus
Organisms: Warmth, Air
Meridians: Lung, Colon, Spleen, Heart
Tri Dosa: increases Vayu & Pitta
GROUND
Krases/temperaments: Melancholic
Biotypes: Sensitive/Tai Yin Metal & Burdened/Shao Yin
Constitutions: Mixed/Phosphoric/Grey-Green Iris & Lymphatic/Carbonic/Blue Iris

Functions and Uses

1   SUPPORTS THE YANG, GENERATES WARMTH AND DISPELS COLD: STIMULATES THE CIRCULATION, CLEARS THE HEAD AND RELIEVES PAIN
    Yang deficiency with *arterial blood & Qi deficiency:* pale face, chilliness, cold limbs, mental depression or dullness
    head damp cold: congested head or sinuses, watery nasal discharge, toothache
    wind damp obstruction: acute neuralgia or rheumatism

2   WARMS AND INVIGORATES THE STOMACH/*SPLEEN* AND INTESTINES, AND RESTRAINS INFECTION; STIMULATES THE UTERUS AND PROMOTES THE MENSES
    intestines cold (Spleen Yang deficiency): fatigue, diarrhea, cold distended abdomen, colic
    CHOLERA, DYSENTERY, typhus

Prickly ash: Class 8

    GASTRIC ULCERS due to deficiency cold
    uterus cold: delayed or no menses with cramps before onset

3   INCREASES THE QI AND REPLENISHES DEFICIENCY: ENHANCES IMMUNE POTENTIAL, RESTORES THE HEART, LUNGS AND NERVE AND CREATES STRENGTH
    heart & lung Qi deficiency: weakness, shortness of breath, chest oppression, spontaneous sweating, palpitations
    nerve deficiency: exhaustion, local numbness or paralysis
    EXHAUSTION or DEBILITY due to overwok, stress, illness or constitution
    LUNG TB

4   CLEARS STASIS, DREDGES THE KIDNEYS, PROMOTES URINATION AND CLEANSING
    kidney Qi stagnation: dry skin, skin rashes, poor appetite
    GENERAL TOXEMIA
    CHRONIC GOUT, rheumatism, arthritis

5   PROMOTES TISSUE REPAIR AND RELIEVES PAIN
    INDOLENT ULCERS, wounds
    TOOTHACHE, sore throat, headache, backache, paralysis
    RHEUMATIC PAIN

Preparation

USE: A DECOCTION or TINCTURE may be made of the bark; the latter will more easily create warmth in **digestive** and **systemic cold** conditions. **Toothache** has been traditionally relieved by chewing on the fresh bark.
DOSAGE: Fairly **small** doses is all that is needed for cold intestinal conditions; the **larger** the dose, the stronger its effect in *restoring the nerve* and *generating strength.*
CAUTION: Avoid use in deficient Yin or excess heat conditions.

Notes

    Although various parts of the Prickly ash tree have long been used by indigenous Americans, Southern Blacks and early White settlers alike for toothache, rheumatic pains and intestinal complaints, we have JOHN KING to thank for its formal introduction into Western medical practice in 1894. With perfect timing and shrewd guesswork his Eclectic practitioners used this remedy from the Southern American States with apparently electrifying effects in the cholera and typhus epidemics of those years. Moreover, Prickly ash has been shown to have *anti-tubercular* as well as *antiseptic properties.* In this connection, it is interesting to note that there **were** suitable *antibiotic* agents such as this one available at the turn of the last century. Had penicillin had not been found, their use could easily have been developed. It is an ironic fact that the distillation of essential oils also saw renewed interest at this time.
    Since then, the bark or berry from the American *Xanthoxyllum,* like the berry of the Chinese variety, *Chuan jiao,* has been mainly considered a *general stimulant,* especially for the peripheral circulation. In generating internal warmth and dispelling cold, it clearly benefits **deficiency cold** syndromes of the circulation, Spleen/intestines and uterus by supporting and mobilizing the body's Yang Qi. Its mild *astringency* is a support in resolving catarrhal conditions of the head and

intestines. In clearing damp cold or wind in the head due to a lack of Yang Qi, and in activating defensive energies, Prickly ash acts like acupuncture point combination GV 14 & 16, Gb 20, TH 5 and LI 4. Moreover, its stimulation extends to renal activities where kidney stagnation is relieved and chronic toxemic conditions involving skin, muscles and joints are improved.

There is yet another slant to this botanical, however, which earns it the title of a *Qi tonic*. Prickly ash is a direct *nervous stimulant* working on the pituitary and hypothalamus, hence having long-range *restoring* effects which probably enhance immune potential. Its *bitter* and *sweet* qualities are the two tonifying tastes in energetic pharmacology and here adress severe deficiencies of the heart, lungs and Spleen/intestines. In Western terms it is also a *nerve tonic*. In short, as a *Yang* and *Qi tonic* in one, Prickly ash bark has as much a place as *Schizandra* and *Astragalus* in *fu zhen* therapy—therapy which aims to "support the authentic vitality."

CINNAMON

Pharmaceutical name: cortex Cinnamomi
Botanical name: Cinnamomum zeylandicum Nees
　　(N.O. Lauraceae)
Ancient names: Cinnamonon (Gr)
　　Canella orientalis (Lat)
Other names: Canelle (Fr)
　　Zimt, Canel, Ceylonzimt (Ge)
Part used: the bark

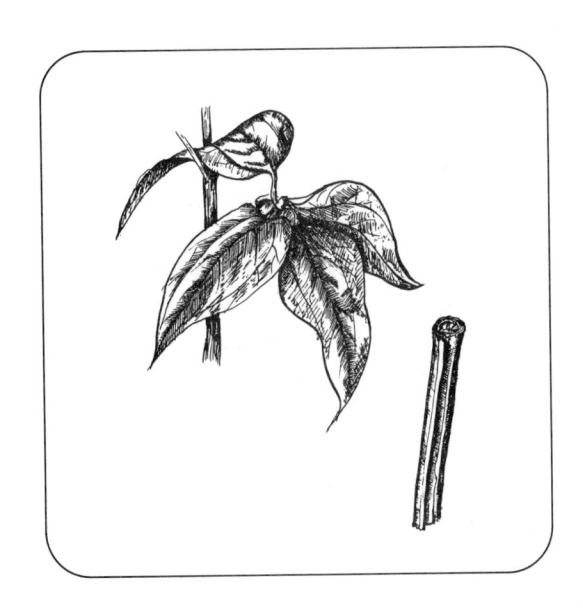

Nature

CATEGORY: mild herb with minimal chronic toxicity
CONSTITUENTS: ess. oil up to 4% (incl. aldehydes, pinenes, eugenol, phellandrenes), tannin, sugar, mannitol, mucilage 3%, calcium oxalate, gum, starch
EFFECTIVE QUALITIES
Primary:　Taste: pungent & astringent & sweet
　　　　　　Warmth: hot
　　　　　　Moisture: dry
Secondary:　Restoring, astringing, solidifying
TROPISM
Organs or parts: lungs, circulation, heart, vascular system, intestines, genitourinary organs
Organisms: Warmth
Meridians: Lung, Spleen, Kidney
Tri Dosas: increases Pita, decreases Kapha
GROUND
Krases/Temperaments: Melancholic
Biotypes: Burdened/Shao Yin
Constitutions: Lymphatic/Carbonic/Blue Iris

Cinnamon: Class 8

Functions and Uses

1. **SUPPORTS THE YANG, GENERATES WARMTH AND CLEARS COLD: STIMULATES THE CIRCULATION, RESTORES THE HEART AND LUNGS AND CREATES STRENGTH**

    heart & lung Qi deficiency: fatigue, shortness of breath, palpitations, melancholy

    arterial blood & Qi deficiency with Yang deficiency: cold limbs and extremities, mental dullness, palpitations

    EXHAUSTION or DEBILITY due to overwork, stress, illness, etc.

2. **CAUSES SWEATING, RELEASES THE EXTERIOR AND SCATTERS WIND COLD; RELIEVES PAIN**

    external wind cold: onset of cold or flu with chilliness, debility, aches and pains, sweating

    wind damp obstruction: acute neuralgias and rheumatism

3. **WARMS AND INVIGORATES THE INTESTINES/*SPLEEN* AND CLEARS FLATUS; PROMOTES THE MENSES**

    intestines cold (Spleen Yang deficiency): fatigue, nausea, no appetite, diarrhea, abdominal distension with flatulence and colic

    Kidney & Spleen Yang deficiency: low vitality, lumbar pain, morning diarrhea, impotence, frigidity

    uterus damp cold: white leucorrhea, no or delayed menses with constant cramps before onset

4. **CREATES ASTRICTION AND DRIES MUCOUS DAMP, ARRESTS DISCHARGE AND STAUNCHES BLEEDING**

    PASSIVE HEMORRHAGE in deficient conditions from lungs or intestines; nasal, urinary & uterine bleeding, intermenstrual bleeding

    LEUCORRHEA in deficiency cold conditions

    CHRONIC DIARRHEA, dysentery

5. **RESTRAINS INFECTION, ANTIDOTES POISON AND CLEARS PARASITES**

    CHRONIC INFECTIOUS DISEASES, e.g. influenza, cystitis, candidiasis, enteritis, bronchitis, upper respiratory infections, cholera, typhoid

    INTESTINAL PARASITES

    ANIMAL BITES & STINGS

    MANGE, lice

Preparation

USE: If a **hot drink** of the Cinnamon bark is prepared using a DECOCTION or TINCTURE, this will stimulate the circulation and *cause sweating*, preventing or resolving **cold** and **flu** due to Wind Cold. Whether taken warm or cool, Cinnamon's effects on the interior are emphasized—*warming, stimulating, astringing* and *relaxing*.

The POWDER or DECOCTION is more efficacious in intestinal conditions, being more *astringent* and *antispasmodic*. The ESSENTIAL OIL has the advantage of being one of the strongest natural *antibacterial* agents known, making it a prime remedy for **chronic infections** when taken internally. It is also certainly the most convenient preparation when it comes to INHALATIONS (**head colds**) and LINIMENTS, for example.

Class 8: Cinnamon

DOSAGE: ESSENTIAL OIL: 2-3 drops three times a day with some olive oil in a gelatin capsule, or 5 drops every two hours at onset of a cold
Others: standard doses

CAUTION: Being a *hot stimulant,* Cinnamon is contraindicated in both full and empty heat conditions, as well as during pregnancy and nursing. Because of its irritant quality (cinnamic aldehydes) which is potentially injurious to the skin and mucosa, oral intake of the ESSENTIAL OIL should only be in a capsule, and external use limited to *counterirritant* LINIMENTS.

NOTE: The twigs and bark of the Cassia cinnamon tree, *Cinnamomum cassia,* are used in virtually the same way as the Ceylon cinnamon.

Notes

When we look at herbals and pharmacopoeias dating as late as the eighteenth century, the age of supposed enlightenment, we note with some amusement that not only the use, but even the geographical origin, of various types of Cinnamon was hotly disputed. No doubt similar disputes took place in Chinese apothecaries, where the comparative effects of *Gui zhi,* the twiglets, and *Rou gui,* the bark were debated—and are still contended even today, with varying clinical uses being given in herbal textbooks. However, although the origins of both Ceylon cinnamon and Cassia, or Saigon cinnamon pose no problem today, we are still free to speculate and argue about the types that were used in Greek medicine, for example. We know that CLAUDIOS GALENOS (GALEN), himself, used **five kinds** of Cinnamon, but none of his extants writings specify their type or origin. At any rate, this is not the burning problem it was during the age of Classical revival, when Greek pharmacology and pharmacy was so avidly emulated.

More relevant today is the issue whether Ceylon cinnamon or Saigon cinnamon should be used and in what preparation form. For medicinal purposes there seems little to choose between these two types, and an almost identical similar essential oil is extracted from both. Ceylonese Cinnamon, with its "indescribable fragrance" (GALEN) is probably more esteemed for this and its superior taste in cooking. If Cassia cinnamon is used, as in the Chinese pharmacy, there is no reason not to adhere to the given indications—although there is as much overlap as differences between the two types. Overall, it is the **usage** of Cinnamon which is of main importance: for example, drunk hot, it will cause sweat in fluish conditions of wind cold; drunk warm or cool, it will support the Yang and warm internally. This, no matter whether the crude bark, the essential oil or the tincture is used.

Cinnamon **can** therefore be used on its own for excellent symptom relief, which includes copious sweating, intestinal or uterine cramps, bleeding and diarrhea. Its functions as a *circulatory stimulant,* however, only come to fruition when used in conjunction with other remedies in the deficiency patterns that it treats. It is a classic assistant herb, boosting the actions of other more directional agents. Like Prickly Ash, Cayenne and Ginger it is also used to give a stimulant tweak to any condition of **cold, deficiency**, and **congestion**—as its ubiquitous addition to Chinese prescriptions for these types of conditions attests. In asthenia or debility it may be combined with *Qi tonics* such as Thyme and Elecampane; in deficient heart or lung conditions with Camphor, Rosemary or Hyssop; in uterus cold patterns with *warm uterine stimulants* such as Angelica, Juniper, Pennyroyal and Blue Cohosh; in deficient Spleen Yang patterns with Calamus, Holy Thistle and the like, where its properties improve every symptom found.

Camphor: Class 8

CAMPHOR

Pharmaceutical name: lignum Cinnamomi camphorae
Botanical name: Cinnamomum camphora Sieb. (N.O. Lauraceae)
Ancient names: Kapur, Kafur (Ar)
Other names: Camphre (Fr)
    Kampfer (Ge)
Part used: the wood

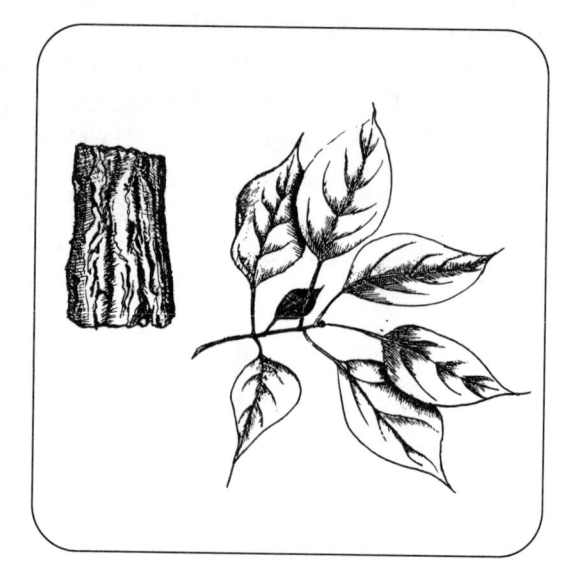

Nature

CATEGORY: medium-strength herb with some toxicity
CONSTITUENTS: ess. oil (incl. geraniol, p-cynol, α-phellandrenes, limonenes, dipentenes), quercetin, sesquiterpencarbohydrocarbon
EFFECTIVE QUALITIES
Primary: pungent & bitter, warm with cooling potential, dry
Secondary: stimulating, restoring, relaxing, calming
TROPISM: cardiovascular system, lungs, kidneys, intestines, reproductive organs, head
    Warmth, Air organisms
    Heart, Pericardium, Lung, Colon meridians
GROUND: Melancholic & Phlegmatic krasis
    Burdened/Shao Yin & Dependant/Tai Yin Earth biotypes
    all three constitutions

Functions and Uses

1. SUPPORTS AND TONIFIES THE YANG, GENERATES WARMTH AND DISPELS COLD; STIMULATES THE HEART AND CIRCULATION, LIFTS THE SPIRIT AND RIDS DEPRESSION

    heart Yang deficiency: tiredness, chilliness, cold extremities, chest oppression, depression
    vanquished Yang: fainting, coma, collapse, heart failure due to shock or trauma
    DEPRESSION in all chronic deficiency conditions

2. CAUSES SWEATING, RELEASES THE EXTERIOR, SCATTERS WIND COLD AND RESOLVES FEVER

    external wind cold: onset of infections with chills, head congestion, possible fever or sore throat
    REMITTENT & LOW TIDAL FEVERS in Shao Yin stage

3. WARMS AND INVIGORATES THE STOMACH AND INTESTINES/*SPLEEN*; DRIES MUCOUS DAMP, ARRESTS DISCHARGE AND CLEARS THE HEAD

    intestines mucous damp (Spleen damp) with Spleen Yang deficiency: tiredness, chilliness, loose mucousy stools, leucorrhea

head damp cold: headache, stuffed head and sinuses, running nasal discharge, sneezing

4   CIRCULATES THE QI AND LOOSENS CONSTRAINT, RELAXES THE NERVE AND FREES SPASMS; CALMS THE SPIRIT AND APPEASES SEXUAL EXCITEMENT

Qi constraint with deficiency: mental or emotional tension, nervous restlessness
kidney Qi constraint: nervous excitement or depression, nausea & vomiting, abdominal colic
uterus Qi constraint: irregular menses with cramps, irritability, PMS
lung Qi constraint: dry spasmodic or nervous coughing, obsessive thinking, worse under tension
SEXUAL ERETHISM in both sexes

5   REDUCES INFLAMMATION, SWELLING AND CONTUSION; RESTRAINS INFECTION, RELIEVES PAIN AND BENEFITS THE SKIN

EAR, NOSE & THROAT INFLAMMATIONS with discharge
SKIN, JOINT & MUSCULAR INFLAMMATIONS
MUSCULAR NEURALGIA, swelling and stiffness
SPRAINS, contusions, chilblains, gout, mastitis, toothache
CHRONIC WOUNDS, ulcers, gangrene
SKIN CONDITIONS and infections generally

Preparation

USE: The ESSENTIAL OIL prepared from Camphor crystals (themselves extracted from the wood) is the most widely available and practical usage form today and may be used like any essential oil. It is made from the lightest fraction of the crystals, and is also called *Camphor white*.
COMPRESSES are excellent in most **skin** conditions, and the INHALATION for **inflammations in the head, head colds with stuffiness** and **congestive** or **spasmodic lung conditions** takes a lot to beat. LINIMENTS are excellent too.

DOSAGE: The **smaller** dose is *stimulant,* whereas the **larger** one is also *relaxant.*
        ESSENTIAL OIL: 2-5 drops in a little warm water

CAUTION: Dosages should not be exceeded, and if used on its own continuously, should be interrupted after ten days by several days' break.
Camphor should not be used in excess heat or excess Yang conditions or with those prone to epilepsy.

Notes

Camphor is one of the very few remedies of the Arab apothecary which escaped the neoclassical expurgation of Renaissance times, and was extensively used by physicians, including the American Eclectics, during the nineteenth century. It originates in the Far East where it is also much in use.

Camphor is very much an agent of opposites, a creator of paradox. Rather than let this distance us from it, it challenges us to look further into its real nature. On the one hand, Camphor is essentially a *Yang supporting warming circulatory stimulant* useful in **deficient cold** conditions of the **intestines, lungs** and **head**, drying any mucous damp in the process, and useful in the onset of fevers as *diaphoretic*. On the other hand, Camphor is an *anti-inflammatory* agent of no mean efficiency, applicable especially to mucosal and skin surfaces, especially in the head; as also a *cooling febrifuge* in all types of fever due to its bitter quality. Plenck's Camphor Vinegar found in

Bayberry: Class 8

the old dispensatories is an example of its use with fevers and infectious inflammations.

And there is another paradox. Camphor is a certain *sympathetic nerve stimulant* and *cardiac stimulant* (for heart Yang deficiency mainly), dispelling gloom and depression, as well as a *nerve relaxant* and *antispasmodic,* especially in larger doses. In this sense, its use "to refresh and restore the fainting and drooping spirits after malignant fevers" (PIERRE POMET, 1694), for example, is balanced by its efficiency in "relieving suffocations of the Womb and procuring sleep" (PITTON DE TOURNEFORT, 1686). The Persian physician IBN SINA's pithy conclusion eight centuries earlier, that Camphor has "a strengthening and calming action," then points to its use in *Qi Constraint* conditions of all kinds where there is underlying **Yang deficiency** or **cold.** This without any doubt is the ideal situation for its use.

In all cases, it is clear that Camphor is an excellent boost for the vital spirit, understood in both the medical and metaphorical sense.

The great Persian clinician AR-RAZI described Camphor as "cold and subtle...cooling the kidneys, bladder and testicles, freezing the sperm and engendering cold diseases in this area", a statement that has provoked much controversy down the ages. While we can resolve the paradox of its warmth by saying that it has both a warming **and** cooling potential in the sense discussed above, we would like to endorse JOHN QUINCY in his dispensatory of 1736 concerning "whether this Drug is prejudicial to Generation by its abating all Desire of Venery, and procuring Barenness," when he concludes: "we shall refer the Decision of this Point to those who have more Leisure and Curiosity for such Inquiries".

BAYBERRY

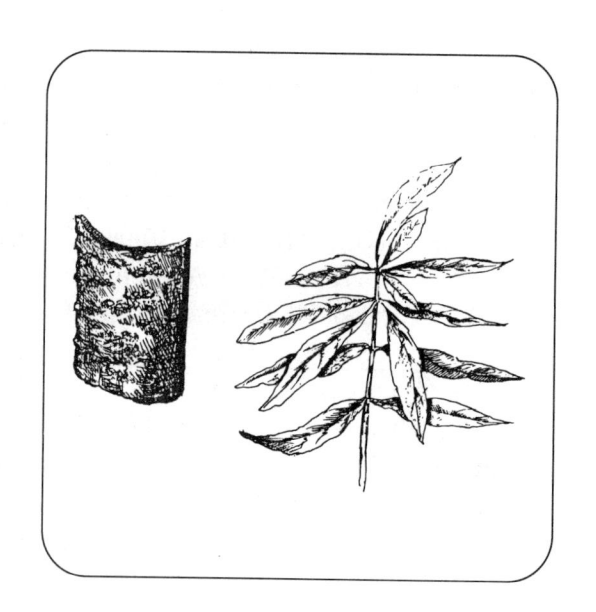

Pharmaceutical name: cortex Myricae
Botanical name: Myrica cerifera L. (N.O. Myricaceae)
Other names: Wax myrtle, Sweet bay, Tallow shrub, Candleberry, Vegetable tallow, Waxberry (Am)
Arbre à la cire, Cirier (Fr)
Wachsmyrte, Wachsgagel, Talgbaum, Amberstaude, Kerzenbeere (Ge)
Part used: the bark; also the berry, *fructus Myricae*

Nature

CATEGORY: mild herb with minimal chronic toxicity
CONSTITUENTS: acrid & astringent resins, myricinic acids, tannic & gallic acids, wax (in berry only)
EFFECTIVE QUALITIES
Primary: astringent, a bit pungent & bitter, warm with cooling potential
Secondary: stimulating, restoring, astringing, decongesting, solidifying
dispersing & stabilizing movement

Class 8: Bayberry

TROPISM: arterial circulation, lungs, head, intestines, liver, uterus
        Warmth organism
        Spleen, Liver, Lung, Colon meridians
GROUND: Phlegmatic & Melancholic krases
        Dependant/Tai Yin Earth & Burdened/Shao Yin biotypes
        Lymphatic/Carbonic/Blue Iris constitution

Functions and Uses

1. SUPPORTS AND TONIFIES THE YANG, GENERATES WARMTH AND DISPELS COLD: STIMULATES THE CIRCULATION AND LUNGS, EXPELS PHLEGM AND CLEARS THE HEAD

   Yang deficiency: weakness, cold limbs and extremities, spontaneous sweating, mental dullness
   arterial blood & Qi deficiency: wheezing, palpitations, fatigue, pale eyelids, face & nails
   head damp cold: congested head & sinuses, thin nasal discharge
   lung phlegm cold: full productive cough with white phlegm

2. CAUSES SWEATING, RELEASES THE EXTERIOR AND SCATTERS WIND COLD; RESOLVES FEVER, REDUCES INFLAMMATION, PUSHES OUT ERUPTIONS AND BENEFITS THE THROAT

   external wind cold: onset of infections with dislike of cold, fatigue, no sweating
   ERUPTIVE FEVERS: chickenpox, measles, scarlet fever
   CHRONIC THROAT conditions: painful, swollen sore throat

3. WARMS AND INVIGORATES THE INTESTINES/*SPLEEN*, LIVER AND GALL BLADDER; CREATES ASTRICTION, RESOLVES MUCUS AND DRIES DAMP; RAISES PROLAPSE, ARRESTS DISCHARGE AND STAUNCHES BLEEDING

   Spleen Yang deficieny with *intestines damp cold:* no appetite, cramping pains, diarrhea
   CHRONIC ENTERITIS
   liver/gall bladder Yang deficiency: frontal or occipital headache worse mornings, flank & midback pain, jaundice, alternating soft & hard stools
   intestines mucous damp (Spleen damp): gurgling bloated abdomen, body and head heaviness, irregular mucousy stool
   CHRONIC DIARRHEA, dysentery, leucorrhea
   HEMORRHAGE from internal organs, incl. intermenstrual and postpartum bleeding
   UTERINE PROLAPSE due to *central Qi sinking*
   SPONGY or BLEEDING GUMS, mouth & gum sores
   COLD BOILS, gangrenous sores, scofulous ulcers, etc.

Preparation

USE: While the DECOCTION is used especially for Bayberry's *astrictive* properties, the TINCTURE is more suited to bring out its *stimulating, warming, sweat inducing* effects. It should be sipped hot at the onset of wind cold. Although a remedy mainly for internal use, its *astringency* makes it an ideal MOUTHWASH, LOTION, etc., in lax tissue states with **pain** or **bleeding**. A SNUFF is used with great success in nasal congestion and adenoids (DIERS RAU, 1972).
DOSAGE: Standard doses throughout. **Large** doses may be used to cause vomiting.
    SNUFF: Use the powdered bark, using fingers or preferably a straw.

Bayberry: Class 8

CAUTION: Due to its *irritant, hot* quality, Bayberry is contraindicated with any acute inflammation and with internal full heat conditions generally.

Notes

Bayberry is a strong *diaphoretic circulatory stimulant*. Like all other herbs in this class it is used for **deficiency cold** conditions due to systemically poor circulation, i.e. Yang deficiency. In his *Natural History of North Carolina* of 1737, the Irish traveller JOHN BRICKELL already noted that "the berries expel Wind and ease all maner of Pains proceeding of Cold, therefore good in Cholick, Palsies...and many other Disorders." Causing sweat as it does, it may also be used in wind cold infectious conditions, with special emphasis on **chronic throat inflammations**.

What sets Bayberry apart from other *pungent hot stimulants*, however, is its *sympathetic nervous stimulation*. As such, it qualifies as a *Yang tonic*, joining Camphor and Basil among others. Global Yang deficiency with fatigue, cold limbs and depression is brilliantly treated by it—depression all the more so as it opens and warms the liver, a function that includes a bile stimulating or *cholagogue* effect. In short, Bayberry is a true reviver of that elusive intangible, the vital spirit.

FINLEY ELLINGWOOD (1898) also emphasizes its use "where **atonic diarrhea**, or persistent diarrhea, accompanies prostrating disease," which puts Bayberry's functions as a *dry astringent* to good use, in addition to its *tonic* ones. **Spleen Yang deficiency** with its fatigue, chilliness and continuous diarrhea cannot fail to spring to mind. Moreover he advises its use "when there is excessive mucus discharge, where catarrhal conditions exist in any locality, especially in the gastrointestinal tract." Here he points to classic damp cold syndromes with systemic deficiency. A similarity in this connection exists with the use of *He zi, fructus Chebulae,* from the Chinese pharmacy, as well as with acupuncture points Bl 20, 21 & 38, Sp 2 & 5, St 41, CV 6 & 8 with moxa.

CLASS 9

Herbs to Restore the Blood, Nourish and Replenish Deficiency

Remedies of this class have a specific function of restoring or building the blood, as well as a more general function of providing substantial nourishment to all tissues. They are used in all **deficiency** conditions involving a nutritional insufficiency resulting in blood deficiency. Being *nutritive* and very concentrated, they are both remedy and food at the same time, variously supplying missing minerals, trace minerals, vitamins, enzymes, and so on. In short, they are both *blood tonics* and *nutritional supplements* and as such work especially on the blood in anabolic processes.[1]

Plant remedies that restore and nourish are even more used in **preventive** medicine than are remedies to restore from Class 8. They are in fact the **similars** mentioned in Hippocratic texts for deficiency conditions. They are ideal preventives, being food and medicine at the same time. They are directed much more at a person's **ground** of disharmony, as seen in their psychosomatic biotype for one thing and in their constitutional tendencies or diatheses to types of illnesses for another. And since nourishment is a universal requirement, the benefit from these herbs actually applies to everyone, irrespective of their biotype or their imbalance, for short or for long-term benefits.

Chinese medicine describes deficiencies of a nutritional nature or that involve aspects of poor nutrition in terms of patterns such as blood deficiency, blood and fluids depletion, liver blood deficiency, uterus blood deficiency and Kidney and Liver depletion. Common symptoms that typify these syndromes are debility and exhaustion, dizziness, a dull white or sallow complexion, dry or withered skin, pale lips, nails and lower eyelids, scanty, delayed, irregular or absent periods, cold extremities, emotional apathy, mental dullness, a thin, weak, rough, hollow or soggy pulse and a short, thin, pale or dry furless tongue. Western medicine recognizes malabsorption syndromes, types of anemia, liver disease and so on in these patterns; or they might be part of other chronic conditions such as autoimmune disease, chronic endocrine imbalance or a metabolic disharmony in general. Their origins lie in either inadequate food intake or in an internal disharmony; often both are found together. Events such as malnutrition, chronic illness, mental or physical overwork, childbirth, excessive sexual acivity and weak constitution can all cause deep deficiencies requiring extended supplementation with herbs of this class, not to mention more specialized supplements such as mineral or vitamin complexes, enzymes, glandular extracts and the various by-products of the apiary such as Royal jelly and Propolis.[2]

On analysis, however, the more specific etiologies of nutritional deficiency in blood deficiency syndromes are more complex. Moreover, they highlight the central role of the blood in anabolic, nutritive processes. There are only two reasons why nutrtional deficiencies occur: either the nutrients themselves are inadequate, or their assimilation is inadequate. In the first case the culprit (at least in the West) is the decreasing quality of food itself, as crops are force-grown chemically with resultant loss of nutrients and as food processing methods further devitalize them through refinement and chemical buffering.[3] The importance of the adoption of "organic", "biodynamic" and "natural" methods of agriculture—for human as well as for planetary survival—is thereby underscored.

In the case of poor assimilation, however, the problems are entirely **internal.** Here nutrient

The Energetics of Western Herbs

transportation, within the context of anabolic processes, simply breaks down. The causes of this may be divided into **hormonal imbalance,** especially of the pituitary, pancreas and pineal glands; and **toxic interference**. Chief among toxemic factors disrupting anabolism are small intestine and liver dysfunctioning, imbalanced fluids PH, and hidden infections (such as candidiasis) of a bacterial, viral, fungal or parasitic nature. Although we are far from understanding all processes involved in some of these disruptions of anabolic efficiency, it is clear that they are potent.

It is in this context of toxic interference that other global patterns of disharmony involving blood deficiency may be understood. Syndromes such as general plethora, general fluids dyskrasia, intestines mucous damp, intestines Qi stagnation, and liver Qi stagnation may all be associated with blood deficiency for this reason. All involve a degree of stagnation and toxicity. Chronic arthritis (a.k.a. cold obstruction), a type of general fluids dyskrasia, is a case in point: it is usually treated in Chinese medicine by formulas that *disperse cold obstruction and nourish the blood.*

Clearly then, the treatment of deficient blood often has to rely on the treatment of contextual disharmonies, whether we broach these analytically or in terms of syndromes, in order to get at its root and provide a real cure.

Herbs in this class are divided into three types. In the first group are *nutritive restoratives,* which increase anabolism and nutrition. Most of these are very high in one or more of the following: minerals, trace elements, vitamins, amino acids and enzymes. They come from a variety of families, and include Flower pollen, Microalgae, Nettle, Artichoke, Alfalfa, Watercress and Kelp.

The second group consists of *blood restoratives,* which increase and regenerate the blood. These botanicals are known empirically and scientifically to have a tropism or affinity for the blood and enhance it in one or more of several ways; chief among them are Parsley, Yellow dock, Red clover and Sarsaparilla.

The third group includes *trophorestoratives,* which nourish certain tissues such as the blood, the nerves, the glands, etc. Of these, the *blood restoratives* just discussed can also be considered *trophorestorative* to that fluid tissue. Specific herbs that nourish and maintain nervous tissue, for example, *nerve trophorestoratives,* include Ginseng (all types), Sage, Valerian and Ho shou wu. Then there are certain remedies that will nourish certain organs, such as Dandelion and Nettle for the liver and Kelp and Bladderwrack for the thyroid. However, too little is known about *glandular trophorestoratives* to make definite claims, and in any event it is clear that the *endocrine gland tonics* of Class 8 will also, in the long run, nourish and regenerate glandular tissue. Certainly the dividing line between a simple *restorative* and a *trophorestorative* is often unclear—and the distinction usually not crucial in actual practice.

All herbs in this class are enhanced by various other types according to the condition presented. Many *tonics* of Class 8, for example, have "anemia", "chlorosis" and the like in their symptomatology, increasing as they do red blood cell count. In traditional physiology the Qi helps build the blood where Spleen Qi deficiency or intestines Qi stagnation is present, not a surprising effect in view of the *bitter/sweet* qualities of most Class 8 *Qi tonics*.

Various *cleansing* remedies from Class 15 may be called for in addition where toxemia or a general fluids dyskrasia is part of blood deficiency.

In conditions of intestines mucous damp with blood deficiency it is neccessary to use *pungent bitter mucolytic* remedies such as Horseradish, Holy thistle, Thyme and Rosemary in addition to blood tonics.

A summary listing of all herbs in this class is found on p. 698.

Notes

1   There are several herb classes in the Materia Medica which affect the blood besides this one. Many *Qi tonic* remedies from Class 7 have some restoring influence on the blood. Class 8 remedies that support the Yang and generate warmth are *circulatory stimulants* which increase arterial circulation. Class 5 botanicals, which are *emmenagogues,* increase menstrual bleeding and frequency. The *astringent venous decongestants* from Class 14 relieve blood congestion and reduce menstrual flow, while *hemostatics* and *styptics* in Class 11 are used to staunch bleeding directly. Clearly, the blood in one or another of its many aspects is involved in a number of treatment strategies.

2   The majority are too specialized for the context of this text, and rightfully require a separate section to do them justice.

3   The pasteurisation of milk reduces the availability of calcium in milk by up to 70%—to give one example out of countless possible ones.

FLOWER POLLEN

Pharmaceutical name: granum floris pollinis
Botanical name: pollen
Other names: Bee pollen (Am)
   Pollen (Fr)
   Blütenpollen, Blütenstaub (Ge)
Part used: the pollen grain

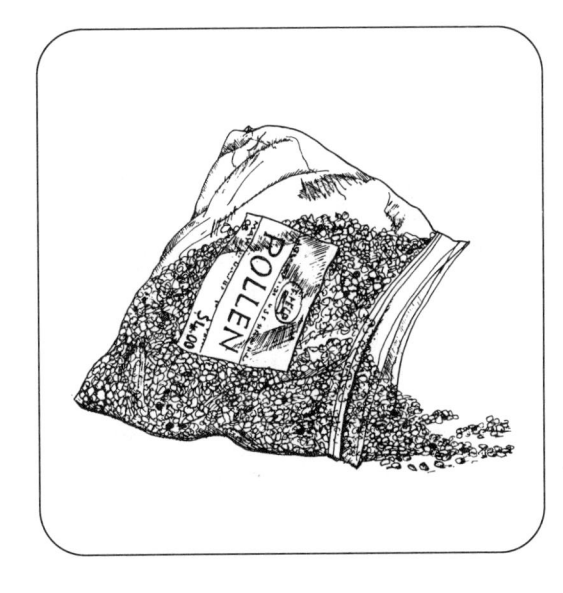

Nature

CATEGORY: mild herb with no chronic toxicity
CONSTITUENTS: 18 proteins 35 % (half in free amino acid form, incl. 8 essentials), saccharides 40%, fats & oils 5%, 16 minerals & trace minerals 3% (incl. calcium, potassium, phosphorus, sodium, sulphur chlorine, magnesium, iron, manganese, copper, iodine, zinc, silica, molybdenum, boron, titanium), 16 vitamins (B1 & 2, thiamin, biotin riboflavin, niacin, B6 complex, pantothenic acid, folic acid, choline, inositol, C, D, E, K, rutin, B12), enzymes & co-enzymes (incl. amylase, diastase, 24 oxidoreductases, 21 transferases, 33 hydrolases, 11 lyases, 5 isomerases, pepsin, trypsin), nucleic acids (DNA & RNA), flavonoids, nucleoside, terpenes, glucose, xanthine, lecithin, lycopin, pentosane, steroid hormones (estrogen & androgen)
EFFECTIVE QUALITIES
Primary: *Taste:* a bit sweet & pungent & salty & sour & bitter
   Warmth: neutral
   Moisture: neutral
Secondary: nourishing, thickening, restoring, dissolving, softening

Flower pollen: Class 9
TROPISM
Organs or parts: all
Organisms: all four
Meridians: all twelve, Chong & Ren
Tri Dosas: increases Kapha & Pitta
GROUND
Krases/temperaments: all four
Biotypes: all eight
Constitutions: all three

Functions and Uses

1 PROMOTES LONGEVITY AND RETARDS AGING; ENHANCES IMMUNE POTENTIAL
   CONSTITUTIONAL WEKNESS; deficient Original Qi
   PREMATURE AGING and senility, insufficient cell regeneration

2 PROVIDES NOURISHMENT AND REPLENISHES DEFICIENCY; RESTORES THE BLOOD AND ESSENCE AND INCREASES THE QI; PROMOTES GROWTH; ENHANCES SEXUAL DESIRE AND GENERATES STRENGTH
   blood and qi deficiency: chronic fatigue, weakness, palpitations, shortness of breath
   ANEMIA
   Kidney Essence deficiency: weak knees, dizziness, backache, poor memory, senility
   EXHAUSTION or debility due to any cause
   SLOW PHYSICAL AND MENTAL DEVELOPMENT in children
   IMPOTENCE, INFERTILITY, poor sexual desire

3 RESTORES THE NERVE, BRAIN AND HEART, BALANCES THE CIRCULATION; BENEFITS THE MEMORY AND LIFTS THE SPIRIT; INDUCES REST
   nerve deficiency: with weakness, oversensitivity, depression
   heart Qi deficiency: palpitations, chest opression
   LOW or HIGH BLOOD PRESSURE
   MENTAL EXHAUSTION due to excessive study, etc.
   POOR MEMORY, MENTAL STUPOR
   CHRONIC DEPRESSION of all types
   INSOMNIA AND UNREST due to heart Yin/blood deficiency, heart and Kidney Yin deficiency

4 RESTORES THE REPRODUCTIVE ORGANS, LENIFIES IRRITATION AND HARMONIZES URINATION
   genitourinary Qi deficiency (kidney Qi infirmity): frequent scangy urination
   PROSTATE ENLARGEMENT with urgent, frequent paincul urination, rectal fullness

5 RESTORES THE INTESTINES/*SPLEEN* AND LIVER AND HARMONIZES METABOLISM: PROMOTES ASSIMILATION, RESTRAINS PUTREFICATION AND PROMOTES BOWEL MOVEMENT
   Spleen Qi deficiency: poor appetitie, fatigue, loose stool
   GASTROENTERITIS

Class 9: Flower pollen

> INTESTINAL FERMENTATION with, e.g., *intestines damp cold* or *intestines Qi stagnation* with flatus and distension
> MALABSORPTION SYNDROME
> IRREGULAR BOWEL MOVEMENT of any kind
> CHRONIC CONSTIPATION in all conditions
> ALL METABOLIC DISHARMONIES

6 **PROMOTES CLEANSING, CLEARS TOXINS AND RESOLVES TOXEMIA; PROMOTES URINATION, SOFTENS DEPOSITS AND DISSIPATES TUMORS; CHELATES HEAVY METALS AND PROMOTS WEIGHT LOSS**
> PREVENTIVE AND REMEDIAL in AUTOTOXICOSIS or *general toxemia,* including heavy metal poisoning
> *general fluids disharmony* with chronic rheumatic or arthritic conditions
> URIC ACID DIATHESIS
> *kidney Qi stagnation:* dry skin, fetid stool, irritability
> *general plethora:* overweight, water retention, cellulite
> HARD DEPOSITS incl. urinary and gallstone, arteriosclerosis
> TUMORS benign and cancerous

7 **ACTIVATES IMMUNITY, RESTRAINS INFECTION, REDUCES INFLAMMATION AND CLEARS TOXINS; PROMOTES TISSUE REPAIR; RELIEVES ALLERGIES**
> PREVENTIVE and remedial in epidemics
> BACTERIAL INFECTIONS of urogenital (e.g. PROSTATITIS, CYSTITIS) digestive (e.g. ENTERITIS) and upper respiratorysystems (e.g. LARYNGITIS), esp. colibacillus amd salmonella
> *fire toxin:* boils, sores, abscesses, fever
> *stomach fire:* fetid breath, thirst for cold drinks, hearburn
> PEPTIC ULCERS due to hyperacidity
> SKIN ULCERS, sores, scabs, eruptions
> BUNS, WOUNDS
> ALLERGIES in general and to light flower pollen in particular

8 **RELIEVES WHEEZING, BENEFITS THE THROAT AND VOICE**
> ASTHMATIC BREATHING in all conditions
> SORE THROAT itchy throat
> VOICE LOSS

9 **PROMOTES ESTROGEN**
> ESTROGEN INSUFFICIENCY with *deficient uterus blood* or *tone* with, e.g., delayed or absent menses

Preparation

USES: Flower pollen is used mainly internally, although it was/is used in COMPRESSES by people in South America, China and Yogoslavia to *promote tissue repair, disinfect* and *cool burns.* Being easy to assimilate, there is no need to tincture, infuse or do anything with it except EAT it. Allowing it to dissolve in the mouth (e.g. under the tongue) ensures fairly rapid influence on the

Flower pollen: Class 9

brain, if this is the desired effect. It is best taken on an empty stomach, on its own or with warm water or herb tea.

DOSES: The normal dose is 1 tsp per day on an empty stomach. This can safely be increased to several times that amount in severe cases, since pollen has no chronic toxicity.

CAUTION: In spite of pollen's success in treating allergies, in some people it can actually cause allergic reactions. To be safe, begin with a small dose at first, e.g. 1/4 tsp. If no reaction occurs, the normal dose can safely be taken.

Notes

If one considers, for a moment, the true nature of this unique substance that has been used in herbal healing throughout recorded history, it becomes clear that the definition flower pollen is actually a far more accurate term for it than bee pollen. These grains are not an animal product, as the name bee pollen suggests: they are a botanical one. The small, orange colored grains found in the stores reveal on close inspection a variety of different colors, and in fact cover every hue of the whole colour spectrum. It is the pollen from untold thousands of wild flowers, herbs, bushes and trees—in which the Mint family plays a major part—that make up these golden granules. Since bees have an intimate relationship with a large segment of flowering plants, notably those which, like them, live in the warmth element, they are privileged to facilitate the accessibility of pollen for their own and for human use (as well as causing pollinization among flowers themselves in so doing). In the process of gathering nectar, which they turn into honey, flower pollen sticks to their bodies. As much as a bee's weight is carried back to the hive, where it is shaped into grains to become nourishment for the bee larvae. These same pollen grains are the substance used as a *nutritive restoring* remedy by humans.

Clearly, the processes involved in making this pollen so easily available to us are the result of a beautiful synergy, in the realm of warmth, between flowers and bees. No other botanical in this Materia Medica is produced in the same way. Propolis, Royal jelly and honey are the other products of the hive. Unlike flower pollen, however, they are substances processed and produced by the bees themselves—hence, actual bee products.

A glance at Flower pollen's function and indications would seem to suggest that it is nature's answer to virtually every malady known. It has the widest spectrum of effects and uses of any herb. It is true that no organ, system or tissue is unaffected by its influence: its tropism is **global**. And certainly, when we let the grains dissolve on the tongue, experientially we can distinctly evaluate all five major tastes—in turn sweet, then a bit spicy, after which some salty, sour and bitter unfold in layers. This also attests to pollen's comprehensive effect from the energetic perspective, since each taste has specific properties.

Taking the modern pharmacological tack, a similar picture results. More chemical constituents—22 in all—are found in flower pollen than in any other botanical, and in higher concentration, on the whole, than in other concentrated nutrients such as royal jelly, microalgae and yeast. The more important of these are ten amino acids, enzymes, a string of minerals, including trace minerals, all known vitamins, antibiotic substances and steroid hormones. In addition, it is thought that as yet unknown ingredients play a part in determining pollen's total effects.

Should we view flower pollen as the ultimate cure-all? As a latter day elixir of longevity?

One thing is certain: It is possibly the finest herb to nourish and supplement in existence. This means that essentially its use is for **deficient** conditions of any kind. Here it goes deeper than any other. It has been touted as a prime *rejuvenating* agent by more than one researcher and more than one gerontologist all over the world. **Endocrine, nervous, organ** and **tissue systems** are all enhanced through its regular use.

Class 9: Microalgae

However, let us be clear: Flower pollen is no cure-all, any more than Microalgae or Nettle. In some conditions it may cure, in many it provides invaluable *nutritive* and *cleansing* support, like all other herbs in this class. But it may do this better than another herb, and it will certainly cover more ground—being the complete rainbow remedy that it is.

Specific uses at which it excels should also be singled out. Conditions involving **weakness** of the **brain**, the **nerves**, as seen in deficient mental conditions, is one of these. **Immune deficiency** and **imbalance** states, with or without **infections**, is another, as is **prostate enlargement**. Nor should flower pollen's *cleansing, detoxifying, resolvent* activities be overlooked. As much as its *restoring* ones, they are applicable to a great variety of conditions involving **toxemia, plethora, sclerosis, tumors** and **infections**.

From the Mayans in Central America to the Slavs in Eastern Europe, flower pollen, along with honey which contains traces of pollen, was considered a medicinal food—indeed, food fit for goddesses and gods. It may have been the Ambrosia of the ancient Greek pantheon. It is not difficult to understand why.

MICROALGAE

Pharmaceutical name: planta tota Microalgae
Botanical name: Aphanizaomenon flos-aquae, vel
　　Spirulina spp. (N.O. Nostocales), *vel*
　　Chlorella spp. (N.O. Chrococcales)
Other names: a) Super Blue-Green™; b)
　　Spirulina c) Chlorella
Part used: the whole plant

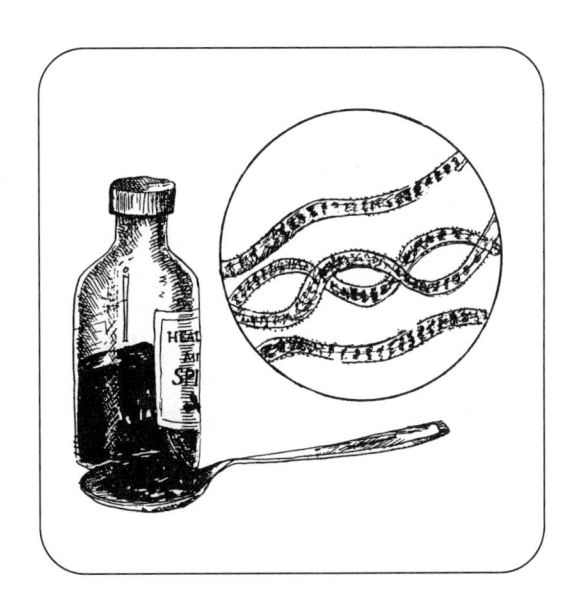

Nature

CATEGORY: mild herb with no chronic toxicity
CONSTITUENTS: protein 50-71%, amino acids (up to 20, incl. 8 essentials), chlorophyll up to 6%, lipids 5%, nucleic acids RNA & DNA, minerals & trace minerals 12-15% (incl. calcium, potasssium, iron, phosphoros, iodine, magnesium, zinc, titanium, copper, cobalt, chlorine, manganese), vitamins (incl.ß-carotene, C, B1, B 2, B6, B12, niacin, choline, folic acid, biotin, pantothenic acid, inositol, ß-tocopherol E), phytol 1%, sterols 2%
EFFECTIVE QUALITIES
Primary: a bit sweet & salty, neutral, neutral
Secondary: nourishing, restoring, dissolving
TROPISM: all organs & parts
　　　　all four organisms
　　　　all twelve meridians
GROUND: all krases, biotypes and constitutions

Microalgae: Class 9

Functions and Uses

1. PROMOTES LONGEVITY AND RETARDS AGING; ENHANCES IMMUNE POTENTIAL

   CONSTITUTIONAL WEAKNESS; deficient Original Qi
   PREMATURE AGING and senility, poor cell regeneration

2. PROVIDES NOURISHMENT AND REPLENISHES DEFICIENCY: RESTORES THE BLOOD AND ESSENCE AND INCREASES THE QI, PROMOTES GROWTH AND GENERATES STRENGTH

   blood & Qi deficiency with fatigue, pale eyelids, face, etc., shallow breathing, palpitations
   ANEMIA
   Kidney Essence deficiency with premature aging & senility, mental dullness, weak knees
   DEBILITY & EXHAUSTION in all conditions, acute and chronic
   SLOW GROWTH or MENTAL RETARDMENT IN CHILDREN
   PROTEIN DEFICIENCY CONDITIONS, PREGNANCY
   DEGENERATIVE DISEASE

3. RESTORES THE NERVE AND BRAIN, BENEFITS THE MEMORY; RELIEVES ANXIETY

   nerve deficiency with weakness, poor memory or concentration
   heart blood & Spleen Qi deficiency with anxiety, unrest, fatigue
   SENILE DEMENTIA

4. RESTORES THE LIVER, PANCREAS AND INTESTINES/*SPLEEN*, HARMONIZES METABOLISM AND REGULATES SECRETIONS: BALANCES INTESTINAL FLORA, RESTRAINS PUTREFACTION AND PROMOTES ASSIMILATION AND WEIGHT-GAIN; BENEFITS VISION

   liver Qi stagnation with constipation, irregular stool, flank pain
   intestines mucous damp (Spleen damp) with no appetite, mucoid diarrhea, epigastric distention, heaviness
   INTESTINAL FERMENTATION, chronic gastritis
   MALABSORPTION SYNDROME
   CHRONIC PANCREATITIS
   LOW BLOOD SUGAR, diabetes (supportive)
   POOR EYESIGHT, cataract, glaucoma, retinitis (nephritic & diabetic)

5. PROMOTES CLEANSING, CLEARS TOXINS AND RESOLVES TOXEMIA; DRAINS PLETHORA AND PROMOTES WEIGHT LOSS; PROTECTS THE LIVER, BENEFITS THE SKIN AND RESOLVES TUMORS; SOFTENS DEPOSITS AND CHELATES HEAVY METALS

   general fluids dyskrasia with chronic arthritic, gouty or rheumatic conditions, incl. rheumatoid and osteo-arthritis
   URIC ACID DIATHESIS
   SKIN CONDITIONS: eczema, dermatitis, acne, warts, cold sores
   HARD DEPOSISTS, incl. atherosclerosis, arteriosclerosis, liver cirrhosis, angiosclerosis
   HEPATITIS (viral, preventive & remedial); liver damage
   HIGH BLOOD CHOLESTEROL, high blood pressure

Class 9: Microalgae

HEAVY METAL AUTOTOXICOSIS (preventive & remedial), e.g. cadmium, lead, copper, mercury

TUMORS benign and cancerous

general plethora with obesity, cellulite, etc.

6 ACTIVATES IMMUNITY, RESTRAINS INFECTION AND REDUCES INFLAMMATION; RESTORES THE LIVER AND RELIEVES ALLERGIES

PREVENTIVE in epidemics and infections

LOCAL & SYSTEMIC INFECTIONS of bacterial, viral or fungal nature, incl. flu, pneumonia, hepatitis, yeast infections, leprosy, herpes, mononucleosis (Epstein-Barr)

PANCREATITIS

ALLERGIES, incl. allergic rhinitis, asthma, dermatitis, mercury; from pesticides and insecticides; from alcohol

7 PROMOTES TISSUE REPAIR AND ARRESTS BLEEDING

ULCERS OF ALL KINDS: peptic ulcer, skin ulcer, leg ulcer, ulcerative carcinoma, diabetic ulcer, bedsore, granuloma

PYORRHEA, gingivitis

WOUNDS, BURNS, etc.

Preparation

USE: A variety of microalgae exist in various preparations and packages in commerce, in POWDER, TABLET, GRANULE and TINCTURE form. They are designed for both internal and external use, e.g. MOUTHWASHES.

Allergic conditions usually need three months of taking Microalgae before any noticeable improvement sets in. Microalgae is safe, and recommended, during pregnancy.

DOSAGE: For maintenence and prevention: 2-5 g per day, in two or three doses, and as directed.

For treatment: 5-10 g per day

There is no upper dosage limit to this entirely nontoxic herb.

CAUTION: With chronic arthritis small doses should be taken to begin with and only gradually increased, since microalgae may initially increase the pain. The same goes for chronic intestinal conditions, where an increase of abdominal flatulence, possibly with cramps, may be experienced. As with miso and Garlic, micro-algae initially increases intestinal fermentation as it destroys noxious bacteria and then, given a balanced wholesome diet, eliminates it entirely.

Notes

The whole subject of microalgae, whether from a botanical, historical, commercial, nutritional or therapeutic point of view, is studded with difficulties. This fact should be clear at the outset, lest any statements made here seem contradictory or nonsensical. Equally clearly, however, microalgae are making an increasing impact on society world wide, such that the obstacles presented to a clear understanding of them by commercial interests, nutritional theories, taxonomic confusion, historical myopia and individual limitations should, and can, be surmounted. Paradoxically, however, as will be suggested below, it is not so much the factual problems that microalgae bring up as the psychological ones which constitute the major barrier to elucidating a rational use for this unique plant.

In simplest terms, microalgae (also known as phytoplankton) are sea plants like the large

Microalgae: Class 9

(macro) algae such as Dulse, Kelp, Iceland moss, etc., but on a miniature scale. Of the three main types defined at top, only Spirulina is visible to naked vision. *Aphanizaomenon* and *Spirulina* belong to the blue-green class of algae, living in saltwater lakes around the world, while *Chlorella* is a freshwater green alga. All are primitive colonial single celled plants without any root, leaf or flower. Indeed, blue-green algae are believed to have been the first form of plant life originating over four billion years ago.

The primal soup, the gestating ocean, which swirled for over two and a half billion years over this planet to lunar rhythms spawned microalgae. As these tiny stirrings of green life absorbed the fluid mineral nourishment and the gaseous carbon dioxide that fostered them, they began to release nitrogenous substances which eventually created oxygen, the basis of all animal and human life. The point here is simply that algae were involved with the very origins of organic life on this planet. The implications for us today, and for our relationship to this primal botanical substance, alga, will be examined below.

There can be no doubt that during the first 30,000 years of the human's existence, microalga was a significant source of food. Washed onto the shores of lakes, it would be collected by women and sun-dried. This is still carried out today by the Kanembu natives along the shores of lake Johann in Chad in the deep African Sahara; they prepare buns with it or drink it as a spicy soup. Historically there is archeological evidence that the Aztecs cultivated Spirulina in several lakes as well as in the intricate Mayan waterways of southern Mexico. In the Near East during Biblical times, the food Manna was prepared with the *Nostoc* species of microalgae, possibly harvested from the Dead Sea. The pattern that emerges is one of recurring forgetting and remembering: time and time again, this simplest form of aquaculture has moved on to agriculture, the cultivation of land plants, with the demise of the former. From time to time, as in times of drought or hardship, this older, lake based farming is inevitably remembered and reintegrated.

Today, with the reality of a dangerous inequality and shortage of distribution of terrestial food sources, the prospects of the aquatic resources that microalgae represent have once again become attractive. Since the First World War several European countries have begun researching and producing a variety of microalgae types, and in the last forty years Japanese companies have expanded this field with characteristic vigor. The only forms of microalgae being produced in commerce today on any scale outside Japan are *Spirulina* and *Aphanizaomenon*. The latter is collected from Upper Klamath Lake, Oregon, where it is fresh freeze-dried for distribution; *Spirulina* is farm grown in monoculture in Thailand and Mexico. Nevertheless, many lakes around the world, both saline and freshwater, naturally contain single strains: *Spirulina,* for example, blooms as the dominant alga in seasonal abundance in many lakes in North and East Africa (Ethiopia, Kenya), Mexico and South America (Peru); while the Oregonian *Aphanizaomenon* itself is an entirely naturally occuring single variety.

While there is little to be gained from comparing the individual merits of these three edible microalgae, a look at their general effects both as food and as remedy is appropriate. The differences between them are not significant enough to warrant quibbling over: this is an exercise given sufficient attention in the available writings on them, which are mostly promotional (or subsidized) literature touting the superiority of one type of microalga over another. There is enough solid evidence from Japan, Mexico and the U.S. that a certain body of effects can be expected from any of these three varieties.

It may be said at the outset that for sheer spectrum and depth of their *nutritive, restoring* and *cleansing* properties, microalgae come a close second to flower pollen. Their *nutritive* content is actually higher, having a much higher protein count than flower pollen (two and a half times that of Kelp and Alfalfa, and highest in *Aphanizaomenon* and *Spirulina,* in fact). This commends their use

Class 9: Microalgae

for children with **slow physical** *and* **mental development**, as an excellent supplement during **pregnancy**, as well as for **chronic** or **degenerative** conditions with **debility** in general. **Anemias** of most kinds are helped, and, in this connection, is well matched to the syndrome Kidney essence deficiency. There is some evidence for an *antiaging* property in microalgae that works via the brain, although the mechanisms involved have as yet only been speculated upon. Certainly in senile dementia, as well as in simple mental exhaustion, microalgae have proved their worth. Interestingly, the amino acid profile of *Aphanizaomenon* is virtually identical as for that of humans.

The benefits of microalgae to the liver are well known and to be expected. Microalgae's *protective, detoxifying* and *restoring* effects on this organ come into their own where **deficiency, stagnation, toxemic** and **hardening** processes affect it, including, in extreme cases, e.g.. hepatitis and liver cirrhosis. As to the pancreas and intestines, conditions as different as intestines damp cold with intestinal fermentation, pancreatitis, diabetes, chronic constipation and diarrhea are successfully addressed. As an *antidyskratic* herb, microalgae redress uric acid imbalances and promote deep, systemic *cleansing,* beneficial in all forms of arthritic, rheumatic and skin conditions. Being *resolvent,* hard deposits are scoured and cholesterol levels lowered. *Antitumoral* effects have been also established and correlated with the acidic polysaccharides (which stimulate immune activity) in their cell walls and their beta carotene and their extremely high chlorophyll content (highest in *Aphanizaomenon* and *Chlorella).* Chlorophyll also explains microalgae's *vulnerary* effects when they are applied to internal and external ulcers as well as wounds and burns.

Not only *anti-infective* properties have been demonstrated in microalgae, but also *antiviral* and *antibacterial* ones. Taken together, they can prevent and treat not only acute bouts of flu, pneumonia, etc., but also chronic debilitating conditions triggered by the Epstein-Barr and the Cytomegalovirus, both of which have definitely been linked to the onset of Aids syndrome.

One may be forgiven for wondering, at this point, why this superbotanical is not used in the West in any way that does it justice. Its strong *immune stimulant* and *antiviral* effects alone should carve it a niche among other herbs such as Lomatium, Echinacea and Astragalus in the treatment of chronic immune deficiency diseases such as candida, infectious mononucleosis and Aids. Clearly, its potential as both a viable high protein and high mineral food and as a therapeutic agent (both preventive and curative) in its own right has simply not been recognized, let alone exploited. This is the exact situation: Microalgae, on the whole, are considered merely one nutritional supplement among many (which of course they are, used for maintenance), with one alga being popular for a few years and then another for the next few years, in faddish succession; but they are hardly considered a serious herb. This is true in spite of the overwhelming evidence of clinical trials, laboratory tests and analyses and the daily experience of countless Japanese physicians. Why is this?

The simplest, most obvious explanation, that microalgae cannot be sold and advertized as a medicine in Western countries, does not really hold water. In Europe, for example, this would be perfectly possible. No, the answer lies quite simply in people, not in the product. Throughout the Far East, algae have always been used as food and medicine, hence the ready acceptance of these miniature varieties. It is we in the West who have not begun to wake up to the real therapeutic significance of microalgae.

Again, there must be a reason for this. The reason is linked to the primal nature, the absolute primordial simplicity of this single-celled organism. Microalga is the substance and emblem of the **embryonic** stage of life on this earth. It represents the **origin of life** within the inchoate, undivided oneness. *Spirulina,* with its endless, undulating spiral filaments swimming in salt water, is perhaps the clearest expression of the embryonic nature of microalgae.

Moreover, this original oneness, however it may be expressed, is a **female** phenomenon. The

Wheatgrass: Class 9

original ocean itself, which gave birth to microalgae, is like female amniotic fluid in the planetary uterus. By contrast, today, at this stage of the evolution of human consciousness, the female principle has been suppressed in favor of the masculine. The individual and society have been moulded by patriarchal values for over 4,000 years.

The point being made here is this: The psyche of the individual today does not consciously accept a substance so evincive of the female principle, so redolent of the holic intrauterine state as microalga. As a result, in the words of scientist and algologist DARYL KOLLMAN, "algae are simply not in the cultural nutritional patterns or in the organic energy identity patterns of most of the human race." That they were, prior to the rise of patristic societies, is clear.

Today, when the female principle is showing signs of renewed stirrings, there is great potential for rediscovering the real power of microalgae. Behind the latest press releases, the advertising hooks and the ever-changing trends lies a universal awakening to their true significance. We may join in this exploration and benefit in more ways than we realized.

WHEATGRASS

Pharmaceutical name: lamina Tritici aestivi
Botanical name: Triticum aestivum L. (N.O. Graminaceae)
Other names: brin de blé (Fr)
Weizenhalm (Ge)
Part used: the leaf

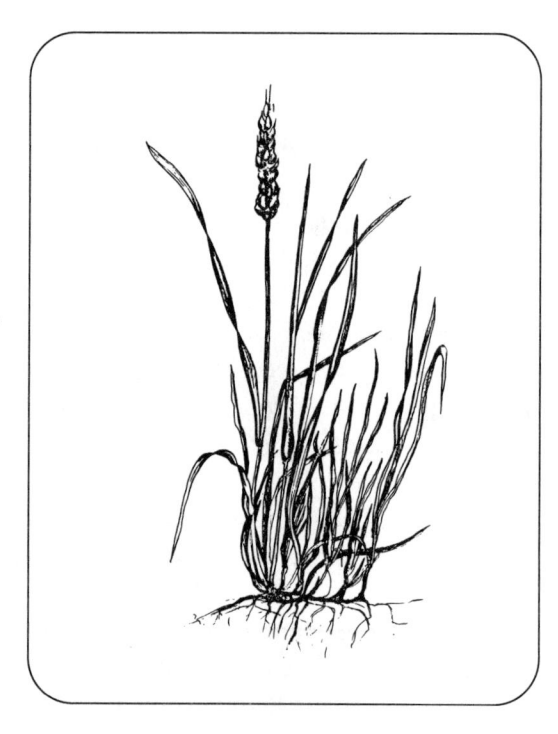

Nature

CATEGORY: mild herb with minimal chronic toxicity
CONSTITUENTS: chlorophyll, choline, enzymes, amino acids, minerals & trace minerals (incl. calcium, iron, chlorine, potassium, zinc, magnesium, phosphorus, sulfur, cobalt), vitamins (incl. C, A, E, F, K, niacin, B1, B2, B6, B17, pantothenic acid)
EFFECTIVE QUALITIES
Primary: sweet, a bit salty & astringent, neutral, neutral
Secondary: nourishing, thickening, restoring, dissolving
TROPISM: blood, fluids, intestines, liver, pancreas, pituitary
Fluid organism
Spleen, Stomach meridians
GROUND: all krases, biotypes and constitutions

Class 9: Wheatgrass

Functions and Uses

1. PROVIDES NOURISHMENT AND REPLENISHES DEFICIENCY: RESTORES THE BLOOD AND FLUIDS, INCREASES THE QI AND GENERATES STRENGTH

    blood & fluids deficiency with fatigue, weakness, pale face, nails & eyelids
    Qi deficiency with fatigue, weakness, shallow breathing
    ANEMIA
    CHRONIC FATIGUE, degenerative disease

2. RESTORES THE LIVER, STOMACH, INTESTINES/*SPLEEN*, PANCREAS AND PITUITARY; HARMONIZES METABOLISM AND REGULATES SECRETIONS; RESTRAINS PUTREFACTION, PROMOTES ASSIMILATION AND WEIGHTGAIN

    liver Qi stagnation with constipation, irregular stool, hemorrhoids
    intestines mucous damp with no appetite, abdominal distention, alternating loose & hard stool
    MALABSORPTION SYNDROME, poor assimilation, malnutrition, chronic *Spleen Qi deficiency*
    GASTRITIS, peptic ulcer
    PANCREATIC INSUFFICIENCY, low blood sugar, diabetes (supportive)
    PITUITARY INSIFFICIENCY

3. PROMOTES CLEANSING, CLEARS TOXINS AND RESOLVES TOXEMIA; DRAINS PLETHORA AND PROMOTES WEIGHT LOSS; CHELATES HEAVY METALS, BENEFITS THE SKIN AND DISSIPATES TUMORS

    general toxemia: breath & body odor, rough dry skin, fetid stool, fatigue
    HEAVY METAL AUTOTOXICOSIS (preventive & remedial)
    general plethora: obesity, cellulite
    HIGH BLOOD PRESSURE
    SKIN CONDITIONS: dermatoses, e.g. eczema
    TUMORS benign & cancerous

4. RESTRAINS INFECTION, REDUCES INFLAMMATION AND PROMOTES TISSUE REPAIR

    MOUTH INFECTIONS, athlete's foot
    SINUSITIS, rhinitis, bronchitis, head colds
    BURNS, gingivitis, stomatitis, pyorrhea
    ULCERS of all kinds: peptic ulcer, ulcerative colitis, skin ulcer, leg ulcer, bedsore
    WOUNDS, cuts, bleeding gums
    INSECT BITES, poison ivy rash

Preparation

USE: The freshly pressed JUICE, or the fresh FREEZE-DRIED extract, of the organically grown wheatgrass is by far the best preparation form; all other dried or powdered preparations are much inferior.

Since it goes off quickly, the JUICE must be drunk within 12 hours of preparing; it may be used internally and externally.

SWABS, POULTICES, etc., should be applied to **external injuries, skin problems, swollen** or **bleeding gums, pyorrhea** and **tired** or **inflamed eyes.** An EYEWASH of the extremely well

Wheatgrass: Class 9

strained JUICE can also be prepared. GARGLES will relieve **sore throat**, and CHEWING the grass directly fights **bad breath**.

Wheatgrass JUICE may be used in ENEMAS and COLONICS for its *cleansing* and *restoring* effect systemically and on the colon itself. As a HAIR RINSE (leave on as long as possible), by strengthening the hair it may help **split ends** and **scalp problems** such as itchy or scaly scalp.

DOSAGE: JUICE: 1-2 ounces taken neat or with water or other juices up to three times a day
 Others: as directed

CAUTION: Overdosing tends to cause malaise, nausea or vomiting.

NOTE: An electric slow-turning juicer made especially for juicing sprouts, wheatgrass, soft vegetables, etc., should be used to extract the juice.

As with other food remedies in this class, wheatgrass should be discontinued for 2-3 days every ten days or so to allow the organism to adapt to changes more easily.

Notes

The preventive and curative uses of juices and extracts from wheatgrass closely follow those of microalgae. The reason for this lies mainly in the element chlorophyll which, more than anything else, is responsible for the general *nutritive, restorative* and *cleansing* effect on the human organism of all grasses.

While we need not analyze the indispensible role of chlorophyll in plant and human ecoloy, we should note its valuable therapeutic effects with both deficiency and excess types of conditions. Since it *nourishes* and *tonifies* with its intensely *sweet* taste, wheatgrass is used on one hand for **blood** and **fluids deficiency** (e.g. anemia), **Qi deficiency** and chronic liver, pancreas and gastrointestinal deficiency—essentialy a **Spleen Qi deficiency** in Chinese medicine. On the other hand, with its generous minerals and trace minerals content, wheatgrass will drain excess conditions characerized by **toxemia** and **plethora**, including those where skin eruptions, overweight and tumors are present, as well as in cases of heavy metal poisoning. Finally, like other grasses and microalgae, wheatgrass has excellent *vulnerary, antiseptic* and *anti-inflammatory* actions that come into their own in the treatment of **ulcers** of any kind. Clearly, it is worth considering using chlorophyll high herbs such as wheatgrass or barleygrass for conditions such as these if their preparation is at all feasible or if a prepared extract from them is in some form available.

ASPARAGUS

Pharmaceutical name: rhizoma Asparagi
Botanical name: Asparagus officinalis L. (N.O. Asparaginae)
Ancient names: Aspharago, Emergo (Gr)
   Asparagus domesticus/segius/sativus/simpliciter (Lat)
Other names: Sparrow grass, Sperage (Eng)
   Asperge (Fr)
   Spargel, Korrallenkraut, Schwammwurz (Ge)
Part used: the rhizome

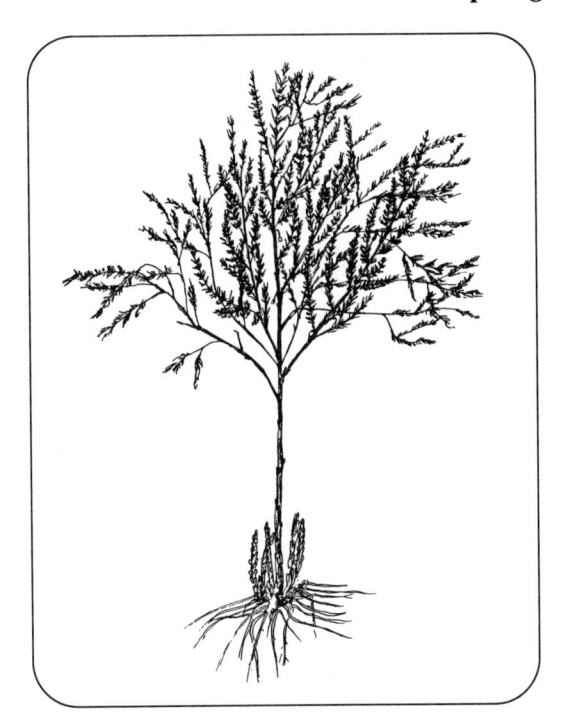

Nature

CATEGORY: mild herb with minimal chronic toxicity
CONSTITUENTS: asparagin, arginin, tyrosin, bernstein acid, methanethiol (methyl mercaptan), asparagose, glycoside (coniferin), chelidonic acid, choline, saponins, flavanoids, purine, calcium, iron, trace minerals 9% (incl. manganese, phosphoros, potassium, copper, fluoride, iodine), vits. A, B, C, vanillin
EFFECTIVE QUALITIES
Primary: a bit sweet & salty, warm, moist
Secondary: nourishing, thickening, stimulating, dissolving, relaxing
TROPISM: urogenital organs, intestines, liver, pancreas, blood, fluids
   Fluid organism
   Kidney, Liver, Small Intestine meridians
GROUND: Sanguine & Phlegmatic krases
   Charming/Yang Ming Earth & Self-Reliant/Yang Ming Metal biotypes
   all constitutions

Functions and Uses

1 PROVIDES NOURISHMENT AND REPLENISHES DEFICIENCY: RESTORES THE BLOOD AND ESSENCE, GENERATES STRENGTH AND BRIGHTENS THE VISION, BENEFITS AND COMFORTS THE SINEWS

   Kidney Essence deficiency: premature senility, white hair, brittle bones, blurred vision, weak knees,
   liver blood deficiency: dry painful eyes, hazy or weak vision, numb limbs, muscle spasms or twitching, stiff tendons, dry skin or hair, dry vagina
   blood deficiency: pale lips, nails, eyelids, shallow breathing, palpitations, fatigue, scanty menses
   DEBILITY in convalescence, due to overwork, childbirth, etc, esp. in childhood

Asparagus: Class 9

2. **RESTORES AND WARMS THE UROGENITAL ORGANS, ENHANCES SEXUAL DESIRE**

    genitourinary cold (Kidney Yang deficiency): lassitude, weak knees and legs, chilliness, lack of sexual desire, impotence, lower backache

3. **PROMOTES CLEANSING, CLEARS TOXINS AND RESOLVES TOXEMIA: SEEPS WATER, PROMOTES URINATION, SOFTENS STONES AND LENIFIES IRRITATION**

    general toxemia and *general fluids dyskrasia:* intermittent pains, chronic skin eruptions, gout, rheumatism, arthritis
    HIGH BLOOD URIC ACID & CHOLESTEROL
    liver fluid congestion: general edema, nausea, fatigue, backache
    CARDIAC EDEMA
    GENERAL BLADDER IRRITATION: obstructed urination, scanty, frequent, dripping or difficult urination, lumbar pain
    URINARY SAND or STONE

4. **MOISTENS THE INTESTINES AND PROMOTES BOWEL MOVEMENT**

    intestines dryness: constipation, dull abdominal pain and swelling, dry mouth & tongue

5. **RESTORES THE PANCREAS AND LOWERS BLOOD SUGAR**
    DIABETES (supportive)

Preparation

USE: The **shoots** of the garden or wild Asparagus, eaten as a vegetable, are not inefficient in *nourishing, restoring* and *cleansing,* as the Italians can attest. They may also be JUICED. It is the **roots** that provide the real medicine, however, with their high mineral and trace elements content. These may be DECOCTED or TINCTURED in the normal way, and serve all purposes. In the past, COMPRESSES were used for chronic or acute painful conditions of all kinds.
DOSAGE: FRESH JUICE: 1 tbsp three times a day
          Others: standard doses
CAUTION: Asparagus is contraindicated with cystitis and in acute joint rheumatism, as it tends to irritate the kidney lining. Moreover, avoid using in infectious heat & damp heat conditions of the kidney & bladder. Being exceptionally high in purine, if used for gout it should be taken in moderation: this applies to the shoots as well as the roots!

Notes

The close connection between the liver and the Fluid organism is indicated when we note that traditional urine inspection was thought to give a better picture of liver condition than of kidney. Hence GALEN considered Asparagus root to be one of the **four opening roots**, which denotes opening the liver and urination in one. However, when SCHROEDER (1611) writes that Asparagus "liberates the liver," he is also pointing to the fact that a range of liver disharmonies are amenable to its influence: we may summarize these here as belonging to its *fluids governing, detoxifying* and *cleansing,* and *synthesizing* and *nourishing* aspects. Each of these would be enough to place it in the appropriate class.

Asparagus deals mainly with **chronic** and **degenerative** stages of illness. As *blood and essence restoring nutritive botanical* it is as important as Alfalfa, Artichoke and flower pollen. It is one of the few remedies that really fits to a T the total possible symptomatology of the Chinese syndrome,

Liver blood deficiency, in the same way as do acupuncture points Bl 17, 18 & 38, Li 3 & 8 and Ki 9. Traditional symptomatology here emphasixes the *vision restoring, eye moistening* and *muscle/tendon softening* and *relaxing* effects of Asparagus root. Here is another Western herb that behaves nicely according to the tenets of Chinese physiology!

Asparagus root should always be thought of as a *moist* remedy: just as it moistens and brightens the eyes like the Yin Qiao extra meridian, so it also provides **internal moisture**, especially in dry intestinal conditions. In this sense it *fosters and protects the Yin* where old age or chronic febrile illness engenders **dryness**. For this reason we could do worse than think of Asparagus as a possible stand-in for a Chinese *Yin tonic* such as *Sang ji sheng, ramulus Visci seu Loranthi*, especially for dry skin conditions and Liver & Kidney Yin deficiency with weak sinews.

Asparagus is also a *seeping diuretic* in liver caused edemas, a *lenitive urinary demulcent* treating urinary irritation, an *antidyskratic cleanser* for general fluids dyskrasia (trace minerals 9%) and, paradoxically perhaps, a *reproductive tonic* à la Damiana with Kidney Yang deficiency patterns. Asparagus in this respect unequivocally lines up with the *Yang tonics Rou con rong, herba Cistanches*, and *Suo yang, herba Cynomorii*, used in Chinese medicine. **Difficult, painful urination**, **backache** and **impotence** are underlined symptoms here.

Its use in acute conditions is relatively minor, being limited to pain relief, muscle spasm and **anuria**.

Like the Chinese Asparagus, *Tian men dong*, with which it has similarities as well as significant differences, this variety was also used for thousands of years B.C.: Egyptian texts and tombs give evidence that Asparagus was treated with the highest respect as a medicinal plant since prehistoric times.

OATS

Pharmaceutical name: herba et fructus Avenae
Botanical name: Avena sativa L. (N.O. Graminae)
Ancient names: Bromos, Symphonion (Gr)
Other names: Avoine (Fr)
    Hafer, Gäbelshaber, Howen (Ge)
Part used: the straw and grain

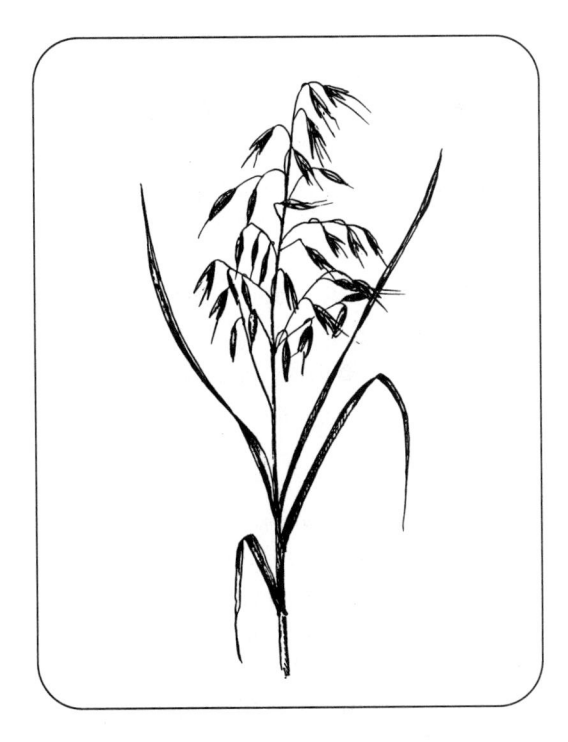

Nature

CATEGORY: mild herb with minimal chronic toxicity
CONSTITUENTS (whole plant): minerals & trace minerals (incl. silica, phosphoros, magnesium, calcium, iron, potassium), vitamins B1 & 2, D, P, Carotene, folliculin-like hormone, alkaloids (incl.

Oats: Class 9

trigonelline & avenine), flavonoid, saponins, sterol, fixed oil, protein, starch
EFFECTIVE QUALITIES
Primary: *Taste:* sweet
         Warmth: warm
         Moisture: moist
Secondary: nourishing, thickening, restoring, solidifying, stimulating, relaxing
TROPISM
Organs or parts: head, nerve, reproductive organs
Organisms: Air, Fluid
Meridians: Spleen, Kidney, Chong & Ren
Tri Dosas: increases Kapha, decreases Pitta & Vayu
GROUND
Krases/temperaments: Melancholic
Biotypes: Sensitive/Tai Yin Metal
Constitutions: all three

Functions and Uses

1   PROVIDES NOURISHMENT AND REPLENISHES DEFICIENCY: INCREASES THE BLOOD, ESSENCE AND QI, PROMOTES GROWTH AND BENEFITS THE BONE; RESTORES THE NERVE, THYROID AND UROGENITAL ORGANS, GENERATES STRENGTH, LIFTS THE SPIRIT AND RIDS DEPRESSION

Liver & Kidney depletion: sore back, heavy knees & legs, dizziness, frequent scanty urination, irregular, scanty or no menses, sterility, impotence
nerve deficiency: weakness, nervous exhaustion, chronic occipital headache, muscular feebleness, local paralysis
blood & Qi deficiency: fatigue, shallow breathing, poor appetite, melancholy, poor thinking
NERVOUS, MENTAL & PHYSICAL DEBILITY or EXHAUSTION due to anorexia, anemia, overwork, excessive sex, chronic illness, chronic addictions, aging
SLOW bone development in children due to essence deficiency
CHRONIC DEPRESSION & ANXIETY
THYROID INSUFFICIENCY with fatigue, poor appetite, cold extremities, constipation, weight gain
ESTROGEN INSUFFICIENCY with delayed, scanty or no menses

2   CIRCULATES THE QI, RELAXES THE NERVE AND FREES SPASMS; RELIEVES PAIN AND INDUCES REST

Qi constraint with nerve deficiency: nervous agitation, unrest, palpitations, insomnia
uterus Qi constraint: delayed, scanty menses with premenstrual tension, cramps, headaches, esp. at vertex, nausea
NEURALGIA, neuritis
PEPTIC ULCERS, gastroenteritis, colic
GOUT, SCIATICA, RHEUMATISM
INSOMNIA

3   CAUSES SWEATING, SCATTERS WIND COLD AND CLEARS THE HEAD

external wind cold: onset of colds with exhaustion, unrest, head congestion
head damp cold: congested head, watery nasal discharge

4	BENEFITS THE SKIN

CHRONIC SKIN conditions: dermatosis, shingles, eczema, herpes
FROSTBITE, chilblains

5	RESTORES THE HEART AND PANCREAS AND LOWERS BLOOD SUGAR

ORGANIC HEART DISEASE
DIABETES (supportive)

Preparation

USE: Oats is the perfect FOOD for babies, children, elderly folk and for those with the deficiency patterns above for whatever reason; also for those who tend to the Sensitive/Tai Yin Metal biotype. Oats is a nutritious prophylactic *pharmakon* (Greek) or *dravya* (Ayurvedic): a food and medicine in one. It should be a major dietary ingredient in conditions of **hyperacidity** with or without **peptic ulcers, jaundice, gall bladder disharmonies, chronic rheumatic, circulatory** and **skin conditions and diabetes.**

The TINCTURE and FLUID EXTRACT should be made from the **entire herb**, i.e. the stalk and the grain. There is little point in tincturing or decocting the "straw", i.e. the stalk alone, since the fruit has most constituents. Long-term use of Oats in any shape or form is advisable in **chronic conditions** where the **nerve, heart, reproductive organs, skin** or **thyroid** is involved.

BATHS of all kinds, on the other hand, can be made using the straw alone, for **run-down or painful** conditions, for **menstrual, urinary** and **intestinal problems** (HIP BATH), for **tired or cold feet**. WASHES will complement internal use in **skin problems, chilblains** and suchlike.

DOSAGE: TINCTURE: 2-3 ml or 50-75 drops
DECOCTION of the straw: standard dose, decoct for 1 hour

For **incipient head colds**: 20 drops of the tincture every few hours, beginning at first sign
For **insomnia**: 30 to 40 drops, or 1/2 tsp of the tincture in a little cold water before retiring.

Notes

Although used by classical Mediterranean cultures, Oats did not flourish as a food until it spread to the more northern parts of Europe with the Roman expansion. Some consider Oats indigenous to the British Isles, in fact. Whatever the truth, it is in northern Europe that over centuries and centuries Oats served to build those extremely robust constitutions which weathered the most extreme climatic and social exiegances—cold, damp, famine, strife and plague, among others. Oats belongs to the North because it is the only grain that is truly *warm* by nature, all others being *neutral* or *cool*. Besides, belonging to the direction North (and hence the Chinese deity Black Warrior or Tortoise) Oats belongs to the element water, restoring as it does the urogenital organs, or the Kidney Qi.

In the Middle Ages oatmeal porridge (from the meal, not the flakes) was the bulwark of the peasant diet. It is difficult to imagine a more *nutritive* and *restoring* grain in existence, nor a remedy with the same broad spectrum and depth of constituents (aside from algae and flower pollen). As a colleague of the writer remarked when acquainted with its functions and uses, taking Oats "is a complete body overhaul from the inside to the outside", since "it goes everywhere." He was speaking from the energetic and bioelectrical point of view, of course.

The comprehensive effect of Oats is rooted in its *sweet* taste, which increases Kapha and thereby promotes substantial solidity, growth and vitality: hence flesh building, weight gain, growth (esp. in children, due to its high protein count), strength and so on. Oats is nothing less than a remedy to help the forces of incarnation (literally "becoming flesh"), of grounding. No wonder it

Parsley root: Class 9

helps with "spaciness", whether due to constitution or due to drugs. (It is successful in *antiaddiction* formulas.) These are clear indications of calcium, silica, fluorine and magnesium bioenergies at work. An archetypal *nutritive restorer* with its sweet warm moistness, Oats serves **deficiency** conditions only: essentially it is a *blood* and *Qi tonic* in one. The Tai Yin Metal/Sensitive biotype will benefit most from its use for preventive or maintenance purpose.

From the analytical perspective we have some interesting details with which to fill out this picture: Oats as a *thyroid, pancreas* and *testis restorative,* as an *estrogen stimulant,* as a *nerve trophorestorative.* Again, a glance at its constituents will corroborate this. Oats clearly has a myriad combination possibilities, all of which are straightforward. Perhaps it excels at rebuilding the **nervous sytem** (with remedies to *restore the nerve* such as Rosemary and Sage); at *restoring* in **genitourinary depletion** (with *urogenital tonics* such as Gravel root, Damiana and Saw palmetto); and at *relaxing* the **nerves** and *inducing rest* (with herbs that circulate the Qi and relax the nerve such as Skullcap and Pasque flower).

PARSLEY ROOT

Pharmaceutical name: radix Petroselini
Botanical name: Petroselinum crispum Hill. *vel P. hortense* Hoffm. (N.O. Umbelliferae)
Ancient names: Petroselinon (Gr)
　　Apium hortense (Lat)
Other names: Persil (Fr)
　　Petersilie, Garteneppich, Bittersilche (Ge)
Part used: the root

Nature

CATEGORY: mild herb with minimal chronic toxicity
CONSTITUENTS: protein 20%, glucoside apiin, ess. oil (incl. apiol, bergapten), terpenes, mucilage, resin, starch, iron, calcium, phosphoros, manganese, trace minerals, volatile alkaloid traces, inositol, sulphur, vit. C, ß-carotene, K
EFFECTIVE QUALITIES
Primary: a bit sweet, warm, moist
Secondary: nourishing, restoring, dissolving
TROPISM: blood, fluids, stomach, liver, kidneys, uterus
　　　　Air, Fluid organisms
　　　　Spleen, Liver, Chong & Ren meridians
GROUND: all krases, biotypes and constitutions

Class 9: Parsley root

Functions and Uses

1 PROVIDES NOURISHMENT AND REPLENISHES DEFICIENCY; RESTORES THE BLOOD AND UTERUS AND RETURNS THE MENSES; PROMOTES HAIR GROWTH

blood deficiency with fatigue, pale eyelids, nails, etc.
ANEMIA, mineral depletion, TB
uterus blood deficiency with delayed or stopped menstruation
AMENORRHEA
HAIR LOSS

2 RESTORES THE LIVER AND STOMACH, STIMULATES THE LIVER AND AWAKENS THE APPETITE

liver & stomach/Spleen Qi deficiency with slow painful digestion, no appetite, fatigue
liver Qi stagnation with right flank pain & distension
LIVER & SPLEEN SWELLING, jaundice, gastritis

3 PROMOTES CLEANSING, CLEARS TOXINS AND RESOLVES TOXEMIA; SEEPS WATER, PROMOTES URINATION AND RELIEVES FLUID CONGESTION; HARMONIZES URINATION AND EXPELS STONES

kidney Qi stagnation with *general toxemia* with skin rashes, fetid stool, fatigue
URIC ACID DIATHESIS
URINARY & GALLSTONES
DIFFICULT or OBSTRUCTED URINATION
liver & kidney fluid congestion with general water retention, fatigue

4 PROMOTES TISSUE REPAIR; ARRESTS LACTATION

FRACTURES
For WEANING

Preparation

USE: This varies with the part used.
The **leaf** *nourishes* and *restores,* feeding blood and tissues, and performs functions 1 & 2 mainly. It should be INFUSED or EATEN straight.
The **root** *nourishes, restores, cleanses* more than anything else, being at work mainly in the blood, liver, spleen and intestines.
It is best used for functions 1, 2 & 3. It should be MACERATED overnight in cold water and briefly heated up before drinking; or a TINCTURE can be made from it.
DOSAGE: standard dosages throughout

Notes

The healing properties of this kitchen herb, of which the use goes back beyond recorded history, demonstrate once again how a remedy can effectively and safely straddle all three main treatment principles: namely, *eliminating, restoring and altering & regulating.* We find it here among the *nutritive* remedies simply because its delicious herb can and should be eaten on a daily basis. With its *sweet warm* qualities it builds the blood and generally nourishes; appropriating to the womb, it will restore womb blood and hence recover long lost menses.

Like many remedies, Parsley has been ticketed *emmenagogue* in the past, a label that should be

Iceland moss: Class 9

used very carefully if at all. Why? Because the causes of **amenorrhea** are varied, and require fundamentally different treatment. As MILLS (1986) rightly points out, many remedies were considered to bring on a period because they were frankly *abortifacient*—pregnancy being a large cause of amenorrhea in the past! Next, periods may cease due to a number of internal disharmonies involving the uterus: if a Qi stagnation is the cause, then the menses are obstructed through retention; if blood deficiency is the cause, the menses are unavailable through insufficiency; if Qi constraint is the cause, the menses are obstructed through spasm. The type of herbal remedy used in the three cases is entirely different. Using Parsley **root**, *radix Petroselini*, we can *nourish* and *restore uterine blood;* using its **seed**, *fructus Petroselini*, we can *relax uterine tone;* using **either** we can *stimulate uterine function*. Parsley is compassionate to woman in that it exceptionally treats three major types of delayed periods.

With the roots of Fennel, Asparagus, Broom and Celery, Parsley belongs to the **five opening roots**—i.e. those used to promote downward water seepage and urination: in this way Parsley is a true *eliminant*. All forms of edema are significantly improved. Also, like Celery, it is an *altering* remedy which *promotes cleansing* through improved renal activity, pulling wastes and toxins out of the blood, and hence indirectly out of the tissues. Its essential oil is most active in this respect and explains the benefits to **chronic toxemic** conditions. Certainly Parsley's *digestive stimulant* and probably *cholagogue* effects offer a good contribution here.

ICELAND MOSS

Pharmaceutical name: thallus Cetrariae
Botanical name: Cetraria islandica Acht. (N.O. Parmeliaceae)
Other names: Eryngo-leaved liverwort (Eng)
　　Mousse d'Islande (Fr)
　　Isländisches Moos (Ge)
Part used: the thallus

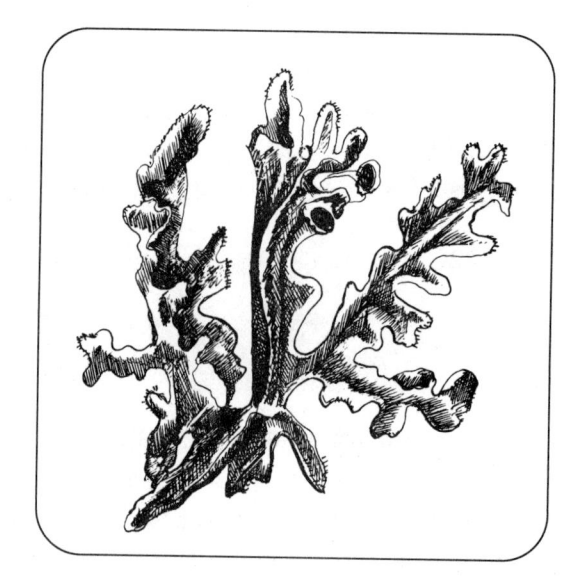

Nature

CATEGORY: mild herb with minimal chronic toxicity
CONSTITUENTS: mucilage (incl. lichenin 30%-40%, isolichenin), bitter acids (incl. fumaric, fumaroprotocetraric, lichesteric & usnic acids), bitter compound (cetrarin & picrolichenin), oxalic acid, carbohydrates, gum, oil, trace minerals incl. iodine
EFFECTIVE QUALITIES
Primary: bitter, a bit sweet & salty & astringent, cool, moist
Secondary: nourishing, thickening, restoring, relaxing
TROPISM: blood, fluids, lungs, stomch, intestines
　　　　Fluid organism
　　　　Spleen, Lung meridians
GROUND: Melancholic krasis

Sensitive/Tai Yin Metal biotype
Lymphatic/carbonic/Blue Iris constitution

Functions and Uses

1. PROVIDES NOURISHMENT AND REPLENISHES DEFICIENCY: RESTORES THE BLOOD AND FLUIDS, INCREASES THE QI, RESTORES THE LUNGS AND *SPLEEN* AND CREATES STRENGTH

   CHRONIC EXHAUSTION due to wasting disease, childbirth, hemorrhage, excessive sexual activity
   blood & fluids deficiency: fatigue, anemia, signs of dryness
   lung Qi deficiency: fatigue, spontaneous sweating, pale complexion
   Spleen Qi deficiency: poor appetite, fatigue, loose stool
   CHRONIC DIARRHEA, gastroenteritis, anorexia
   ATONIC LUNG TB
   INSUFFICIENT BREAST MILK

2. FOSTERS THE YIN, PROVIDES MOISTURE AND CLEARS HEAT, SOOTHES AND LENIFIES DRYNESS; LIQUIFIES VISCOUS PHLEGM, RELIEVES WHEEZING AND COUGHING

   lung Yin deficiency: night sweats, feverishness, dry unproductive cough, emaciation
   lung dryness: dry tickling cough, head & body aches
   CROUP, whooping cough, pneumonia
   lung dry phlegm: coughing up scanty viscous phlegm, asthmatic breathing
   stomach & intestines dryness: abdominal distension & lumpiness, dry vomiting, hunger without appetite
   INSUFFICIENT or EXCESSIVE GASTRIC ACIDITY
   GASTRITIS, PEPTIC ULCER

3. REDUCES INFLAMMATION, RESTRAINS INFECTION AND CLEARS TOXINS

   intestines damp cold/heat: diarrhea with mucousy stool, possibly with blood; exhaustion
   GASTROENTERITIS, dysentery

4. SETTLES THE STOMACH, QUELLS NAUSEA AND CHECKS VOMITING

   NAUSEA & VOMITING in all conditions

Preparation

USE: There are two basic ways of preparing Iceland moss. The one is to make a bitter tasting DECOCTION, which is especially effective with deficient Spleen or lung Qi, vomiting and night sweats, while being strengthening at the same time.
The other is to remove its bitter substance, *cetrarin,* by a quick boiling and discarding of the water, followed by a standard DECOCTION. This preparation is suitable where its *demulcent* and antiseptic properties are needed.
DOSAGE: Standard doses apply; a sweetener may be used.
CAUTION: Do not use with fever present, as Iceland moss is highly nutritious.

Kelp: Class 9

Notes

Iceland moss is an underrated remedy that has only been given adequate "press" by the herbalist EDWARD SHOOK in his original and informative writings on botanicals. An effective *nutritive restorer* and *sweet cool demulcent* in one, it finds equal application with **deficient blood**, **fluids** and **Qi** conditions, and in **dry** or **deficient Yin** conditions. Its focus is very much the lungs and intestines: lung Qi deficiency and Spleen Qi deficiency need Iceland moss where exhaustion, diarrhea and the like manifest; its *bitter* and somewhat *sweet* taste make for immediate *digestive activation,* as for deeper, long-term *tonification*. On the side of the blood and fluids, it strongly *increases Kapha* like Alfalfa, Oats, flower pollen and the seaweeds, *nourishing, building blood, fluids* and *tissues* (including breast milk) in so doing. In this sense Iceland moss is a remedy for **chronic atonic** conditions with **dryness**; as well as where hemorrhage, childbirth, etc. have depleted the fluids.

On the other hand, Iceland moss also has uses in **acute** conditions: its *sweet moist astringent* effects (the result of mucilage and acids in synergy) help resolve acute **dry** and **Yin deficient** conditions of the lungs and stomach—here it may be reinforced by other *cold moist demulcents* such as Borage, Chickweed, Purslane and Mallow. In this context it is a good remedy for any type of **gastric ulcer**, and should be selected in preference to *astringents* for those tending to the above-mentioned overall conditions.

KELP

Pharmaceutical name: thallus Laminariae
Botanical name: Laminaria spp. (N.O. Laminariaceae)
Other names: Kombu (Jap)
  Kun bu (Ch)
  Laminaires (Fr)
Part used: the thallus

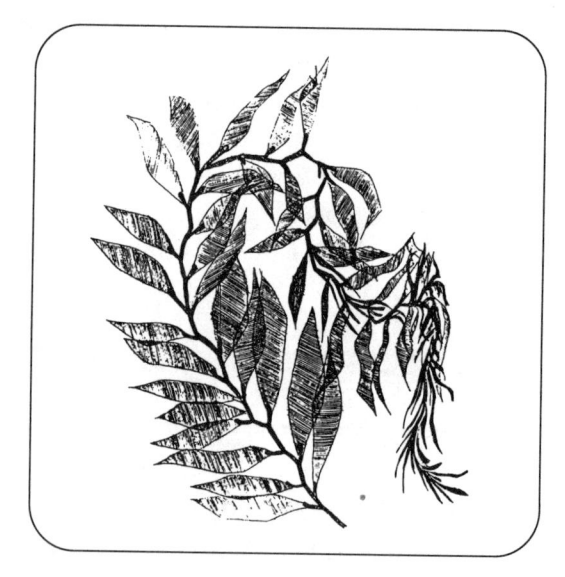

Nature

CATEGORY: mild herb with minimal chronic toxicity
CONSTITUENTS: minerals & trace minerals (incl. iodine, potassium, sodium, magnesium, calcium, iron, manganese, germanium, zinc, bromium, silica), ergosterol, ess. oil, mannitol alcohol, mucilages, bitter, vits. incl. A, B's (incl. B_{12}), C, D's, E
EFFECTIVE QUALITIES
Primary: salty, cool, moist
Secondary: nourishing, restoring, decongesting, softening, dissolving
TROPISM: blood, fluids, liver, stomach, intestines, kidneys, bladder
  Fluid organism
  Liver, Stomach, Kidney, Bladder meridians
GROUND: all krases, biotypes and constitutions

Functions and Uses

1. **PROVIDES NOURISHMENT AND MOISTURE, REPLENISHES DEFICIENCY AND ENHANCES IMMUNE POTENTIAL; RESTORES THE BLOOD, LIVER AND STOMACH AND HARMONIZES METABOLISM; PROMOTES GROWTH AND RESTORES STRENGTH**

   CONSTITUTIONAL WEAKNESS, deficient Original Qi
   blood & fluids deficiency with fatigue, palpitations, pale eyelids
   ANEMIA, signs of dryness
   liver & stomach Qi deficiency with slow, painful digestion
   intestines dryness with constipation
   FATIGUE, EXHAUSTION in all conditions
   SLOW MENTAL & PHYSICAL DEVELOPMENT in children
   RICKETS

2. **PROMOTES CLEANSING, CLEARS TOXINS, RESOLVES TOXEMIA AND DRAINS PLETHORA; SEEPS WATER, PROMOTES URINATION AND RELIEVES FLUID CONGESTION; CHELATES HEAVY METALS, SOFTENS DEPOSITS, DISSIPATES TUMORS AND BENEFITS THE SKIN**

   general fluids dyskrasia with chronic rheumatism, arthritis, i.e. cold obstruction; gout, chronic skin eruptions
   liver & kidney fluid congestion with generalized or local water retention
   general plethora and *general toxemia* with overweight, cellulite, malaise
   ARSENIC & MERCURY POISONING
   OBESITY, inability to loose weight
   SKIN CONDITIONS in general, incl. psoriasis
   SCROFULOUS & LYMPHATIC DIATHESIS with congestion and swelling, syphilis
   CATARRHAL DIATHESIS
   FATTY HEART DEGENERATION
   HARD DEPOSITS, arteriosclerosis, fibrous tumors

3. **CLEARS HEAT, LENIFIES IRRITATION, RELIEVES PAIN AND PROMOTES URINATION**

   bladder damp heat with painful urination, thirst
   PAIN in all conditions
   ACUTE NEPHRITIS with obstructed urination
   stomach fire with thirst, bleeding gums
   ADENITIS

4. **HARMONIZES THE HORMONES AND RESTORES THE PITUITARY, THYROID, AND ADRENALS**

   HORMONAL IMBALANCE in general
   THYROID INSUFFICIENCY, goitre
   MENOPAUSAL SYNDROME
   HIGH BLOOD PRESSURE

5. **RELIEVES ASTHMA**

   ASTHMA, wheezing in any condition

Kelp: Class 9

Preparation

USE: The main use of Kelp is as a FOOD. It is a sea vegetable after all, and has been used as such in Oriental cultures especially: it is the Japanese *Kombu* and the Chinese *Kun bu*. Kelp may also be taken as a nutritional supplement as POWDER and derivatives thereof (such as capsules, tablets), and should be taken **with meals**. A TINCTURE made from the whole or powdered thallus is equally effective.

BATHS of all types are an extremely effective way of absorbing Kelp or Bladderwrack, especially whole body baths. The nodulus or bag of the seaweed should firstly be placed in a bath with **hot** running water for a few minutes, after which the temperature can be adjusted. 20 minutes is a sufficient soak, and soap should not be used. (It is best to take a shower before taking a seaweed bath.) Skin brushing the whole body before will also enhance mineral absorption.

If a course of BODY BATHS is undertaken, two or three per week for 10 to 20 weeks is sufficient. In severe conditions, courses may be done every two or three months.

DOSAGE: POWDER: 1/2-2 g
                          TINCTURE: 6-26 drops, or 1/2-2 ml

CAUTION: Seaweed BATHS should not be taken with the following conditions: acute inflammations and infections, including acute joint inflammations, weeping eczema, lung abscess or TB, hyperthyroidism, cardiac decompensation, cardiorenal conditions.

Notes

A true understanding of Kelp and its medicinal effects can only be gleaned by looking at the elements that it carries and by an appreciation of these as the result of nature's creative "ideas". Among the numerous **bioenergies** that go to make Kelp the astonishing *nourishing, cleansing* and *regulating* remedy it is, the one that results in the formation of iodine in both land and sea plants figures foremost in the nature of Kelp. Of course Kelp contains a gamut of minerals of both the substantial and trace kind, which accounts for its broad and systemic *regulating* function on processes within the metabolic and fluid environment. Here *nourishing, cleansing* and *decongesting* effects are uppermost. Kelp, after all, is an important *antidyskratic* remedy with positive results in many types of general fluids dyskrasia, from scrofulous, lymphatic, catarrhal and uric acid diatheses, chronic skin conditions, plethoric and overweight conditions, to hot, inflammatory conditions (*salty cool moist* energetics) of the stomach and bladder mainly.

However, it is **iodine** as both bioenergy and trace substance in one that gives Kelp a therapeutic or, better still, a healing depth not found in other plants. Iodine connects us to the source of physical and spiritual existence—this is its essence. Its influence through the thyroid gland, and from there throughout the organism, is all-pervasive, inescapable. It has been described as that which ignites and maintains the fire of life, the living flame itself (FUNKE, 1980). In this sense it is comparable to what Chinese medicine describes as *ming men huo* (literally, "karma gate fire"), and to the "innate warmth" of Hippokratic medicine. In other words, iodine bioenergy initiates, maintains and regulates all living human processes—physiological, emotional, mental and spiritual. (An example of this on the physiological level is iodine's key role in maintaining the chemical balance in electrolytic dissociation.)

This pervasive influence is easy to see in practice, since as little as a few micrograms' difference in weight of this element in the system can mean the difference between a hyperthyroid and a hypothyroid condition, with its ineluctable physical, emotional and mental changes on the individual. In other words, more than anything else, iodine bioenergy determines **ground** and **temperament**. A slight excess will produce a Tough/Shao Yang or a Expressive/Jue Yin type of individual, with the familiar retinue of **spasmodic, sclerotic, neurotic** and **congestive** symptoms of the Hematic/Brown Iris variety, and the typical intense, dramatic extrovert personality; while a slight insufficiency will tend to produce a Dependant/Tai Yin Earth or a Sensitive/Tai Yin Metal biotype with their **deficiency/atonic damp/catarrhal** and **cold** conditions of the Lymphatic/Blue Iris type and their laid-back, sluggish, introvert character.

It becomes clear that Kelp's very high iodine content is influential in **harmonizing** very basic living processes. Specifically, for example, it works in *regulating metabolism, acid-base levels* and *insulin metabolism,* as well as in *stimulating leukopoiesis* and *antibody production*, especially in those conditions where the thyroid is weak or iodine uptake simply lacking. All chronic infections, chronic metabolic illnesses (deficient & excess) benefit from its inclusion in prescriptions. If this were insufficient reason to regard Kelp, like all marine algae or sea vegetables, as a good maintenance supplement as well as a remedy, we should consider the fact that iodine counteracts **chronic mercury** and **arsenic poisoning**: given the ubiquitous presence of these two environmental pollutants due to amalgam tooth fillings on one hand and chemical products of all kinds on the other, a daily intake of seaweed in *any* form becomes a necessary preventive measure at the present time.

BLADDERWRACK

Pharmaceutical name: thallus Fuci
Botanical name: **Fucus vesiculosus** L. (N.O. Fucaceae)
Other names: Quercus marina (Lat)
 Varech vésiculeux, Chêne marin, Laitue marine (Fr)
Part used: the thallus

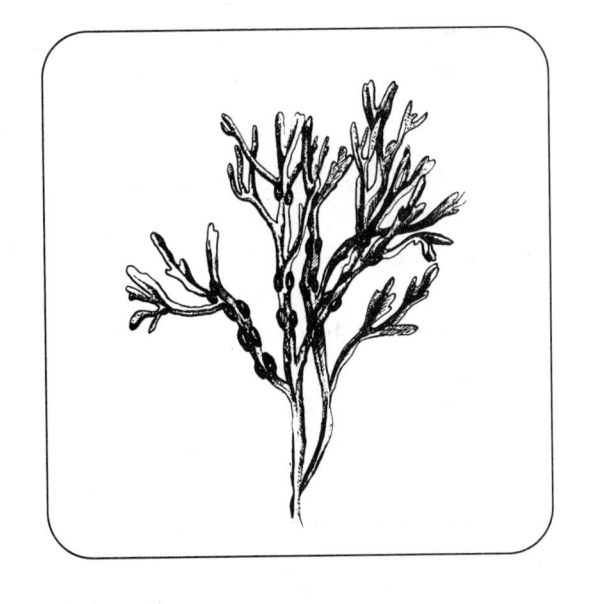

This herb is virtually identical in its constituents, functions and uses to KELP, Laminaria spp., (p. 366) but is possibly slightly less strong.

Alfalfa: Class 9

ALFALFA

Pharmaceutical name: herba Medicaginis
Botanical name: Medicago sativa L. (N.O. Papilionaceae)
Ancient names: Lazwardija (Per)
 Medica vera, Lucerna (Lat)
Other names: Lucerne, Purple medic, Burgundy hay, Spanish clover (Eng)
 Buffalo herb (Am)
 Lucerne, Médoise, Trèfle de Bourgogne, Sain-foin (Fr)
 Luzerne, Hoher Klee, Dreijähriger Klee, Spanischer Klee (Ge)
Part used: the herb

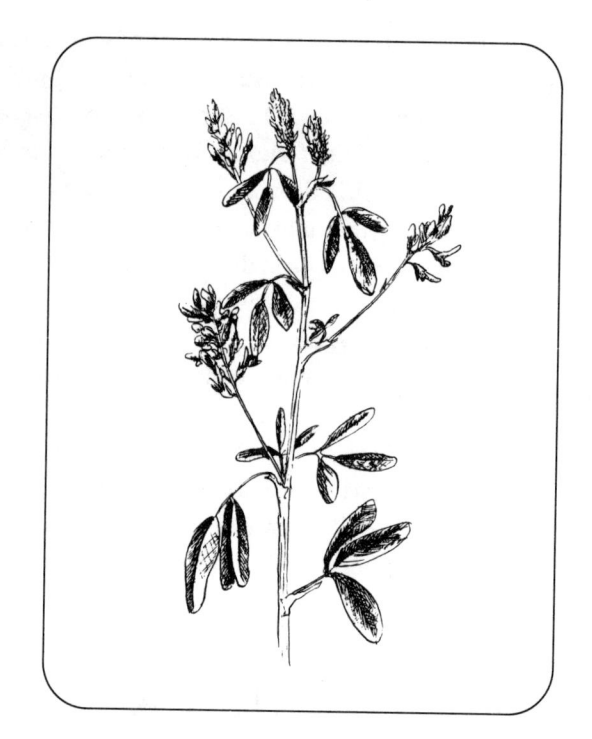

Nature

CATEGORY: mild herb with minimal chronic toxicity
CONSTITUENTS: eight digestive enzymes, protein, mucilage, minerals & trace minerals (incl. calcium, magnesium, phosphoros, iron, potassium), chlorophyll, vitamins A,B,D,E,K,P, folic acid, niacin, saponins, sterols, flavonoids, coumarins, alkaloids, amino acids, organic acids
EFFECTIVE QUALITIES
Primary: salty, a bit bitter, neutral, moist
Secondary: nourishing, thickening, restoring, dissolving
TROPISM: stomach, liver, pancreas, blood, fluids
 Fluid organism
 Spleen, Stomach meridians
GROUND: all krases, biotypes and constitutions

Functions and Uses

1 PROVIDES NOURISHMENT AND REPLENISHES DEFICIENCY: RESTORES THE BLOOD, STOMACH/*SPLEEN* AND PANCREAS, PROMOTES WEIGHT GAIN AND LACTATION AND GENERATES STRENGTH

blood deficiency: weakness, palpitations, dizziness, shallow breathing, white complexion
ANEMIA
INSUFFICIENT BREAST MILK

stomach & Spleen Qi deficiency: fatigue, poor appetite, slow or difficult digestion, despondency
DEBILITY & WEIGHT LOSS due to constitution, pregnancy, chronic disease, malabsorption syndromes
GASTRIC & DUODENAL HYPERACIDITY and ulcers
DIABETES (supportive)

Class 9: Alfalfa

2   PROMOTES CLEANSING, CLEARS TOXINS AND RESOLVES TOXEMIA; PROTECTS THE LIVER AND PROMOTES URINATION

general toxemia and *general fluids dyskrasia:* intermittent muscle or joint pains, fetid stool, scanty urine, irritability, fatigue
CHRONIC UREMIA, arthritis, sciatica, gout, rheumatism
HIGH BLOOD CHOLESTEROL, atherosclerosis
LIVER TOXICOSIS (preventive and remedial)

3   RIDS DEPRESSION, RELIEVES PAIN AND INDUCES REST

DEPRESSION, unrest, pain in any condition

4   STRENGTHENS THE BLOOD VESSELS

FRAGILE CAPILLARIES, spontaneous bleeding

Preparation

USE: INFUSION, POWDER and TABLETS are the main forms found today.
Taken **before** eating, Alfalfa assists in preparing digestion by ensuring appropriate gastric secretions; taken **with** or **after** a meal, it will promote absorption, especially of calcium and protein, and in the long run increase colonic peristalsis. However, its benefits other than those connected with digestion will unfold better if taken **in between** meals. It can and should be taken **continuously** for those conditions it is best at remedying, to wit, chronic deficiencies involving the blood and Qi.
Alfalfa is both a nutritional supplement and a medicinal herb. It may be taken throughout pregnancy and is especially valuable during the last month of the term to ensure adequate vit. K provision to the baby, and also during the first week or two postpartum.
DOSAGE: INFUSION: 1 to 2 tsp per cup of water
              Others: as directed; twice that amount in severe cases

Notes

The beauty of Alfalfa's luminous azure flowers prompted ancient Persians to call it *lazwardija, azure blue,* with reference to the blue glaze used in their ceramic work. Their physicians and pharmacists brought this "father of all foods" to Spain with the medieval Islamic expansion, whence it spread to Europe. Since then, Alfalfa has been more important as cattle fodder than as a medicine, simply because of the neglect that **nourishing** and **altering and regulating** as treatment strategies suffered.

Galenic medicine in its later European development clearly favored **elimination** by whatever means to treat illness, as evinced by the progressively stronger *purgatives, diaphoretics, emetics* that were used from the sixteenth century onwards. Even when it aspired to **regulate** the fluids in the face of a blatant fluids dyskrasia, it sought to do so in terms of eliminant techniques and the resultant **quantity** of injurious wastes that could be evoked. Little thought was given to the possibility of regulating a fluids dyskrasia by purely **qualitative** means, by **altering** injurious processes. As a result, Alfalfa with its slow, undramatic effects had no place in the evacuant arsenal.

Alfalfa is recognized today as an agent for **functional**, **chronic**, and **degenerative metabolic** conditions. Yet even now it is not recognized as a serious medicine, since nourishing is supposed to be the function of food uniquely. It is only when nourishing is accepted as a treatment method in its own right that the function of remedies in this class becomes meaningful.

Nettle: Class 9

Even though Alfalfa by *increasing Kapha* promotes solidity, weight gain and strength, all typical of an increase of Spleen Qi, it is not an oily remedy and hence cannot possibly produce Qi stagnation like some Chinese blood and Yin tonics. The large and trace minerals, digestive enzymes, amino acids and vitamins it contains ensure this adequately. On the contrary, as described above, Alfalfa is an important *digestive* remedy in several ways, including the regulation of gastric acidity.

Alfalfa's wide gamut of substances also ensures a *resolvent, cleansing* and hardness *dissolving* effect, which goes hand in hand with its primary *nutritive* ones. In this sense it is the inverse of Celery. Its saponins decrease lipid levels in the blood, and one of its proteins is *antitumoral,* while it has also been shown to protect the liver and small intestine from chemical damage. These are just some examples of the complexities involved in the mechanisms of its *antidyskratic* and *diuretic cleansing* functions, which, by causing systemic **altering** and **regulating** changes for the better, once again address **chronic metabolic** disturbances.

NETTLE

Pharmaceutical name: folium Urticae
Botanical name: Urtica dioica L. (N.O. Urticaceae)
Ancient names: Akalyphe, Analypse (Gk)
    Acantum (Lat)
Other names: Stinging nettle, Scaddie (Eng)
    Ortie, Ortie piquante (Fr)
    Brennessel, Donnernessel (Ge)
Parts used: the leaf; also the seed, *semen Urticae*

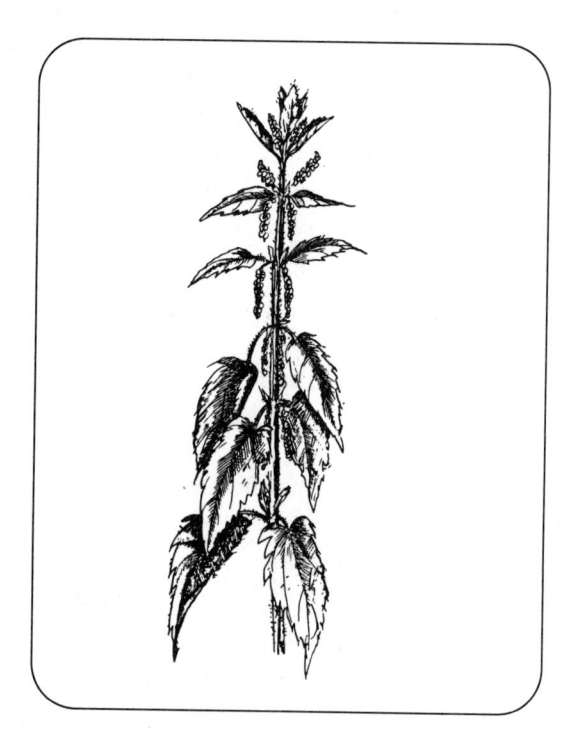

Nature

CATEGORY: mild herb with minimal chronic toxicity
CONSTITUENTS: formic acid, histamine, chlorophyll, xanthophyll, enzyme secretin, tannin, carotine, glucoquinone, iron, trace minerals (incl. silicon, phosphorus, chlorine, sodium, magnesium, sulphur, potassium), vitamins (esp. C, B, ß-carotene), lecithin, protein (up to 24%), mucilage, tannic & gallic acid, glycoside, hormones
EFFECTIVE QUALITIES
Primary: astringent, a bit bitter, cool, dry
Secondary: nourishing, restoring, astringing, stimulating dissolving
    stabilizing movement
TROPISM: blood, fluids, lungs, intestines, spleen, liver, kidneys, bladder, uterus, connective tissue
    Air, Fluid organisms

Class 9: Nettle

Liver, Spleen, Bladder, Chong & Ren meridians
GROUND: Choleric & Phlegmatic krases
Tough/Shao Yang & Dependant/Tai Yin Earth biotypes
all three constitutions

Functions and Uses

1. PROVIDES NOURISHMENT AND REPLENISHES DEFICIENCY: RESTORES THE BLOOD AND RETURNS THE MENSES; PROMOTES LACTATION AND BENEFITS THE HAIR

   blood & fluids deficiency and *liver blood deficiency:* weakness, exhaustion, dizziness, amenorrhea
   ANEMIA, tuberculosis, rickets, hemophilia
   uterus blood deficiency: delayed, scanty or absent menstruation
   AMENORRHEA
   CHRONIC & DEGENERATIVE DISEASE
   CONNECTIVE TISSUE DEGENERATION
   INSUFFICIENT BREAST MILK
   HAIR LOSS and general hair care

2. RESTORES THE INTESTINES/*SPLEEN* AND LUNGS, STIMULATES THE LUNGS AND RELIEVES WHEEZING; RELIEVES ALLERGIES

   Spleen Qi deficiency: diarrhea, flatulence, fatigue
   CHRONIC GASTRIC DEGENERATION & ULCERS
   DIABETES (supportive)
   lung phlegm damp: shortness of breath, coughing up thin white phlegm
   CHRONIC BRONCHITIS, bronchial asthma, TB
   HAYFEVER, allergic asthms

3. CREATES ASTRICTION, DRIES DAMP AND ARRESTS DISCHARGE; RESTRAINS INFECTION AND STAUNCHES BLEEDING

   genitourinary damp cold: leucorrhea, urethritis
   bladder damp heat: frequent urgent urination, cloudy urine
   ACUTE & CHRONIC URINARY INFECTIONS
   MOUTH & THROAT INFECTIONS, sores, ulcers, catarrh
   HEMORRHAGE internal or external, including menstrual & intermenstrual
   LUNG TB with coughing up blood
   BURNS, BITES & STINGS, WOUNDS

4. PROMOTES CLEANSING, CLEARS TOXINS AND RESOLVES TOXEMIA: STIMULATES THE LIVER, DREDGES THE KIDNEYS, BENEFITS THE SKIN AND RESOLVES TUMORS

   liver Qi stagnation: constipation, abdominal distension, jaundice
   kidney Qi stagnation: skin eruptions, malaise, cystitis
   general toxemia and *general fluids dyskrasia:* chronic arthritis, gout, rheumatism, eczema, urticaria, scrofulosis
   URIC ACID DIATHESIS with chronic skin, joint & gouty conditions
   SKIN CONDITIONS in general
   TUMORS, CANCERS (incl. spleen)

Nettle: Class 9

5   SEEPS WATER, PROMOTES URINATION AND RELIEVES FLUID CONGESTION; LENIFIES IRRITATION, SOFTENS DEPOSITS AND EXPELS STONES
liver & kidney fluid congestion: general or ankle swelling, puffy eyes in morning
ASCITES, hemorrhoids
HARD DEPOSITS: urinary stones, gallstones
BLADDER IRRITATION in all conditions; scanty, difficult, frequent urination, lumbar pains

Preparation

USE: The freshly expressed JUICE of the entire plant is probably the most efficient use of this herb as a medicine, bringing out the entire range of its actions to best advantage. Virtually as good is the FREEZE DRIED product. The standard INFUSION, TINCTURE and FLUID EXTRACT act in the same way, but not quite as well as the juice.

An effective SYRUP can be made for **lung** conditions outlined above —on its own or combined with Mullein, Elecampane, Coltsfoot, etc.)—while SMOKING the dried plant may bring relief in wheezing and **asthma.** Externally GARGLES, WASHES, COMPRESSES, etc., are used in **degenerative** and **arthritic** conditions of muscles, tendons and joints, providing **pain relief** as well as deep-level treatment. A HAIR RINSE for **weak or falling hair** is excellent. (A VINEGAR DECOCTION of Nettle root with Rosemary or Birch leaves is traditional). Nettle OINTMENT is superb for dealing with **skin** conditions, singly or with say Marigold, Burdock or Figwort.

DOSAGE: Standard doses are used throughout; these may be safely increased *ad libitum*.

Notes

Nettle is one of those remedies that have either been praised to the skies for its beneficial effects or totally ignored as a bothersome weed: the Nettle definitely inspires partisanship of one kind or another. Among its acolytes was the Greek philosopher PHANIAS, the Greek physician DIOSKURIDES, the Roman poet CATULLUS, the German painter ALBRECHT DÜRER and his contemporaries, the physician-herbalists OTTO BRUNFELS and HIERONYMUS BOCK and, in this century, the philosopher RUDOLPH STEINER. In the introduction to his herbal of 1532, for example, BOCK notes that "our doctors and pharmacists are ashamed to fetch such a common weed from behind the fences and include it in their formulas, although both in cookery and in medicine it has proven its mighty, impressive effects." Although much the same could be said today, biochemistry has nevertheless made the use of remedies such as Nettle acceptable.

Nettle's excellent *blood building* effects depend largely on its trace minerals, chlorophyll and the enzyme secretin and are only partly due to causing an increase in red blod cells. Blood and fluids generally are increased, and both liver blood and uterus blood are nourished. In uterus blood deficiency with oligo- or amenorrhea, Nettle acts in a way that acupuncture points Bl 17, 18 & 20, Sp 6 & 10, CV 3 & 4, and St 29 together would. Moreover, Nettle is **generally** *nutritive,* and should be chosen when **blood deficiency** is compounded with other conditions such as **toxemia, Spleen Qi deficiency** and **general metabolic stagnation**. In other words, its *cleansing, digestive* and *urinary stimulant* activities provide excellent back-up, for example, where complex conditions such as gout, arthritis and skin eruptions arise out of underlying insufficiencies of all the internal organs, notably the liver, kidneys, spleen and intestines. It is Nettle's very comprehensive *antidyskratic* as well as *restoring* effects which make it so useful in general fluids dyskrasia. Like all other remedies in this class it also provides deep, all-round support to other remedies addressing almost *any* condition of excess or deficiency.

Since working primarily on the blood level, Nettle is also a medium-strength *hemostatic* and *astringent* for **hemorrhages** and bleeding. With its *lung strengthening* properties it should also be

Class 9: Watercress

included in formulations for tuberculosis and all lung Yin deficieny syndromes: as a silica containing plant it will duplicate Horsetail's effect on this organ, as well as on connective tissue in general.

WATERCRESS

Pharmaceutical name: herba Nasturtii
Botanical name: Nasturtium officinale R.Br.
    (N.O. Cruciferae)
Ancient names: Kardamon (Gr)
    Sisymbrium, Rorippa, Nasturtium (Lat)
Other names: Poor man's bread, Well grass, Teng tongues, Billers (Eng)
    Cresson, Cresson de fontaine, Santé du corps (Fr)
    Brunnenkresse, Garten/Wasserkresse, Quellranke, Wassersenf (Ge)
Part used: the herb

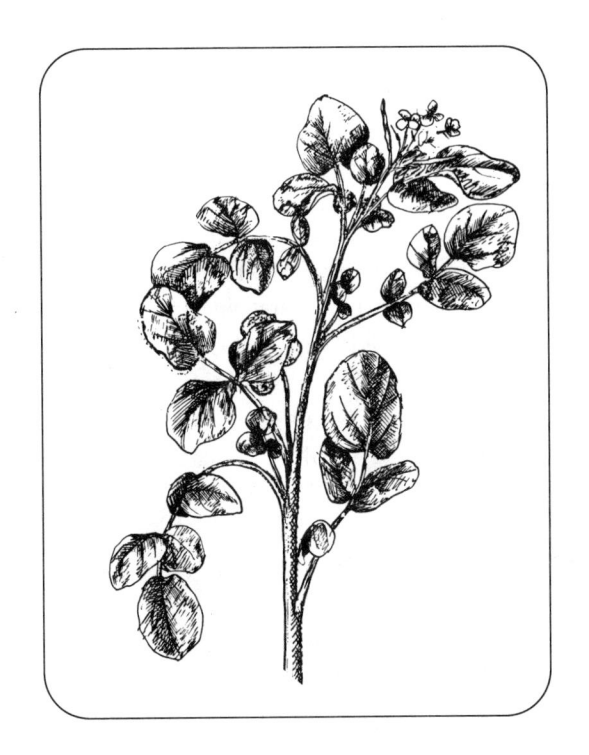

Nature

CATEGORY: mild herb with minimal chronic toxicity
CONSTITUENTS: raphanolide raphanol, diastase, ferment, gluconasturiin, bitter, ess. oil (incl. phenyl ethyl-mustard oil), vits. A,C,D, calcium, iron, iodine, chlorine, fluorine, phosphorus, sulphur, manganese, silica, arsenic, niacin, zinc, copper, chlorine, germanium
EFFECTIVE QUALITIES
Primary: pungent, a bit bitter, warm, dry
Secondary: nourishing, restoring, stimulating, softening, dissolving
TROPISM: blood, fluids, lymph, nerves, liver, stomach, lungs, intestines, brain, thyroid, pituitary, pancreas
    Air & Fluid organisms
    Spleen, Lung, Stomach, Colon meridians
GROUND: Phlegmatic, Sanguine & Melancholic krases
    all eight biotypes
    all three constitutions

Functions and Uses

1   PROVIDES NOURISHMENT, REPLENISHES DEFICIENCY AND ENHANCES IMMUNE POTENTIAL; RESTORES THE BLOOD, GLANDS, NERVE AND BRAIN; PROMOTES LACTATION

    blood deficiency with fatigue, pale eyelids, face & nails
    ANEMIA
    INSUFFICIENT BREAST MILK

Watercress: Class 9

    PITUITARY & THYROID DEFICIENCY
nerve deficiency with weakness, fatigue, depression
DEBILITY, exhaustion, physical or mental, due to any cause

2   RESTORES THE LIVER, GALL BLADDER, STOMACH AND PANCREAS
liver & stomach Qi deficiency with slow painful digestion
BILIARY INSUFFICENCY
DIABETES (supportive)

3   PROMOTES CLEANSING, CLEARS TOXINS AND RESOLVES TOXEMIA; ENLIVENS THE LYMPH, SOFTENS DEPOSITS AND PROMOTES URINATION
general toxemia and *general fluids dyskrasia* with chronic skin eruptions, painful urination, prostate irritation, vaginal pruritus, rheumatism
LYMPH CONGESTION with SKIN ERUPTIONS
SCURVY, SCROFULA
HARD DEPOSITS: urinary & gallstones
INTESTINAL PARASITES

4   STIMULATES THE LUNGS, EXPELS VISCOUS PHLEGM AND CLEARS THE HEAD; CLEARS MUCOUS DAMP
lung phlegm damp with thin white phlegm, wheezing
BRONCHITIS
head damp cold with head congestion; head colds
intestines mucous damp (Spleen damp) with mucousy stool, gurgling distended abdomen

Preparation

USE: The best preparation is the freshly pressed JUICE. Eaten in salads, it is a medicinal FOOD, combining well with other spring tonic greens such as Lamb's lettuce, Dandelion and Nettle leaves. The JUICE is used externally in **skin diseases**, blemishes, hair loss, etc. A good TINCTURE can be made from the fresh plant.

DOSAGE: JUICE: 2 tsp (10 ml) diluted in a glass of water three times a day.
               TINCTURE: generous standard doses apply.

CAUTION: The preferably **organically grown** Watercress should be carefully washed before eating or juicing. If a course is taken, three days' break every eight days should be made, to prevent irritation of the cystic mucosa. Use with care during pregnancy.

Notes

    Watercress is another one of several supererior food-remedies with a strong *cleansing* as well as *nourishing* function. Its plethora of analyzable constituents is typical of a plant that comes into being as a result of a number of different bioenergetic activities whose interplay in a **fluid environment** finally produce Watercress as we know it—growing in the cold running waters of streams and fountains. Its iron and iodine content, for example, are the direct result of levels of those elements found in its environing water.

    Like other remedies that provide nourishment, Watercress is a prime anabolic *blood builder*. It restores every aspect of the blood, both in a structural and a functional sense: as a bearer of oxygen, as a fluid tissue, as an immune vehicle. This is mostly due to its amazing range of minerals and trace elements. In this connection, Watercress should prove excellent for balancing the calcium constitutional phase in Carbonic and Phosphoric types, like the homeopathic Calc. carb. and Calc. phos., regulating **calcium metabolism** and **levels**. Closely connected to this is its *antidyskratic diuretic* activities which not only cleanse fluids, blood and tissues, but also exert a global *regulating* effect on these. The sage PARACELSUS provides a helpful image when he says that Watercress draws all toxin to itself and transforms it, in the human body as in nature. **Mucus accretion** in the **lymphatic** and **digestive** system is scoured and removed, for example. Every aspect of the body's fluid organism is overhauled and regenerated in a harmonious way.

On an **endocrine** level, too, Watercress's effects display the same seamless interconnection between *restoring, nourishing, cleansing* and *eliminating*. Here pituitary and thyroid deficiencies are adressed above all, again proving that this is a remedy for **chronic** and **degenerative** states in the main—aside from its maintenance use as dietary supplement.

MALVA SYLVE
STRIS PVMILA

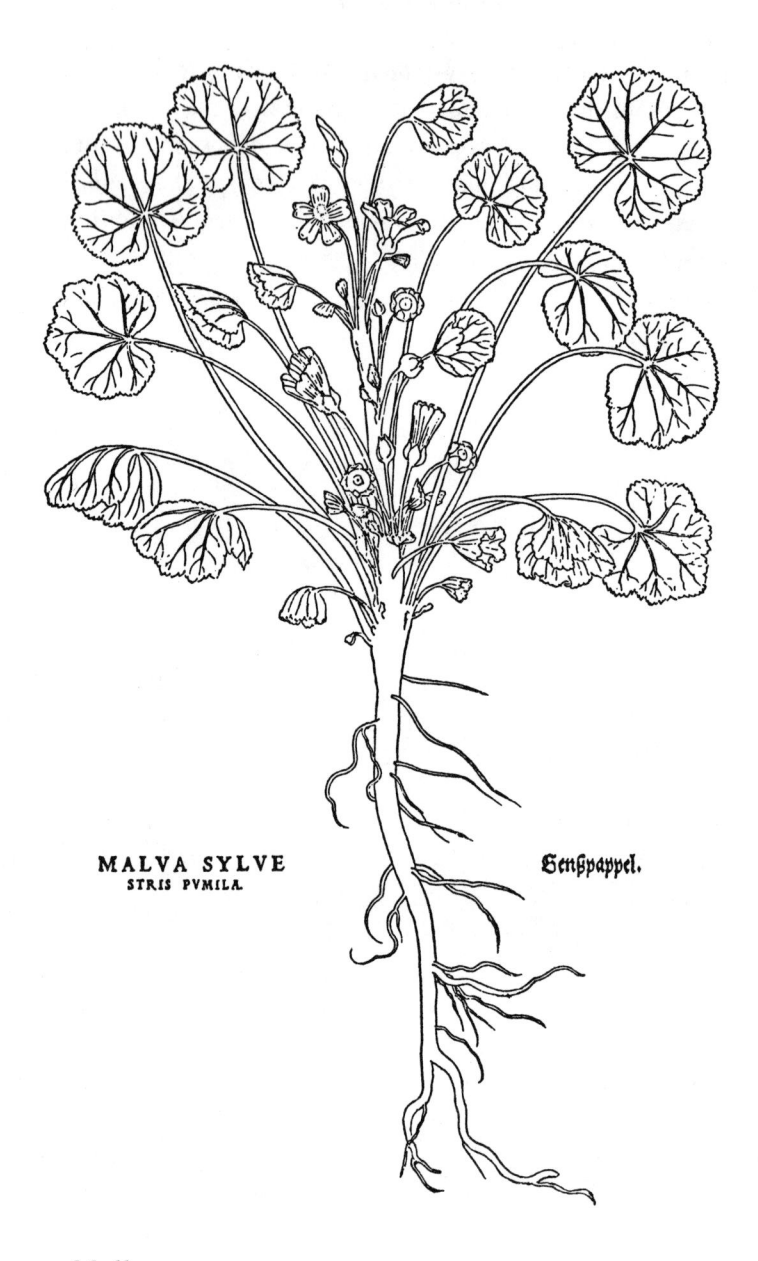

Senffpappel.

Mallow

CLASS 10

Herbs to Foster the Yin, Provide Moisture and Lenify Dryness

Botanicals in this class are used to provide moisture in conditions of internal **dryness**. These conditions are also known as Yin deficiency in Chinese medicine, since fluids and moisture are considered part of the body's Yin as a whole. Whatever their origins, and whether found locally or systemically, dry conditions always entail a lack of fluid and are characterizd by dryness, irritation and roughness. By substantially lubricating dry tissue, these herbs lenify and soothe irritation caused by dryness, relax any local tension and recreate moisture.

There is a variety of conditions and symptoms in which normal moisture or fluids need recreating. The moistening method therefore is used when a dry climate causes dryness in the lungs, for example, or in cool dry autumns or hot dry summers, or when dryness is simply caused by air onditioning or atmospheric city pollution. In addition, moisture needs providing when dryness is generated purely due to endogenous physiological reasons. Fluids are either unavailable or lost due to factors such as poor nutrition, an excessive consumption of hot, spicy food, excessive activity of any kind, childbirth, low estrogen secretion, hemorrhage, diarrhea, vomiting and fevers.

The conditions involving dryness as part of their overall profile essentially divide into deficiency and excess kinds. Dryness due to deficiency occurs when any aspect of the body's Yin, namely fluids or blood, becomes injured. Dryness due to excess, on the other hand, results when heat or Qi constraint affect the Yin. In all these conditions the moist aspect of the body's Yin may be injured. Moreover, a dry condition may present as a systemic condition or as a purely local one. In this case dryness is often found along the hollow organs lined with the mucous membrane, such as mouth, stomach, intestines, sinuses and lungs. They generate typical symptom patterns well known to both Chinese and Greek medicine.

When the lungs suffer from dryness, syndromes such as lung Yin deficiency, lung dryness and lung heat dryness may present. They are similar enough to single out their common symptoms, which are dry, irritative, unproductive coughing, sometimes with scanty sticky phlegm; chest pains; dry mouth, nose and throat; headache; and a thin pulse. (Lung Yin deficiency often entails tuberculosis.) If the stomach is affected it is called either stomach dryness or stomach Yin deficiency and presents an uncomfortable, lumpy sensation in the epigastrium, a feeling of hunger without any desire to eat, scanty urine, constipation, a dry mouth and tongue and a thin pulse.

Blood and fluids depletion is an example of a systemic syndrome creating dry symptoms such as dry mouth, throat and tongue, constipation, debility, exhaustion and a rough, hollow or soggy pulse. Systemic Yin deficiency is another, and typically presents feverishness especially in the late afternoon only, dry throat, mental and physical unrest, heat in the soles, palms or sternum, a dry red tongue and a thin, fast pulse. Yin deficiency, of whatever kind, may or may not present signs of heat and, if only affecting a particular organ, may not entail the systemic neurovascular changes described in Class 16.

The types of dry conditions involving excess as opposed to deficiency, namely Qi constraint and heat, are described in Classes 12 and 13 respectively since, involving as they do more than simple primary dryness, they require more than simply moisturizing.

In all dry conditions it is clearly neccessary not only to assess predisposing, perhaps

The Energetics of Western Herbs

constitutional, etiologies as well as triggering ones, but also to determine the nature of the overall syndrome that is causing the dryness. This allows for more specific, comprehensive and therefore effective treatment.

Herbs that foster the Yin, provide moisture and lenify dryness are mainly found in the *Plantaginaceae, Malvaceae* and *Gramineae* families. (Most cereal grains are naturally moist, for example.) Most have a *sweet* or *bland* taste, a *thick, smooth, moist* texture, and a *cooling* effect. They are called *demulcents* when used internally and *emollients* when applied to the skin surface. Some also have *restorative* or *nutritive* qualities or properties. Since addressing the fluid, moist element in the body, which belongs to the body's Yin as a whole, these remedies are known as *Yin tonics* in Oriental medicine. It is in this sense that they are variously said to *foster* or *cultivate the Yin (yang yin)* or to *water* or *moisten the Yin (zhi yin)*.[1]

These *demulcent Yin tonics* produce their effect through their mucilage (such as pectin, gums and polysaccharides) and sometimes through their saponin content. They coat the digestive canal with a fine protective layer of mucilage. This not only glosses and feeds but also soothes, slows down and relaxes the mucosa topically. These moisture bearing herbs are therefore able to deal with dryness due on the one hand to damaged mucosa and fluid insufficiency (e.g. due to fluid or blood loss, poor nutrition or Qi constraint), and on the other due to local overactivity (e.g. due to infection, inflammation or Qi constraint). Hence their application in both **deficiency dry** conditions, such as fevers, ulcers and TB, and **excess dry** conditions such as gastritis, diarrhea, irritable colon, bladder irritation and allergic asthma. Moreover, these mucilagenous herbs not only provide a local effect; they also have a reflex action at a distance, hence the *relaxant* effect at a distance created by *demulcents* such as Marsh mallow and Comfrey on the lungs, bladder and colon.

Demulcents such as Borage, Mullein, Ribwort plantain and Red clover appropriate to the lungs, whereas Licorice, Iceland moss and Slippery elm have a greater affinity for the stomach and intestines. Most are also used externally for their *emollient* effect in dry or itchy (pruritic) skin conditions, as well as for inflammations, wounds and bleeding. Another group of *demulcents* focuses on the urinary system, *relaxing* and *soothing* irritation of the cystic membrane, Couch grass, Asparagus, the Mallows and Cornsilk being prime examples.

Whetever the condition treated, *demulcents* are rarely used on their own, unless it is for immediate symptom relief. They are usually combined with other herbs addressing the specific and systemic pattern of disharmony involved in creating dryness. For example, if dryness is caused by blood & fluids deficiency, *demulcents* are joined by Class 9 *nutritives* in creating a formula to treat both the symptom and the overall condition in one.

The **syrup** as a preparation form is an excellent way of enhancing the *moistening, glossing* properties of these herbs, especially when applied to chest conditions.

Caution: *Demulcent* remedies should be avoided in severe and chronic cases of Spleen Qi deficiency, where they may inhibit digestion and assimilation of nutrients.

A summary listing of all herbs in this class may be found on p. 699.

Notes

1 Since *demulcents* moisten the Yin of certain organs, they are the true equivalents of the Chinese herbs that are said to foster the Yin *(yang yin)*. Like *demulcents,* the Chinese *Yin tonics* do not redress systemic Yin imbalance (as would be expected), but rather only certain aspects of the Yin such as lung Yin, Kidney Yin, etc. As a result, although it is fair to equate *demulcents* with *Yin tonics,* it is important to distinguish these mucilage loaded herbs from the deeper acting systemic

Yin tonics of Class 16. The latter tonify the organism's Yin as a whole by strongly increasing parasympathetic and inhibiting sympathetic nerve functions.

MARSH MALLOW

Pharmaceutical name: radix Althaeae
Botanical name: Althaea officinalis L. (N.O. Malvaceae)
Ancient names: Althaia (Gr)
    Ibiscus (Lat)
Other names: Mallards, Mauls, Cheeses (Eng)
    Sweetweed, Mortification root, Wymote (Am)
    Eibisch, Weisse Malve, Weisse Pappelblume, Attichkraut, Samtpappel, Schleimwurzel, Heilwurz (Ge)
    Guimauve (Fr)
Part used: the root; also the leaf, *folium Althaeae*

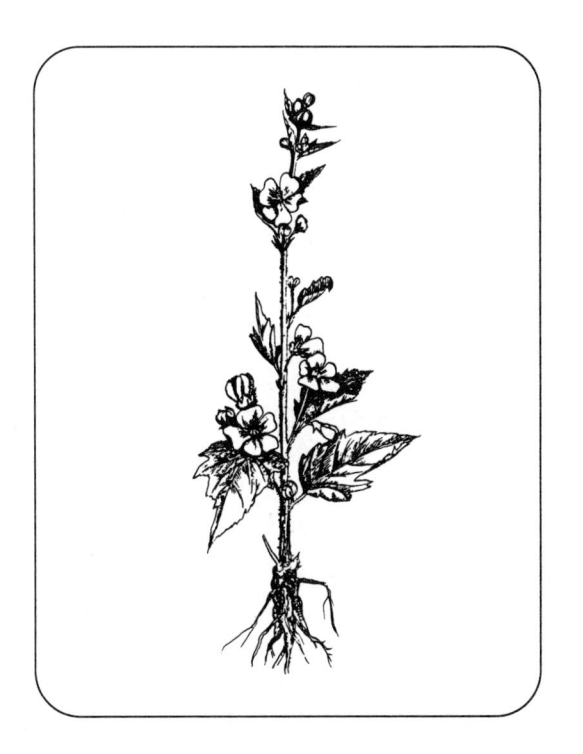

Nature

CATEGORY: mild herb with minimal chronic toxicity
CONSTITUENTS: starch, mucilage (up to 35% in root), pectin, tannins, fixed oil, sugar, asparagin, calcium, phophorus, trace minerals, phytosterol, malic acid
EFFECTIVE QUALITIES
Primary: sweet, cool, moist, with a secondary drying effect
Secondary: softening, thickening, relaxing
TROPISM: lungs, stomach, intestines, bladder, kidneys
    Warmth, Fluid organisms
    Lung, Stomach, Colon, Bladder meridians
GROUND: Choleric & Sanguine krases
    Tough/Shao Yang & Charming/Yang Ming Earth biotypes
    Hematic/Sulphuric/Brown Iris constitution

Functions and Uses

1 FOSTERS THE YIN, PROVIDES MOISTURE, LENIFIES DRYNESS AND CLEARS HEAT; PROMOTES EXPECTORATION AND URINATION

lung dryness: headache, dry mouth, nose and throat, tickling dry cough
WHOOPING COUGH, pneumonia
lung Yin deficiency: dry unproductive cough or with blood-tinged sticky sputum, night sweats
PLEURISY
stomach & intestines dryness: abdominal distention with lumpy sensation, hunger without eating, constipation

Marsh mallow: Class 10

    GASTRITIS, hiatus hernia
stomach fire: great appetite, fetid breath, swollen painful gums
GASTRIC & DUODENAL ULCERS due to hyperacidity
NEPHRITIS, kidney colic

2   ACTIVATES IMMUNITY, RESTRAINS INFECTION AND PUTREFACTION, REDUCES INFLAMMATION AND CLEARS TOXINS; SOFTENS BOILS AND DRAWS PUS, PROMOTES TISSUE REPAIR

intestines damp heat: urgent burning passing of fetid stool with blood and mucous; enteritis, dysentery
bladder damp heat: frequent painful urination, dry mouth;
MUCOUS CYSTITIS, URETHRITIS
GENERAL BLADDER IRRITATION
URINARY GRAVEL & STONES
skin damp heat: boils, furuncles; insect stings
CHRONIC LOCAL INFECTION & putrefaction: of mouth, throat
SLOW HEALING WOUNDS, ulcers, abscesses, gangrene
BREAST lumps or swelling, mastitis
DRY SKIN ERUPTIONS, cuts, burns

3   MOLLIFIES AND COMFORTS THE SINEWS

BRUISES, sprains, aches or stiffness in muscles and tendons

4   PROMOTES LACTATION

INSUFFICIENT BREAST MILK

Preparation

USE: Marsh mallow as a remedy is equally at home in internal and external uses. The ideal preparation is a COLD MACERATION for several hours, e.g. overnight in a fridge; the TINCTURE is mainly applicable to function 2 above. Both these preparations can be used externally in DOUCHES, WASHES, POULTICES, etc. Marsh mallow OINTMENTS were still popular in the 1820's for mellowing stiff or **painful sinews** and can be combined with Asparagus root or Chickweed for this purpose. MATTIOLI (1611) commends it for ENEMAS with the addition of other *cool astringent* herbs, as well as a HIPBATH recipe for **urinary stones**. In SYRUPS with other lung remedies Marsh mallow comes into its own.

Only when used as a GARGLE should Marsh mallow be DECOCTED in the normal way, as its starch is beneficial here.

DOSAGE: standard doses throughout

Notes

    The root of the Marsh mallow, with its unalloyed *sweet* taste is perhaps the most important remedy for *providing moisture* and *lenifying dryness* in this class: it is moisture made substantial. This is due to its high content of mucilage, as well as to the variety of its uses. Greek medicine made extensive use of Althaia, and the earliest record goes back to the ninth century B.C.

    There are two types of *demulcents:* one that is also *nutritive* and deals with **chronic deficient** conditions, such as Iceland moss, Irish moss, Comfrey, Slippery elm and Purslane; and another that is a *demulcent* pure and simple. The first also tends to restore the blood, nourish and engender fluids, while the other simply moistens and soothes by its sheer substance. Marsh mallow definitely belongs to the latter kind.

In contrast to those botanicals whose local *calming* and *relaxing* effects result from a very energetic action, *demulcents* such as the Mallows work by their very presence. Their *sweet* taste, which belongs to Kapha, has *heavy, cold* properties, and is responsible for their *moistening, soothing, slowing, calming* presence. It is very much needed in conditions of **gastric** and **intestinal dryness, inflammation** and **hyperactivity,** where syndromes such as stomach fire, intestines dryness and intestines damp heat evolve. Their presence in the gut even goes so far as to evoke sympathetic reactions in the lungs and bladder: hence the same effects obtained in conditions such as lung dryness or Yin deficiency and bladder damp heat and general irritation. Like several others in this class, both Marsh mallow root and Blue mallow flower can be likened to the *sweet bland moist Yin tonics* from the Chinese repertory. They compare favorably with a *cool demulcent* such as *Bei sha shen, radix Glehniae.*

Marsh mallow is a remedy for **acute** conditions where **pain**, **irritation** and **redness** present on skin or mucosa. In chronic conditions of this type, and in full heat syndromes, other remedies are appropriate: nevertheless, in these a good *emollient* influence such as this is often needed for underlying support.

BLUE MALLOW

Pharmaceutical name: flos seu folium Malvae
Botanical name: Malva sylvestris, seu
 rotundifolia L. (N.O. Malvaceae)
Other names: a) Blue Mallow, High mallow,
 Common mallow, Cheeseflower, Country
  mallow (Eng & Am)
 Grande mauve, Mauve sauvage, Fouassier,
  Fromageon (Fr)
 Wilde Malve, Grosse Käsepappel,
  Rosspappel (Ge)
 b) Dwarf mallow, Low mallow, Cheeseplant
  (Eng & Am)
 Petite mauve (Fr)
 Kleine Käsepappel (Ge)
Part used: the flower or the leaf

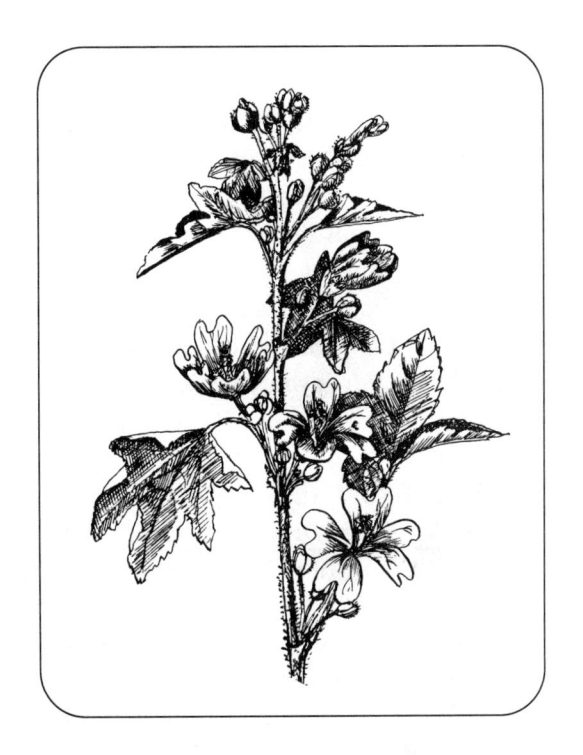

*Both these types of Mallow are virtually identical in nature and are used in a similar way to Marsh mallow, but are considered less effective overall. Their main strength lies in **external usage** in all skin conditions with dryness, heat or damp heat; in mouth, gum and throat inflammations and for insect stings.*

USE: The standard infusion for WASHES, GARGLES, etc., as well as for internal use.

Slippery elm: Class 10

SLIPPERY ELM

Pharmaceutical name: cortex Ulmi
Botanical name: Ulmus fulva Michx. (N.O.
	Ulmaceae)
Other names: Red elm, Indian elm, Moose elm,
	Sweet elm, Rock elm (Am)
Part used: the bark

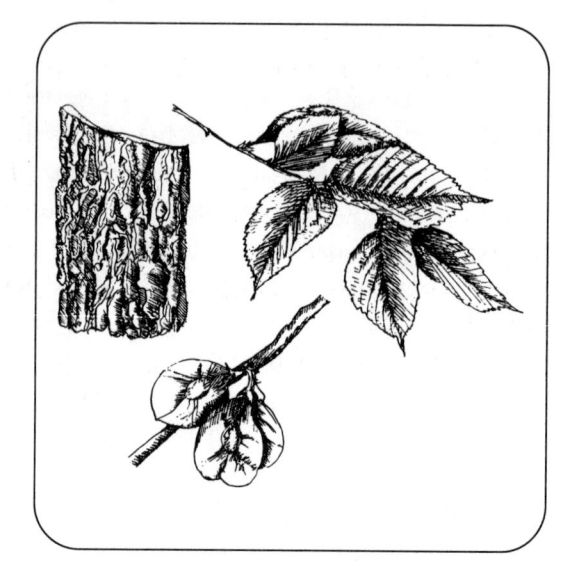

Nature

CATEGORY: mild herb with minimal chronic toxicity
CONSTITUENTS: polysaccharides, mucilage up to 50%, starch, tannins, calcium oxalates, calcium, vit. C
EFFECTIVE QUALITIES
Primary: sweet & bland, cool, moist
Secondary: nourishing, thickening, astringing
	stabilizing movement
TROPISM: lungs, stomach, bladder
	Fluid, Warmth organisms
	Lung, Stomach meridians
GROUND all for symptomatic use

Functions and Uses

1 FOSTERS THE YIN, PROVIDES MOISTURE, LENIFIES DRYNESS AND CLEARS HEAT; PROVIDES NOURISHMENT AND SUPPORTS STRENGTH
   DEBILITY with global or local DRYNESS from hot illness (e.g., Shao Yin stage fevers), old age, childbirth, etc.
   lung dryness with dry cough & sensitivity
   lung Yin deficiency with coughing up blood
   stomach dryness with distaste for eating, abdominal discomfort
   PEPTIC ULCERS, high gastric acidity
   bladder damp heat with chronic inflammation, irritation
   THROAT INFLAMMATION
   skin damp heat with boils, furuncles
   BURNS, skin inflammation, dry skin eruptions

2 CREATES ASTRICTION, RESTRAINS INFECTION AND ARRESTS DISCHARGE
   DIARRHEA with intestines damp cold or chronic damp heat conditions
   CHILDREN's CHOLERA
   LUNG HEMORRHAGE due to *lung Qi deficiency*

HEMORRHOIDS
INJURIES of all kinds, sores

Preparation

USE: Slippery elm bark may be DECOCTED, or its powder made into a PASTE, gruel, etc., e.g. with raw Goat's milk for **lung** or **stomach dyness**. Its mild *astringent* property may be increased by adding some honey; as a *demulcent* it combines well with Licorice or Comfrey root. Externally, COMPRESSES or simple APPLICATIONS of the paste should be used.
DOSAGE: standard generous doses throughout
CAUTION: If the stomach is weak and Slippery elm causes stagnation, *digestive stimulants* such as Clove, Fennel or Ginger should be added to this herb.

Notes

Although Slippery elm has been described as the American Marsh mallow, it would be more accurate to call it the terrestrial Irish moss: a *nutritive demulcent* and *emollient*. Native Americans were more skilled than any in its use, and they found many more types of Elms besides the main ones listed above. The most pertinent conditions for its use, however, are **weakness** with **dryness**, such as is found while convalescing from a long fever. It is nutritious enough to count as a survival food and moist enough to increase the fluids globally.

Since bedecking the respiratory and gastric mucosa more than adequately, Slippery elm will provide welcome relief in **Yin deficiencies** of either **lung** or **stomach**, relieving **irritation**, **dryness** and even **ulceration** in so doing. In many respects, it resembles the Chinese Yin tonifying remedies that also clear empty heat, generate fluids and recoup lost forces, such as *Mai men dong, radix Ophiopogonis, Xuan shen, radix Panacis quinquefolii,* and *Shi hu, herba Dendrobii*. It is definitely a good North American equivalent of these. This, together with its gentle astringency, makes Slippery elm a good choice in not too severe conditions of infectious damp heat of the intestines or bladder.

COMFREY

Pharmaceutical name: radix Symphyti
Botanical name: Symphytum officinalis
Ancient names: Symphyton (Gr)
    Confirma, Solidago, Consolida maior (Lat)
Other names: Boneset, Knitbone, Walwort,
    Bruisewort, Consound, Knitback (Eng)
    Consoude, Oreille d'âne, Herbe aux
    coupures, Sain-foin (Fr)
    Beinwell, Wallwurz, Schwarzwurz,
    Schmerzwurz, Blutwurz (Ge)
Part used: the root; also the leaf, *folium Symphyti*

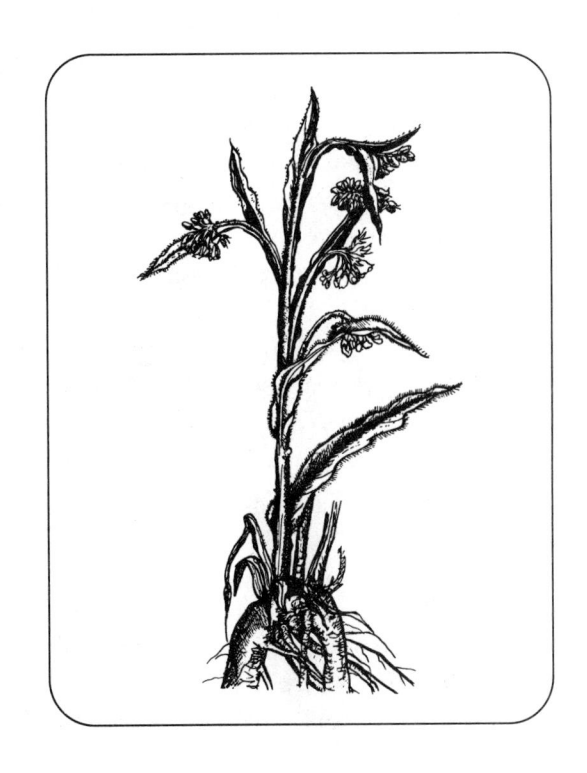

Comfrey: Class 10

Nature

CATEGORY: mild herb with minimal chronic toxicity
CONSTITUENTS: mucilage, tannin, allantoin, asparagin, inulin, alkaloids (incl. consolidin, consolicin), cholin, ess. oil, protein, trace minerals, iron, calcium, phosphorus, vitamins (incl. B 12), nicotinic & pantothenic acid
EFFECTIVE QUALITIES
Primary: *Taste:* a bit sweet & bland & astringent
Warmth: cool
Moisture: moist with a secondary drying effect
Secondary: softening, astringing, solidifying, restoring, nourishing
TROPISM
Organs: lungs, skin, stomach, intestines, bladder, genitals
Organisms: Fluid
Meridians: Lung, Stomach, Bladder
Tri Dosas: increases Kapha
GROUND
krasis/temperament, biotype & constitution: all for symptomatic use

Functions and Uses

1 FOSTERS THE YIN, PROVIDES MOISTURE AND LENIFIES DRYNESS; CLEARS HEAT AND PROMOTES BOWEL MOVEMENT; SOFTENS BOILS AND DRAWS PUS
lung dryness: dry cough with no phlegm, dry mouth & nose, headache, sore throat
PNEUMONIA, LARYNGITIS, BRONCHITIS
lung Yin deficiency: afternoon fever, dry cough
WHOOPING COUGH, TB
stomach dryness: dry mouth, dry vomiting
GASTRIC & DUODENAL ULCER, ulcerative colitis, castric cancer
intestines dryness: difficult bowel movement, dry stool, chronic constipation
BLADDER & KIDNEY ULCERS, urinary spasms & irritation
NEPHRITIS, acute or chronic
PERIOSTITIS, tendinitis, mastitis
skin damp heat: boils, carbuncles
ECZEMA, ACNE
LOW TIDAL FEVERS in Shao Yin stage

2 PROMOTES TISSUE REPAIR, CREATES ASTRICTION, REDUCES INFLAMMATION AND CLOTTING; ARRESTS BLEEDING AND DISCHARGE; RELIEVES PAIN
BONE FRACTURES
WOUNDS & RUPTURES, internal & external, incl. chronic ones
BRUISES, contusions, sprains, burns, swelling
CHRONIC ULCERS of all types; abscesses, varicoses veins
HEMORRHAGE internally, or externally, from any orifice
bladder damp heat: blood in urine, back pain
ACUTE URINARY INFECTIONS
ARTHRITIS, RHEUMATISM
BONE & TENDON PAIN

3   RESTORES THE BLOOD AND FLUIDS, STRENGTHENS THE LIVER AND UROGENITAL ORGANS

Liver & Kidney depletion: scanty, irregular or no menses with pale flow, weakness, lower backache, scanty urine

blood & fluids deficiency: (as above) with dry skin

ANEMIA, wasting disease

Preparation

USE: While the **entire plant** is *emollient, astringent* and *vulnerary,* the **root** is also *nourishing* and *restoring.* The **leaf** is the strongest for *tissue healing.* Both **root** and **leaf** are equally used internally and externally.

Comfrey's reliability in most **bone fractures, hemorrhages, wounds** and **ulcers** (including perineal tears) have always been in the limelight. For these, the FRESH HERB, PLASTER, POULTICE, WARM COMPRESS or OINTMENT is used. The base for these may be a cold water overnight MACERATION or a short DECOCTION of the **root**, or an INFUSION of the **leaf**. The TINCTURE is preferable when LINIMENTS for **painful** conditions are required.

Country bonesetters and town barber-surgeons used to make elaborate PLASTERS which often included Camphor, Turpentine, various gums and resins, as well as other good wound herbs such as Arnica, Plantain and St. John's wort. WILHELM RYFF (1573), for example, gives four separate PLASTER formulations. Internal use will only accelerate healing in any injury.

As an internal remedy, the DECOCTION of the **root** as well as the GLYCERINE EXTRACT is preferable to any alcoholic extract. Since Comfrey is a major lung herb, a thick, soothing SYRUP is just what **dry** or **hot lung** conditions need. Being *nutritive*, the **root** was CANDIED in the past. The **leaves** may also be eaten: in parts of Switzerland they are baked in dough to make COMFREY CAKES, while COMFREY TEMPURA is a Japanese-style treat.

DOSAGE: Large doses are used for injuries and bleeding and where a *bulk laxative* effect is needed. Otherwise, **standard** doses apply to this safe, nontoxic plant for internal use.

Notes

There is no doubt that Comfrey has always held pride of place as the foremost botanical for promoting tissue healing. All its names throughout the ages attest to this: Boneset, Knitbone and Knitback are self-explanatory, while the Greek root-word *symphein* itself means "to grow together", as does the German *wallen* and the French *soudre*. Both the Latin names *Confirma* and *Consolida maior* (the latter HILDEGARD VON BINGEN's appellation) speak for themselves. Today we have the benefit of knowing that its ability to literally weld tissue together, whether bone, flesh or sinews, is mainly due to its *allantoin* content. Allantoin has a calcium type of effect, bioenergetically speaking, which stimulates cell production for repairing connective tissue, bone, collagen, etc., leaving the injury often scarless. Its tannins moreover cause sufficient astriction not only to staunch bleeding but also to make stitches unneccessary.

Nevertheless, in spite of its use among past European women country healers solely for traumas, Comfrey is also a remedy for syndromes. How could it not be, with its ample mucilage content evincing a *moist* nature ideal for **dry, irritated** conditions, its *cool* quality which clears **heat** and **inflammation**, its *astringent* taste which soothes, calms and relieves **pain**? The final outcome of these its primary qualities is a botanical that *calms, restores* and *nourishes*. Its mucilage bedecks whatever tissue it contacts with a slimy mucilagenous coat, *protecting, soothing* and *cooling* the mucous membranes or skin: hence its use not only in ulcers, but also in irritable or acute inflammatory conditions, burns (even 3rd degree), swelling and ecchymosis. Secondary effects of its *demulcent* qualities include the drawing of boils and abscesses to the surface and the

Mullein: Class 10

reflex *relaxation* of lung and urinary tissues.

In short, Comfrey is a prime botanical for **deficient Yin** and **dry** conditions of various kinds, whether due to blood & fluids depletion, wind heat, internal heat or Qi constraint—like other herbs in this class, both in this and in the Chinese materia medica. Furthermore, its *nutritive* content makes it useful in any type of **depletion**, e.g. due to prolonged illness. On the other hand, the traditional use of Comfrey for arthritis, gout, etc., cannot be rationally explained—but is none the less effective for that.

The historical use of this plant is interesting in that it demonstrates the increasing primitiveness of Western medicine in eighteenth and nineteenth century America, and the superior skill of Native American healers in their use of plants. The latter apparently received various types of Comfrey from the earliest white settlers in the sixteenth century; by the time of the great migrations westwards, having realized its amazing potential, they were found to be applying it with far greater skill than the current medics—probably as skillfully as the Greek *rhizomatai* had done two milleniums earlier. They were effectively able to make redundant the primitive and septic surgery and amputation carried out by Western physicians, thus saving countless lives that would otherwise have been lost.

MULLEIN

Pharmaceutical name: flos Verbasci
Botanical name: Verbascum thapsiforme L., *seu phlomoides* L. (N.O. Scrofulariaceae)
Ancient names: Phlomos, Phlegouro, Lychnitis (Gr)
    Candela regia, Lanaria, Candelaria, Th(l)apsus (Lat)
Other names: Jupiter's staff, Haire's beard, Bullocks lungwort Blanket herb, Woolwort (Eng)
    Bouillon blanc, Molène, Oreille de loup, Herbe de St-Fiacre (Fr)
    Grosse Königskerze, Weisser Andorn, Kerzenkraut (Ge)
Part used: the flower; also the leaf, *folium Verbasci*

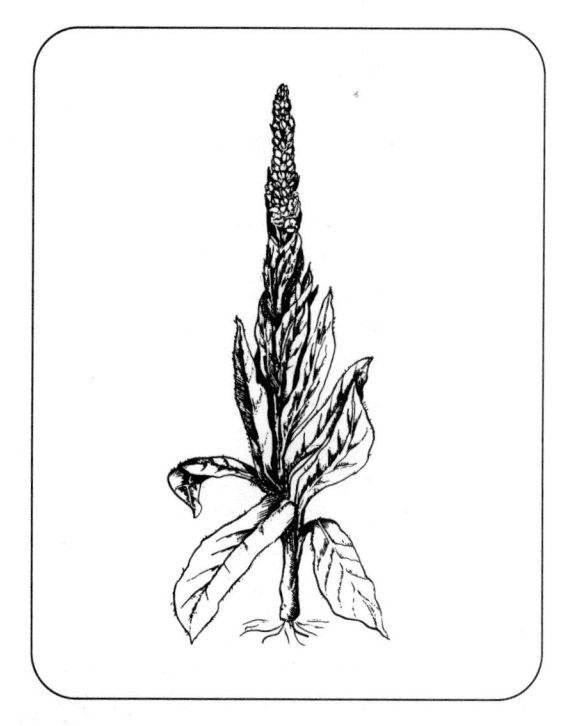

Nature

CATEGORY: mild herb with minimal chronic toxicity
CONSTITUENTS: mucilage, gum, saponins, ess. oil, flavonoids (incl. hesperidin and verbascoside), glycoside (incl. aucubin), carotene, bitter amaroid, resin
EFFECTIVE QUALITIES
Primary: a bit sweet & astringent & bland, cool, moist with a secondary drying effect
Secondary: thickening, restoring, astringing, softening, relaxing
TROPISM: lungs, stomach, intestines, bladder
    Warmth, Fluid organisms
    Lung, Stomach, Bladder meridians
GROUND: all krases, biotypes and constitutions

Class 10: Mullein

Functions and Uses

1 FOSTERS THE YIN, PROVIDES MOISTURE AND LENIFIES DRYNESS; RELIEVES COUGHING

   lung heat dryness: feeling of heat and dryness in chest, fever, dry cough
   lung phlegm dryness: dry hacking cough with scanty phlegm
   TRACHEITIS, laryngitis, tonsilitis
   lung Yin deficiency: weak dry cough, coughing up blood and sputum
   LUNG TB
   ALLERGIES of all types

2 STIMULATES THE LUNGS, LIQUIFIES AND EXPELS VISCOUS PHLEGM; RELAXES THE BRONCHI, OPENS THE CHEST AND LEVELS ASTHMA

   lung Qi constraint: rasping or tickling dry cough, wheezing
   SPASMODIC ASTHMA, whooping cough
   lung phlegm damp/heat: coughing up thin white or viscous yellow phlegm, full cough, sore throat, chest fullness

3 CREATES ASTRICTION, DRIES MUCOUS DAMP, RESTRAINS INFECTION AND REDUCES INFLAMMATION; ARRESTS DISCHARGE AND BLEEDING; HARMONIZES URINATION AND LENIFIES IRRITATION

   head damp cold: nasal and head congestion, watery discharge, head or body aches
   HAYFEVER
   intestines damp cold/heat: urgent passing of liquid stool, abdominal pain
   ACUTE & CHRONIC intestinal infections
   bladder damp heat: frequent, urgent painful urination, thirst, backache
   ACUTE & CHRONIC CYSTITIS
   bladder Qi constraint: suppressed urination, scanty and frequent urination, bedwetting
   GENERAL BLADDER IRRITATION due to any cause
   HEMORRHAGE internal or external, esp. from lungs, intestines

4 SOFTENS BOILS AND DRAWS PUS; RESOLVES SWELLING AND DISSIPATES TUMORS

   SKIN INFECTIONS, ECZEMA, dermatosis, scurf
   skin damp heat: boils, furuncles, abscesses
   WOUNDS, open sores, ulcers, esp. with swelling
   TUMORS, swollen glands, scrofula, swollen testicles or scrotum
   EARACHE, TOOTHACHE RHEUMATISM
   HEMORRHOIDS
   MOUTH AND EYE INFLAMMATIONS
   SPLINTERS & THORNS

Preparation

USE: The **flower** should be used if a *relaxant* effect is intended, while the **leaf** is equally good, if not better, for *soothing* and *leniating* through Mullein's mucilage content. A short DECOCTION is generally recommended, unless a GLYCERINE EXTRACT is preferred. If used for **intestinal damp** conditions, a short DECOCTION in goat's milk may be used to enhance its *astringent* effects.

Various preparations for Mullein's **external uses** may be made or had, such as the OIL (for **painful**,

Borage: Class 10

swollen conditions,) the SALVE (for **inflammatory** and **irritable infectious** conditions), and the CREAM.

Drunk **hot**, Mullein tea *causes sweating*.

Damp, **catarrhal intestinal** conditions will also benefit from ENEMAS with Mullein, while a SYRUP containing it will enhance all the indicated lung syndromes.

DOSAGE: generous standard doses throughout

Notes

Mullein, like Coltsfoot, is almost an all-purpose lung remedy, and, like Comfrey, was eagerly taken up by Native Americans into their repertoire (which already counted giants like Pleurisy root and Blood root). In Greek classical times it was apparently one of DIOSKURIDES's most favorite remedies, and certainly has always had a reputation in keeping with its reliability.

It is Mullein's high mucilage content which finds it a place among botanicals that provide moisture—considered *Yin tonics* in Chinese medicine. And it is very much a *cool demulcent* with *anti-inflammatory* and *antibacterial* effects—always directed to the lungs and chest. All manner of hot lung syndromes with **fever(ishness)**, **dryness** and **irritation** respond well to it, as do **asthmatic** and **spasmodic** conditions, for similar reasons. Mullein clearly deserves a place among herbal bedfellows of a *sweet bland cool moist* quality such as *Bei sha shen, radix Glehniae,* and *Shi hu, herba Dendrobii,* from China. Indeed, we could do worse than view this Western *Yin tonic* as a replacement for these or as an addition to acupuncture points BL 13, LU 10 & 5 and TH 5 in dry heat conditions of the lungs.

In addition, Mullein contains some essential oil and saponins. Together these ensure a *secretolytic stimulant* loosening of hardened mucous and a productive cough, useful not only in lung Qi constraint situations but also in **chronic catarrhal** conditions.

Likewise, **spasmodic**, **irritative** and **damp heat** infectious conditions of the **urinary passages** also find relief from the use of Mullein. Here as in the lungs and intestines, the synergy of its *soothing, relaxing* and *astrictive* effects are most welcome and should find support from other appropriate remedies according to the exact syndrome presenting.

BORAGE

Ph*armaceutical name: folium Borraginis*
Botanical name: Borrago officinale L. (N.O. Boraginaceae)
Ancient names: Euphrosine (Gr)
    Lingua bovis, Libanion, buglossa domestica (Lat)
Other names: Burrage, Levant, Star flower, Bee bread (Eng)
    Bourrache (Fr)
    Borretsch, Herzblumen, Wohlgemuth, Liebäuglein, Gurkenkraut (Ge)
Part used: the leaf

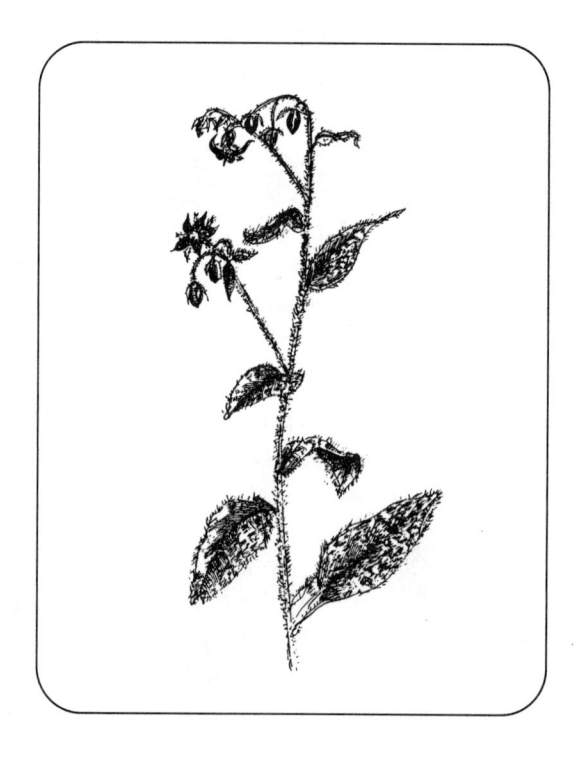

Class 10: Borage

Nature

CATEGORY: mild herb with minimal chronic toxicity
CONSTITUENTS: saponins, potassium nitrate, cyanogenic substances, mucilage 30%, asparagin, lactic/acetic/malic acids, tannins 3%, trace minerals, resins, ess. oil traces
EFFECTIVE QUALITIES
Primary: a bit sweet & salty, cold, moist
Secondary: restoring, astringing, calming, softening
TROPISM: lungs, heart, kidneys, bladder
　　　　　Warmth, Fluid organisms
　　　　　Lung, Heart, Kidney meridians
GROUND: Sanguine & Choleric krases
　　　　　Charming/Yang Ming earth, Industrious/Tai Yang & Tough/Shao yang biotypes
　　　　　all three constitutions for symptomatic use

Functions and Uses

1 FOSTERS THE YIN, PROVIDES MOISTURE AND LENIFIES DRYNESS; CLEARS HEAT, INFLAMMATION AND TOXINS; SUPPORTS THE HEART AND LIFTS THE SPIRIT

   lung Yin deficiency with afternoon fever, emaciation
   lung heat/wind dryness with dry throat, rasping cough, fever
   PLEURISY, TB, whooping cough, pneumonia (initial stages)
   heart Yin deficiency with mental unrest, palpitations, anxiety
   kidney fire with fever, obstructed urination
   LOW TIDAL FEVERS with empty heat in Shao Yin stage
   CHRONIC NEPHRITIS
   THROAT & MOUTH INFLAMMATIONS (stomatitis, laryngitis)
   fire toxin with hot swellings, boils, sores, running ulcers
   DRY SKIN CONDITIONS (dermatoses) of all kinds
   DEPRESSION, GRIEF

2 CAUSES SWEATING, RELEASES THE EXTERIOR AND SCATTERS WIND HEAT; RESOLVES FEVER, PUSHES OUT ERUPTIONS AND BENEFITS THE THROAT

   external wind heat and *lung wind heat* onset of infections with fever, red sore swollen throat, coughing
   LARYNGITIS, tracheitis
   ERUPTIVE FEVERS, e.g. measles, chickenpox

3 DREDGES THE KIDNEYS, PROMOTES URINATION AND CLEANSING AND BENEFITS THE SKIN

   kidney Qi stagnation & general toxemia with skin eruptions, chronic rheumatism
   bladder & kidney damp heat with burning red urine, colic, frequent scanty urination
   LIVER CIRRHOSIS

Borage: Class 10

Preparation

USE: The long INFUSION, DECOCTION or FLUID EXTRACT are the most suitable preparations. The SYRUP for lung complaints and the Borage flower CONSERVE were traditional preparations. EYEWASHES, MOUTHWASHES, GARGLES, POULTICES are strongly recommended too.
DOSAGE: standard doses throughout

Notes

Borage has always been cultivated in herb gardens not only for its lovely sky blue flowers, but for its excellent medicinal and culinary uses. It was in fact traditionally considered a good heat clearing plant, whether partaken of in summer salads with other cooling greens such as Endive and Purslane or in the form of a medicinal preparation for various types of hot conditions. Borage definitely qualifies as member of the Forgotten Cooling Herbs Club, alongside others such as Grapevine, Rose, Selfheal, Purslane, Artichoke, Chicory and the Sorrels.

The two essential conditions which Borage straddles are **Yin deficiency** and **wind heat**. First, like its *cool moist cool Yin fostering* companions in this class, Borage specializes in deficiency heat conditions manifesting tissue **dryness, irritation** and **inflammation**. Borage specifically addresses the organs of the Upper Warmer, however, and is therefore used for all deficient, hot and dry conditions of the lungs and heart. In the past it was very much thought of as supporting the heart: together with Violet, Rose and Sweet woodruff, it belonged to the four heart tonics. In this respect, Borage resembles *Mai men dong, radix Ophiopogonis,* from the equivalent Chinese category of *Yin tonics*. Particular to Borage, in this connection, are its *antidepressant* properties. "It strengthens the Heart and Vital Spirit, takes away anxiety, depression and grief," begins MATTIOLI's entry of 1611. Scientific pharmacology has a hard time explaining this—but does that invalidate over two and a half thousand years of actual experience?

Secondly, since it affects the Upper Warmer and the lungs, Borage is a good **wind heat** herb where *sweating* and *cooling* need to be initiated. Addressing mainly lung wind heat at the onset of upper and lower **respiratory infections**, Borage excels with painful, swollen sore throats, dry hacking coughs and fever. Through a combination of *astringent, demulcent* and *cleansing* properties, it acts as a *detoxifying disinfectant,* clearing the fire toxin of toxemia, boils, infections and fever, including damp heat of the bladder. From this perspective Borage is clearly a therapeutic equivalent to the Chinese Chrysanthemum flower, *Ju hua, flos Chrysanthemi morifolii,* minus the liver component.

Borage is considered *antipyretic* in addition to *diaphoretic,* and its reliable *diuretic* effect not only helps clear heat, but also contributes to speedily resolving children's eruptive fevers.

CHICKWEED

Pharmaceutical name: herba Stellariae
Botanical name: Stellaria media Villars (syn. Alsine media L.) (N.O. Caryophyllaceae)
Ancient names: Alsine (Gr)
   Marona, Morsus gallinae, Hippia (Lat)
Other names: Stitchwort, Starwort, Adder's mouth, Satin flower, Tongue grass, Winterweed (Eng & Am)
   Mouron blanc, Mouron des oiseaux, Stellaire, Morgeline (Fr)
   Vogelmiere, Hühnerdarm, Sternmiere, Mäusedarm, Gänsekraut (Ge)
Part used: the herb

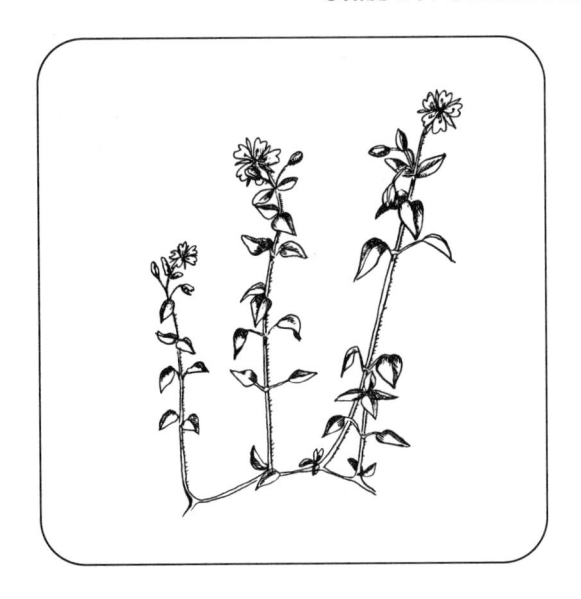

Nature

CATEGORY: mild herb with minimal chronic toxicity
CONSTITUENTS: mucilage, oil containing linoleic, silicic & other acids, rutin, saponins, fixed oil, starch, ascorbic acid, calcium, trace minerals (incl. silica, potassium, magnesium), ferrous phosphate, lime, vitamins A, B, C,
EFFECTIVE QUALITIES
Primary: a bit sweet & salty, cold, moist
Secondary: restoring, nourishing, softening
TROPISM: stomach, intestines, heart, lungs, kidneys, blood
   Warmth, Fluid organisms
   Stomach, Colon, Heart, Lung meridians
GROUND: Choleric krasis
   Tough/Shao Yang & Industrious/Tao Yang biotypes
   all three constitutions

Functions and Uses

1. **FOSTERS THE YIN, PROVIDES MOISTURE, LENIFIES DRYNESS AND CLEARS HEAT**

   stomach dryness with worry, inordinate hunger & thirst
   intestines dry heat with dry hard stools, constipation
   heart Yin deficiency with palpitations, dry mouth & throat
   lung Yin deficiency with dry unproductive cough, insomnia, low afternoon fever
   LUNG TB, whooping cough, bronchitis
   HEMOPTYSIS

2. **REDUCES INFLAMMATION AND CLEARS TOXINS; SOFTENS BOILS AND DRAWS PUS; SOOTHES AND BENEFITS THE SKIN**

   skin damp heat with boils, furuncles
   EYE, KIDNEY & BLADDER INFLAMMATIONS with heat & damp heat, e.g. conjunctivitis, nephritis, cystitis, etc.

Chickweed: Class 10

    ACUTE joint rheumatism
    SKIN ERUPTIONS, e.g. dermatitis, scabies

3   <u>DREDGES THE KIDNEYS AND PROMOTES URINATION AND CLEANSING</u>
    kidney Qi stagnation with skin eruptions, rheumatism, gout
    HEMORRHOIDS

4   <u>RESTORES THE BLOOD AND GENERATES STRENGTH; RELAXES AND COMFORTS THE SINEWS</u>
    blood deficiency with fatigue, palpitations, pale complexion
    ANEMIA
    FATIGUE due to overwork, illness, anemia
    CRAMPED, tight muscles
    LOCAL CONGESTION

Preparation

USE: A short DECOCTION or a GLYCERINE EXTRACT of the fresh herb works best for Chickweed. Chickweed is used both internally and externally. WILLIAM SALMON (1710) gives a nice *drawing* POULTICE for boils, etc., made of Chickweed, Mallow, Linseed and Fenugreek, and local muscle or blood congestions will also benefit from these.

DOSAGE: generous standard doses throughout

Notes

Like many a seemingly inert botanical abandoned during the onslaught of experimental pharmacology, Chickweed has finally re-emerged as a significant *cold nutritive demulcent* remedy. But its neglect predates the second half of the nineteenth century by far. It is significant that its Yin, structive and substantial medicinal effects were obscured from the Renaissance onwards when Yang, active and directional remedies won the day—when active routing of disease with minerals such as mercury was standard procedure, no matter what the nature of the condition or the vitality of the patient. Let us speak plainly: Chickweed is a **feminine herb** which could not survive this masculine phase of declining Galenic medicine.

It is significant that today, when increasingly a balance between the masculine and the feminine principles is being sought on every level, apparently "inactive "weeds like Chickweed appeal to us once again. Once more we can imagine its uses by lineages of wise women in times past, and hear the echoes of the many similar remedies still used in China today. In Chinese medicine Chickweed would be classed as a *Yin tonic,* appropriately enough. Its *moist, mucic* and slightly *sweet* effective qualities makes it "nourish the Yin," clear heat and provide moisture. Its use is mainly for lung and heart Yin deficient conditions (where it supports cardiac functions), and secondarily for stomach and intestinal dryness, Dealing with the **dryness**, **heat** and **irritation**, it closely resembles *Sha shen, radix Glehnia littoralis,* in its functions.

Like some other moisturizing herbs in this class, Chickweed also has a significant *nutritive* component, clearly a benefit in chronic Yin deficiency syndromes with exhaustion, as well as providing systemic support for dry or hot constitutions such as the Choleric.

IRISH MOSS

Pharmaceutical name: thallus Chondri
Botanical name: **Chondrus crispus** Stackh. (N.O. Algae)
Other names: Carrageen, Carrahan, Pearl moss (Ir)
　　Mousse d'Irlande (Fr)
　　Irländisches Moos (Ge)
Part used: the thallus

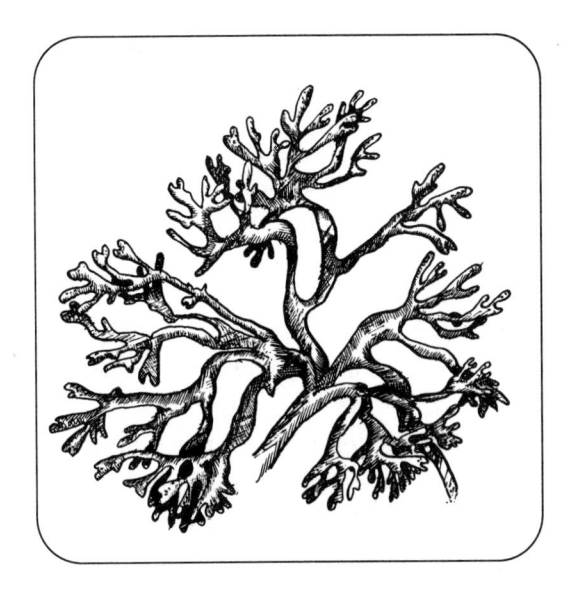

Nature

CATEGORY: mild herb with minimal chronic toxicity
CONSTITUENTS: mucilage, minerals, trace minerals
EFFECTIVE QUALITIES:
Primary: a bit sweet & salty & bland, cool, moist & dry
Secondary: nourishing, restoring, relaxing

This remedy is virtually identical to ICELAND MOSS (p. 364) in all its functions and uses, except that it does not have a bitter taste, hence is not restoring to stomach & Spleen Qi. Its other functions and uses, based on its moistening and nourishing qualities, are the same.

Preparation

USE: A DECOCTION is prepared by steeping 1/2 oz of the moss in cold water for about 15 minutes, then simmering it in 3 pints of water for 10 or 15 minutes. For lung conditions, goat's milk may be used instead of water. It may be drunk freely, plain or sweetened.

Carageen, as it is also known, is also used much like its Japanese relative KANTEN (AGAR-AGAR) for making jellies, puddings, pies and such. It can be used in any recipe calling for Kanten.

Lungwort lichen: Class 10

LUNGWORT LICHEN

Pharmaceutical name: lichen Stictae
Botanical name: **Sticta Pulmonaria** Ach. (syn. **Lobaria pulmonaria** Hoffm. (N.O. Lichenes)
Ancient names: Pulmonaria arborea (Lat)
Other names: Mossy lungwort, Tree lungwort (Eng)
Lichen pulmonaire, Pulmonaire du chêne, Herbe aux poumons (Fr)
Lungenflechte, Lungengrass (Ge)
Part used: the lichen

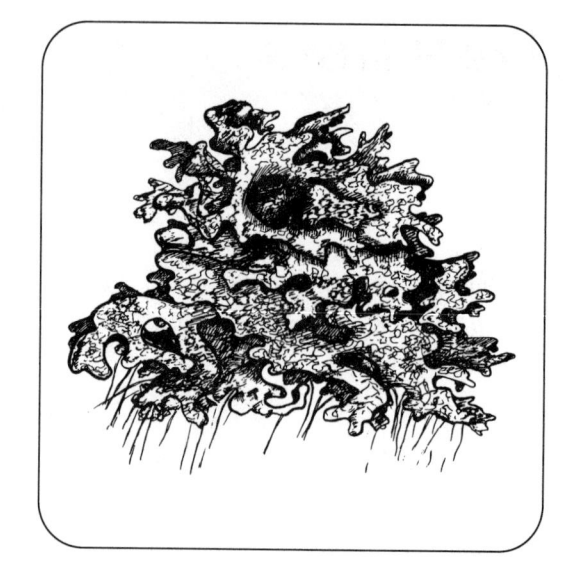

Nature

CATEGORY: mild herb with minimal chronic toxicity
CONSTITUENTS: mucilage, trace minerals, tannin
EFFECTIVE QUALITIES
Primary: a bit sweet & salty & bland & astringent, cool, moist & dry
Secondary: restoring, relaxing, softening

This herb is virtually identical to ICELAND MOSS (p. 364) in all its aspects. The only difference is that it does not have a bitter taste like the latter and therefore does not increase the Qi by restoring Spleen and lung Qi as Iceland moss does. Lungwort lichen is used in addition for **rheumatism** of the **muscles** and **small joints**; and in **hayfever**, **head colds** or **flu** with severe **frontal headache** and **watery nasal discharge**.

Preparation

USE: The INFUSION and TINCTURE is used in standard doses.
NOTE: The herb LUNGWORT, *Pulmonaria officinalis* (N.O. Boraginaceae), containing mucilage, tannins, silicic acid, minerals, resins and saponins, is used interchangeably with Lungwort lichen. Its slightly more *stimulating* quality, however, means that, like Borage, it can be used to cause sweating for (**lung**) **wind heat** onsets of cold and catarrh.

ALOE GEL

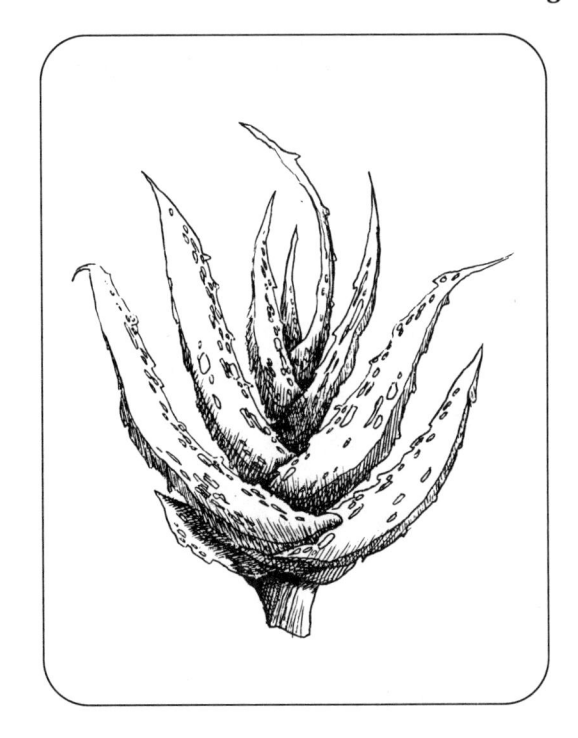

Pharmaceutical name: liquamen folii Aloidis
Botanical name: Aloe vera L. (N.O. Liliaceae)
Other names: Gel d'aloès (Fr)
   Aloe-Gel (Ge)
Part used: the leaf gel

Nature

CATEGORY: mild herb with minimal chronic toxicity
CONSTITUENTS: polysaccharides (incl. fructose, glucose, mannose, arabinose, galactose, xylose), 18 amino acids (incl. serin, salin, asparagin, glutaminic acid), calcium, magnesium, sodium, manganese, zinc, magnesium lactate, pradiciminase & aloctin-A, glycoproteins, tannins, steroids, enzymes (incl. oxydase, catalase, amylase), organic acids, antibiotic substance, glucuronic acid, calcium oxalate, hormones, saponins, vitamins, chloride, sulphate, lignin, amylase-like enzyme, alpha amylase, cholin
EFFECTIVE QUALITIES
Primary: bland, a bit salty, cool, moist
Secondary: restoring, softening
TROPISM: skin, stomach
   Fluid organism
   Stomach meridian
GROUND: all krases, biotypes and constitutions for symptomatic use

Functions and Uses

1   PROVIDES MOISTURE AND LENIFIES IRRITATION; REDUCES INFLAMMATION, RESTRAINS INFECTION AND PROMOTES TISSUE REPAIR; BENEFITS THE SKIN
   DRY SKIN ERUPTIONS simple or infective, irritation, rashes, incl. eczema, poison ivy rash, diaper rash
   BURNS, sunburn, radiation damage
   INFLAMMATIONS of all kinds, incl. mouth, gums, eyes & skin
   SKIN ULCERS, varicose ulcers, sores, gangrene
   PEPTIC ULCER of any kind
   DENTAL ABSCESS, periodontitis, caries
   NAIL FUNGUS, athlete's foot

Aloe gel: Class 10

       OILY SKIN, dandruff, hair loss
       SKIN BLEMISHES, spots, freckles, rough skin
       As INSECT repellent

2   RESOLVES MUCUS AND DRIES DAMP
       head damp cold with sinus congestion
       BRONCHITIS, ASTHMA

3   ARRESTS BLEEDING AND LACTATION
       MINOR CUTS, scrapes, etc.
       FOR WEANING

Preparation

USE: The bland-tasting **gel** is obtained from the tubular inner cells found in the central pulp of the Aloe leaf. It can be applied neat or with a COMPRESS. Internal use (mainly for **ulcers**) is enhanced when the gel is emulsified. **Head** and **nasal congestion** is relievd by placing some in each nostril or sniffing it diluted, and bronchial conditions are improved with INHALATION using a vaporizer.

DOSAGE: up to tbsp for internal use

Notes

Aloe gel presents a very different remedy from that obtained from the outer cells of the plant, namely the *laxative* Aloes discussed in Class 3. Here we have a supremely effective agent for external use mainly where *moisture, protection, cooling, lenifying* and *antisepsis* are needed externally—a good household and first aid remedy. In addition, serious dermatitis, burns, leg ulcers and a variety of dental problems respond admirably to its influence, as fairly recent experience has shown.

Biochemically Aloe gel has a lot of ingredients to account for its effects, notably polysaccharides, *vulnerary* hormones and amino acids, *anti-inflammatory* zinc and manganese—and many more that are not understood. It would be amazing to get a glimpse of the architecture of its constituents, so that an understanding of its biochemical form might complement that of its substance. If this were possible, then the nature of the bioenergies that created it would become evident. Only then would the reasons become clear why its constituents on their own, not built up in any particular structure, have proved experimentally to have none of the properties of the same constituents in the gel itself.

BALM OF GILEAD

Pharmaceutical name: gemma Populi
Botanical name: Populus balsamifera L. (N.O. Salicaceae)
Other names: Balsam poplar, Tacamahac, Hackmatac (Am)
Baumier, Liard (Fr)
Balsamespe, Balsampappel, Tacahamacpappel, Falscher Sattelholzbaum (Ge)
Part used: the bud; also the bark, *cortex Populi*

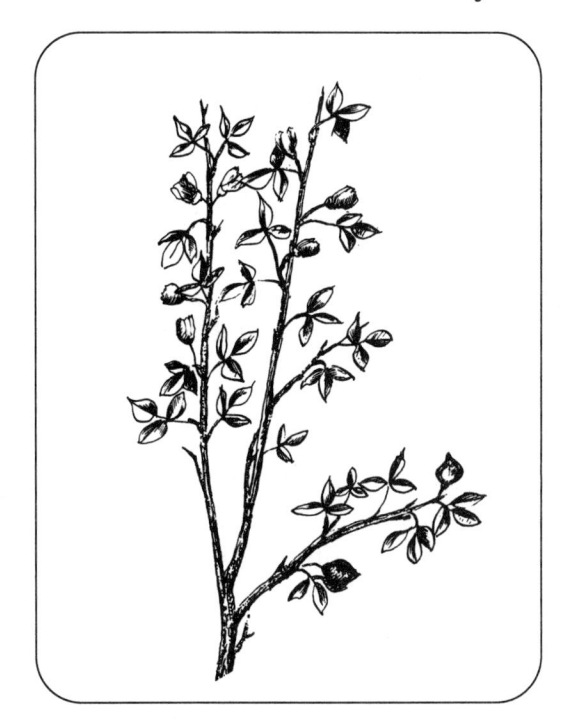

Nature

CATEGORY: mild herb with minimal chronic toxicity
CONSTITUENTS: populin (which becomes salicia), benzoic acid (which becomes salicylic acid), ess. oil, tannins, resins, gallic acids, mannitol
EFFECTIVE QUALITIES
Primary: bitter, a bit pungent, cool, moist
Secondary: restoring, softening, dissolving
TROPISM: stomach, intestines, lungs, kidneys, blood
Warmth, Fluid organisms
Stomach, Colon, Lung meridians
GROUND: all krases, biotypes and constitutions

Functions and Uses

1. PROVIDES MOISTURE, LENIFIES DRYNESS, CLEARS HEAT AND REDUCES INFLAMMATION, PROMOTES BOWEL MOVEMENT

    stomach dryness with epigastric discomfort or lumpiness, dry mouth & tongue
    intestines dryness with distended, abdomen, constipation
    PEPTIC ULCERS due to high acidity
    lung dryness with dry unproductive cough, dry mouth, nose or throat, sore throat
    lung phlegm dryness with difficult coughing or mucous production
    DRY CHRONIC BRONCHITIS
    DRY COUGH, SORE THROAT
    GALL BLADDER & URINARY INFLAMMATION, irritation or ulceration

2. COOLS, MOISTENS AND SOOTHES THE SKIN, PROMOTES TISSUE REPAIR

    skin damp heat with boils, furuncles
    BURNS, dermatitis, pimples

Balm of Gilead: Class 10

>SKIN CONDITIONS with dryness, irritation, itchiness; eczema, dermatosis, dermatitis, psoriasis, dry scaling skin, chaps, hemorrhoids
>CUTS, bruises, sprains
>MUSCULAR ACHES & SORENESS

3   DREDGES AND SOOTHES THE KIDNEYS, PROMOTES CLEANSING AND URINATION

kidney Qi stagnation & general toxemia with gout, rheumatism, scurvy
HIGH BLOOD CHOLESTEROL & uric acid

Preparation

USE: The Balsam poplar, or Tacamahac poplar, is the main source of this remedy. However, it is possible to substitute the buds or bark of the Black poplar *(Populus nigra),* and the Cottonwood tree *(P. candicans):* these will certainly cover its main functions. The Black poplar was much used in European pharmacy until the ninteenth century; a SALVE for hemorrhoids might be still available as a last relic of its extensive past use.

The full spectrum of uses is only obtained by the **buds**, while the **outer bark** may be used for its *restoring, moistening and soothing* qualities described in function 1. Ideal preparations are the short DECOCTION, the TINCTURE or FLUID EXTRACT, and the OLEORESIN itself with which the buds are impregnated, known as *Tacamahac,* a Native American appellation. It is possible to extract this oneself, but is hardly worth the trouble. Excellent OINTMENTS and CREAMS, and OILS for LINIMENTS, may be prepared from the **buds** or its **resin**, all for their *lenifying and pain-relieving* effects.

In **bronchial** troubles with any dryness or tough, viscous phlegm with difficult or tickling coughs, the steam INHALATION works admirably; according to Ojibwa Indian practice, so does the SALVE pasted into the nose. A SYRUP might also be tried for these symptoms.

The **buds** of the Balsam poplar should be used if diuertic *cleansing* effects are required in **chronic rheumatic** and such like complaints.

DOSAGE: Short DECOCTION: 1 or 2 tbsp as required, or three times daily.
TINCTURE: 2 tsp or 10 ml

Notes

Balm of Gilead stood in good repute as an external remedy among Native Americans and early settlers, and in Europe already finds a mention by NICOLAS MONARDES in his descriptions of American botanicals of 1577. Its resins, essential oil, benzoic acid and populin all contrive to create a cool *emollient, lenitive, anodyne* botanical used mainly in **dry**, **irritative** and vaguely **painful** conditions of the **skin** and **muscles**. Similar results are achieved internally when Balm of Gilead is brought into contact with **dry** and **inflammatory** conditions involving the **respiratory** and **gastric mucosa**, such as is found with lung, stomach or intestinal dryness. Dry, unproductive tight coughs are especially relieved, in this context.

In outright acute infections, however, Balm of Gilead should be combined with *cold disinfectant* botanicals from Class 4 (if the chest is affected) or Class 13 (in the case of the intestines). Its mild *cleansing effects* through the kidneys is an added asset whenever it is used.

CLASS 11

Herbs to Cause Astriction, Dry Mucous Damp, Arrest Discharge and Stop Bleeding

The purpose of botanicals in this class is to cause an astriction, tightening or shrinking of tissue for the treatment of **mucous damp** conditions. They tighten muscle and connective tissue as well as soft tissue such as mucosa and skin. Causing astriction is a Restoring type of treatment since it results in local and overall restorative effects.

Mucous damp conditions are catarrhal conditions involving excessive mucus secretion. In all traditional medical systems mucus accumulation is considered undesirable. It is called *phlegma* in Greek, *tan yin* (mucous fluid) and *tan shi* (mucous damp) in Chinese and *ama* in Ayurvedic medicine. The origins of these conditions can be as varied as the symptoms they give rise to and include old age, chronic illness, excessive purging treatment and predisposing constitutional factors. Typically, a weak mucous membrane is found in the context of deficient, run-down conditions such as deficient Spleen Qi or Spleen Yang, and will produce intestinal damp cold with irregular mucoid stools, abdominal gurgling, etc., or genitourinary damp cold with white leucorrhea. These on turn may lay the ground for infectious damp heat conditions. In the head, chest or digestive tract accumulated mucus becomes thicker and more viscous, causing stagnation and congestion.

Treating mucous damp has two aspects: first, ridding the body of any mucus that has accumulated by expelling it upward or downward with *eliminating* herbs; secondly, resolving it to prevent its reoccurence.[1]

Removing stagnant mucus is a matter of eliminating a substantial excess. Since the mucosa is found from the head to the colon, loosening and eliminating mucus requires different tactics and remedies, depending on where it is found. When non-infectious, or with mild or chronic infections, it is a damp cold condition, as in genitourinary cold, intestines damp cold and head damp cold. In these conditions, mucosal tissue looses its normal tone and oversecretes. When mucus stagnates in the lungs it is called phlegm and is eliminated by stimulating the coughing reflex with Class 4 *expectorants*. When overproductive in the gut, it is treated with *astringents* from this class according to the guidelines set out below and in Class 19. Over many years mucus also tends to congeal and adhere to the walls of the colon, forming the dark viscous lumps and strings sometimes eliminated in colonic therapy. This chronic type should be eliminated not only with the help of colonics, but also with the judicious use of Class 3 *laxative* herbs (both *bulk* and *stimulant laxatives*), as well as with suitable essential oils.

Preventing excessive mucus from being generated is the more fundamental and difficult task, requiring treatment of the ground of the whole individual and using *restoring* rather than *eliminant* herbs. Specifically, the tone of the mucous membrane must be restored if chronic oversecretion is to be ameliorated. Botanicals able to do this are *tonic astringents,* or *anticatarrhal* remedies, which actually resolve mucus and dry damp. It is in this sense that causing astriction is a Restoring rather than an Eliminating method of treatment.

Here as elsewhere it is important to support local treatment by rebalancing whatever global pattern of disharmony presents. Damp cold catarrhal conditions due to a "weeping" mucosa are

The Energetics of Western Herbs

usually found with excess conditions such as Yin excess, and blood congestion, or with deficient conditions such as Qi deficiency and Yang deficiency.

Astriction is also the method of choice when blood return is sluggish causing **venous blood stagnation** with internal varicosis, hemorrhoids, copious periods, etc., for which Class 14 *decongestant astringents* are used; when there is a **Qi** or **Yin deficiency** entailing fluid spillage, such as diarrhea and excessive sweating, for which Class 7 and 10 *restoratives* and the present class's *tonic astringents* should be adopted; when there is passive or active **bleeding**, for which the *hemostatic* remedies of this class are used; when there is premature or involuntary **seminal discharge**, and when there is **soft tissue inflammation**, **infection** or **swelling**, for which *astringents* from this class and from Class 13 are used; and when a **deficiency** of **central Qi** causes intestinal, rectal or uterine prolapse.

Botanicals that cause astriction do so by virtue of their high tannin, tannic acid or gallic acid content, which causes an *astringent* taste. Some also possess a *sour* taste, a second sensory proof of their ability to astrict and shrink. Their *restoring* effect is directed both to **chronic** deficient conditions with mucous damp, where they treat the underlying tissue state, and to **acute** discharges and hemorrhage, where they deal with the immediate situation. Moreover they are useful for inflammation of the skin or mucosa in the mouth, throat, lungs and digestive tract: here they are used to prepare mouthwashes, gargles, douches and enemas in addition to their internal use.

Astringents vary a great deal not only in strength, but also in the focus of their work. Some, like Bilberry, Purple loosestrife, Walnut, Tormentil and Geranium, work best with **chronic diarrhea** (both simple and infectious); while others such as Eyebright, Thyme, Elder and Pleurisy root are more suited to upper respiratory discharges with **head damp cold** ("cold phlegmatic fluids in the brain," according to Galenic theory). Some such as Sage, Cypress and Cranesbill, can stop excessive perspiration specifically *(anhydrotics),* while others, like Grapevine, Chasteberry, Yarrow and Tormentil, arrest urogenital discharges (including seminal emission). Others, called *hemostatics* (or *styptics* when used externally), specialize in putting an end to *bleeding* through capillary shrinkage in one area or another; among these are Ribwort plantain, Shepherd's purse, Lady's mantle and Nettle. Some *hemostatics* are also *coagulant* in that they speed up blood clotting and hence the termination of bleeding.

There are two further types of *astringent* herbs which paradoxically are used for Draining, not Restoring, purposes. The first type is the *astringent venous tonic* from Class 14 which homes in on the venous circulation, enlivening the blood and relieving blood stagnation by toning the veins: Yarrow, Horse chestnut, Red root and Cypress belong to this group, found mainly in Class 14.

The second type is the *astringent bitter cold antiseptic* of Class 13 employed for restraining infection and resolving inflammation on both external and internal skin surfaces, e.g. in damp heat conditions such as acute intestinal or urogenital infections.

Concerning the tissue mechanics of *astringents,* two distinct actions can be distinguished. The first is that of the *tonic astringent,* which tightens up mucus membrane cells, thereby preventing excessive mucus production. The second is that of the *dry astringent* which simply curdles the mucus proteins and so stops discharge.

The first type of *astringent* clearly merits the title of a *tonic,* in this case a *mucosal tonic:* by toning the mucus producing cells themselves it effectively *resolves mucus,* thereby drying damp. The *tonic astringent,* such as Yarrow, Elder flower, Tansy, Goldenseal, Ribwort, Thyme and Eyebright, has also been called *anticatarrhal* for this reason. The *dry astringent,* on the other hand, simply dries damp without any deeper toning. It rightfully belongs to the symptom treatment herb classes and is only discussed here alongside the *tonics* for practical reasons.

Unless used for mild conditions, or externally, or with hemorrhage or other discharge, remedies from this class are most frequently combined with *astringent cold herbs* from Class 13 to clear infections and *bland moist* herbs from Class 10 to soothe and relax.

A summary listing of all herbs in this class is found on p. 699.

Notes

1   In traditional Greek medicine all excess mucus was called phlegm *(phlegmon);* it is one of the four fluids that can cause injury (see appendix A). It arises from a combination of the *damp* and *cold* effective qualities *(dynameis)*. It was recognized that a phlegm injury, no matter where the phlegm was actually detected, formed a certain pattern of disharmony with typical symptoms of retention or excretion. It was usually treated by drawing it to the intestines or the stomach, "preparing" it by softening it, and then evacuating it through bowel movement or vomiting—a procedure still favored by Greek and Ayurvedic medical practice today.

TORMENTIL

Pharmaceutical name: rhizoma Potentillae
Botanical name: Potentilla erecta Raeuschel (syn.
    Potentilla tormentilla Necker), *vel*
    Potentilla anserina L., (N.O. Rosaceae)
Ancient names: Heptaphullon, Chrysogonon (Gr)
    Tormentilla, Septifolium (Lat)
Other names: a) Setfoil, Seven leaves, Shepherd's
        knot, Blood root, Ewe daisy, Biscuit
        (Eng)
    Blutwurz, Ruhrwurz, Siebenfünffingerkraut,
        Abbiss, Retterwurzel, Birkwurz,
        Gewaltskraut, Heydecker (Ge)
    b) Cinquefoil, Silverweed/feather, Goose
        tansy, Wild agrimony, Marsh corn, Moss
        crops, Crampwort (Eng)
    Argentine, Cameroche (Fr)
    Gänsefingerkraut, Krampfkraut, Gänserich (Ge)
Part used: the rhizome

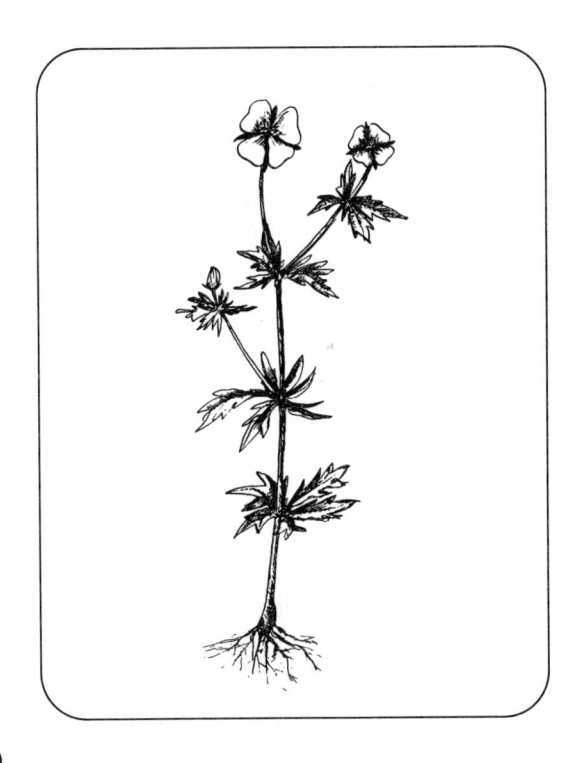

Nature

CATEGORY: mild herb with minimal chronic toxicity
CONSTITUENTS: catechin tannins 17-25%, tormentoside yielding termantinic acid & glucose, catechindimers, glycoside, organic acids, resin, gum, ess. oil, calcium oxalate
EFFECTIVE QUALITIES
Primary: *Taste:* astringent, a bit sweet & bitter
        Warmth: cool
        Moisture: dry
Secondary: astringing, restoring, solidifying
        stabilizing movement

Tormentil: Class 11

TROPISM

Organs or parts: stomach, intestines, skin, blood
Organisms: Fluid
Meridians: Spleen, Heart
Tri Dosas: decreases Kapha & Pitta

GROUND

All krases, biotypes and constitutions

Functions and Uses

1. CREATES ASTRICTION: DRIES MUCOUS DAMP, STAUNCHES BLEEDING AND ARRESTS DISCHARGE; RAISES CENTRAL QI

    HEMORRHAGE from lungs, uterus, bleeding from mouth or nose, or from wounds
    CHRONIC DIARRHEA in damp heat & damp cold conditions, esp. with alternating diarrhea & constipation; dysentery
    CHRONIC LEUCORRHEA in damp heat/cold conditions
    URINARY INCONTINANCE, seminal and urethral discharge
    HEMORRHOIDS
    MENORRAGIA, METRORRHPIA
    PROLAPSE of uterus or bowels due to *central Qi sinking*

2. RESTRAINS INFECTION AND CLEARS TOXINS; ANTIDOTES POISON, RELIEVES PAIN, PROMOTES TISSUE REPAIR AND BENEFITS THE SKIN

    PREVENTIVE in epidemics
    MOUTH, THROAT, GUM & tonsil infections, loose, spongy or bleeding gums (stematitis, gingivitis, etc.)
    EYE INFLAMMATION, sore eyes
    BURNS, sunburn
    WOUNDS, CUTS, abrasions, atonic ulcers, running sores, poison oak, skin eruptions
    skin damp heat: boils, inflammations, dermatoses
    SKIN ERUPTIONS, DRY or WEEPING (dermatoses)
    SEPTICEMIA, venereal infections
    POISONING from food or herb
    HEADACHE
    JOINT RHEUMATISM, GOUT, DIABETES, URINARY STONES

3. RESTORES THE *SPLEEN*/INTESTINES AND THE HEART

    Spleen Qi deficiency: poor appetite, loose stool, fatigue, indigestion
    Heart Qi deficiency: mental confusion, palpitations & shortness of breath worse on exertion

Preparation

USE: The DECOCTION is as efficient as the TINCTURE for all purpo-ses. Tormentil lends itself to the whole variety of external preparations: MOUTHWASHES, GARGLES and DOUCHES where the upper and lower mucous membrane is inflamed or infected; WASHES, LOTIONS, FOMENTATIONS, OINTMENTS where external surfaces are concerned. For internal conditions with **bleeding** or **discharge** it should be taken internally.

SILVERWEED, *Potentilla anserina,* is especially efficacious in the above conditions with **spasms** and **cramps.**

DOSAGE: standard doses throughout
CAUTION: In the unlikely case that Tormentil is used more than three weeks at a stretch, it should be discontinued for a week, due to its high tannin content.
NOTE: The three types of Five-finger grass, *Potentilla reptans seu canadensis seu grandiflora,* are all considered very inferior to the above two varieties of Potentilla.

Notes

Tormentil is another botanical which arrives to us laden with a history of *anti-infective* uses from the Middle Ages when epidemics were rife. Today, knowing that this is one of the most ideal tannin containing remedies for causing tissue astriction, Tormentil is used rather for localized **mucosal infections**. Containing condensed tannins rather than hydrolysable ones, it is absolutely safe and reliable. **Chronic infections** of the **digestive tract** with subacute or chronic **inflammation** is where it excels; its *antiseptic* and *anti-inflammatory* properties through lenifying and calming the intestines will bring both **damp heat** and **damp cold** conditions with discharges to an end, while relieving the attendant discomfort. Genital discharges and urinary incontinence are also helped.

Moreover, Tormentil has another reason for being preferred over other *astringents* with intestinal damp conditions: its *bitter sweet* taste makes for a *liver/stomach/Spleen tonic* which only enhances the functions of its astrictive properties. As an *astringent tonic,* therefore, Tormentil should be used for chronic constitutional Spleen Qi deficiency patterns with tendency to loose stool, flaccid tissues and fatigue, along the lines of acupuncture points Bl 20 & 38, Sp 3, St 36 and CV 12.

Scientifically speaking, this plant has more mysteries to reveal. The Dutch Renaissance botanist MATHIAS DE LOBEL (1570) reported that the French physician RONDELET from Lyons had in the previous century successfully used Tormentil for **rheumatoid arthritis**, a use that survives in European country areas even today. **Diabetes** is another traditional indication on purely empirical grounds, suggesting that at one time, and for thousands of years past, it must have been a very versatile, popular healing remedy indeed.

CRANESBILL

Pharmaceutical name: radix Geranii
Botanical name: Geranium maculatum L., seu robertianum L. (N.O.Geraniaceae)
Other names: a) Wild Geranium, Crowfoot, Chocolate flower, Wild alum root (Am)
b) Herb Robert, Bloodwort, Dragons blood (Eng)
Herbe Robert, Bec de grue, Aiguille du berger (Fr)
Ruprechtskraut, Rotlaufkraut, Kranich-schnabel (Ge)
Part used: the root

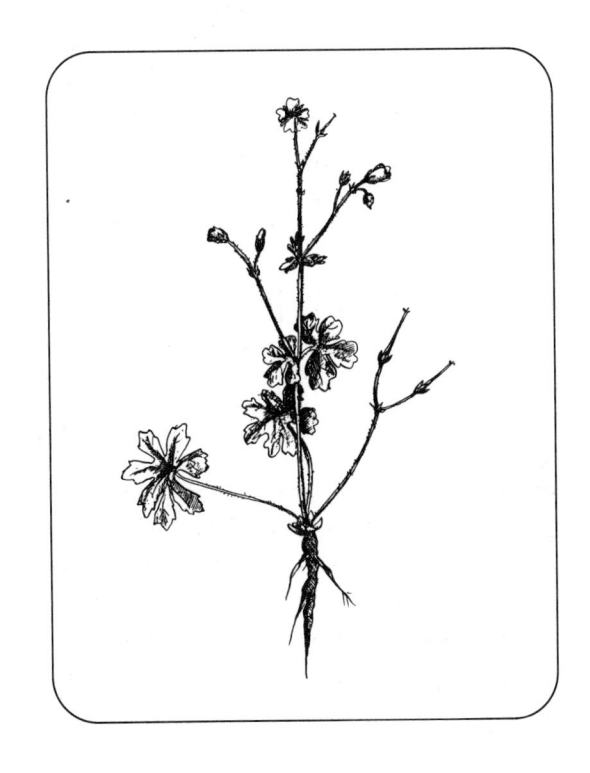

Cranesbill: Class 11

Nature

CATEGORY: mild herb with minimal chronic toxicity
CONSTITUENTS: tannins (10 to 25%) gallic acid, potassium sulfates, calcium, resin, pectin
EFFECTIVE QUALITIES
Primary: astringent, a bit sweet, cool, dry
Secondary: astringing, restoring, solidifying stabilizing movement
TROPISM: stomach, intestines, urogenital organs, kidneys
        Fluid organism
        Small Intestine, Colon meridians

Functions and Uses

1. **CREATES ASTRICTION, RESOLVES MUCUS AND DRIES DAMP; ARRESTS DISCHARGE AND STAUNCHES BLEEDING**
   intestines damp cold with loose mucousy stools, chronic diarrhea, constant need to pass stool
   SUBACUTE or CHRONIC ENTERITIS, dysentery, cholera
   genitourinary damp cold with thin white leucorrhea
   MUCOUS CYSTITIS, urethritis
   PASSIVE HEMORRHAGE from nose, mouth, internal organs, copious menses (menorhagia) or intermenstrual uterine bleeding (metrorrhagia), blood in urine
   HEMORRHOIDS

2. **RESTRAINS SECRETIONS, LOWERS ACIDITY AND RELIEVES PAIN**
   GASTRIC ULCERS due to hyperacidity
   INDOLENT ULCERS of mouth, bladder, intestines
   EXCESSIVE BREAST MILK
   EXCESSIVE PERSPIRATION during day or night

3. **PROMOTES URINATION**
   kidney fire with obstructed urination, kidney pain, diarrhea
   BRIGHT's DISEASE

Preparation

USE: The TINCTURE and FLUID EXTRACT are the most useful forms, unless a DECOCTION of Cranesbill **root** or an INFUSION of Herb Robert **herb** is prepared.
ENEMAS are used for **bleeding hemorrhoids**.
DOSAGE: Up to three times normal doses may be used in severe cases. Use with care if there is a tendency to constipation.
NOTE: Herb Robert is another Cranesbill type common in Europe, and one out of many in the Geranium family. Along with most other Cranesbills such as Common dovesfoot, it may be used interchageably with the American Cranesbill.

Notes

    Cranesbill is a reliable, average strength *astringent* remedy with a long history of Native American use behind it. Although having some *cooling* effects in acute damp heat inflammatory conditions, it is nevertheless more suited to **chronic infections** of the **mucosa**. Its best application is with chronically lingering cases of **damp cold** with non suppurative **discharges** of the **urogenital** or **digestive** organs, especially those involving gastric acidity, ulcers or hemorrhoids. It treats simple damp cold type diarrhea, for example, in much the same way that, say, acupuncture points Sp 4 & 9, CV 9, St 25 and Bl 20 treat it.

Interestingly, both Cranesbill and Herb Robert are additionally used in much the same way that *Wu bei zi, Galla Rhi chinensi* is used: namely to stop excessive sweating and passive bleeding in deficiency conditions.

OAK BARK

Pharmaceutical name: cortex Querci
Botanical name: Quercus alba et spp. L. (N.O. Cupuliferae)
Other names: Chêne (Fr)
    Eiche, Eichenrinde (Ge)
Part used: the bark

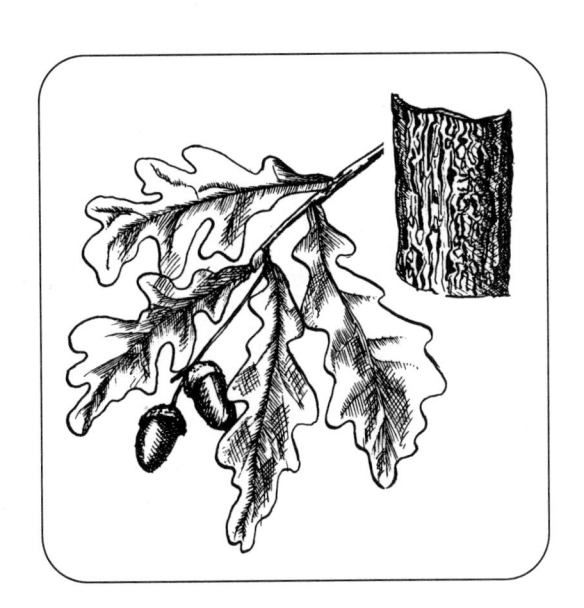

Nature

CATEGORY: mild herb with minimal chronic toxicity
CONSTITUENTS: tannin 10-20%, quercin
EFFECTIVE QUALITIES
Primary: astringent, cool, dry
Secondary: astringing, restoring, solidifying
    stabilizing movement

This remedy is virtually identical in its nature, functions and uses to CRANESBILL, *radix Geranii, (p. 405) with the following differences:*

1   In addition to addressing **damp cold** conditions with "relaxed mucous membranes with profuse discharges" (ELLINGWOOD, 1898), as Cranesbill does, Oak bark is also used for **damp heat** conditions of the **digestive tract**, including acute infectious enteritis, dysentery, etc.

2   Oak bark is also particularly used for "profuse, exhausting night sweats" (ELLINGWOOD) found in **deficient Yin** conditions of all kinds.

3   Used externally, Oak bark preparations are applied to **skin ulcers, dry** and **weeping eczemas, eye inflammations** and **hemorrhoids**.

4   Oak bark does not treat kidney fire like Cranesbill.

DOSAGE: TINCTURE: 0.5-1.5 ml or 14-35 drops
        DECOCTION: 1-2 tsp per 1/2 l (or pint) of water

Geranium: Class 11

GERANIUM

Pharmaceutical name: herba Pelargonii
Botanical name: Pelargonium odorantissimum
  Soland, seu roseum L'Her (N.O.
  Geraniaceae)
Ancient names: Geranion (Gr)
Other names: Sweet/Rose/Nutmeg scented
  geranium (Eng)
  Géranium (Fr)
  Geranie (Ge)
Part used: the herb

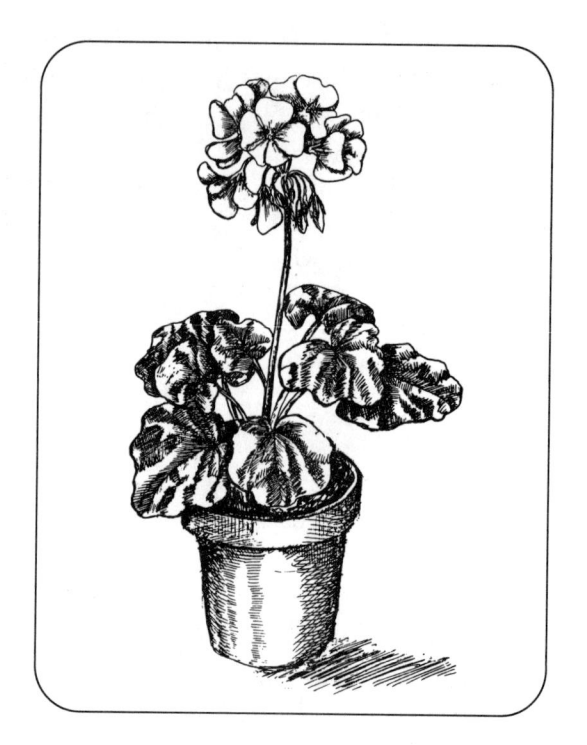

Nature

CATEGORY: mild herb with minimal chronic toxicity
CONSTITUENTS: ess. oil (incl. geraniol, citronellol, linalol, terpineol, phenylethylic alcohol), tannins, resin
EFFECTIVE QUALITIES
Primary: astringent, a bit sweet & pungent & bitter, warm with cooling potential, dry & moist
Secondary: astringing, restoring, stimulating, decongesting, softening
  stabilizing movement
TROPISM: stomach, intestines, urogenital organs, liver, kidneys, adrenals, gonads
  Fluid, Warmth organisms
  Spleen, Liver, Kidney, Chong & Ren meridians
GROUND: Phlegmatic, Melancholic & Sanguine krases
  Self-Reliant/Yang Ming Metal, Burdened/Shao Yin, & Charming/Yang Ming Earth
    biotypes
  all three constitutions

Functions and Uses

1. CREATES ASTRICTION, DRIES MUCOUS DAMP AND ARRESTS DISCHARGE; RESTRAINS SECRETIONS AND STAUNCHES BLEEDING, RESTRAINS INFECTION, REDUCES INFLAMMATION AND CLEARS TOXINS

    intestines damp cold: loose stool, chronic diarrhea, no appetite
    genitourinary damp cold: white leucorrhea
    MUCOUS CYSTITIS
    PASSIVE HEMORRHAGE: from nose, mouth, internal organs; menorrhigia, metrorrhagia
    EXCESSIVE BREAST MILK, congested breasts
    EXCESSIVE SWEATING during day or night
    INTESTINAL INFECTIONS at subacute or chronic stage, incl. enteritis, typhus, cholera

Class 11: Geranium

INFLAMMATIONS of mouth, throat, eye & breast
lung Yin deficiency: lung TB with night sweats stomach fire: great appetite and thirst, heartburn

2 **PROMOTES TISSUE REPAIR, RESOLVES CONTUSION AND RELIEVES PAIN; DISSIPATES TUMORS, BENEFITS AND MOISTENS THE SKIN**
CHRONIC WOUNDS, ulcers, abscesses, boils, burns
INTERNAL RUPTURES and injuries
PEPTIC ULCER,
CANCEROUS tumors, incl. stomach cancer
PAIN in the face, in lumbar region
DRY SKIN conditions, incl. rashes, eczema, herpes, ringworm, shingles, scurf
PARASITIC skin conditions, lice
INSECT REPELLANT

3 **RESTORES THE INTESTINES/*SPLEEN*, PANCREAS, ADRENALS AND GONADS; PROMOTES ESTROGEN, LIFTS THE SPIRIT AND RIDS DEPRESSION**
Spleen Qi deficiency: diarrhea, abdominal pain, fatigue
GASTROENTERITIS
DIABETES (supportive)
ADRENAL INSUFFICIENCY with weakness, fatigue, depression
ESTROGEN INSUFFICIENCY with liver blood deficiency or uterus blood deficiency with dry skin, hair or nails, delayed, scanty or absent emnses
MENOPAUSAL SYNDROME, STERILITY

4 **CLEARS STASIS, SEEPS WATER, PROMOTES URINATION AND SOFTENS STONES**
liver Qi stagnation: right flank soreness, jaundice
kidney Qi stagnation: malaise, skin rashes, mucous cystitis,
liver fluid congestion: local or general water retention
URINARY STONE or sand

Preparation

USE: This Geranium type is only generally available in ESSENTIAL OIL form, which is extracted from the whole plant. Both internal and external uses are appropriate. Externally, the sweet, fragrant oil may be MASSAGED into the skin with a base oil, or a 2% water dilution made for SWABS, WASHES, COMPRESSES, GARGLES and the like. DOUCHES and ENEMAS are suitable for **gynecological** and **intestinal** conditions.

A long INFUSION using the fresh or dried herb also goes a long way to fulfilling the above applications. A TINCTURE may be made from the fresh plant for greater *astringent* effects.
DOSAGE: ESSENTIAL OIL: 2-4 drops three times a day in a little warm water
Others: standard doses
CAUTION: Avoid using Geranium for acute infections of any kind, i.e. with damp heat with discharges.

Notes

The warming, delicate, rose scented Geranium is an unusual *astringent* remedy for several reasons. First, it is an essential oil, relying not on tannin mediated topical astrictive effects on skin

Eyebright: Class 11

cells, but probably on its action on nerve endings behind the cells. As a result, when treating essentially **damp cold** conditions with discharges such as diarrhea and leucorrhea, Geranium has the distinct advantage of not drying out the tissues while performing its astriction. Its *astringency* is stronger than that of Witch hazel or Purple loosestrife, but less strong than Oak bark or Walnut leaf.

Secondly, while doing virtually everything that is required of any good *astringent,* it also restores Spleen Qi with its fragrant and somewhat *sweet, pungent* and *bitter taste* qualities. As a *restorative* herb Geranium is a useful adjunct for Qi deficiency conditions with adrenal deficiency causing symptoms such as depression, exhaustion, excessive daytime sweating, etc., and will also replenish pancreatic or gonadal insufficiency with their ensuing symptoms. In addition, its *stimulant* edge mobilizes stagnant fluids through liver, adrenal and kidney activation.

Thirdly, Geranium evinces *demulcent* qualities as well as *astringent* ones, topically soothing and calming while gently *restoring*. Its *sweet moist* taste qualities guarantee a protective effect on fluid surfaces internally and a moisturizing effect on the skin externally—clearly ideal complements to its primary action—whence its application for all **dry skin** conditions, simple, eruptive or infectious. Geranium in fact will *regulate* skin conditions and, therefore, as and important cosmetic agent is applicable to all skin types. Where **internal dry conditions** are generated by hormonal imbalance, resulting in syndromes such as liver blood deficiency and uterus blood deficiency, Geranium through its *estrogenic and demulcent* effects combined, will also provide moisture, lenify irritation and gloss dryness. Here also, Geranium is clearly a woman's friend.

EYEBRIGHT

Phaeutical name: herba Euphrasiae
Botanical name: Euphrasia rostkoviana Hayne,
    vel spp. (N.O. Scrophulariaceae)
Ancient name: Frasia, Luminella, Ambrosia,
    Eufragia (Lat)
Other Name: Euphrasy, Adhib, Ewfras (Eng)
    Euphraise, Brise-lunettes (Fr)
    Augstenzieger, Wiesenaugentrost, Schabab,
    Hirnkraut, Weisses Ruhrkraut, Zwang-
    kraut (Ge)
Part used: the whole herb

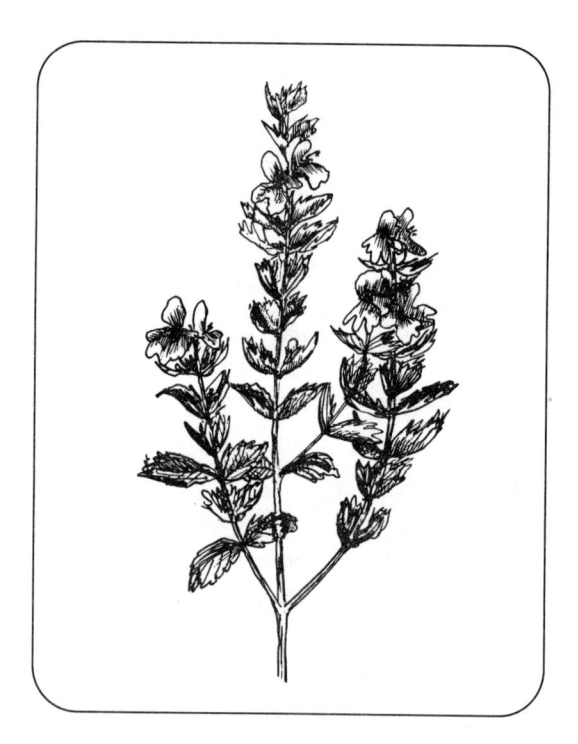

Nature

CATEGORY: mild herb with minimal chronic toxicity
CONSTITUENTS: resins, tannins, ess. oil, glycosides (incl. aucubin, aneobin, rhynanthin), bitter, trace elements, euphrastanic acid
EFFECTIVE QUALITIES
Primary: a bit astringent & pungent & bitter, cool, dry
Secondary: astringing, restoring, decongesting, dissolving

Class 11: Eyebright

TROPISM: eyes, lungs, stomach, intestines, kidneys
            Fluid organism
            Lung, Spleen, Colon meridians
GROUND: all krases, biotypes and constitutions

Functions and Uses

1. **CREATES ASTRICTION, RESOLVES MUCUS, DRIES DAMP AND ARRESTS DISCHARGE; REDUCES INFLAMMATION, RESTRAINS INFECTION AND CLEARS THE HEAD**

    head damp cold & lung wind cold: headache, earache, stuffed sinuses, watery nasal discharge, general aches and pains, chills, possible slight fever
    CORYZA, RHINORRHEA, FLU, HAYFEVER
    EAR, NOSE and THROAT INFECTIONS and CATARRH with profuse watery discharge, with or without acute inflammation.
    intestines damp cold: indigestion, loose stool
    CHRONIC GASTROENTERITIS
    EYE INFECTIONS with red, swollen, stinging or burning eyes & eyelids, thin watery or thick yellow discharge
    STYES, conjunctivitis, blepharitis, keratitis, iritis
    LEUCORRHEA

2. **RESTORES AND STRENGTHENS THE EYES; CLEARS THE EYES AND ENHANCES VISION**

    POOR or FAULTY EYESIGHT due to strain of close work, reading, etc.
    MUCOUS FILM, CLOUD or DUST in eyes; bloodshot eyes; glaucoma, corneal macula

3. **DREDGES THE KIDNEYS, SOFTENS STONES AND HARMONIZES URINATION; ANTIDOTES POISON**

    kidney Qi stagnation: tiredness, headaches, pus in urine, painful urination
    URINARY STONES or sand
    BLADDER IRRITATION in general
    ALCOHOL & NICOTINE autotoxicosis

4. **STRENGTHENS THE *SPLEEN*/INTESTINES; INDUCES REST**

    Spleen Qi deficiency: poor appetite, tiredness, swollen painful abdomen, diarrhea
    UNREST, nervous headaches, insomnia

Preparation

USE: Eyebright is meant for internal as well as external use, and the INFUSION and TINCTURE are equally good. In many if not most cases that profit from its use, internal and external treatment will go hand in hand. LOTIONS, EYEWASHES, cotton wool SWABS and DOUCHES are the main external applications.

DOSAGE: standard doses throughout
For an EYEBATH, infuse (some say shortly decoct) 1.5 g, or about 1/2 tsp, in 50 ml (or 1 cup) of water for 10 minutes, and strain. Refrigerate the liquid in an airtight (and if possible sterilized) container. Use over two days, no more.

Turpentine: Class 11

Notes

With its pretty eye-like flowers Eyebright is a plant that is the sheer delight of those addicted to the doctrine of signatures. True enough, Eyebright is perhaps the most specific eye remedy known, dealing beneficially with every conceivable condition that may beset those very delicate organs. The neoplatonic radical ARNALD DE VILLANOVA in the early 1300's wrote a good booklet on this *Luminella,* and eminent natural physicians from BOCK, FUCHS, HALLER, HOFFMAN through to KING and FELTER have recorded their successes with it. Even the medic WOODVILLE in the nineteenth century epitomized it as the *verum oculorum solamen* in the style of the twelfth century Schola Salernita poem! However, Eyebright is not intrinsically superior to any other efficient remedy; it just seems like a miracle producer when relieving eye conditions that are exquisitely painful.

Eyebright not only restores poor vision (possibly through its renal/urinary *cleansing* action, but let us not be reductionist), but also removes surface matter from the eyes. In inflammations or infections it *cools* and *dries,* gently *astringing* and *disinfecting,* while resolving catarrh and exudate—and makes more expensive herbs like Goldenseal quite superfluous. BOCK (1532), ever the ardent spokesman for common garden plants, recommends combining it with crushed Fennel seeds and Vervain herb in all catarrhal eye conditions; nor can this simple formula be improved upon for eye inflammations today.

There is another application for this herb, popular in traditional wise woman medicine right up to the present day: as a *tonic astringent* or *mucosal restorer* of the upper respiratory tract in particular. As such, it is effective for **catarrhal head colds** with **wind cold** type aches and pains, chills, thin watery discharges from nose and eyes, and complete misery. (It has a reputation for some *sedative* effects as well). Hayfever, coryza and bronchitis qualify as Western entities in this context. Its effect in the intestinal tract is similar, resolving what is essentially **damp cold**. Here its bitter component, in promoting digestion and boosting forces via Spleen Qi, is ideal in chronic deficiency conditions of this type.

TURPENTINE

Pharmaceutical name: oleum Terebinthinae rectificatae, seu oleum aethereum Terebinthinae
Botanical name: Pinus spp. *vel Abies* spp. (N.O. Coniferae)
Ancient names: Terminthon (Gr)
Other names: Térébenthine (Fr)
 Terpentin (Ge)
Part used: the turpentine or essential oil from the pitch

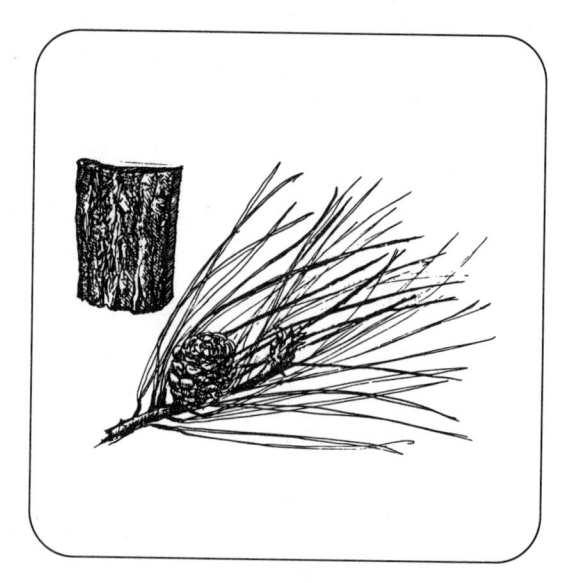

Nature

CATEGORY: medium-strength herb with slight chronic toxicity
CONSTITUENTS: ess. oil 15-32%, resin 70-85% (incl. resinic [diterpenic] acids 65%), bitters

EFFECTIVE QUALITIES
Primary: astringent & pungent & bitter, warm with cooling potential, moist & dry
Secondary: astringing, restoring, stimulating, decongesting, dissolving
TROPISM: upper & lower respiratory organs, stomach, intestines, urogenital organs, kidneys
  Fluid, Warmth organisms
  Lung, Spleen, Colon meridians
GROUND: Melancholic & Phlegmatic krases
  Sensitive/Tai Yin Metal, Dependant/Tai Yin Earth, & Self-Reliant/Yang Ming Metal biotypes
  Lymphatic/Carbonic/Blue Iris & Mixed/Phosphoric/Grey-Green Iris

Functions and Uses

1 CREATES ASTRICTION, RESOLVES MUCUS AND DRIES DAMP; ARRESTS DISCHARGE AND BLEEDING AND LENIFIES IRRITATION

   head damp cold with acute or chronic nasal catarrh
   lung phlegm damp with coughing up white phlegm
   CHRONIC BRONCHITIS
   intestines mucous damp (Spleen damp) with gurgling abdomen, flatus, heaviness
   INTESTINAL FERMENTATION
   genitourinary damp cold with white discharges
   PASSIVE HEMORRHAGE from intestines (incl. ulcers), lungs, uterus (incl. postpartum), esp. in deficient & cold conditions

2 WARMS AND INVIGORATES THE STOMACH/*SPLEEN* AND INTESTINES, REMOVES STAGNANCY, ABATES DISTENSION AND PROMOTES BOWEL MOVEMENT

   stomach & intestines cold with Qi stagnation with epigastric pain & swelling, chronic constipation

3 DREDGES THE KIDNEYS, PROMOTES URINATION AND EXPELS STONES

   kidney Qi stagnation with skin rashes, cystitis, dribbling urination
   URINARY STONES and gallstones, esp. with pain

4 CLEARS HEAT, REDUCES INFLAMMATION AND FEVER AND RELIEVES PAIN

   lung heat dryness with dry coughs, headache
   PLEURISY, PNEUMONIA, WHOOPING COUGH TB, CROUP (all types)
   intestines dry heat with constipation, thirst
   ACUTE FEVER, esp. in Shao Yin stage
   INFLAMMATION with CONGESTION of any type in deficient conditions
   RHEUMATISM, ARTHRITIS, NEURITIS with pain, swelling, heat
   EARACHE, deafness

5 RESTRAINS INFECTION, PROMOTES TISSUE REPAIR AND BENEFITS THE SKIN; CLEARS PARASITES, ANTIDOTES PHOSPHORUS

   ATONIC, INDOLENT WOUNDS, abscesses, ulcers, sores
   TYPHUS, TYPHOID FEVER
   INFECTIONS of lungs, intestines, bladder, kidneys & reproductive organs (esp. cystitis)
   SKIN ERUPTIONS dermatoses and dermatitis of all types incl. parasitic; skin blemishes

Turpentine: Class 11

INTESTINAL PARASITES, esp. tapeworm
ACCIDENTAL PHOSPHORUS INTAKE

Preparation

USE: Turpentine is extracted from the gummy pitch of a variety of Pine or Fir and sometimes Spruce or Larch trees all over the world; their uses are virtually identical for all practical purposes. Only the **rectified turpentine** or the ESSENTIAL OIL distilled thereof should be used, whether externally or internally.

PLASTERS, POULTICES, LINIMENTS and SALVES and the like are excellent for **injuries, infections** and **pain.** COMPRESSES and PLASTERS should be removed after about 1/2 hour and only applied once a day. Longer than that they produce **counter-irritation**—a treatment method in its own right for all painful conditions (see p.). In addition, INHALATIONS (for all lung and head conditions), DOUCHES, SQUATTING INHALATIONS, ENEMAS and SYRUPS are some other effective methods of using this versatile remedy.

DOSAGE: ESSENTIAL OIL: 6-10 drops in some warm water three or four times a day.
 RECTIFIED TURPENTINE: 10-20 drops (i.e. up to 1/4 tsp) in warm water or honey.
 Small doses are sufficient for function 2 above.

CAUTION: Turpentine is toxic in much larger doses, although rarely fatal; nevertheless, it should not be used continuously internally or externally. Exceptional individuals may be oversentitive to even therapeutic doses. Turpentine is contraindicated in kidney inflammation.

Notes

The fact of Turpentine's early and almost universal use for healing is shown, for example, in a recipe for a *balsam* set out by the woman physician and midwife TROTULA in her *De morbis mulierum* of 1059. This salve, which was both healing and cosmetic, consisted of "thrice distilled Turpentine, Wood aloes, Ambergris and Musk," and the author goes on to claim that it "preserves youth, heals all wounds, marvellously clears the eyes." This recipe incidentally goes to show, as do countless later still-room books, all penned by women in beautiful italic writing, that as far as the majority of healers in those days were concerned—namely women—there was no real division between beauty care and medecine: in all their extant writings, receipts for medicinal salves, juleps and diet drinks jostle those for cosmetic lotions, creams and the like.

However, Turpentine had to await the nineteenth century American Eclectic medical movement to receive full therapeutic analysis as a botanical medicine. Only then did it reveal itself a supremely effective, if rather paradoxical, remedy. In first place, it was recognized as a good *astringent* and *hemostatic,* with definite *anticatarrhal* effects on the mucosa. As such, Turpentine is a universal herb for **damp cold** conditions "especially if there be relaxed, enfeebled, atonic mucous membranes" (ELLINGWOOD, 1898). Secondly, it was discovered excellent for **dry heat** conditions (with inflammation, persistent fevers) "when the tongue is dry, glazed and dark red, the temperature persistently high, the pulse small, wiry, rapid and feeble . . . the urine scanty and dark." Here Eclectic physician FINLEY ELLINGWOOD accurately describes deficient Yin conditions in the best observational style of early nineteenth century French hospital medicine. This conclusion is reinforced by HARVEY FELTER (1922) two decades later when he writes that "it is always a remedy for atony and debility, never for active and plethoric conditions".

In short, Turpentine emerges as an *astringent tonic* for when the vital spirits (i.e. defense responses) are weakened, causing either a **catarrhal diathesis** (damp cold) or a **hot** one (empty heat). In either case its *antiseptic* and *antifermentative* properties, equal to those of Garlic, are clearly an asset, whether **gastrointestinal, urogenital** or **respiratory** disharmonies present. It is

Class 11: Walnut

unavoidably clear that Turpentine forces us to live with the paradox of a *stimulating, pungent warming* herb that is also used for deficiency heat and inflammatory conditions.

Turpentine should also be thought of as a **lung** remedy in a variety of syndromes (with **dryness, heat** and **phlegm damp** mainly), including tuberculosis. Again paradoxically, its *vulnerary* and *anodyne* effects complete the profile of a remedy as important in **acute situations** as it is in **chronic** ones.

WALNUT

Pharmaceutical name: folium seu cortex fructi Juglandis
Botanical name: Juglans regia L. (N.O. Juglandaceae)
Ancient names: Karya, Basilika (Gr)
    Nux persica/regia, Jovis glans (Lat)
Other names: Noix (Fr)
    Walnuss, Welschnuss, Steinnuss (Ge)
Part used: the leaf or the fruit rind

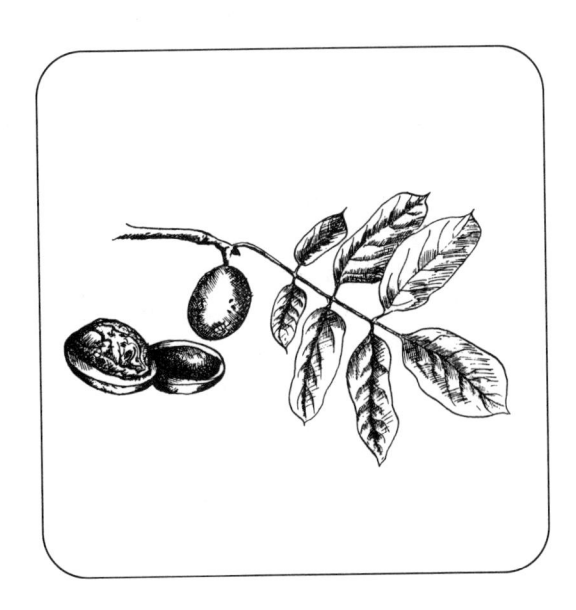

Nature

CATEGORY: mild herb with minimal chronic toxicity
CONSTITUENTS: flavonoids, tannins, bitter (juglone), ellagic, tannic & gallic acids, ess. oil, serotonin, protein, vitamins, trace minerals (incl. magnesium, iodine, copper, silicon, zinc), calcium, potassium, sulphur, sulphur iodide, calcium phosphate & oxalate, potassium & calcium chloride, magnesium phosphate, potassium sulphate, alkaloids, vit C
EFFECTIVE QUALITIES
Primary: astringent & bitter & pungent, a bit warm with cooling potential, dry
Secondary: astringing, solidifying, stimulating, dissolving stabilizing movement
TROPISM: stomach, intestines, pancreas, skin, veins, bones, nerves
    Warmth, Fluid organisms
    Spleen, Small Intestine meridians
GROUND: Phlegmatic & Melancholic krases
    Dependant/Tai Yin Earth, Self-Reliant/Yang Ming Metal, Sensitive/Tai Yin Metal & Burdened/Shao Yin biotypes
    Lymphatic/Carbonic/Blue Iris & Mixed/Phosphoric/Grey-Green Iris

Functions and Uses

1 CREATES ASTRICTION, RESTRAINS SECRETIONS AND DRIES MUCOUS DAMP; ARRESTS DISCHARGE, STAUNCHES BLEEDING AND RAISES CENTRAL QI

HEMORRHAGE in any part
intestines mucus/damp cold (Spleen damp) with splashing abdomen, loose mucousy stool
CHRONIC DIARRHEA, dysentery, mucous colitis
SPONTANEOUS SWEATING from palms & soles

Walnut: Class 11

central Qi sinking with uterine or intestinal prolapse
DIABETES (supportive)

2   WARMS AND INVIGORATES THE STOMACH/*SPLEEN* AND INTESTINES AND CREATES STRENGTH; MOVES STAGNANCY, PROMOTES BOWEL MOVEMENT AND EXPELS PARASITES

stomach & intestines cold (Spleen Yang deficiency) with diarrhea, no appetite, weakness, fatigue
ANEMIA, chronic fatigue
intestines Qi stagnation with abdominal distention & pain, constipation
INTESTINAL PARASITES, esp. tapeworm & ringworm

3   BENEFITS THE SKIN, HAIR AND BONE AND DISSIPATES TUMORS; REDUCES INFLAMMATION, RESTRAINS INFECTION AND PROMOTES TISSUE REPAIR

CHRONIC ECZEMA (dry or suppurative), dermatosis, pruritus, herpes, ringworm, dandruff, scrofulosis, lymph swelling, wrinkles
SYPHILIS, tuberculosis
VARICOSE VEINS
WEAK HAIR, hair loss
CARIES, bone degeneration or swelling
TUMORS benign & cancerous
CHRONIC INFLAMMATORY INFECTIONS of intestines & urogenital organs
MOUTH, GUM, THROAT & EYE INFLAMMATIONS
WOUNDS, ulcers, boils, abscesses, esp. the atonic cold type

Preparation

USE: A long INFUSION and the TINCTURE are used internally of either/both leaf and rind. Externally, BATHS, DOUCHES, WASHES, GARGLES and such are used with excellent results for the variety of conditions listed under function 3.

The **dried leaf** contains an essential oil, an alkaloid and a bitter substance in addition to tannins, minerals, etc.: it is more *warming* and *antispasmodic,* and better used for Spleen Yang deficiency and intestines Qi stagnation patterns, especially where weakness and discharge are present.

The **mature rind** contains trace minerals, malic, citric & oxalic acids, and hydrojuglone in addition to tannins, etc.: it is *cooling* and better applied to **inflammatory** conditions. Used in a hair rinse, the Walnut rind will darken hair as well as discourage hair loss.

DOSAGE: TINCTURE: 1-2 ml or 25-50 drops
              INFUSION: standard doses.

CAUTION: Avoid with tinnitus (ringing in the ears) present. If used internally over about ten days, alternate weekly with a complementry astringent remedy such as Geranium, Tormentil, Oak bark or Blackberry.

Notes

The Walnut tree has Asian origins, and has always been revered not only for cultish reasons, but also for the many practical uses that its wood, fruit, leaf and flower may be put to. Greeks and Romans especially estimated the products of this "imperial nut", and Walnut oil and meat were extensively used for both culinary and medicinal purposes.

As intense as the Walnut tree is in its very earthy, concentrated and enduring type of vitality (evident in its dense, hard wood, for example), so *strengthening* on the whole organism are its therapeutic effects. The meat of the nuts has always been considered highly nutritive, being full of minerals and trace minerals as it is, and was said to feed the **brain**, based on the suggestion or omen given by its appearance, including the hard shell. By the same token however, a similarity to the **intestines** is just as evident, and is actually more relevant from the therapeutic vantage point.

While sidestepping any need to endorse a doctrine of signatures at this point, it is worth considering for a moment that the mind does not create links of this kind gratuitously: the essentially spontaneous synmorphous nature of such associations should be recognized. Whether we go on to deduce natural laws from repeated observation of such things, as did many Renaissance scientists and physicians, is another matter entirely. In any case, when it comes to actual practice, noticing such links first hand is often very useful therapeutically and should not be rejected offhand on principle—any more than they should be accepted without reservation, without the screening of the rational mind, in fact.

Like Geranium, then, Walnut is an important warm *astringent tonic* with medium- strength astringency. Like a few others also it raises prolapsed conditions, stops excessive sweating and bleeding *(hemostatic* and *styptic),* in addition to relieving the more usual **catarrhal damp cold** conditions of the intestines, reproductive organs and skin. In addition, Walnut definitely increases peristalsis with a net *laxative* effect, and eliminates intestinal parasites besides.

The bitter substance found in Walnut leaves has *antifungal* properties and represent a useful adjunct to their *anti-inflammatory, antiseptic* and *detergent* actions on surface tissues such as skin and mucus membranes. Walnut's beneficial influence on a large range of **skin** disorders arouses the suspicion of internal *cleansing* effects, which in European folk healing has always been considered fact rather than surmise. We must leave this an open question at the present time. Certainly, Walnut is often combined with plants such as Hearstease in chronic skin eruptions, for example. Finally, Walnut's tropism for deficiency conditions of the **bone**, **nail** and **hair**, again due to its generous amounts of mineral and trace elements, must be considered outstanding.

Canadian fleabane: Class II

CANADIAN FLEABANE

Pharmaceutical name: herba Erigerontis
Botanical name: Erigeron canadensis L.
   (N.O.Compositae)
Other names: Horseweed, Butterweed, Coltstail,
   Prideweed, Scabious (Am)
   Vergerette du Canada (Fr)
   Kanadisches Berufskraut, Hexenbesen,
   Wilder Hanf (Ge)
Part used: the herb

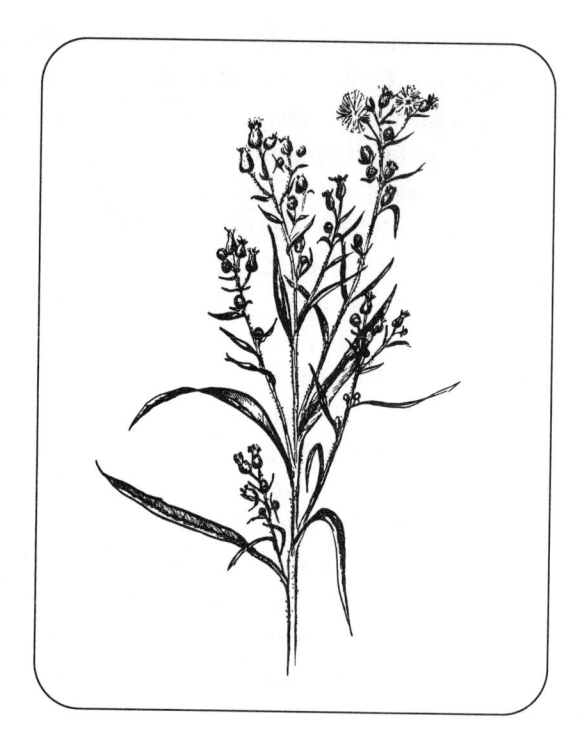

Nature

CATEGORY: mild herb with minimal chronic toxicity
CONSTITUENTS: bitter, tannic & gallic acids, ess. oil, flavones, choline
EFFECTIVE QUALITIES
Primary: a bit astringent & bitter & sour, cool, dry
Secondary: astringing, solidifying, simulating, relaxing
   stabilizing movement
TROPISM: lungs, kidneys, bladder, intestines, nerves
   Fluid, Air organisms
   Lung, Spleen, Kidney meridians
GROUND: all krases, biotypes and constitutions

Functions and Uses

1 CREATES ASTRICTION, DRIES MUCOUS DAMP, ARRESTS DISCHARGE AND STAUNCHES BLEEDING; RAISES CENTRAL QI
   PASSIVE BLEEDING from all internal parts; coughing or vomiting blood
   INTERMENSTRUAL BLEEDING, menorrhagia, postpartum hemorrhage
   CHRONIC INTESTINAL & GENITOURINARY DISCHARGES due to damp heat or cold,
      incl. diarrhea, enteritis, dysentery, children's cholera, chronic urethritis, cystitis, gonorrhea
   central Qi sinking with uterine, rectal or intestinal prolapse

2 PROMOTES CLEANSING AND RESOLVES TOXEMIA, DREDGES THE KIDNEYS, PROMOTES URINATION AND EXPELS STONES
   kidney Qi stagnation & general toxemia with cystitis, skin rashes, painful urination
   URIC ACID DIATHESIS with chronic arthritis, gout, rheumatism
   NEPHROSIS, chronic nephritis, albuminaria
   BLADDER STONES

Class 11: Canadian fleabane

3   STIMULATES THE LUNGS AND CIRCULATION, OPENS THE CHEST AND EXPELS PHLEGM

lung phlegm damp with coughing copious white phlegm, wheezing, cold extremities, fatigue
CHRONIC BRONCHITIS

4   RELAXES THE NERVE AND FREES SPASMS

Qi constraint with unrest, irritability, intestinal colic

Preparations

USE: The INFUSION and TINCTURE are used. DOUCHES & ENEMAS may be prepared for external use. If available, the ESSENTIAL OIL may be used alone internally or, alternatively and equally good, massaged topically with a base oil.
DOSAGE: INFUSION & TINCTURE: standard doses
                 ESSENTIAL OIL: 4-6 drop doses (not oftener than every hour in acute situations)
NOTE: There is a similar plant that was used interchangeably with Canadian fleabane up to the eigteenth and nineteenth centuries. This is FLEAWORT, *Pulicaria dysenterica* L. (N.O. Compositae), known as Kunuza in Greek, Conyza, Cunilago, Pulicaria, etc. in Latin; Fleabane or Cammock in English; Herbe des puces in French; and Dürrwurz, Hundsauge, Flohkraut and Ruhrkraut in German.

Notes

Both the various Fleabanes, of which the Canadian one is the most common type, and the European Fleawort *(Pulicaria dysenterica)* have the same uses. Nature's permutations of plants and therapeutic effects in this respect is uniquely playful. Whereas the same botanical will often find different uses on different continents, (e.g. Cleavers, Shepherd's purse, Raspberry), here we have an example of the exact inverse: two entirely different plants from different continents with identical uses. It proves that the natural forces which engender plant life care nothing for botanical classification, let alone accuracy: they will create similar and identical constituents, qualities and effects wherever and whenever they please. These **bioenergies,** being active and configurative and therefore **Yang** by nature, will latch on to any susceptible plant family or class—being structive, passive and **Yin—in** order to fulfill their creative fantasies through plant types. And this can occur anywhere on the planet. Humans merely join in the game unconsciously: they employ these different plants in exactly the same way, and even go as far as giving them similar names—in this case Fleabane and Fleawort.

Fleabane is not only a gentle *astringent,* but also a good *hemostatic* and *uterine decongestant,* in the vein of acupuncture points Sp 1, 8 & 10, Li 2 and St 29, when used in gynecology for **heavy periods** and **intermenstrual bleeding.** Hemorrhages as well as discharges of all kinds are controlled by its use, therefore. Where infection and inflammation are severe, however, more *antiseptic* and *cooling* remedies should be combined with it. With uterine bleeding, other *hemostatics* such as Shepherd's purse, Lady's mantle and Nettle spring to mind as suitable combinations.

Fleawort, on the other hand, was espoused by Italian natural physician PIERANDREA MATTIOLI (1611) as an important *urogenital restorer* and *stimulant,* not unlike Goldenrod. He advises it for chronic deficiency and **stasis** with **painful urination** and **stone formations** as well as for **menstrual retention.**

Both Fleabanes should find use at the present time, since they are mild *nerve relaxants* besides.

Sumac: Class 11

SUMAC

Pharmacological name: cortex radicis Rhudis
Botanical name: Rhus glabra L. (N.O. Anacardiaceae)
Ancient names: Rhous (Gr)
   Rhus, Coggyria (Lat)
Other names: Smooth/Mountain/Upland/Scarlet/ Sleek sumac (Am)
   Sumac, Pincentroyale (Fr)
   Sumach, Gerberbaum, Galgel (Ge)
Part used: the root bark

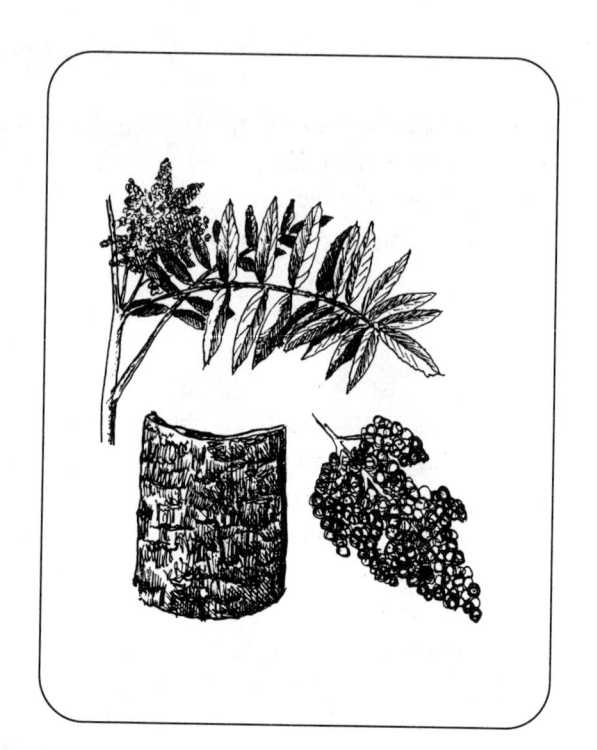

Nature

CATEGORY: mild herb with minimal chronic toxicity
CONSTITUENTS: gallotannic acid, calcium bimalate, fixed oil, resin, gum, starch
EFFECTIVE QUALITIES
Primary: a bit astringent & sour, cold, dry
Secondary: astringing, restoring
   stabilizing movement
TROPISM: urogenital organs, lungs, throat
   Fluid organism
   Kidney, Bladder, Lung meridians
GROUND: all krases, biotypes and constitutions

Functions and Uses

1 CREATES ASTRICTION, RESTRAINS SECRETIONS AND DRIES MUCOUS DAMP; ARRESTS DISCHARGE AND BLEEDING
   CATARRHAL DISCHARGES from lungs, genital organs in cold damp conditions
   DIARRHEA & NIGHT SWEATS in deficiency conditions
   PASSIVE HEMORRHAGE from uterus, lungs
   BLEEDING or spongy GUMS, sore throat, aphthous sores
   THROAT soreness, throat ulcers with fetid scretion
   TISSUE flabbiness or ulceration

2 RESTORES THE URINARY ORGANS, MODERATES AND REGULATES URINATION
   COPIOUS URINATION, BEDWETTING (enuresis) esp. in diabetes, & interstitial nephritis
   INCONTINENT or frequent scanty urination due to *genitourinary Qi deficiency*

Preparation

USE: Sumac requires the DECOCTION, TINCTURE or POWDER, whether the root bark, tree bark or berry is used. External uses include GARGLING, MOUTHWASHES, SWABS, etc., where a good *astringent* effect is required.

DOSAGE: TINCTURE: 1-4 ml or 25-100 drops
DECOCTION: 5-20 g
POWDER: 1-30 g

Notes

Sumac is another of many botanicals from the Native American repetoire, which was adopted into the U.S. pharmacopoeia during the last century. Specific and outstanding in its functions as an herb that causes astriction is its **moderating effect** on **urination.** This is underpinned by a *restoring* influence on the tone of the bladder and resultant greater urinary control. Sumac root bark is an excellent adjunct, as a result, not only to reinforce other remedies in this class in a variety of more acute conditions, but also to achieve specific urinary results in the treatment of **deficiency** syndromes such as Kidney Qi infirmity and Qi deficiency. It achieves the same as F*u pen zi, fructus Rubi,* and *Qian shi, semen Euryales,* in the same category of Chinese botanicals, or as acupuncture point formulation Sp 6, Bl 28, St 28 and CV 3.

The **berries** of the Purple sumac tree are more *sour cold* by quality than the bark and may be helpful in mild cases of damp heat in the bladder or intestines.

GENERAL INDEX

For medical and herbal terms see also the Glossary of Terms (p. 745)

Abu Hanifa, 41
adaptogenics, 233, 696
adrenal restoratives, 697
adrenocortical hormones inhibitors, 706
adrenocortical hormones stimulants, 706
adrenomedullary hormones inhibitors, 706
adrenomedullary hormones stimulants, 706
Agamede, 643
Agrimony, 522
Air organism, 425
Aktuarios, Ioannes, 19
Al-Abbas, ali ibn, 57
Al Israili, 496
Al Kindi, 24, 27
Alder buckthorn, 178
Alfalfa, 370
Alkmaion of Kroton, 24
Aloe gel, 317
Aloes, 180
Alpini, Prospero, 41
Altering, 101, 573
Amenorrhea, 210
American ginseng, 241
American mandrake, 166
American senna, 179
analeptics, 660
Analytical approach, 3, 5, 9, 23, 25, 32, 33, 63, 95
anesthetics, 711
Angelica, 275
anhydrotics, 402, 700
Animal remedies, 212, 579
Aniseed, 468
anodyne, 665-667, 710, 711
anthelmintics, 689, 713
anti-allergics, 701
Anti-arthritics, 709
anti-ascaris remedies, 713
antibacterials, 713
anticatarrhals, 401, 700
anticoagulants, 552, 553, 703
anticontusion remedies, 552, 712
antidepressants, 659, 660, 710
antidyskratics, 577, 666, 703
antifungals, 713
anti-infectives, 671, 672, 712

anti-inflammatories, 477, 480, 702
anti-oxyuris remedies, 713
antilipemics, 705
antilithics, 578, 704
antipyretics, 701
antirheumatics, 711
antiseptics, 480, 672, 702, 713
antispasmodics, 647, 700, 704
anti-taenia remedies, 714
antitumor herbs, 578, 704
antitussives, 185, 694
antivenom remedies, 713
antivirals, 713
aperitives, 696
Aretaios, 19
Aristotle, 13, 24, 41, 60, 609
aromatics, 694
Artemis, 8
Arterial blood and Qi deficiency, 727
arterial resolvents, 705
astringents, 401, 403, 699
Archigenes, 19
Arnica, 254
Ar-Razi (Rhazes), 7, 20, 27, 42, 57, 58, 60, 79, 145, 482, 497
Artichoke, 583
Aschner, Bernhard, 209, 225, 327, 482, 667
Asparagus, 357
Avicenna (see ibn Sina)
Bacon, Roger, 24
Balance, 16, 27
Balm, 494
Balm of Gilead, 399
Balmony, 170
Baptisia, 684
Barberry, 287
Barham, Henry, 109, 602
Barrough, Phillip, 42
Barton, William, 167, 556
Bartram, John, 193
Basil, 660
Bateson, Gregory, 37
Bath, 90
Bauhin, Jean, and Gaspard, 41, 62, 662
Bayberry, 340
Bearberry, 528
Bergamot, 466
Bergzabern, Johann von, 41, 42, 62, 515, 530

The Energetics of Western Herbs

Bethroot, 640
Betony, 451
Bichat, Xavier, 25, 42
Bigelow, James, 193
Bilberry, 533
Bingen, Hildegard von, 7, 27, 41, 139, 387, 314, 535, 644
Bioenergies, 48, 73, 81
Biotypes, 4, 16, 50
Birch, 592
Birthroot, 640
Birthwort, 642
Bitter orange flower, 657
Bitter orange rind, 466
bitter tonics, 696
Black cohosh, 436
Black haw, 632
Black pepper, 328
Black walnut, 415
Blackberry, 531
Bladder and kidney damp heat, 480, 723,
Bladder Qi constraint, 426, 723
Bladderwrack, 369
Blessed thistle, 278
Blood deficiency, 153, 344, 379, 726
Blood heat, 479, 481, 482, 727
Blood root, 192
blood congestion, 481, 551, 552
blood tonics, 343, 627, 698
Bloodletting, 481
Blue cohosh, 637 Blue flag, 163
Blue mallow, 383
Bock, Hieronymus, 7, 9, 41, 61, 248, 374, 412, 581
Boerhaave, Hermann, 153, 482, 617
Bogbean, 485
Bohm, David, 35
Boneset, 130
Borage, 390
Boyle, Robert, 24, 25,
Brickell, John, 169, 342
Broussais, François, 481
Brunfels, Otto, 7, 9, 43, 61, 76, 79, 109, 332, 374, 435
Buckthorn, 178
Bugleweed, 449
Buchu, 296
Butterbur, 116
Caesalpino, Andrea, 41
Cajeput, 678
Calamint, 125
Calamus, 272
Calendula, 565
Camomile, 462
Camphor, 338
Canada snakeroot, 216

Canadian fleabane, 418
Capra, Fritjof, 35
Capsule, 83
Caraway, 470
Cardamom, 252
cardiac tonics, 234, 648, 659, 696, 697
carminatives, 645, 708
Carrichter, Bartholomeus, 43, 96, 456
Carver, Jonathan, 93, 605
Cascara sagrada, 176
Castaneda, Carlos, 35
Categories, three, 48, 52, 53
Catnip, 124
Cayenne, 322
Celandine, 156
Celery, 599
Celsus, Cornelius, 19, 43
Centaury, 487
Central Qi sinking, 726
Cereus, 260
Chaparral, 686
Chasteberry, 471
Chickweed, 393
Chicory, 492
childbirth preparers, 629, 708
choleretics, 152, 692
cholagogues, 152
Christopher, John, 320
cicatrisants, 669, 711
Cinnamon, 335
circulatory stimulants, 104, 319, 665, 698, 710
Cleavers, 584
coagulants, 402, 700
cleansers, 482, 575-579, 703
Cleansing, 101, 575
Clinical medicine, 62
Clutterbuck, Henry, 481
CNS regulators, 706
Cold, 29, 320
Cold obstruction, 576, 665, 725
Cole, William, 42, 67, 113, 141, 175, 212, 253, 264, 445
Congealed blood, 481, 552
Constantine the African, 472
Constituents, 48
Coltsfoot, 206
Comfrey, 385
Compress, 87
Coneflower, purple, 681
Constituents, 48
Constitution, 4, 50
Constraint, 425
Cornsilk, 536
Couch grass, 148
counterirritants, 180, 666, 711

General Index

Cowslip flower, 269
Cowslip root, 613
Cramp bark, 634
Cranesbill, 405
Cream, 89
Croll, Oswald, 25, 55
Culpeper, Nicholas, 1, 58, 64, 96, 141
Culver's root, 161
Cypress, 567
Damiana, 300
Damp, 29, 401, 645, 665
Damp heat, 225, 480
Dandelion leaf, 146
Dandelion root, 580
De la Boë, Frans (Sylvius), 25, 27
De L'Ecluse, Charles Clusius, 41, 61, 515, 530
De L'Obel, Mathias, 41, 405
Decoction, 80
decongestants, 479, 551-553, 702, 703
Deficiency, 29, 227, 343
Delivery, 629
demulcents, 380, 427, 699
dermatropics, 577, 704
Derivation, 666
detergents, 669, 712
diaphoretics, 103-106, 665, 691, 710
Diathesis, 16
digestives, 645, 646, 696, 708, 709
Dinand, Alfred P., 43
Dioskurides, Pedanios, 5, 43, 57, 59, 60, 61, 374, 390, 526
discutients, 705
diuretics, 135, 578, 692, 704
Dodoens, Rembert, 27, 43, 515, 527
Douche, 84
Draining, 423
Dryness, 29, 153, 379, 425
Dürer, Albrecht, 374
Dwarf elder, 147
Dysfunction, 25, 27, 34
Dyskrasia, 16, 22
Echinacea, 681
Eclectic medicine, 62, 95, 97, 155
Effective qualities, 15-17, 22-24, 33, 48, 59, 60
Einstein, Albert, 37
Elder bark, 146
Elder flower, 121
Elecampane, 243
Eliminating, 99
Ellingwood, Finley, 19, 27, 62-64, 217, 243, 259, 262, 414, 432, 636, 685
emetics, 225, 695
emmenagogues, 209-212, 628, 694
emollients, 380, 699

Empirical approach, 5
endocrine restoratives, 697
Enema, 85
Essence, 17, 18
Essential oil, 80, 672
estrogen inhibitors, 707
estrogen stimulants, 236, 706
Ettmueller, Michael, 43
Eucalyptus, 128
Excess, 29
Excess heat, 153, 226, 478, 479, 481
expectorants, 185, 693,
External/internal, 30
External treatments, 212, 666
External wind cold (see wind cold)
External wind heat (see wind heat)
Eye preparations, 91
Eyebright, 410
False unicorn, 308
Félicie, Jacobie, 644
Felter, Harvey, 62, 64, 556, 564, 575
Feminine principle, 13, 259, 353, 394
Fennel, 291
febrifuge, 477, 701, 709
Fernel, Jean, 19, 543
Fever, 103, 476, 478, 479, 647
Feverfew, 286
Figwort, 594
Filth pharmacy, 212
Fire toxin, 480, 702
Five elements, 15
Fleawort, 419
Flower pollen, 345
Floyer, John, 21, 23, 37, 93, 94, 319
Fluid extract, 82
Fluid organism, 135
Fluid congestion, 135, 154
Fluids depletion, 153, 343, 379
Fluids, four, 15
Fomentation, 87
Four elements, 15, 17,
Four fluids, 15, 16
Fringe tree, 168
Fuchs, Leonhardt, 27, 42, 61, 62, 109
Fumitory, 170
Gabir (Jafar al sufi), 24
galactagogues, 697
Galen, 2, 7, 13-18, 22, 24, 33, 42-45, 50, 58-62, 99, 109, 145, 153, 209, 224, 225, 229, 293, 337, 482, 497, 546, 573
Gargle, 83
Garlic, 473
gastric stimulants, 645
General fluids dyskrasia, 576, 577, 666, 727

The Energetics of Western Herbs

General plethora, 105, 154, 727
General toxemia, 105, 154, 481, 575
Genitourinary damp cold, 723
Genitourinary damp heat, 480, 723
Genitourinary Qi deficiency, 235, 723
Gentian, 483
Geranium, 408
Gerard, John, 548
Gerard of Cremona, 27
Gesner, Conrad, 41
Ghee, 82
Giles de Corbeil, 19
Ginger, 110
Ginseng, American, 241
Glauber, 25, 27
Goethe, Johann W., 37, 257, 614
Goldenrod, 140
Goldenseal, 553
gonadotropic hormones regulators, 707
Grapevine, 508
Gravel root, 303
Grindelia, 202
Ground, 4, 16, 50
Hahnemann, Samuel, 25, 37, 50, 229, 644
Hamilton, James, 153, 154
Harig, Georg, 229
Hawthorn, 257
Hazelwort, 218
Head damp cold, 725
Head damp heat, 726
Heart blood congestion, 716
Heart blood deficiency, 715
Heart blood and Spleen Qi deficiency, 648, 715
Heart fire, 427, 716
Heart fluid congestion, 716
Heart & Kidney Yang deficiency, 715
Heart & Kidney Yin deficiency, 715
Heart & lung Qi deficiency, 715
Heart Qi constraint, 426, 648, 715
Heart Qi deficiency, 234, 715
heart restoratives (see *cardiac tonics*)
Heart Yang deficiency, 234, 659, 715
Heart Yin deficiency, 715
Heat, 475
Heisenberg, Werner, 35
Helonias, 308
Helvetius, Johann F., 27
hemostatics, 402, 628, 700
Hense, 50
hepatic stimulants, 234
Herbals, 59-64
Herb classes, 26, 41-46
Herb combining, 76
Herb duration, 70

Herb selection, 67-70
Herb dosage, 74, 75
Hermbstaedt, S.F., 24
Herophilos, 94
Herring, Constantine, 63
Hervieu, Placide, 94
Hippokrates, 8, 15, 27, 43, 45, 60, 100, 102, 143, 209, 225, 229
Hoffman, Friedrich, 27
Holy thistle, 278
Homeopathy, 62, 63, 73, 95, 97
Hops, 652
Horehound, white, 203
hormonal regulators, 623, 706
Horse chestnut, 561
Horseradish, 325
Horsetail, 517
Horstius, Johann D., 27
Hot, 29
Hufeland, Wilhelm C., 28, 102, 153, 209, 225, 268, 482
hydragogues, 154
Hydrangea, 606
hypertensives, 234, 696
hypnotics, 647, 709
hypoglycemiants, 707
hypotensives, 427, 701
Hyssop, 187
ibn al-Baitar, 42, 60, 205, 500
ibn Sina (Avicenna), 7, 24, 27, 42, 56, 57, 58, 60, 97, 340, 482, 493
Iceland moss, 364
Immunity, 232
immunity potentizers, 233, 696
immunostimulants, 672, 712
Infection, 671
Infusion, 80
Inhalation, 84
Inmortal, 196
insulin stimulants, 707
insulin inhibitors, 707
Integrative thinking, 35, 36, 60, 65
Internal, 30
Internal wind, 722, 647
Intestines cold, 719
Intestines damp cold, 151, 719
Intestines damp heat, 480, 720
Intestines dry heat, 152, 478, 720
Intestines dryness, 153
Intestines mucous damp, 645, 646, 719
Intestines Qi constraint, 426, 719
Intestines Qi stagnation, 151, 645
Irish moss, 395
Ishak ibn Amran, 521
Jasmine, 298

General Index

Juniper, 213
Kalm, Peter, 605
Kelp, 366
Kevran, Louis, 37
Kidney/endocrine disharmony, 722
Kidney Essence deficiency, 722
Kidney fire, 723
Kidney fluid congestion, 135, 722
Kidney Qi constraint, 426, 647, 722
Kidney Qi infirmity, 235, 723
Kidney Qi stagnation, 722
Kidney wind, 722
Kidney Yang deficiency, 551, 722
Kidney Yin deficiency, 721
King, John, 27, 28, 62-64, 155, 334, 682
Klaproth, Michael, 24
Krasis, 4, 50
Kratevas, 62
Kurtz, Ron, 50
Labor, 629
labor promoters, 708
Lady's mantle, 513
Lady's slipper, 457
Lavender, 498
Lavoisier, Antoine, 24, 27
laxatives, 151-155, 692, 693
Leary, Timothy, 35
Leclerc, Henri, 55, 526
Lémery, Nicolas, 25, 27, 43
Lemnie, Levine, 18,
Lemon, 538
Leung Kok Yuan, 621
Li dong yuan, 102, 229
Li shi zhen, 19,
Li zi, 42
Libavius, 25
Licorice, 238
Life root, 34
Lily of the valley, 263
Linden, 119
Liniment, 90
Linnacre, Thomas, 22
Linnaeus, Carl, 458
Liu wan su, 102
Liver and gall bladder damp heat, 721
Liver and gall bladder Yang excess, 721
Liver and Kidney depletion, 343, 720
Liver and stomach Qi deficiency, 234, 720
Liver blood deficiency, 343, 720
Liver cold stagnation, 720
Liver/endocrine disharmony, 647
Liver fire, 152, 478, 647, 721
Liver fluid congestion, 135, 721
liver protectives, 696

Liver Qi stagnation, 152, 551, 720
Liver/Spleen disharmony, 426, 646, 719
liver restoratives, 697
Liver Yang deficiency, 720
Liver Yang rising, 427, 647, 721
Lloyd, John, 27, 62, 63, 434, 435, 556
Lobelia, 429
Localization, 40
Lonicer, Adam, 57
Loosestrife, 526
Lotion, 89,
Lovage, 137
Lung dryness, 379, 717
Lung heat dryness,
Lung and Kidney Yang deficiency, 716
Lung fluid congestion, 718
Lung phlegm cold/damp, 185, 717
Lung phlegm dryness, 186, 718
Lung phlegm heat, 185, 717
Lung Qi constraint, 186, 717
Lung Qi deficiency, 233, 426, 716
lung tonics, 695
Lung wind cold, 716
Lung wind heat 716
Lung Yin deficiency, 379, 716
Lungwort lichen, 396
lymphatic cleansers, 579, 705
lymphatic restoratives, 697
mammary restoratives, 697
Magendie, François, 6, 13, 43, 100
Mao ze dong, 95
Marigold, 565
Marjoram, 444
Marsh mallow, 381
Masterwort, 115
Mattioli, Pierandrea, 7, 41, 143, 164, 222, 264, 293, 392,
  419, 470, 590
May apple, 166
Meadowsweet, 547
Melilot, 501
Melissa, 494
Microalgae, 349
Milk thistle, 159
Mineral remedies, 579, 648
Minerals, liquid trace, 703
Miscarriage, 728
miscarriage preventers, 708
Mistletoe, 649
Mithridates, 95
Moench, Conrad, 682
Monardes, Nicolas, 113, 400, 602, 656
Morning sickness, 628
Motherwort, 441
Mouthwash, 82

The Energetics of Western Herbs

Mucus, 401
Mugwort, 315
Mullein, 388
Multi-paradigm thinking, 34, 36
Myrrh, 676
narcotics, 709
Native American tradition, 5, 62, 96, 159, 162, 165, 169, 303, 312, 388, 602, 693, 641
Nedham, Marchamont, 31
Neroli, 657
Nerve deficiency, 659, 727
Nerve excess, 647, 727
nerve relaxants, 700
nerve stimulants, 660, 710
nerve tonics, 233, 659, 695, 710
nerve trophorestoratives, 234, 659, 710
Nettle, 372
Neuman, 24
nutritives, 343, 699
Oak bark, 407
Oats, 359
Ointment, 88
Oregano, 221
Oregon grape root, 290
Oshá, 114
ovary restoratives, 697
oxytocics, 708
pancreas restoratives, 698
Paracelsus, 24, 25, 496, 590
Paradigms, 2, 12-15, 21, 31-40
Parasites, 689
parasiticides, 689, 714
parasympathetic inhibitors, 620, 606
parasympathetic stimulants, 620, 706
parathyroid restoratives, 698
Parkinson, John, 62, 286, 287, 489
Parsley root, 362
Parsley seed, 439
parturients, 427, 629, 708
partus preparators, 708
Pasque flower, 433
Passionflower, 655
Pasteur, Louis, 100, 102
Patin, Guy, 481
Paul of Aegina, 19
Paullini, Christian, 248
Pelikan, Wilhelm, 257, 262
Pennyroyal, 219
Peppermint, 107
Petrus de Crescentis, 259
Pharmaceutical name, 48
Pharmacognosy, 21-24
Phenomenological approach, 11, 12, 21-23, 24, 25, 32, 33, 63, 93

Phlegm, 185, 186, 647
Physical organism,
Physis, 4, 16, 50
Pierrakos, John, 50
Pine, 190
pineal restoratives, 698
Pipsissewa, 588
pituitary hormone regulators, 707
pituitary restoratives, 698
Plantain, 543
Plaster, 86
Pleurisy root, 198
Plinius secundus, 41, 61, 472
Poke root, 603
Pollen, 345
Pomet, Pierre, 47, 145, 340
Poplar, 302
Porkert, Manfred, 35
Postpartum, 628, 629
Potentilla, 403
Poterius, 27
Poultice, 86
Pregnancy, 627
pregnancy enhancers, 708
Premature delivery, 628
Preparation, 52, 71, 70-72
Prickly ash, 333
Priessnitz, Vinzenz, 102
progesterone stimulants, 707
prostate restoratives, 698
Pseudo-Yuhanna (Ioannes Mesuë), 7, 42, 145, 512
Pulsatilla, 433
Pulse diagnosis, 19, 94
purgatives, 152, 693
Purslane, 541
pustulants, 666, 667, 711
Pythagoras, 143
Qi, 4, 16, 18, 29, 93
Qi constraint, 106, 226, 425-428, 481, 645, 646, 726
Qi deficiency, 233, 659, 726
Quincy, John, 42, 43, 45, 46, 183, 218
Rafinesque, Constantine, 641
Raspberry, 630
Ray, John, 41
Red clover, 610
Red elder, 147
Red root, 557
refrigerants, 475-482, 701
Regulating, 573
relaxants, 427, 647, 700
resolvants, 577, 579, 704
Requena, Yves, 50,
restoratives, 231-237, 695
Restoring, 227-229

General Index

Rhazes (see Ar-Razi)
Rhineberry, 178
Rhubarb, 173
Ribwort plantain, 543
Rivière, Lazarus, 27, 153, 209, 225
Rose, 510
Rosemary, 330
Röszlin, Eucharius (Rhodion), 42, 57, 97, 491, 497
rubefacients, 666, 669, 711
Rue, 223
Rufus of Ephesos, 19,
Rush, Benjamin, 481
Ryff, Walther H., 57, 58, 61, 62, 96, 97, 109, 117, 277, 332, 446, 500, 512, 662
Sage, 246
Salmon, William, 42, 57, 58, 96, 117, 218, 293, 497, 543, 545
Salve, 88
Sandalwood, 520
Sanicle, 515
Sarsaparilla, 601
Sassafras, 112
Savory, 662
Saw palmetto, 294
Scabious, 200
Schatz, Jean, 35
Schoepf, Johann D., 199
Schroeder, Johann, 42, 240, 282, 323, 358
Scudder, John, 27, 62, 435, 453
Sea holly, 305
sedatives, 647, 709
seeping diuretics, 135, 692
Selfheal, 503
Senna, 178
Serapio Junior, 43, 472
Sheldon, William, 50
Shepherd's purse, 559
Shook, Edward, 366
Silverweed, 404
Simonis, Werner C., 43, 237
Skin damp heat, 726
Skullcap, 447
Slippery elm, 384
Smoke, 85
Sources, 55-65
spasmolytics (see *antispasmodics*)
Spearmint, 126
Specific symptoms, 33, 34, 97
Speedwell, 591
Spirit deficiency, 659, 660
Spirit excess, 647, 648
Spleen damp, 645, 646, 719
Spleen damp cold, 151, 719
Spleen and Kidney yang deficiency, 719
Spleen Qi deficiency, 233, 234, 645, 718
Spleen Qi sinking, 719
Spleen Yang deficiency, 645, 719
spleen restoratives, 698
Sprengel, Curt, 94
Squatting inhalation, 84
Squaw vine, 635
Squills, 142
Stearn, Samuel, 200
St. John's wort, 454
Stahl, Ernst, 25
Stahl (homeopath), 50
Steiner, Rudolf, 37, 236, 374, 428, 443, 621, 698
stimulants, 319
Stomach cold, 718
Stomach dryness, 379, 426, 718
Stomach fire, 426, 718
Stomach Qi reflux, 718
Stomach Qi stagnation, 645, 646, 718
Stomach Yin deficiency, 718
Stone root, 570
Strabo, Walafried, 248, 491
Struthius, Joseph, 19
styptics, 402, 700
Sumac, 420
Swab, 88
Sweet flag, 272
Sydenham, Thomas, 23, 28, 37, 153, 225, 226, 482
sympathetic inhibitors, 620, 706
sympathetic stimulants, 620, 706
Symptom treatment, 625
Symptomatology, 64
Syrup, 83
Tamarind, 182
Tansy, 283
Tea tree, 680
Temperament (see *krasis*)
testis restoratives, 698
testosterone stimulants, 707
Therapeutics, 24-26, 43,
Theriac, Roman, 95
Theophrastus, 41, 59,
Thomson, Samuel, 320, 324, 431
Three treasures, 17
Thurston, 320
Thyme, 249
thymus restoratives, 698
thyroid restoratives, 698
thyroxine inhibitors, 707
thyroxine stimulants, 707
Tincture, 72, 81, 99b
tonics, 231-237, 695
Tormentil, 403
Toxemia, 575, 641, 672

The Energetics of Western Herbs

Tournefort, Pitton de, 43, 117, 340, 491, 497
Trace minerals, liquid, 703
Treichler, Rudolf, 428
Tropism, 49
trophorestoratives, 344
Trotula of Salerno, 139, 414, 644
Tryon, Thomas, 22
Turpentine, 412
Unschuld, Paul, 35
Urine diagnosis, 19
urogenital tonics, 235, 697
uterine decongestants, 552
uterine tonics, 235, 629, 697
Uterus blood deficiency, 236, 343, 724
Uterus blood congestion, 552, 724
Uterus cold, 211, 724
Uterus Qi constraint, 426, 724
Uterus Qi deficiency, 235, 724
Uterus Qi stagnation, 210, 724
Uva ursi, 528
Valentine, Basil, 24
Valerian, 265
Van Helmont, Jean-Baptiste, 25, 27, 145
Venous blood stagnation, 551, 727
venous tonics, 552, 703
vermicides, 689, 713
vermifuges, 713
Vervain, 132
vesicants, 667, 711
Vikings, 509
Villanova, Arnald de, 109, 412
Violet, 609
Virchow, 25, 100
Virginia snakeroot, 118
Vital spirit(s), 4,
Vogel, Virgil, 96
Von Grauvogel, 50
vulneraries, 669, 711
Walnut, 415
Wang Shu Ho, 94
Warmth organism, 319, 475
Watercress, 375
Watts, Alan, 35
Wash, 88
Webster, Herbert, 27, 28, 62, 155, 225
Weiss, Rudolf, 52
Wheatgrass, 354
White deadnettle, 313
White oak, 407
White horehound, 203
Whitmont, Edward, 37
Wholeness, 14, 16
Wilber, Ken, 35
Wild carrot, 144

Wild cherry, 459
Wild ginger, 216
Wild indigo, 684
Wild yam, 460
Willow, 524
Wind/cold, 104, 725
Wind/damp obstruction, 105, 665, 725
Wind/heat, 104, 725
Wintergreen, 588
Wise woman tradition, 5, 8, 9, 22, 55, 59, 61, 96, 139, 307, 442, 644
Witch hazel, 563
Woehler, Friedrich, 23
Wood betony, 451
Wood sorrel, 505
Wormwood, 489
Yarrow, 280
Yellow dock, 586
Yellow Emperor, 11
Yerba santa, 194
Yang, 28, 476, 619
Yang deficiency, 320, 620, 659
Yang drainers, 620, 706
Yang excess, 620
Yang tonics, 620, 706
Yin, 28, 619
Yin deficiency, 102, 153, 379, 479, 610
Yin drainers, 620, 706
Yin excess, 320, 620
Yin tonics, 380, 620, 706
Yin and Yang regulators, 620
Zhang zi he, 100,
Zhu dan xi, 102

Inquiries about courses in herbal medicine incorporating the principles and methods on which this text is based should be addressed to:

Artemis Institute
P.O. Box 4295
Boulder, Colorado 80306
U.S.A.

The institute offers classes, correspondence courses and seminars. It also provides database programs and herbal products.

Information will be sent on request.

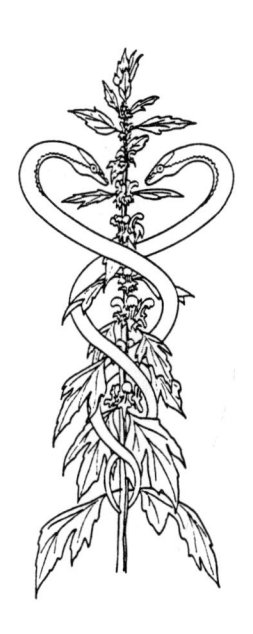